THE AMERICAN ACADEMY OF ORTHOPAEDIC SURGEONS

Instructional
Course
Lectures

Volume XXX 1981

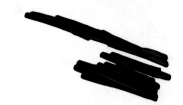

THE AMERICAN ACADEMY OF ORTHOPAEDIC SURGEONS

Instructional Course Lectures

Volume XXX 1981

Edited by

David G. Murray, M.D.

Chairman, Department of Orthopaedic Surgery,
Upstate Medical Center College of Medicine,
Syracuse, New York

With 727 illustrations

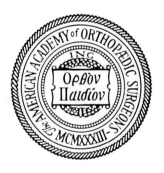

The C. V. Mosby Company

ST. LOUIS · TORONTO · LONDON   1981

MOSBY

1906 **75** 1981
YEARS

A TRADITION OF PUBLISHING EXCELLENCE

Editor: Eugenia A. Klein
Assistant editor: Kathryn H. Falk
Manuscript editor: Carl Masthay
Design: Staff
Production: Jeanne A. Gulledge

Printed in the United States of America

International Standard Book Number 0-8016-0048-0

Library of Congress Catalog Card Number 43-17054

The C.V. Mosby Company
11830 Westline Industrial Drive, St. Louis, Missouri 63141

C/CB/B   9   8   7   6   5   4   3   2   1   03/C/321

Contributors

Harlan C. Amstutz, M.D.

Professor and Chief, Division of Orthopaedic Surgery, UCLA School of Medicine, The Center for Health Sciences, Los Angeles, California

Fred Behrens, M.D., F.R.C.S.(C)

St. Paul–Ramsey Medical Center; Assistant Professor, Department of Orthopaedic Surgery, University of Minnesota, St. Paul, Minnesota

James B. Bennett, M.D.

Assistant Professor, Division of Orthopedic Surgery, Baylor Affiliated Hospitals, Houston, Texas

James D. Black, M.Sc.

Research Associate, Cleveland Research Institute, Cleveland, Ohio

Richard S. Bryan, M.D.

Consultant, Department of Orthopedic Surgery, Mayo Clinic and Mayo Foundation; Professor of Orthopedic Surgery, Mayo Medical School, Rochester, Minnesota

S. Terry Canale, M.D.

Assistant Clinical Professor, Department of Orthopaedic Surgery, University of Tennessee Center for the Health Sciences; Chief of Pediatric Orthopaedics, LeBonheur Children's Hospital; Staff, The Campbell Clinic, Memphis, Tennessee

Robert H. Cofield, M.D.

Consultant, Department of Orthopedic Surgery, Mayo Clinic and Mayo Foundation; Assistant Professor of Orthopedic Surgery, Mayo Medical School, Rochester, Minnesota

Mark B. Coventry, M.D.

Consultant, Department of Orthopedics, Mayo Clinic and Mayo Foundation; Professor of Orthopedic Surgery, Mayo Medical School, Rochester, Minnesota

Alvin H. Crawford, M.D.

Director of Pediatric Orthopaedics, Children's Hospital Medical Center, Cincinnati; Associate Professor of Pediatrics and Orthopaedic Surgery, Department of Pediatrics and Orthopaedic Surgery, University of Cincinnati College of Medicine, Cincinnati, Ohio

Thomas B. Dameron, Jr., M.D.

Raleigh Orthopaedic Clinic, Raleigh; Clinical Professor, Department of Orthopaedic Surgery, University of North Carolina, Chapel Hill, North Carolina

Lorraine J. Day, M.D.

Assistant Professor of Orthopaedic Surgery, Department of Orthopaedic Surgery, University of California–San Francisco, San Francisco, California

W. Thomas Edwards, M.S.

Massachusetts Institute of Technology, Cambridge; Department of Orthopaedic Surgery, Beth Israel Hospital–Harvard Medical School, Boston, Massachusetts

David A. Fischer, M.D.

Hennepin County Medical Center; Clinical Assistant Professor, Department of Orthopaedic Surgery, University of Minnesota, Minneapolis, Minnesota

Gary E. Friedlaender, M.D.

Associate Professor, Department of Surgery (Orthopaedics) and Division of Oncology, Yale University School of Medicine, New Haven, Connecticut

v

Adrian Graff-Radford, M.D.

Clinical Instructor in Surgery/Orthopaedics, Department of Surgery, Division of Orthopaedics, UCLA, Los Angeles, California

A. Seth Greenwald, D. Phil. (Oxon)

Executive Director, Cleveland Research Institute, Cleveland, Ohio

Sigvard T. Hansen, Jr., M.D.

Professor and Chairman, Department of Orthopaedic Surgery, University of Washington, Seattle, Washington

Marion C. Harper, M.D.

Assistant Professor, Division of Orthopaedic Surgery, University of Missouri Medical Center; Chief of Orthopaedic Services, Harry S Truman Veterans Administration Hospital, Columbia, Missouri

Wilson C. Hayes, Ph.D.

Associate Professor, Department of Orthopaedic Surgery, Beth Israel Hospital–Harvard Medical School, Boston, Massachusetts

Anthony K. Hedley, M.B., B.Ch., F.R.C.S.

Assistant Professor, Division of Orthopaedic Surgery, UCLA School of Medicine, The Center for Health Sciences, Los Angeles, California

John Nevil Insall, M.D.

Attending Orthopaedic Surgeon, The Hospital for Special Surgery and New York Hospital; Clinical Professor of Surgery (Orthopaedics), Cornell University Medical College, New York, New York

Renner M. Johnston, M.D.

Associate Professor of Orthopaedics, Department of Orthopaedic Surgery, University of Colorado Medical Center, Denver, Colorado

Richard E. Jones III, M.D.

Associate Professor, Division of Orthopaedic Surgery, University of Texas Health Sciences Center, Dallas, Texas

Herbert Kaufer, M.D.

Professor, Department of Surgery, Section of Orthopaedic Surgery, University of Michigan, Ann Arbor, Michigan

Donald B. Kettelkamp, M.D., M.S.

Professor and Chairman, Department of Orthopaedic Surgery, Indiana University School of Medicine, Indianapolis, Indiana

A.J.C. Lee, B.Sc., Ph.D.

Senior Lecturer, Department of Engineering Science, University of Exeter, Exeter, Devon, United Kingdom

R.S.M. Ling, M.A., B.M. (Oxon), F.R.C.S.

Senior Consultant Orthopaedic Surgeon, Princess Elizabeth Orthopaedic Hospital, Exeter, Devon, United Kingdom

G. Dean MacEwen, M.D.

Medical Director, Alfred I. duPont Institute, Wilmington, Delaware

Henry J. Mankin, M.D.

Chief of Orthopaedics, Edith M. Ashley Professor of Orthopaedic Surgery, Department of Orthopaedic Surgery, Massachusetts General Hospital–Harvard Medical School, Boston, Massachusetts

Mary-Blair Matejczyk, M.D.

Clinical Instructor in Orthopaedic Surgery, Case Western Reserve University School of Medicine; Orthopaedic Research Associate, Cleveland Research Institute, Cleveland, Ohio

Larry S. Matthews, M.D.

Professor, Department of Surgery, Section of Orthopaedic Surgery, University of Michigan, Ann Arbor, Michigan

Dana C. Mears, M.D.

Associate Professor, Department of Orthopaedic Surgery, University of Pittsburgh, Pittsburgh, Pennsylvania

Robert W. Metcalf, M.D.

Assistant Clinical Professor, Orthopaedic Surgery, University of Utah, College of Medicine, Salt Lake City, Utah

Robert J. Neviaser, M.D.

Professor of Orthopaedic Surgery, George Washington University Medical Center, Washington, D.C.

Thomas J. Neviaser, M.D.

Assistant Clinical Professor of Orthopaedic Surgery, George Washington Medical Center, Washington, D.C.

Manohar M. Panjabi, Dr. Tech.

Associate Professor and Director of Biomechanics, Section of Orthopaedic Surgery, Yale University School of Medicine, New Haven, Connecticut

Ira Posner, M.D.

Resident, Department of Orthopaedic Surgery, Harvard Medical School, Boston, Massachusetts

Chitranjan S. Ranawat, M.D.

Professor of Orthopaedic Surgery, Department of Orthopaedics, Cornell University Medical Center; Director of Hand Services and Attending Physician, Hospital for Special Surgery, New York, New York

Lee H. Riley, Jr., M.D.

Professor and Director, Department of Orthopaedic Surgery, Johns Hopkins University School of Medicine, Baltimore, Maryland

Gregory Schwab, M.D.

Assistant Instructor, Division of Orthopedic Surgery, Baylor Affiliated Hospitals, Houston, Texas

Irwin M. Siegel, M.D.

Associate Professor, Departments of Orthopaedic Surgery and Neurological Sciences, Rush–Presbyterian–St. Luke's Medical Center; Lecturer, Department of Orthopaedic Surgery, University of Illinois, Abraham Lincoln College of Medicine; Senior Attending Surgeon, Department of Orthopaedic Surgery, Louis A. Weiss Memorial Hospital, Chicago, Illinois

Taylor K. Smith, M.D.

Professor and Chief, Division of Orthopaedic Surgery, Department of Surgery, University of Texas Medical School at Houston, Houston, Texas

Hugh S. Tullos, M.D.

Associate Professor and Head, Division of Orthopedic Surgery, Baylor College of Medicine, Houston, Texas

Augustus A. White III, M.D., Dr. Med. Sc.

Professor of Orthopaedic Surgery, Harvard Medical School, Orthopaedic Surgeon-in-Chief, Beth Israel Hospital–Harvard Medical School, Department of Orthopaedic Surgery, Boston, Massachusetts

Alan H. Wilde, M.D.

Chairman, Department of Orthopaedic Surgery, Cleveland Clinic Foundation, Cleveland, Ohio

G. William Woods, M.D.

Assistant Professor, Division of Orthopedic Surgery, Baylor Affiliated Hospitals, Houston, Texas

Preface

As with previous volumes in the Instructional Course Series, Volume XXX represents an attempt by the Instructional Course Committee to bring together material that will serve as a lasting reference source for the orthopaedic surgeon, along with other individuals in medical and allied fields. The annual presentations at the Academy meeting provide an excellent opportunity for the evolution and refinement of educational subject matter. Frequently a specific course represents a unique synthesis of the opinions of several experts in the field brought to bear on a single problem. Although such summaries are based as much as possible on established principles, current thought and innovative practices are unusually well integrated.

Out of the extensive schedule of Instructional Courses produced at the annual meeting in 1980, the Committee has attempted to select a representative cross section of topics. Such a selection process is difficult because it must take into account not only the subjects listed but also the contents of previous Instructional Course volumes, existing publications by the faculty members, and in many instances the ability of an author to take the time out of a busy schedule to prepare a manuscript. This year we are particularly pleased with the variety of the subject matter and with the high quality of the contributions. The authors have ex-

ceeded themselves in providing the substance for a first-class publication.

Each contribution represents the thoughts—practical and philosophical—of a single author or group of authors. Since part of the lasting value of this series lies in the preservation of the unique characteristics of some of the foremost teachers in the field of the musculoskeletal system, the editing process has been softened to retain an individual flavor in each chapter. It is hoped that the readers will excuse any inconsistencies in style that may have resulted and, in turn, enjoy the personalities of the contributors as mirrored in their writing.

Anyone who has attempted to compile a book requiring manuscripts from many sources can appreciate the problems that can arise. The Instructional Course Committee is very fortunate to have had the outstanding cooperation of so many persons at every level from start to finish. To those who contributed so greatly we express our sincere appreciation and are confident that Volume XXX of the Instructional Course Series provides a fitting tribute to their efforts.

Committee on Instructional Courses

David G. Murray, *Chairman*
Hanes H. Brindley
Joseph A. Kopta
Victor H. Frankel
C. McCollister Evarts

Contents

Section I   GENERAL ORTHOPAEDICS AND PEDIATRIC ORTHOPAEDICS, 1

1   Diagnosis, management, and orthopaedic treatment of muscular dystrophy, 3
Irwin M. Siegel, M.D.

2   Bone banking: current methods and suggested guidelines, 36

     A   Background and current methods, 36
Gary E. Friedlaender, M.D.
Henry J. Mankin, M.D.

     B   Guidelines for banking of musculoskeletal tissues, 52
Gary E. Friedlaender, M.D.
Henry J. Mankin, M.D.

3   Neurofibromatosis in childhood, 56
Alvin H. Crawford, M.D.

4   Treatment of Legg-Calvé-Perthes disease, 75
G. Dean MacEwen, M.D.

5   Biotrigonometric analysis and practical applications of osteotomies of tibia in children, 85
S. Terry Canale, M.D.
Marion C. Harper, M.D.

Section II   TRAUMA

6   Management of multiply injured patient, 105
Taylor K. Smith, M.D.
Lorraine J. Day, M.D.
Sigvard T. Hansen, Jr., M.D.
Renner M. Johnston, M.D.

7   External skeletal fixation, 112

     A   Introduction to external skeletal fixation, 112
Fred Behrens, M.D., F.R.C.S.(C)

     B   Basic concepts, 118
Fred Behrens, M.D., F.R.C.S.(C)

C External fixator application, 125

Fred Behrens, M.D., F.R.C.S.(C)
Richard E. Jones III, M.D.
David A. Fischer, M.D.

D Soft-tissue coverage, 143
Richard E. Jones III, M.D.

E Bone grafting: general principles and use in open fractures, 152
Fred Behrens, M.D., F.R.C.S.(C)

F External fixation in open fractures, 156

1 Tibia, 156

Fred Behrens, M.D., F.R.C.S.(C)

2 Femur, 162

Dana C. Mears, M.D.

3 Pelvis, 164

Dana C. Mears, M.D.

4 Upper extremity, 169

Richard E. Jones III, M.D.

G Treatment of infected nonunions and failed septic joints, 176
Dana C. Mears, M.D.

H Complications of external skeletal fixation, 178
Fred Behrens, M.D., F.R.C.S.(C)

Section III   FRACTURES ABOUT THE ELBOW

8 Factors influencing elbow instability, 185
Hugh S. Tullos, M.D.
Gregory Schwab, M.D.
James B. Bennett, M.D.
G. William Woods, M.D.

9 Fractures about the elbow in adults, 200
Richard S. Bryan, M.D.

10 Transverse fractures of distal humerus in children, 224
Thomas B. Dameron, Jr., M.D.

A Supracondylar humeral fractures, 224

B Transverse distal humeral epiphyseal fractures, 235

Section IV   SHOULDER

11 Lesions of musculotendinous cuff of shoulder: diagnosis and management, 239

A Tears of rotator cuff, 239

Robert J. Neviaser, M.D.
Thomas J. Neviaser, M.D.

B Lesions of long head of biceps tendon, 250

  Thomas J. Neviaser, M.D.
  Robert J. Neviaser, M.D.

12 Tears of rotator cuff, 258

  Robert H. Cofield, M.D.

Section V KNEE

13 Reconstruction of the difficult arthritic knee, 277

A An articulated knee prosthesis for treatment of severe mechanical knee joint disease, 277

  Larry S. Matthews, M.D.
  Herbert Kaufer, M.D.

B Treatment of the difficult arthritic knee, 284

  Donald B. Kettelkamp, M.D., M.S.

C Place of nonconstrained total knee replacement unit in reconstruction of the difficult arthritic knee, 297

  Lee H. Riley, Jr., M.D.

14 Total knee replacement, 301

A Stability characteristics of total knee designs, 301

  A. Seth Greenwald, D. Phil. (Oxon)
  James D. Black, M.Sc.
  Mary-Blair Matejczyk, M.D.

B Evaluation of patients for knee arthroplasty, 313

  Richard S. Bryan, M.D.

C Technique of total knee replacement, 324

  John Nevil Insall, M.D.

D Complications after knee replacement: prevention and management, 334

  Alan H. Wilde, M.D.

15 Patella pain syndromes and chondromalacia patellae, 342

  John Nevil Insall, M.D.

16 Operative arthroscopy of the knee, 357

  Robert W. Metcalf, M.D.

17 Fixation failure of tibial component: causes and prevention, 397

  Chitranjan S. Ranawat, M.D.

Section VI TECHNIQUES OF REVISION SURGERY AND CONTROVERSIES IN TOTAL HIP

18 Indications for surface replacement of hip, 405

  Mark B. Coventry, M.D.

19   Improved cementing techniques, 407

A.J.C. Lee, B.Sc., Ph.D.
R.S.M. Ling, M.A., B.M. (Oxon), F.R.C.S.

20   Fixation failure and techniques of revision surgery in total hip replacement, 414

Harlan C. Amstutz, M.D.

21   THARIES approach to surface replacement of hip, 422

Harlan C. Amstutz, M.D.
Adrian Graff-Radford, M.D.

22   Complications of surface replacements, 444

Anthony K. Hedley, M.B., B.Ch., F.R.C.S.

Section VII   THE SPINE

23   Spinal stability: evaluation and treatment, 457

Augustus A. White III, M.D., Dr. Med. Sc.
Manohar M. Panjabi, Dr. Tech.
Ira Posner, M.D.
W. Thomas Edwards, M.S.
Wilson C. Hayes, Ph.D.

THE AMERICAN ACADEMY OF ORTHOPAEDIC SURGEONS

Instructional
Course
Lectures

Volume XXX 1981

GENERAL ORTHOPAEDICS
AND PEDIATRIC ORTHOPAEDICS

Chapter 1

Diagnosis, management, and orthopaedic treatment of muscular dystrophy

IRWIN M. SIEGEL, M.D.
Chicago, Illinois

Muscular dystrophy is the general designation for a group of chronic diseases whose most prominent characteristic is a progressive degeneration of skeletal musculature, leading to weakness, atrophy, contracture, deformity, and progressive disability.

These diseases are, for the most part, hereditary conditions, although spontaneous occurrence as a result of point mutation is not uncommon. The genetic pattern and therefore the mechanism of transmission vary in the different types of dystrophy. Although any voluntary muscle can be affected, axial musculature and that of the limb girdles is most frequently and most severely involved (Fig. 1-1). As a rule, it can be said that the earlier clinical symptoms appear, the more rapidly the disease progresses. The primary pathologic condition in all types of dystrophy appears to lie in the muscle cell itself, with the nervous system involved only indirectly, if at all.[114] It is estimated that there are approximately 350 cases of all forms of muscular dystrophy for each million live births. Currently, there are over 10,000 children with Duchenne muscular dystrophy living in the United States.

The early diagnosis of muscular dystrophy is essential so that vital genetic counseling and sometimes important therapy are not delayed. Although presently incurable, many of the muscular dystrophies are treatable. Supportive and symptomatic aids are available and—with appropriate orthopaedic therapy—comfort, functional capacity, and perhaps even life expectancy can be significantly increased.

DIAGNOSIS

The diagnosis of muscular dystrophy is made on the basis of the following:
1. Clinical history
2. Physical examination
3. Genetic background
4. Serum muscle enzyme elevation
5. Electromyographic changes
6. Muscle biopsy

Muscular weakness can result from a variety of causes. Neoplastic, toxic, inflammatory, nutritional, and metabolic conditions can cause primary or secondary abiotrophy of muscle. Diseases of muscle should be distinguished from those of nerve. This differential diagnosis is usually not difficult. With some exceptions, neuropathies occur with distal involvement, whereas weakness in most myopathies is, at least initially, proximal in location. In neuropathies, atrophy exceeds weakness. The opposite is true in most myopathies. Fasciculations and spasticity can be seen in neuropathy, never in myopathy. Defects of neuromuscular transmission, such as myasthenia gravis, exhibit fatigue and ptosis, which responds to cholinergic drugs.[56] Serum muscle enzymes are usually normal or only slightly elevated in neuropathy. Electromyographic and biopsy changes also assist in differentiating neuropathic from myopathic processes.

Common muscular dystrophies

Duchenne muscular dystrophy. Boys with Duchenne muscular dystrophy (DMD) often have a normal birth and developmental history.[145] They

A
B
C

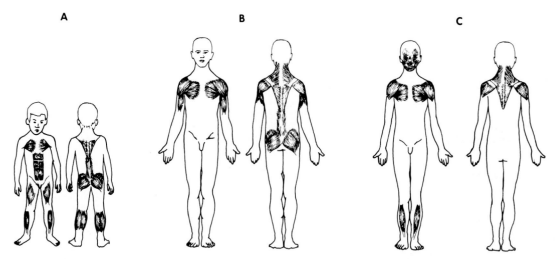

Fig. 1-1. Early distribution of muscle weakness in three major forms of muscular dystrophy: **A,** Duchenne dystrophy, **B,** limb-girdle dystrophy, and **C,** facioscapulohumeral dystrophy. (From Siegel, I.M.: The clinical management of muscle disease, London, 1977, William Heinemann Medical Books, Ltd.)

are commonly asymptomatic until 3 to 5 years of age, at which time a significant enough mass of muscle is lost to impair function.[37] Prompt diagnosis is often missed in these patients and important genetic counseling is delayed. The following are early signs[124]:
1. Flatfeet (secondary to heel-cord contracture)
2. Weak shoulder extension
3. Hesitance when ascending stairs
4. Slight lateral pelvic shift when arising from floor in seated position
5. Acceleration during final stage of sitting down
6. Poor standing jump
7. Waddling run

Later the full clinical picture includes the following:
1. Waddling gait
2. Frequent falling
3. Difficulty ascending stairs
4. Slipping through
5. Positive Gowers' sign (Fig. 1-2)
6. Lordosis
7. Progressive equinus
8. Calf hypertrophy
9. Weak neck flexion
10. Depression of deep tendon reflexes, except those of Achilles tendons

Weakness and contracture prevent independent ambulation in approximately 45% of such patients by 9 years of age and the remainder by 12 years. As a general rule, the child has difficulty rising from the floor, ascending stairs, and, finally, walking at yearly intervals, in this sequence.[141] The Becker form of childhood dystrophy presents with a similar distribution of muscular weakness but is of later onset and slower progression.

Limb-girdle dystrophy. Weakness in limb-girdle dystrophy (LGD) is mainly confined to the pelvic or shoulder girdle. Whereas DMD affects only boys, LGD can be found in either sex. Pseudohypertrophy is unusual. The brachioradialis muscle is often preserved, and contractures are slow to develop. LGD occurs from late in the first to the fourth decade of life. Although the disease progresses slowly, most patients are incapacitated within 10 to 20 years after onset.[10]

Facioscapulohumeral dystrophy. Facioscapulohumeral dystrophy (FSH, Landouzy-Déjerine disease) is characterized by weakness of the facial musculature, the shoulder girdle (the deltoid usually being spared), the muscles of the pelvic girdle, and the peroneals and tibialis anticus. Patients with the disease have difficulty walking on their heels. Weakness is commonly asymmetric in distribution and degree. *Formes frustes* are seen in

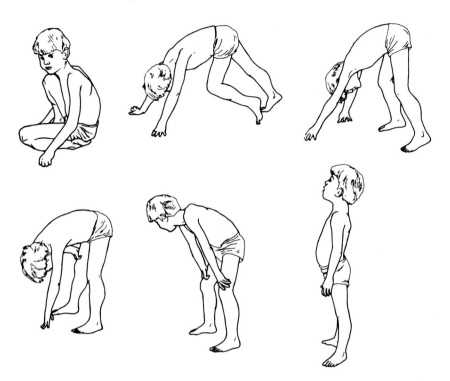

Fig. 1-2. Gowers' sign. (From Siegel, I.M.: The clinical management of muscle disease, London, 1977, William Heinemann Medical Books, Ltd.)

FSH, even with full penetrance of the defective gene. Onset is usually in adolescence or adulthood. Cervical spondylosis as well as cauda equina syndrome (secondary to lumbar hyperextension) can be seen late in the disease. When FSH occurs in early childhood, it runs a rapidly disabling course.

Dystrophia myotonica. Dystrophia myotonica is distinguished by myotonia as well as weakness (often distal).[21] Although most cases are of adult onset, where a mother has the disease, neonatal dystrophia myotonica can occur in her offspring.[62] Such infants are "floppy" at birth, have a typical "inverted-V" oral configuration, and frequently present with dislocated hips and talipes equinovarus (secondary to contracture of the Achilles and posterior tibial tendons).

Dystrophia myotonica is a disease of membrane. Although genetic penetrance is complete, expressivity may be limited to the minimal genetic discriminant. In addition to myotonia (both effort and percussion) and weakness, the complete syndrome is as follows:

1. Stellate cataract and retinal alterations
2. Gonadal atrophy
3. Faulty tolerance to carbohydrate
4. ECG abnormalities
5. Frontal and parietal alopecia in males
6. Thyroid dysfunction
7. Low IgG level
8. Cardiac conduction defects
9. Impaired pulmonary function
10. Progressive psychosocial deterioration
11. Low basal metabolic rate
12. Cerebral ventricular dilatation
13. Skull abnormalities including hyperostosis cranii, decrease in sella turcica size, prognathism, hyperostosis frontalis interna, and enlargement of the paranasal sinuses

The disease is characterized by a typical (lugubrious) facies, footdrop, and facial diplegia. Differential diagnosis includes paramyotonia (precipitated by exposure to cold) and myotonia congenita (Thomsen's disease, generalized muscle hypertrophy). Although the weakness in dystrophia myotonica is untreatable, a variety of drugs (such

Table 1-1. Working classification of the common diseases of muscle

Type	Age of onset	Sex	Symptoms	Course	Miscellaneous
Childhood dystrophy Severe (Duchenne) Benign (Becker) Later onset, slower progression	1 to 4 years	Male primarily	Clumsiness, toe-walking, lordosis, Gowers' sign, pseudohypertrophy	Increasing weakness with contracture, wheelchair by 9 to 12 years of age, death in late teens	Cardiomyopathy, mental retardation
Limb-girdle dystrophy	Any; commonly first to fourth decade	Equal	Extensor weakness in shoulders and hip	Slow progress with late disability	Occasional pseudohypertrophy
Facioscapulo-humeral dystrophy (Landouzy-Déjerine)	First to third decade	Equal	Paucity of facial expression, variable speech defects, difficulty in abducting arms, scapular winging, Bell's sign, shoulder, neck, pelvis and ankle dorsiflexion weakness	Progressive weakness, very late disability except with onset in childhood	Variable life expectancy; little tendency to develop contractures
Dystrophia myotonica	Birth to 50 years	Equal	Myotonia, lugubrious facies, severe fatigability, dropfoot gait	Slowly progressive weakness, temporal baldness, cataracts, gonadal atrophy, sterility, impotence, hypothyroidism, diabetes, acromegaly, hyperostosis cranii, cardiac, central nervous system and endocrine abnormalities	Progressive social and mental retardation

From Siegel, I. M.: The clinical management of muscle disease, London, 1977, William Heinemann Medical Books, Ltd.

as quinine, Dilantin, procainamide, corticosteroids) can alleviate the myotonia.

A classification of the most common muscular dystrophies of orthopaedic interest is presented in Table 1-1.

Less common diseases of muscle

Congenital myopathies. The congenital myopathies are a group of primary diseases of muscle, which can be symptomatic at birth, presenting with weakness and hypotonia, or may not appear until later in childhood. A positive family history is often elicited. These variations in onset may reflect a disease spectrum of a single genetic abnormality.[16]

Congenital absence of a muscle (especially pectoralis and sternocleidomastoid), though often present as an isolated abnormality, is sometimes associated with a congenital myopathy such as myotubular myopathy.[35] The congenitally dystrophic child generally has a dysmorphic appearance (unusually long face, long, narrow fingers, high-arched palate, kyphoscoliosis, pectus excavatum or carinatum, pes cavus).

Diagnosis is aided by special histochemical techniques and electron microscopy.[36] The morphologically distinct myopathies are as follows:

1. Central core disease
2. Megaconial myopathy
3. Pleoconial myopathy
4. Nemaline myopathy
5. Myotubular myopathy
6. Congenital disproportion of fiber types
7. Multicore disease
8. Minicore disease
9. Reducing body myopathy
10. Fingerprint myopathy
11. Sarcotubular myopathy

Both central core disease and nemaline myopathy show dominant inheritance and are nonprogressive.[33] Motor skills are slow to develop. Serum muscle enzymes are usually normal. These conditions are of particular interest to orthopaedic surgeons because congenital dislocation of the hip is often present[8] and difficult to treat because of associated muscle weakness.[105]

Metabolic myopathies. The chemical defect in these diseases of muscle relates to disorders of the storage of glycogen or other metabolites, defects in lipid metabolism, or a variety of enzymatic abnormalities. Some examples are listed below:

Disorder	*Basic defect*
Pompe glycogenosis II in infantile, juvenile, and adult forms	Acid maltase deficiency (α-1,4-glucosidase)
McArdle glycogenosis V	Muscle phosphorylase deficiency
Phosphofructokinase deficiency	—
Carnitine palmityl transferase deficiency	—
Myoadenylate deaminase deficiency	—
Acute intermittent porphyria	Uroporphyrinogen I synthetase

Medical myopathies. Myopathy may accompany a host of medical diseases. Weakness can occur secondary to anemia, infection, diuretic-induced hypokalemia, or antacid-produced hypophosphatemia. Many endocrinopathies cause muscle wasting. The most common of these are as follows:

1. Hyperthyroidism
2. Hypothyroidism
3. Hyperparathyroidism
4. Addison's disease
5. Cushing's syndrome

Appropriate workup will allow diagnosis of myopathy secondary to these conditions.

Polymyositis. Polymyositis is a rare, nonsuppurative, inflammatory disease of unknown cause (though presumed to belong to the group of autoimmune responses).[11] Approximately 50% of all cases of polymyositis are linked either with a collagen or connective tissue disorder or with a malignant tumor. Such neoplastic disease is usually carcinoma (bronchogenic or prostatic in males; uterine, ovarian, or mammary in females). However, neoplasm is seldom found in the child with polymyositis. The remainder develop as primary myopathies or demonstrate a heliotropic rash (dermatomyositis).[85]

The diagnosis of polymyositis is of more than academic interest, as the disease is often responsive to steroid[12,38] or immunosuppressive therapy[60] or plasmaphoresis. In contrast to classic Duchenne muscular dystrophy, polymyositis has no familial tendency. It is more common in the black race, and females are more frequently affected than males in a ratio of approximately two to one. Initial symptoms may be abrupt and febrile. The disease follows a variable acute, subacute, or chronic course.[99]

Generalized proximal muscle weakness is noted and, with acute onset, muscular pain and stiffness are common. Inflammation may lead to muscle calcinosis. Atrophy is minimal, pseudohypertrophy rare, but dysphagia frequent. Serum muscle enzymes are elevated, as occasionally are the sedimentation rate and white blood cell count. Fifty percent of patients with polymyositis have a positive latex test, and 50% have a rise in antinuclear antibodies.

Genetics

The muscular dystrophies are pedigree specific. Fig. 1-3 and Table 1-2 illustrate the patterns of genetic determination and risk factors.

DMD demonstrates sex-linked recessive heritability. It is carried only by the female and passed only to the male. A Duchenne-like dystrophy has been described in females.[72] In such cases, polymyositis, juvenile spinal muscular atrophy (Kugelberg-Welander disease), and gonadal dysgenesis (Turner's syndrome) should be ruled out. An autosomal recessive childhood myopathy, the incidence of which is increased with consanguineous matings, can affect girls as well as boys.[101] Mating of an affected male with a carrier female can pro-

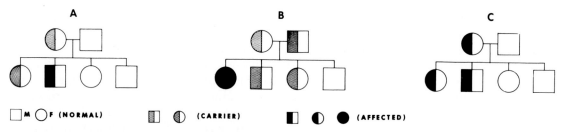

$$\square \text{M} \quad \bigcirc \text{F (NORMAL)} \qquad \boxminus \quad \varnothing \quad \text{(CARRIER)} \qquad \blacksquare \quad \bullet \quad \bullet \quad \text{(AFFECTED)}$$

Fig. 1-3. Patterns of genetic determination for the most common types of muscular dystrophy. **A,** Sex-linked heredity (classic Duchenne dystrophy) carried only by females and transmitted only to males, with 50% risk of each male child having the disease and 50% risk of each female being born a carrier. (Were a male with sex-linked dystrophy to procreate, none of his sons could have the disease and all his daughters would be carriers, unless of course his mate were a carrier, in which case each son would stand a 50% risk of inheriting the disease.) **B,** Autosomal recessive heredity (limb-girdle dystrophy). Both parents carry the defective gene, with 25% risk (regardless of sex) of transmitting the disease and 50% risk (again regardless of sex) of transmitting carrier state. **C,** Autosomal dominant heredity (facioscapulohumeral dystrophy). Either parent has the disease (there is no carrier state), with 50% risk for any child (regardless of sex) inheriting the disease. (From Siegel, I.M.: The clinical management of muscle disease, London, 1977, William Heinemann Medical Books, Ltd.)

Table 1-2. Risk factors for most common types of muscular dystrophy

Type	Genetic pattern	Affected risk	Carrier risk	Miscellaneous
Duchenne	Sex-linked Recessive	Each male 50%	Each female 50%	One third or more of all cases caused by sporadic mutation
Limb girdle	Autosomal recessive	Each child 25%	Each child 50%	Affected rise 100% if both parents exhibit clinical disease
Facioscapulohumeral	Autosomal Dominant	Each child 50%	0	Fully penetrant trait
Dystrophia myotonica*	Autosomal dominant	Each child 50%	0	Variable expressivity *formes frustes* occur

From Siegel, I.M.: The clinical management of muscle disease, London, 1977, William Heinemann Medical Books, Ltd.
*If the mother has the disease, it can appear in an affected child at birth. If the father has the disease, it usually appears in an affected child in adolescence or young adulthood.

duce an affected female. Lyonization with mosaic abiotrophy may result in a female myopathy. Finally, some females exhibiting Duchenne-like dystrophy are manifesting carriers.[95]

Limb-girdle dystrophy presents with an autosomal recessive pedigree. Facioscapulohumeral dystrophy is autosomal dominant in its hereditary pattern. Dystrophia myotonica is usually autosomal dominant but may be autosomal recessive.

Serum enzymes

The level of a number of muscle enzymes is elevated in the serum in muscular dystrophy. These include aldolase, SGOT, SGPT, and lactate dehy-rogenase.[97] Creatine phosphokinase (CPK), because of its specificity and sensitivity, provides the best biochemical index for the diagnosis of diseases of skeletal muscle. It is the function of this enzyme to catalyze reversibly the transfer of an energy-rich bond from creatine phosphate to adenosine diphosphate, forming creatine and adenosine triphosphate (CP + ADP ⇋ Creatine + ATP).

Creatine phosphokinase elevation in the muscular dystrophies is greatest in the Duchenne type and not so striking in the less rapidly progressive forms. In DMD, the highest levels are often found at birth and during the first years of life, well before the disease is clinically evident. With increasing age, diminished muscle mass, and decreased functional ability, serum enzyme levels fall.

Creatine phosphokinase is occasionally elevated in chronic denervating disease and is higher after exercise, myocardial infarction, intramuscular injection, and muscular injury.[98] Elevation of creatine phosphokinase activity is also seen in cerebrovascular disease, hypokalemia, hypothyroidism, severe anoxia, alcoholism, and acute psychoses.

Electromyography

An electromyogram (EMG) is a valuable adjunct in the diagnosis of muscle disease. The examination is noninvasive, relatively simple and well tolerated by most patients. Single motor unit potentials are elicited and interpreted.

Electromyography is useful in the differentiation of diseases of the anterior horn cell and peripheral nerves and muscles. Important components are amplitude, frequency, and duration of the evoked potential. Normal muscle (except for insertional activity secondary to needle stimulation) is electrically silent at rest.

The myopathic EMG is characterized by increased frequency, decreased duration, and decreased amplitude of action potentials.[140] This contrasts with a neuropathic EMG in which frequency is decreased and amplitude and duration are increased (Fig. 1-4). Additionally, the myopathic EMG reveals increased insertional activity, short polyphasic potentials, and a retained interference pattern. The neuropathic EMG shows frequent fibrillation potentials, a group polyphasic potential, and a reduced interference pattern (Fig. 1-5).

The EMG in dystrophia myotonica is characterized by trains of spiked potentials and positive waves fired at a high frequency, which then wax and wane until they die out, the so-called divebomber sound pattern, which is specific for myotonia.[138] Electromyographic myotonia, without clinical myotonia, may be found in acid maltase deficiency, denervation, and certain toxic neuropathies.

The EMG in polymyositis combines both neuropathic and myopathic features.

Muscle biopsy

A well-performed and expertly interpreted muscle biopsy can usually distinguish a neuropathy from a myopathy, diagnose an inflammatory myopathy, and, through the use of special histo-

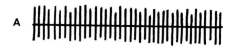
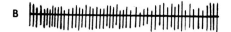
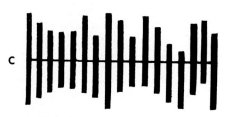

Fig. 1-4. Schematic diagram of features of electrical response in electromyogram for, **A,** normal; **B,** myopathic (increased frequency, decreased duration, decreased amplitude); and **C,** neuropathic (decreased frequency, increased duration, increased amplitude) states. (From Siegel, I.M.: The clinical management of muscle disease, London, 1977, William Heinemann Medical Books, Ltd.)

chemical staining, frequently differentiate the congenital myopathies. Muscle biopsy is not useful when one is determining the prognosis, assessing the degree of involvement, evaluating therapy, or distinguishing between the common muscular dystrophies.[55]

The biopsy site should be carefully determined.[76] The muscle selected should be only moderately involved clinically. The value of a biopsy is decreased if a muscle not at all affected or one totally destroyed is chosen. In early disease, choose a weak muscle; in late disease, one relatively strong. The gastrocnemius is usually a poor site for muscle biopsy. If the lower limb is favored, the vastus lateralis is often the best muscle available. Ordinarily, the rectus abdominus is the preferred site, as it is usually in an early stage of weakness, and biopsy here does not even minimally impair ambulation. Muscle recently traumatized by EMG needles sould not be biopsied because such testing produces histologic artifacts.

Biopsy can be performed open or with a special biopsy needle. If local anesthesia is used, direct trauma to the muscle under biopsy, by the needle or by infiltration of muscle tissue with the anesthetic agent, should be avoided. Muscle removed for histologic examination can be kept at its original in situ length when one of several special bi-

MINIMAL CONTRACTION   **MAXIMAL CONTRACTION**

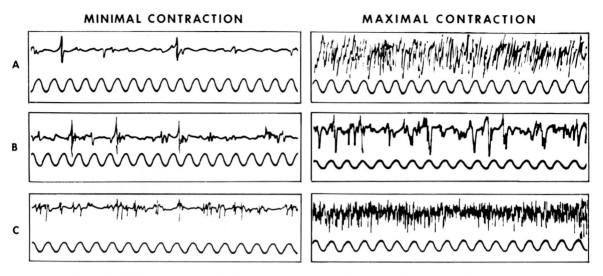

Fig. 1-5. EMG in, *A,* normal, *B,* neuropathic, and, *C,* myopathic muscle. (From Siegel, I.M.: The clinical management of muscle disease, London, 1977, William Heinemann Medical Books, Ltd.)

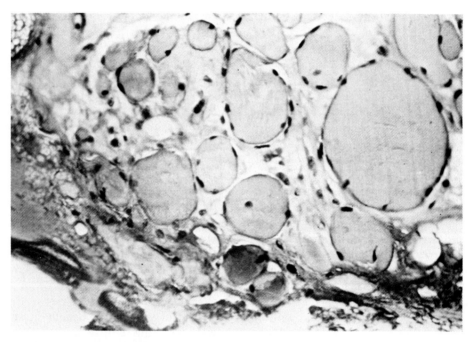

Fig. 1-6. Myopathy. (From Siegel, I.M.: The clinical management of muscle disease, London, 1977, William Heinemann Medical Books, Ltd.)

opsy clamps available is used.[106] Removal of several adjacent superficial strips of muscle is preferable to biopsy of deep tissue. It is unnecessary to take a massive specimen.

On hematoxylin-and-eosin sections, myopathy is characterized by fiber necrosis, connective tissue proliferation, hyalin, granular and fatty degeneration, and an increased number of nuclei with nuclear migration to the center of muscle fibers (Fig. 1-6).[58]

Neuropathy typically shows small angulated fibers on cross section, bundles of atrophic small fi-

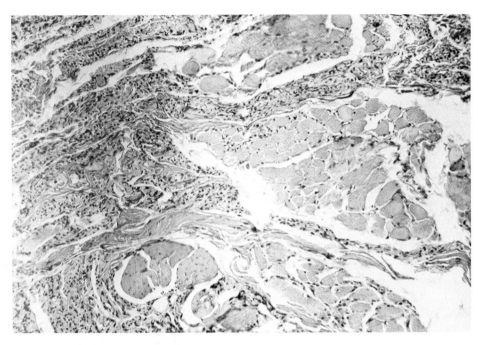

Fig. 1-7. Neuropathy. (From Siegel, I.M.: The clinical management of muscle disease, London, 1977, William Heinemann Medical Books, Ltd.)

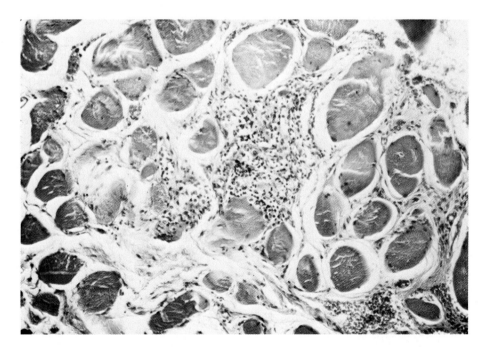

Fig. 1-8. Polymyositis. (From Siegel, I.M.: The clinical management of muscle disease, London, 1977, William Heinemann Medical Books, Ltd.)

bers interspersed with groups of normally innervated fibers of normal size, and little increase in connective tissue (Fig. 1-7).

Aggregates of inflammatory cells are seen in polymyositis, as well as segmental necrosis with fiber degeneration and regeneration, interstitial edema, perivasculitis, and perifascicular muscle fiber atrophy (Fig. 1-8).

Histochemical methods are of value in the study of muscle biopsies because they demonstrate specific fiber types on the basis of various enzyme reactions, thus indicating selective fiber type involvement in certain diseases. They may also reveal absence of a particular enzyme or an excess or deficit of a particular storage product. Various structural changes in the muscle, which would not be revealed with routine histologic stains, become apparent with special histochemical analysis. Histochemical study and the investigation of ultrastructural muscle change with the electron microscope are particularly valuable in the diagnosis and investigation of the metabolic and congenital myopathies.

Carrier state

Genetic counseling is an important part of the total treatment of the patient with muscular dystrophy. Although approximately one third of all cases of Duchenne dystrophy are sporadic neomutations, mothers of afflicted children should know if they are carriers of the disease so that future pregnancy can be planned. Additionally, female siblings of such patients should be tested for the carrier state and counseled (informed, not advised) concerning the risk of bearing a child with Duchenne muscular dystrophy.

Women "at risk" are categorized as follows:
1. *Definite carriers.* Mothers of an affected son who also have dystrophic male relatives in the female line of inheritance. Also included are mothers of two affected sons by different nonconsanguineous fathers.
2. *Probable carriers.* Mothers of two or more sons with muscular dystrophy who have no other affected relatives.
3. *Possible carriers.*
   a. Mothers of those who are isolated cases.
   b. Sisters or other female relatives of affected males. Possible carriers may have a known risk (such as the daughter of a definite carrier where the risk is 50%) or an unknown risk (sister of a sporadic case).

Bayesian statistical tables are available for calculation of the jeopardy for a mother or sister with, respectively, an affected son or brother. Risk is based on the number of normal males in the family and the serum creatine phosphokinase of the concerned female as well as that of her mother.[40]

Identification of carriers depends on the fact that they carry a microcosm of the full-blown disease, which may be detected by appropriate investigation. Careful physical examination can indeed reveal slight weakness of limb-girdle musculature[113] and even calf enlargement in DMD carriers. Serum creative phosphokinase is elevated in approximately 70% of carriers of Duchenne dystrophy. However, the test is less useful in relatives of patients afflicted with any of the less acute, usually autosomal hereditary forms of myopathy (limb-girdle, facioscapulohumeral, and myotonic). A carrier's creatine phosphokinase is most consistently elevated during childhood and adolescence. By the time most carriers reach adulthood, all myopathic cells are fully degraded and serum creatine phosphokinase has returned to normal.

In addition to biochemical screening, DMD carriers will occasionally show changes in EMG and ECG, as well as a muscle biopsy revealing minimal myopathic changes. If a known carrier elects to have children, it is possible to identify fetal sex by examination of amnionic fluid (there are risks to this procedure, including a 1 in 1000 rate of infection and a 1 in 200 incidence of spontaneous abortion), and therapeutic abortion can be performed if the fetal cells indicate a male chromosomal pattern. Determination of the creatine phosphokinase of fetal blood, utilizing fetoscopy, has up to now not proved reliable for prenatal diagnosis.

The following outline shows the techniques reported as helpful in DMD carrier detection*:

1. *Genetic*
   Pedigree analysis
   Linkage analysis
   Markers
   Particular (bayesian) analysis combining data from several sources
2. *Clinical*
   Manual muscle testing

*Courtesy S. Phipps, M.S., Department of Genetics, Milwaukee Children's Hospital, Milwaukee, Wisconsin.

Quantitative EMG changes
Qualitative biopsy changes in skeletal muscle
Electron microscopy of skeletal muscle[a]
Relaxation time (adductor pollicis)[b]
3. *Blood chemistry*
Creatine phosphokinase, aldolase, SGOT, SGPT
Pyruvate kinase[c]
Lactate dehydrogenase[d]
Hemopexin[e]
Myoglobinemia[f]
4. *Others*
In vitro ribosomal protein synthesis,[g,h]
Endogenous phosphorylation of red blood cell membranes[i]
Electron microscopy of red blood cell membranes[j]
Lymphocyte capping[k]

X-ray features

Roentgen features of muscular dystrophy, though not pathognomonic, are the following[41,51,87]:

1. Osteoporosis
2. Talipes equinocavovarus
3. Vertebral caninization
4. Decreased tibial diameter (Fig. 1-9)
5. Overtubulation of long bone shafts
6. Symmetric diminution in size of the scapulas
7. Small pelvis with flaring iliac bones and prominent ischial spines
8. Increased soft-tissue shadows in areas of hypertrophy and pseudohypertrophy
9. Valgus hip deformity
10. Lordosis (early) and scoliosis (late)

[a]Ionasescu, V., Radu, H., and Nicolescu, P.: Arch. Pathol. **99**(8):436, 1975.
[b]Oepkes, C.T., and van Weerden, T.W.: Neurology **29**(4):523, 1979.
[c]Alberts, M.C., and Samaha, F.T.: Neurology **24**:462, 1974.
[d]Roses, A.D., Roses, M.J., Nicholson, G.A., et al.: Neurology **27**(5):414, 1977.
[e]Danieli, G.A., and Angeline, C.: Lancet **2**:90, 1976.
[f]Adornato, B.T., Kagen, L.J., and Engel, W.K.: Lancet **2**:499, 1978.
[g]Ionasescu, V., Zellweger, H., and Burmeister, L.: Acta Neurol. Scand. **54**(5):442, 1976.
[h]Ionasescu, V., Zellweger, H., Shirk, P., and Conway, T.W.: Neurology **23**(5):497, 1973.
[i]Roses, A.D., Roses, J.J., Miller, S.E., et al.: N. Engl. J. Med. **294**(4):193, 1976.
[j]Matheson, D.W., and Howland, J.L.: Science **184**:165, 1974.
[k]Pickard, N.A., Gruemer, H.D., Verril, H.L., et al.: N. Engl. J. Med. **299**(16):841, 1978.

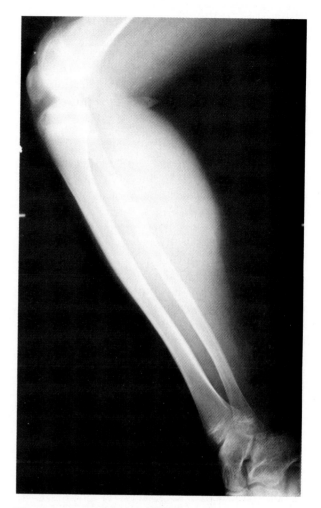

Fig. 1-9. Lateral roentgenogram of leg in Duchenne muscular dystrophy showing *1*, osteoporosis; *2*, decreased tibial diameter; *3*, overtubulation of long bone shafts; *4*, increased soft-tissue shadow. (From Siegel, I.M.: The clinical management of muscle disease, London, 1977, William Heinemann Medical Books, Ltd.)

GENERAL TREATMENT

Optimal therapy for the patient with a muscle disease should be prospective and aggressive and conducted in an atmosphere of intelligent concern. Management is best administered by a team that includes pediatric, neurologic, genetic, and physiatric as well as orthopaedic consultants. In addition, physical therapists, occupational therapists, and medical social workers or psychologists can assist the patient and family. Dietary and speech therapy, as well as subspecialty consultation, where indicated (such as in the areas of gastrointestinal and cardiopulmonary care), provide a thoroughgoing approach to the problems of total management. The patient with muscular dystrophy often develops multisystem complaints during the course of his illness. Skill in diagnosing and treating such nonmotor complications can prolong independent function. Some major nonorthopaedic complications are as follows.

Cardiac

The heart is a muscle, and cardiac involvement is common in most forms of muscular dystrophy.[102] It is said to be present in over 80% of patients with Duchenne muscular dystrophy. Such children frequently suffer posterobasal fibrosis of the left ventricle, and electrocardiographic changes are noted during all stages of the disease, even when overt clinical evidence of cardiomyopathy is lacking because restricted activity maintains a precarious status quo.[103] Patients with advanced myopathy, particularly those in wheelchairs, sometimes develop a straight back syndrome that may mimic organic heart disease by causing systolic murmer with pseudocardiomegaly or with an abnormal electrocardiogram.[28,30,54] The most common ECG findings of cardiomyopathy consist of tall right precordial R waves and deep left precordial Q waves (Fig. 1-10).[131]

Cardiac disorder is not characteristic of limbgirdle, FSH, or Becker's dystrophy. In dystrophia myotonica, heart disease usually occurs late in the course of the disease and most commonly appears as a disturbance of atrioventricular conduction. Such patients may require cardiac pacemakers.

Where indicated, treatment of cardiac complications in the muscular dystrophies is along conventional lines.

Respiratory

Pulmonary problems are frequently encountered in the advanced stages of the muscular dystrophies.[1] Decreased pulmonary function with poor respiratory toilet, compounded by weakness of deglutition, which increases the danger of aspiration penumonitis, lays fertile ground for respiratory complications, especially hypostatic pneumonia.[20] Long-term inadequate ventilation can result in chronic CO_2 narcosis (blood pressure increase, nightmares, sleeplessness) and secondary polycythemia in any of the muscular dystrophies.[57] Alveolar hypotension with a gross reduc-

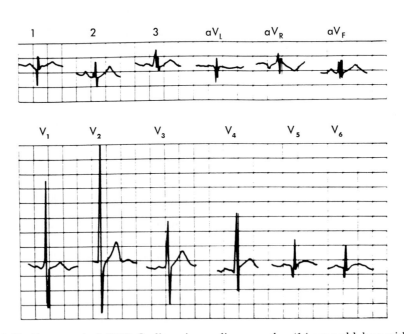

Fig. 1-10. Some typical ECG findings in cardiomyopathy (14-year-old boy with Duchenne muscular dystrophy). Note narrow but deep Q waves in leads 1, aV_L, V_5, and V_6; RSR pattern in aV_R; and dominant (R) waves in V_1 and V_2. (From Siegel, I.M.: The clinical management of muscle disease, London, 1977, William Heinemann Medical Books, Ltd.)

tion in the maximal expiratory pressure are common pulmonary findings in dystrophia myotonica.[17]

Periodic evaluation of pulmonary function to monitor restrictive pulmonary disease must be an integral part of any treatment program for patients with muscular dystrophy.[123,142] Reduction of vital capacity, forced expiratory ability, and maximal voluntary ventilation are common findings.[71] Thirty percent vital capacity in the chronic phase of restrictive ventilatory insufficiency can maintain tidal volume in the minimally active patient. As ventilation drops, the accessory respiratory muscles (such as the sternocleidomastoid and platysma) are brought into play. Decreased respiratory function can lead to cor pulmonale with right heart failure and cardiomyopathy.[26] Diminished vital capacity secondary to a weakened chest bellows decreases the ability to cough.[142]

Reduction in chest compliance and progressive weakness of the respiratory musculature require an ongoing program of pulmonary rehabilitation,[2] including diaphragmatic breathing exercises,[116] postural drainage, proper humidification, chest percussion, and training in the use of various respiratory aids.[3,67] Vigorous treatment of upper respiratory infections to avoid serious pulmonary disease can include pharyngeal suction and intermittent positive-pressure breathing therapy.[26] Mechanical ventilation of patients in the terminal stages of DMD can be managed at home without a tracheostomy. Apparatus available includes the rocking bed, plastic wrap ventilator, pneumobelt, and chest-abdomen cuirass respirator.[5]

Dietary

Obesity hastens functional disability, and nutrition should be carefully monitored throughout the course of DMD but particularly after wheelchair confinement. A well-balanced vitamin-supplemented diet of no less than 1200 calories is provided. Patients are encouraged to choose fruits and vegetables as alternatives to high-caloric snacks. High-fiber foods and fruit juices aid in maintaining normal elimination. Only small amounts of milk products are offered because of their mucus-producing tendency. Wheelchair-bound patients often reduce fluid intake and, reluctant to ask for toileting assistance, retain urine as long as possible. Such urinary stasis predisposes to infection. In addition to assuring adequate fluid intake, foods such as cereals, meats, poultry, fish, and cranberry juice, which lower urinary pH because of their acid residues, are advised.

Patients in the later stages of muscular dystrophy find deglutition difficult because of posterior pharyngeal and upper esophageal weakness. Oculopharyngeal myopathy (a rare autosomal dominant muscle disease) is characterized by dysphagia. Instruction in proper positioning (head flexion), eating slowly, introducing soft and pureed foods into the diet, and sitting upright for a time after meals can assist the patient with the task of swallowing. Patients with myotonic dystrophy should avoid cold foods or fluids because they may provoke pharyngeal myotonia.

Dysfunction of smooth muscle, particularly that of the gastrointestinal tract, has been noted in muscular dystrophy.[50,70,88] Both acute megacolon and gastric dilatation[111] have been reported. Treatment of these conditions is no different from that in the patient without muscle disease.

Psychosocial

Muscular dystrophy is a disease of the psyche as well as the soma. The importance of psychosocial care cannot be ignored.[137] Children with Duchenne muscular dystrophy face the same problems of body image, peer interaction, family adjustment, and sexuality that all normal children must resolve in the process of maturing.[147] Needless to say, the dystrophic child has increased difficulty establishing emotional independence from his parents.[129] His social contacts are limited, and he frequently uses fantasy and denial as mechanisms of adjustment. Hopeful but realistic feedback, not pity, is required if he is to develop a capacity for lasting interpersonal relationships and establish the meaningful and stable identity that leads to self-acceptance. The home should provide appropriate role models, opportunity for learning, and privacy. Sexual needs must be recognized and accepted.

Supportive psychiatric intervention, made available at times of psychologic crisis, can avert critical emotional damage. Intelligent and empathic counseling of both the patient and his family throughout the course of the illness is an important part of the total management of muscular dystrophy. This includes early discovery of carriers and appropriate genetic counseling of both the patient's parents and female siblings.

In the treatment of muscular dystrophy, the

family is the patient. Group therapy has been found valuable in assisting parents of children with muscular dystrophy by helping them develop insight and increasing communication through sharing of experiences.[83]

Mental retardation has been observed in 30% to 50% of patients with Duchenne muscular dystrophy.[79,90] Verbal and performance I.Q.'s are equally affected. The intellectual subnormality is present from birth and is nonprogressive.[32] In families containing two or more patients, the affected members often have a similar I.Q.[149] This suggests that mental retardation may be genetically determined.

Decreased intellectual functioning does not occur in patients with limb-girdle or FSH dystrophy. Mental defects, intellectual deterioration, and lack of initiative are often present in varying degree in dystrophia myotonica. Nonspecific electroencephalographic abnormalities, cerebroventricular enlargement, and heterotopias have also been described in this disease.

Miscellaneous

Problems with speech are frequent in the muscular dystrophies.[6,96] Weakness of the facial musculature in FSH, tongue hypertrophy in DMD, changes in the jaws, and orthodontic deformity lead to decreased vocal intensity, reduced breath support, nasality, and the open-mouth posture. Speech therapy may be beneficial as well as morale-building.

There is evidence that, in addition to muscle involvement, DMD may cause changes in the collagen vascular system. A subcutaneous reticular vascular pattern, accentuated by exercise, is seen in these patients. Additionally, nonspecific changes in subcutaneous fat have been reported. Another skin condition, erythema ab igne, and seborrheic dermatitis are also common in Duchenne dystrophy.[125]

Pressure decubiti in the wheelchair- or bed-bound patient seldom occur, even though special seating pads or mattresses never relieve compression below capillary closing pressure of 32 mm Hg. Areas of skin irritation can be toughened with the daily application of a moist tea bag.

Patients with Duchenne muscular dystrophy do not procreate. In the adult forms of muscular disease (limb-girdle dystrophy, FSH) pregnancy is usually uneventful, though there is occasional increased loss of muscle power during the third trimester. Because the myometrium is not af-

fected in these diseases, labor is usually normal. However, in dystrophia myotonica, assistance is often required during the second stage of labor.

MOTOR-RELATED TREATMENT
Physical therapy

The physical therapist plays several important roles in the management of the patient with muscular dystrophy.[66] The first role is that of an assessor who measures specific muscle weakness, imbalance, and contracture.[39] The distribution of weakness and pathokinetic sequence are similar in all the major muscular dystrophies. For instance, although cervical extensors, tibialis posterior, and toe flexors are commonly spared in all types, all groups show involvement of lower and middle trapezius muscles. Differences lie in the degree and rapidity of progression of weakness and contracture. In Duchenne muscular dystrophy, the anterior cervical flexors (particularly sternocleidomastoid) are involved early and severely. Strength in the hamstring muscles is usually preserved in DMD (lateral hamstrings are spared the longest), whereas the brachioradialis is commonly strong in limb-girdle dystrophy. The sternal portion of the pectoralis major is spared in FSH, though the tibialis anticus and peroneals are frequently involved early in this disease.

The pattern of loss is proximal to distal in all the common dystrophies. Distal myopathies are rare autosomal dominantly inherited diseases, here weakness is present in the hands or feet, with slow, or no, progression. DMD and limb-girdle dystrophy are symmetric in distribution, FSH may be asymmetric. Flexors are usually weaker than extensors in the neck and trunk, but extensors are usually weaker in the shoulders and hips.[133] Triceps brachii may be stronger than biceps brachii in the Becker form of muscular dystrophy. One of the earliest signs of FSH can be finger- or wrist-extensor weakness.

Most major axial or appendicular musculature requires at least 30% to 50% anatomic loss before critical clinical weakness becomes obvious. This accounts for the apparent normal functioning of children with DMD during the first several years of life (the abiotrophic half-life of muscle in DMD is 4.8 years).[132] Improvement of some patients from 5 to 7 years of age can be explained by the processes of normal development, which, utilizing residual muscle strength and increased motor coordination, outstrip the progress of the disease during this period. However, even though the mechanical efficiency of the skeleton probably doubles as bone matures (the skeletal mass increases 20 times from the newborn to the adult, whereas the muscle mass increases 40 times), a greater proportion of muscle is required as the limbs grow, since the work necessary to move an appendage is proportional to the fourth power of its length, whereas that achieved by a muscle is proportional to the cube of its length.[4] This explains why a patient with a condition limiting his ultimate muscle mass may eventually lose the ability to ambulate, even though he had been able to do so when small and the disease remained inactive with no increased loss of strength.

Gradient measurement of strength and functional ability falls within the purview of the physical therapist.[92] From a rehabilitation standpoint, the sum of muscle weakness, contracture, and imbalance determines a patient's ability to perform the activities of daily living. Standard muscle testing, which follows changes in strength in individual muscles, is not sensitive enough to evaluate the functional status of muscle groups, depending as they do on a delicate agonist-antagonist balance.[93] Muscle activity is a complex operation, consisting of a prime mover working in concert with antagonists, synergists, and stabilizers. Attempts to define the specific action of a single muscle is academic and impractical. Also to be considered are the relative activities of those muscles essentially stabilizing position (tonic) and those mostly activating movement (phasic).

Muscle testing grades key muscles both as to their strength and range of motion against gravity.[152] Any change in range is interpreted as indicating a change in strength. Muscle imbalance is as important a factor as specific muscle weakness in compromising motor function. This method enables the prescription of exercise programs (both active and passive) designed to relieve such imbalance.

A patient's ability to perform a number of standard tasks is also assessed, both as to time required and method employed to complete the task. Subtle alterations in method as well as slight changes in time required for any given task, objectively reflect changes in strength.[69]

Patients are rated on a functional 10-step scale[141]:

1. Walks and climbs stairs without assistance.
2. Walks and climbs stairs with aid of railing.
3. Walks and climbs stairs slowly with aid of railing.
4. Walks but cannot climb stairs.
5. Walks unassisted but cannot climb stairs or get out of chair.
6. Walks only with assistance or with braces.
7. In wheelchair, sits erect and can roll chair and perform bed and wheelchair activities of daily living.
8. In wheelchair, sits erect but is unable to perform bed and chair activities without assistance.
9. In wheelchair, sits erect only with support and able to do only minimal activities of daily living.
10. In bed, cannot perform activities of daily living without assistance.

This system provides a treatment format for the physical therapy program.[143] In stages 1 to 3, the patient is ambulating independently, though with a disturbed gait pattern, and passive stretch of early lower extremity contracture is necessary. However, functional activities of daily living and ambulation are sufficient exercise, and a special exercise program is unnecessary in stages 1 to 3. Somewhere between stages 5 and 6, lower extremity surgery is indicated because of increased difficulty with antigravity activities, secondary to contracture.

Well-meaning caretakers sometimes encourage ambulant patients in stages 5 or 6 to avoid activity and use wheelchairs. Patients so treated lose strength rapidly, becoming permanently wheelchair-bound within a relatively short period of time. In some cases, there is an unfortunate tendency to avoid the wheelchair entirely in stage 7, condemning the patient to stage 10 immediately. Patients can usually be taught wheelchair transfer techniques and allowed wheelchair independence for a significantly longer period of time. When the patient reaches stage 7, routine conditioning exercises are prescribed to retard disuse atrophy and maintain independence in wheelchair activities as long as possible. Prophylactic treatment of scoliosis is also initiated at this time. It is essential that patients after stage 7 be given care befitting their physiologic means. This includes use of a tilt or standup table or appropriate bracing and continued contracture stretching. Cardiac and pulmonary problems become more severe during and after stage 7. Obesity is usually a problem when a patient becomes wheelchair-confined. The closer a patient is to bed confinement, the more assistive devices he requires.

The second role of the physical therapist is that

of an instructor who teaches exercises, stretching, and gait training, directed toward improving muscular strength, preventing and correcting contracture, and increasing efficiency in the functional activities of daily living.[22] At the same time, one should avoid overenthusiastic stretching of contractures because it causes pain, stimulates the stretch reflex strengthening the deforming muscle or muscles, and prompts the patient to fight the passive force by an active effort of his own. Disability from weakness must be distinguished from that caused by contracture. The essential tenodesis effect of contracture in the face of severe loss of muscular support should be monitored by the physical therapist.

Muscular activity enhances contractile protein synthesis. The dangers of inactivity in the patient with DMD are well documented. At complete rest, strength is lost at a rate of approximately 3% a day.[84] Until a specific cure is discovered for muscular dystrophy, all attempts to treat the disease will be palliative. Nonetheless, it is desirable to preserve maximal physical function through an aggressive program of therapy, pending such discovery, because when it is possible to arrest the disease process, those patients ambulatory will be much better off than those comfined to a wheelchair or bed.

Three processes contribute to the deformities of muscular dystrophy:

1. Muscle weakness
2. Muscle imbalance

3. Specific muscle contracture (secondary to gravity and compensatory postural habitus)

An aggressive program of physical therapy provides submaximal exercise,[29] gait training, and contracture stretching (particularly hip flexors, tensor fasciae latae, and heel cords).[7] Although the benefits of active exercise in the management of muscular dystrophy are still debated,[74,144] it is generally agreed that nonexhausting functional exercise is helpful in maintaining strength.[31] Passive stretching of contractures, by balancing agonist against antagonist, can prolong function, decrease the energy cost of muscular activity to the patient, and preserve balance necessary for maintenance of the upright posture and proper seating when wheelchair confinement becomes necessary.[44,75]

Standing and walking are the best functional physical therapy for the patient with DMD. Two to 3 hours a day of such activity is encouraged. If the patient feels rested after a full night's sleep, he is not being overexercised. Stretch positioning (proning) to stretch hip flexors and vigorous, active assisted exercise can significantly lengthen the period of functional ability.[63]

Night splints are sometimes also effective in preserving joint posture,[135] but such appliances are of little value after deformities have occurred and should be used in addition to, and not instead of, manual contracture stretching. Where lower extremity night splints are used, knee-ankle-foot orthoses (KAFO) are advised because AFO night

Table 1-3. Exercises for stretching key musculature

Muscles	Active	Passive
Hip flexors	Lying supine at edge of bed or table, hold opposite knee and hip flexed, drop leg over edge, and allow weight of extremity to extend hip	Patient prone with knees extended; while stabilizing hip from behind, elevate knee from table
Tensor fasciae latae (iliotibial band)	Stand with one side toward wall and feet about 8 to 12 inches from wall, keep knees straight, and lean near hip toward wall	Patient prone with thigh extended and abducted; stabilizing hip posteriorly, adduct hip to maximum stretch position
Hamstrings	Toe-touching in standing or seated position with knees straight	Patient supine, hip flexed, knee extended; elevate leg to maximum stretch position
Heel cords	Stand arm's length from a wall; supporting body with hands on wall and keeping knees extended and *heels on floor,* attempt to lean chest to wall, thus dorsiflexing ankles	Patient supine, knees extended; cup heel in palm maintaining foot in neutral position and supporting sole to avoid bending foot at tarsal joints; dorsiflex ankle to position of maximal stretch

From Siegel, I. M.: The clinical management of muscle disease, London, 1977, William Heinemann Medical Books, Ltd.

splints for ankle equinus may initiate or increase knee flexion contracture because of the tendency of patients to flex their knees in order to relieve discomfort from triceps surae tightness.

Patients with DMD suffer severe disuse atrophy when put to bed. They should not be bed or chair confined for more than a day at most. Alternate haunch standing is encouraged to avoid heel-cord contracture. Although weakening is symmetric in many of the muscular dystrophies, joint contractures are not so. Unequal contracture occurs secondary to habitually maintained postures, both awake and asleep, and also to increased activity in the dominant extremities. Two-joint muscles contract the earliest and the most. Although one cannot prevent primary weakness, atrophy of disuse and excessive contracture are controllable. Table 1-3 describes exercises for stretching key musculature.

Occupational therapy

As the patient with muscular dystrophy finds it increasingly difficult because of progressive weakness and disability to attend to his tasks of daily living, the occupational therapist can aid in assessing and assisting him. A variety of techniques and aids can be used.[94] Patients with weak quadriceps muscles require chairs and toilet seats that are elevated. A bathtub stool, used with a shower spray, allows the patient to bathe with decreased back strain. Assistive devices, lift and transfer equipment, clothing adaptations,[61] special mattresses, and so on, are available.

Wheelchair care

When ambulation is no longer possible, wheelchair confinement becomes necessary. This is a critical incident, both physiologically and psychologically, in the life of the patient with muscular dystrophy[139]; thus every effort should be devoted to making the wheelchair the passport to more, rather than less, activity.[48,49]

Special wheelchair adaptations can increase comfort, while providing spinal support.[47,91] Where indicated, balanced forearm orthoses (enabling weakened upper extremity musculature to operate across rather than against the field of gravity) facilitate use of the hands for self-feeding, writing, and other utilitarian tasks.[23] Wheelchairs sometimes permit the home-confined walker the benefits of community travel, and electric wheelchairs are available for patients with in-

sufficient strength to manage the standard model.

Adequate trunk support positions the patient upright, enabling him to use the wheelchair more effectively. A firm seat and back and a wide safety belt are provided. When neck extension is weak, an extended back rest is fitted to support the head.[52]

A wheelchair of proper size is prescribed. This incorporates large rear wheels, hand brakes, swinging, adjustable foot rests with heel straps, and upholstered, removable desklike arms. A zippered back permits obese patients to be easily placed supine for part of the day to stretch out hip contractures. A combination wheelchair commode eliminates the problem of difficult transfer from wheelchair to toilet, and families with limited space prefer this combination to a separate commode. Daily passive stretch of hips, knees, and ankles, augmented by wedges for the feet, holding the ankles in neutral or dorsiflexion, and extended leg rests, used to prevent flexion contracture of the knees, can delay disabling contractures of the lower extremities in wheelchair-confined patients. As long as the legs are kept supple through stretching, long leg braces can be applied and the patient easily tilted from his chair. This is a considerably easier task than lifting a flail, obese adolescent. Standing erect for at least several hours a day, with help from a tilt or standing table, provides considerable psychologic and physiologic value to the patient. Such activity reduces the frequency of static urinary complications and lessens the degree of disuse osteoporosis. Wheelchair complications include the following:

1. Scoliosis.
2. Obesity.
3. Acceleration of cardiopulmonary difficulties.
4. Decrease in general rate of all metabolic processes.
5. Reduction of circulation to lower extremities with dependent edema.
6. Accelerating decrement of muscle mass, which reduces potassium stores; sudden stress (such as infection) may result in sufficient loss of potassium to cause paralytic ileus.
7. Increase in weakness and contracture.
8. Sometimes mental and emotional problems secondary to confinement and almost complete lack of mobility.
9. Functional problems of transfer, feeding,

recreation, and so on, both for the patient and his family.

10. Possibility of superior mesenteric artery obstruction ("cast syndrome") secondary to constrictive torso bracing or (in thin individuals) when the patient with paralytic disease is moved to the sitting position.

Although care at this stage of muscular dystrophy is truly supportive, the preservation of maximal residual motor power and the maintenance of the ability to attend to the tasks of daily living are important to both the patient's physical and emotional well-being.

Orthopaedic management

Pathomechanics. Although all skeletal muscle is affected in Duchenne muscular dystrophy clinical weakness is first noted and ultimately most severe in those antigravity muscles serving a postural role.[13] This includes the muscles of the limb girdles, the knee extensors, and the dorsiflexors of the ankle. Management of patients with DMD requires an understanding of the pathomechanics involved in the natural evolution of this process so that orthopaedic or physiatric intervention can be appropriately staged.

Postural dynamics. The pattern of muscular wasting in DMD bears a direct relationship to muscular function, determined by the muscle's location in the body. As postulated by Bonsett,[14] regional differences relate to postural, supportive, and traumatic factors. The dynamic postural role of muscle is served by reflex contractile responses. As the disease advances, reflex function is lost, functional muscle mass is reduced, pseudohypertrophic degeneration occurs, and the muscle deteriorates to a passive, supportive role. With the decline of elasticity and the ability to contract reflexly, such muscle is now vulnerable to deforming forces imposed by a postural or supportive traumatic stress.

Although physiologically at rest, a muscle is physically in a state of tonic stretch. Muscle spindles protect against overstretch. Loss of the deep tendon reflex marks the regression of a muscle from a kinetic to a purely static state. The Achilles reflex is lost last because of the long stretch range of its tendon, which places the spindle environment in a receptive tension state. With absence of the stretch reflex, passive stretch can occur, leaving an inadequately responsive muscle excessively vulnerable to ordinary strain.

Work hypertrophy is seen in antigravity mus-

cles maintaining pelvic femoral alignment. These muscles are the buttocks, thighs, and calves in the lower extremities and the shoulder stabilizers in the upper. The serratus anterior is a major postural fixator of the shoulder and is affected early. The psoas (postural) is more severely involved than the iliacus (nonpostural); the abdominal portion of the pectoralis major is more than its clavicular part; the clavicular head of the sternocleidomastoid is more than the sternal head of that muscle; cervical flexors are more than cervical extensors because of the increased need for head flexion to balance advancing lordosis. Postural overwork (hypertrophy) weakens the dystrophic muscle.

Biokinetics. Alterations of the dynamics of postural maintenance in DMD, secondary to the pattern of muscular involvement necessary to compensate for weakness or as a result of imbalance between opposing muscle groups, lead to hip-and knee-flexion contracture, ankle equinocavovarus, and spinal distortions in the sagittal plane (lordosis) in the still ambulatory patient and in the coronal plane (scoliosis) in the patient who is wheelchair confined.

Normal locomotion requires modulation of the center of gravity just anterior to the lumbosacral junction. The center of gravity is elevated in the stance phase of gait, thus building potential energy, which is converted to kinetic energy during the swing phase. Although some vertical center-of-gravity displacement is necessary to achieve this potential-kinetic energy tradeoff, unproductive movement is balanced off by certain coordinated joint motions, including (1) pelvic rotation, (2) pelvic tilt on the swing side, and (3) knee flexion on the stance leg. Coupling of knee extension with ankle dorsiflexion, and of knee flexion with ankle plantar flexion, maintains equal leg length throughout gait. Physiologic knee valgus places the foot under the center of gravity without excessive lateral torso shift during stance.[104] These postural adaptations enable the body to remain upright by maintaining the line of the center of gravity within its base of support. They also serve Newton's third law well as the torque of ground contact during gait passes upward through the center of gravity, avoiding undue angular acceleration of the body when in motion. In muscular dystrophy, such adjustments become increasingly difficult as weakness and contracture progress.

Clinical correlation. In DMD, the hip flexors, ten-

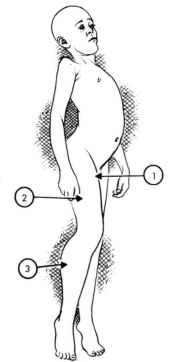

Fig. 1-11. Ambulation-limiting contractures occur in, *1*, hip flexors; *2*, tensor fasciae latae; and, *3*, triceps surae. (From Siegel, I.M.: The clinical management of muscle disease, London, 1977, William Heinemann Medical Books, Ltd.)

sor fasciae latae and triceps surae develop ambulation-limiting contractures (Fig. 1-11). With progress of quadriceps weakness and increasing contracture in the above muscle groups, the base of support decreases, the patient can no longer utilize normal mechanisms for efficient balance, and he must walk with a wide gait, characterized by equinus, heel varus, knee flexion, hip flexion, and hip abduction.

Exaggerated lumbar lordosis is a functional deformity noted early as the child attempts to compensate for pelvic force imbalance secondary to weakened hip extension, accompanied by hip-flexion contracture. The center of gravity is shifted posteriorly in lordosis, and he adjusts by rising on the balls of his feet and ultimately on his toes. Abdominal and low back extensor weakness contribute to this awkward and effortful posture as loss of scapular stabilizer strength draws the shoulders forward, requiring increased lumbar lordosis to achieve torso balance. The hips are further abducted in a desperate effort to widen the base of support so that the line of gravity will fall within its confines. Several biarticular muscles of the lower extremity reverse their usual roles in response to the antigravity needs of this postural crisis. With fixed equinus, the soleus (and sometimes gastrocnemius) functions as an extensor of the knee, and if the ankle is fixed in equinus by

external resistance, and the knee flexed and its extension prevented by superincumbent body load, the hamstring muscles will contract in a vain attempt to extend the knee and keep the body upright.

Although the long arch is obliterated secondary to early minimal heel-cord contracture, it is reconstructed with initiation of the inevitable equinovarus deformity. As the ankle is held in plantar flexion, the narrow portion of the talus is brought into the mortise, rendering this joint vulnerable to forces that shape a rotatory deformity.

The center of hip rotation shifts medially during standing. Thus the psoas major functions as an external hip rotator in the swing phase and an internal rotator in the stance phase. The tensor fasciae latae internally rotates the hip. Reasonable agonist-antagonist rotation balance is maintained at this joint, and severe rotational deformities of the hip are not usually seen in ambulatory DMD.

Energetics. The pathokinetics of DMD have been outlined elsewhere.[119] Progression of weakness, contracture, and deformity in various muscle groups is not entirely sequential because these morbid events overlap and some occur concurrently. So long as the patient can maintain his line of gravity behind his hips, in front of his knees, and within his base of support, the upright posture can be sustained (Fig. 1-12).

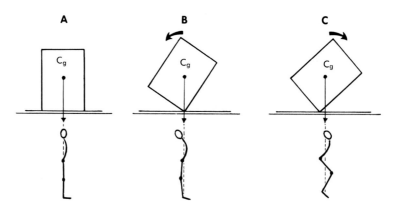

Fig. 1-12. A, Line of gravity maintained behind hips, in front of knees, and within base of support. **B,** Lumbar lordosis, equinus, and knee extension permit upright posture. **C,** Line of gravity no longer as in **A** or **B.** Standing no longer possible. C_g, Center of gravity.

Initiation of gait requires body unbalancing through coordinated activity of the tibialis anticus, quadriceps, hip abductors, and peroneal muscles,[89] a process the advanced Duchenne dystrophic patient finds difficult to perform. To execute the swing phase of gait, two conditions seem necessary: the hip must extend and the extensor muscles must unload.[100] Progressive hip flexion contracture in DMD interferes with both requisites. Incapacity to properly modulate the center of gravity during gait, and so utilize normal compensatory mechanisms to minimize energy expenditure in forward motion, and inability to balance the ground reaction through proper control of angular acceleration lead to excessive rolling of the body for balance in DMD at a severe expenditure of metabolic energy during ambulation.

The earliest musculature to show clinical weakness in DMD is that appearing first in the embryo. Principal functional loss is noted in the limb girdles. The most severe contractures occur in postural muscles spanning two joints. Muscular weakness, tendon contracture, and mechanical malposture contribute to ultimate deformity.

An outline of the biomechanical sequence leading to the typical dystrophic picture follows:
1. Weakness of hip extensors and shoulder stabilizers.
2. Hip flexor contracture forcing trunk forward.
3. Compensatory lumbar lordosis.
4. Because of forward shift of center of mass, patient rises on his toes, thus shortening ankle-to-toes lever arm and shifting center of gravity forward.
5. Hip abduction increases equilibrium by widening body's base of support.
6. Tensor fasciae latae contracture.
7. External tibial torsion; thus ankle and knee axes are no longer in same plane.
8. Ankle varus (an effort to bring ankle into better postural alignment).
9. Knee flexion for balance.
10. Quadriceps weakens; equinus required to lock knees for stability.
11. With foot fixed in equinus and knee flexed, combination of gastrocnemius and soleus now acts to extend knee.
12. True exercise hypertrophy of calf as it overworks to maintain knee in extension.
13. Widening of base of support with concomitant increase of those forces causing equinocavovarus.
    a. Unopposed heel-cord contracture acting upon eccentric medial insertion of Achilles tendon.
    b. Tarsal slide in an anterior medial direction.
    c. Increase of toe-flexion action for grasp stability.
    d. Secondary intrinsic foot muscle contracture.
    e. Unopposed action of tibialis posticus against weak peroneals and tibialis anticus.
    f. Unopposed action of toe flexors against weakened toe extensors.
14. Triceps surae overwork stress with "pseudohypertrophy."

The net result of these events is a stance and

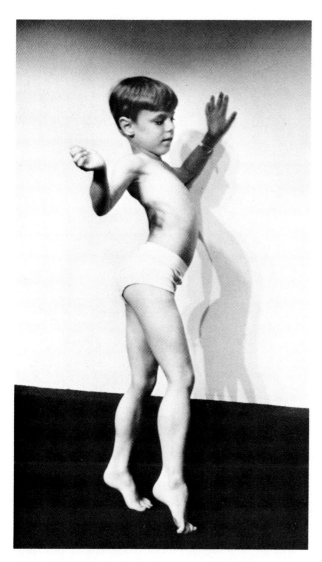

Fig. 1-13. Posture in Duchenne muscular dystrophy.

gait typified by hip flexion and abduction, increasing lumbar lordosis and foot equinocavovarus (Fig. 1-13). Mediolateral subtalar instability secondary to muscular imbalance (strong posterior tibial, weak peroneals, and so on) allows the foot to invert during the swing phase of gait. Initiation of stance in this insecure position may cause falling. Generalized weakness makes it increasingly difficult to attain alignment stability when the trunk is balanced over unstable lower extremities. Proprioceptive abilities are also affected. Sufficient strength to execute postural adjustments necessary to compensate for selective weakening and contracture is lacking. In this regard, small nonmuscular changes assume significance. A slight weight gain or a period of several days of bed rest can decrease strength enough to prohibit ambulation.

Surgical treatment. The aim of operative therapy is to release ambulation-limiting contractures sufficiently to bring the body into adequate standing and walking equilibrium so as to enable the application of appropriate orthoses that offer satisfactory support without undue weight.[130] Orthopaedic intervention should occur at appropriate times in the natural progression of the disease. Surgical management must permit early postoperative mobilization, as even brief restraint can lead to rapid loss of strength in the dystrophic patient. Once one is wheelchair confined, it is difficult, if not impossible, to recoup the ability to stand and walk.[125]

Anesthesia. Patients with muscular dystrophy are poor anesthetic risks because of inadequate pulmonary reserve and the possibility of malignant hyperthermia, which is significantly increased in patients with muscle disease.[24] Depolarizing agents cause a sharp rise in serum potassium, which places the neuromuscular patient at increased risk for cardiac arrest. The creatine phosphokinase is also elevated in the intraoperative period. Incidents of respiratory failure increase with exposure to depressive drugs. Anesthesia must be closely monitored, with particular attention being paid to adequate ventilation being assured, gastric dilatation being prevented, and potassium overload being prohibited.[151]

The clinical manifestations of malignant hyperthermia (muscular rigidity, hyperthermia, and myoglobinuria) are the result of an excessive release of calcium into the myoplasm. This occurs when muscle cell membranes are exposed to general anesthetic agents such as halothane, cyclopropane, chloroform, methoxyflurane, diethyl ether, succinylcholine (suxamethonium) chloride, ketamine, and enflurane. The condition is caused by an underlying membrane disorder of muscle, particularly that of the sarcoplasmic reticulum. Myoplasmic calcium levels are reduced by drugs such as procaine, procainamide, and dantrolene.

A high index of suspicion is aroused by the history of a hyperthermic response to anesthesia in the patient or a relative. The safest anesthetic agent for patients with muscular dystrophy is nitrous oxide. Rectal temperature during surgery should be constantly monitored. In the case of an unexplained, uncontrollable rapid rise in temperature (as high as 107° F has been reported), anesthesia should be discontinued, followed by the ad-

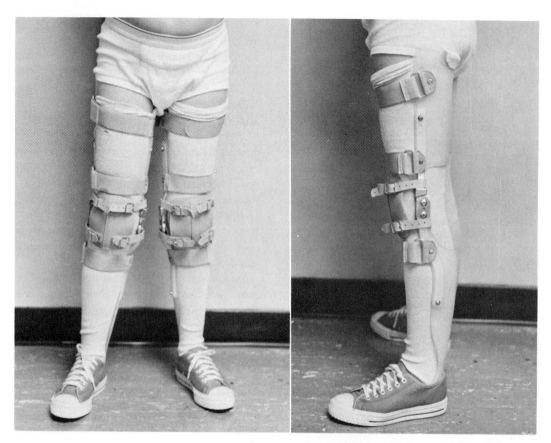

Fig. 1-14. Plastic KAFO (knee-ankle-foot orthosis). **A,** Frontal view. **B,** Lateral view.

ministration of 100% oxygen by endotracheal tube, and surgery terminated as rapidly as possible. The patient is cooled by the application of external ice or a hypothermic blanket, by gastric, bladder, rectal, or wound lavage with cold fluids and by the intravenous administration of cooled Ringer's solution. Calcium gluconate is given to correct hypocalcemia and bicarbonate to control metabolic acidosis. Corticosteroids may help prevent cerebral edema. Dantrolene is now considered the drug of choice for the prevention and treatment of the malignant hyperthermia syndrome. The patient recovering from an expisode of malignant hyperthermia should be monitored for bleeding diathesis from disseminated intravascular coagulopathy, brain damage, renal failure, and cardiac complications, since massive myoglobinuria often accompanies an acute attack.[16]

Lower extremity surgery and bracing. In selected patients, a variety of orthopaedic surgical procedures have proved successful in reestablishing balance and maintaining mobility.[46] Spencer and Vignos were able to extend independent ambulation an average of 24 months in a series of 15 boys with DMD through a program of heel-cord tenotomy, release of the iliotibial bands, and long leg bracing.[136] Apparently the additional energy required for brace ambulation did not cause significant cardiovascular complications and enough residual power for walking with braces remained even when muscle weakness, complicated by contracture, prevented independent walking.[141]

The development of vacuum-molded petroplastic orthoses, which are considerable lighter but as sturdy as their steel or aluminum counterparts, has proved particularly useful in the postsurgical rehabilitation of muscular dystrophy[150] (Figs. 1-14). The plastic brace incorporates a molded footplate, which obviates the need for an attached orthopaedic shoe. Any style of footwear, even tennis shoes (the most desirable shoe for such patients because of their lightness and soles, which grip the floor), can be comfortably worn with the brace. One can regulate ankle mobility by varying the width of the posterior strut connecting the calfpiece to the footplate. The plastic is molded with the ankle in slight dorsiflexion, and the strut is then trimmed until slight plantar flexion and rotation are possible. Because the appliance is form fitted from plastic, it is less bulky than a standard brace, more comfortable, and quite cosmetically acceptable. Velcro fittings can be used for closure and the entire legpiece hidden underneath a long stocking. All materials (including the kneepad, which can be fabricated from Plastazote and Velcro) are nontoxic, radiolucent, unaffected by oils or ultraviolet light, and completely waterproof. The appliance can be washed and dried with ease, a characteristic that contrasts with the difficulty of cleaning the leather utilized in the ordinary brace. Because of their lightness, ease of application, cosmetic acceptablity, choice of footwear, and other desirable features, there is strong patient compliance and parent satisfaction with these orthoses.[122]

Spencer and Vignos suggest that 4 to 5 additional years of independent ambulation can be granted the patient with DMD through a comprehensive treatment program, which includes bracing after correction of lower extremity contractures. Spencer concluded that surgery is contraindicated until long leg braces are required for continued ambulation.[134]

Reports by Winters and McLaughlin,[148] by Curtis,[25] and by Bowker (paper presented at the American Congress of Rehabilitation Medicine, 1972), using techniques like those described by Spencer and Vignos,[136] confirmed the latter authors' impression that patients continuing to walk in braces maintain better alignment of weight-bearing joints and suffer less sedentary osteoporosis and disuse muscular atrophy.

Similar results were reported by Hsu,[68] who presented a series of 12 patients undergoing tensor fasciae latae and Achilles tendon tenotomies with posterior tibial transfers. Bowker and Halpin do not transfer the posterior tibial but simply weaken this muscle by transection at the musculotendinous junction.[15]

Siegel, Miller, and Ray noted that with ankle equinovarus, when the sum of the extension lag of the hip and knee was greater than 90 degrees, ambulation terminated.[130] These patients had stopped walking or, by clinical assessment, were about to stop at the time of operation. They reported on 21 patients who underwent bilateral subcutaneous hip flexor, bipolar tensor fasciae latae, and bilateral heel cord tenotomies, followed by lower extremity bracing. They continued to ambulate 10 to 22 months postoperatively. They accomplished subcutaneous tenotomy of hip flexors (including sartorius and straight head of rectus femoris) by introducing the tenotome at the antero-superior iliac spine and sweeping it distally and posteriorly. The knife is kept close to the bone, and the procedure is performed while the contralateral hip is fully flexed. Flexion contracture was usually decreased by at least 50%, with remaining contracture existing in the deeper hip flexors (such as iliopsoas), as well as in the anterior hip capsule. Through the same stab wound, the tenotome severs the origin of the tensor fascia latae at the lateral aspect of the anterior portion of the iliac crest. Bipolar tensor fasciae latae tenotomy is completed by subcutaneous release of the iliotibial band just proximal to the lateral aspect of the knee joint. Section of the lateral intermuscular septum is assured when this incision is carried to bone. Separation of approximately 1 inch in the palpable ends of the transected iliotibial band, accompanied by correction of tensor fasciae latae contracture, is thus accomplished. Finally, percutaneous tenotomy of the heel cord is performed in its distal third (Fig. 1-15). It is important to tenotomize the Achilles tendon without a tourniquet because a hematoma forms quickly in this area and skin does not fall into the space created by separation of the cut ends of the tendon. The entire bilateral percutaneous procedure should take less than 5 minutes. Toe-to-groin, light plaster casts are applied, with the ankles at neutral and the knees in 5 degrees of flexion. For assurance of plantigrade position in the casts, the plantar surfaces are flattened on a board during application. Heels are fish mouthed to avoid pressure, the bottoms are pounded soft, and adhesive tape is applied to the soles for friction. This is more stable than rubber walkers and provides firmer floor contact, reinforcing the kinesthetic supporting response. Casts are worn for 3 weeks, and knee-ankle-foot orthoses then fitted. As the child grows, braces require lengthening, and care must be taken not to bring the proximal support higher than 2 cm below the ischial tuberosity or else the orthosis will not permit the ischial seating necessary for ambulation.

Preoperative knee contractures of more than 20 degrees are corrected in serial casts to 5 degrees

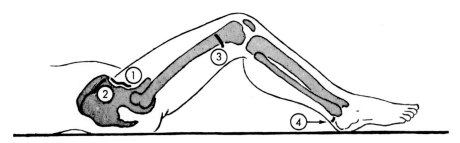

Fig. 1-15. Sites for percutaneous tenotomy release: *1*, Hip flexors; *2* and *3*, bipolar tensor fasciae latae; *4*, achilles tendon.

or less. Surgical correction of knee contractures has not been found necessary, though release of the tensor fasciae latae incidentally corrects some knee flexion. Heel-cord legthening as an isolated procedure will not succeed if the quadriceps is weak, unless accompanied by long leg bracing. Tensor faciae release with posterior tibial transfer can be performed "prophylactically" in the younger patient and isolated heel-cord release carried out if the quadriceps is graded fair or better, and an AFO splint, modified for floor reaction, applied, as indicated.

Postoperative care includes the brief use of nasal oxygen and intermittent positive-pressure breathing. A CircOlectric bed permits the patient to stand with his feet resting on the footboard attachment the afternoon of surgery. When he is in bed, the attendant positions him to stretch the hips into extension and adduction by binding the legs together at the knees and elevating the sacrum when on his back and the knees when on his abdomen. Because subcutaneous tenotomy minimizes pain and the possibility of wound dehiscence, physical therapy can be initiated the afternoon of surgery, with treatment consisting of standing and passive hip exercise. The patient is walked the first postoperative day. Initially the use of a light aluminum walker may be necessary until he adjusts to his rediscovered balance. During walking, torso shift over the supporting limb is still necessary, but the exaggerated posture of head-and-shoulder extension, as well as the severe lumbar lordosis, which were a preoperative necessity for body alignment, are not longer required. Lumbar lordosis disappears when these children sit, and they walk sitting on their braces with a penguin type of gait. Hospitalization is necessary for a week or less, after which a program of physical therapy, including hip stretching and walking, is continued at home. Braces may be worn as night splints, if tolerated.

Eyring and associates operated on 17 patients (54 operations) whose average age was 9 years.[42] Surgery (heel-cord lengthening and posterior tibial transfers) was performed early in an attempt to prolong nonbraced ambulation. Orthoses were applied as the degree of weakness required. The total hospital stay for all procedures averaged 1.5 days, with all patients beginning ambulation within 48 hours after surgery.

Johnson concluded that interference, surgical or otherwise, with passive stabilization of the hip or the knee will result in a loss of ambulation.[73] Because iliotibial tract tightness causes premature loss of ambulation in DMD, surgical release can prolong ambulation, permitting orthotic support of the knee joint when nonbraced passive and active stabilization are compromised.

Equinus was noted as the most common deformity by Roy and Gibson in reviewing 30 patients undergoing orthopaedic procedures.[115] In addition, these investigators observed that early surgical correction of equinus was not only followed by rapid rehabilitation but also slowed further heel-cord contracture, often permitting brace-free ambulation. One can break the vicious cycle of events in muscular dystrophy (weakness-imbalance-contracture-deformity), thus delaying progression of disability. Roy and Gibson also commented that posterior tibial transfer slowed the recurrence of equinus.

Even in patients confined to bed, the tibialis posticus has been graded as "fair plus" and has remained a continuing deforming force. A variety of techniques for relocation of this muscle have been suggested. Spencer transfers it through the interosseous membrane, inserting the tendon through a drill hole in the third cuneiform by means of an 0-chromic suture, tied over a bolster on the bottom of the foot.[134] Hsu uses a modified procedure.[68] The transfer, however, does not work in phase but on command because the tibilis posticus is a stance-phase muscle and, when transferred to the dorsum, is called upon to act in swing phase. However, relocation of its insertion removes an overactive tendency to inversion, providing an active eversion tenodesis effect. This operation is best performed early as a prophylactic procedure before severe plantar soft-tissue contracture or bony deformity in the foot have occurred.

Although more than half a dystrophic patient's total muscle mass is lost by the end of independent ambulation, by which time he is sometimes too weak to stand alone, he is often able to walk again after correction of contractures and bracing. The reason is that other factors are also influential in preventing ambulation. Muscular atrophy secondary to decreased physical activity, obesity, emotional problems, and wheelchair immobilization imposed for the convenience of others all play a role in limiting walking potential.

Complications of lower extremity surgery include heel decubitus ulcer, transection of superficial nerves, or any of the usual postoperative problems occuring after even short anesthesia and relatively bloodless surgery in a patient with poor respiratory toilet and generalized weakness. Fortunately, the incidence and degree of these complications have been minimal.

After surgery and bracing, the patient can usually handle his toilet needs with minimal help, and chair transfer is facilitated when he locks his braces at the knees and uses his legs as a long lever to tilt him to the standing position. The additional period of independent ambulation may represent up to 20% of the life-span of these children and is thus a highly significant benefit to both them and their caretakers as maintenance of the upright posture has extended their ability to attend to the tasks of daily living for a significant portion of their lives.

Surgical treatment of foot deformity. Correction of lower extremity instability is mandatory because even minor degrees of contracture in weight-bearing joints can interfere with balance and comprimise ambulation.[107] Where possible, all foot surgery should be bilateral, so that symmetric posture can be maintained.

Foot drop, secondary to tibialis anticus weak-

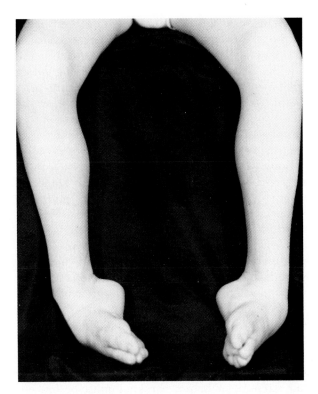

Fig. 1-16. Equinocavovarus deformity in Duchenne muscular dystrophy. (From Siegel, I.M.: The clinical management of muscle disease, London, 1977, William Heinemann Medical Books, Ltd.)

ness in facioscapulohumeral dystrophy, and steppage gait, caused by weak dorsiflexion in dystrophia myotonica, can both be managed with light wire-spring drop-foot bracing or a floor-reaction orthosis.[86] Patients with peroneal muscular atrophy (Charcot-Marie-Tooth disease) will not usually tolerate plastic floor-reaction orthoses because these block the kinesthetic input they require for balance. If a spring-loaded dorsiflexion assist will not suffice, such cases are best managed with posterior tibial transfer or, where bony deformity is severe, triple arthrodesis.[59]

In DMD, a rapidly progressive weakening of foot musculature with contracture occurs, and although this may respond temporarily to conservative measures, such as passive stretch and the use of corrective shoe inserts (such as the UCB model), surgical correction is ultimately necessary. Equinocavovarus advances because of selective weakening of foot musculature (Fig. 1-16). Once the foot is inverted beyond the tibiotalar sagittal midline, almost all dorsal and volar musculature, intrinsic and extrinsic, works to invert it further.[128] Progression of this deformity makes standing and walking uncomfortable and difficult. Equinocavovarus is particularly disabling when combined with flexion abduction hip contracture. Despite correction of the hip, the foot deformity can progress. Pressure decubiti sometimes develop, and equinocavovarus will eventually prevent maintenance of the upright posture.

Bony deformation precludes the use of soft-tissue release alone for correction. The standard techniques of triple arthrodesis or midtarsal wedge resection are contraindicated as DMD patients suffer rapid loss of stregth when inactive, and operations such as these require prolonged postoperative immobilization to assure bone fusion. Early in the disease, when equinus alone is the major deforming factor and little cavus or varus is present, isolated heel-cord tenotomy can be performed, if one keeps in mind that heel-cord lengthening removes the stabilizing equinus force, which hyperextends and locks the knee during stance, so that, unless the quadriceps is graded as fair strength or better, the knee must be braced. Later, when all elements of the deformity are present, a more extensive surgical procedure is necessary. Percutaneous tarsal medullostomy of the talar head and anterior portion of the calcaneus are carried out. This enucleation of cancellous bone is accompanied by percutaneous plantar fasciotomy and tenotomy of the tibialis posticus, also performed percutaneously. Correction is obtained by manipulation of the foot with collapse of the curetted bones.[126] As an alternative procedure, Falewski de Leon has recommended percutaneous tarsal osteoclasis.[43] Appropriate plaster casts are applied, and the patient is encouraged to stand the evening of surgery and ambulate the next day. Casts are worn for 3 weeks. For wheelchair-confined patients, advanced equinocavovarus is treated by the simple expedient of midtarsal dorsolateral closing wedge osteotomy.

A variety of other orthopaedic procedures has been suggested, including percutaneous metatarsal osteotomy to correct forefoot adduction, and dorsolateral transfer of the tibilis anticus tendon in polymyositis to remove a deforming inversion force, creating an active dorsiflexor working in the neutral or eversion direction.[121]

Relatively simple surgical procedures are available, and a judicious choice among them, followed by immediate postoperative mobilization, can pro-

long ambulation. As the patient's ability to stand and walk diminishes, one must determine whether this is the result of contracture or weakness. Experience has shown that, where indicated, the earlier surgery is done, the better the ensuing result. The indications for surgery (except for early prophylactic transfer of the posterior tibial muscle) are contractures sufficient to threaten walking. The conditions are enough strength to motivate braced extremities postoperatively and cardiorespiratory reserves adequate to survive general anesthesia.

Upper extremities. Except in the rare primary distal myopathies, hand weakness is not a problem until late in the course of muscular dystrophy. Contractures about the wrist most often occur in flexion, and these can usually be managed with proper splintage. Elbow-flexion contracture, with pronation of the forearm and the wrist in flexion and ulnar deviation, is seen in wheelchair dystrophic patients. This position is the one in which the elbow and forearm are held most of the time for functional activity. Severe progression of contracture can be retarded by appropriate passive stretching exercises. Patients with neuromuscular diseases (particularly peripheral neuropathy) are predisposed to compression neuropathies. Most commonly seen in the wheelchair muscular dystrophic patient is ulnar neuritis secondary to wheelchair arm pressure on the elbow and forearm.

Shoulder weakness and instability in DMD or limb-girdle dystrophy does not usually become severe enough to interfere with function until the patient is wheelchair confined, at which time it can be treated with assistive appliances. However, in FSH, shoulder weakness can early on significantly interfere with upper extremity function, especially with such tasks as eating and overhead dressing. Because of the lack of scapular stability, the deltoids lose their mechanical advantage, particularly in forward flexion of the arms. In selected cases, the following several surgical procedures are available for scapular stabilization:

1. Screw fixation of scapula to posterior ribs
2. Interscapular fascial transplant
3. Fusion through bone graft between posterior ribs and deep scapular surface, augmented by wire-loop fixation of scapula to ribs[18]
4. Scapular fixation to posterior ribs through fascial ties[81]

After scapular fixation, patients no longer require a "thrown" movement to elevate the arm. Even slight improvement in abduction is useful when a stabilized scapula provides a firm base for this motion. However, the scapula should not be fixed with its vertebral border more than 20 degrees from the vertical, and it is necessary to allow at least one upper extremity the freedom to attend to toileting tasks.

Scoliosis. Paralytic scoliosis, one of the most serious complications of muscular dystrophy, occurs with increasing age and advancing disability. Its presence depends on the type of dystrophy; its progress relates to the severity of the disease.[120]

The onset of limb-girdle dystrophy typically occurs near the time when spinal growth has been completed. Progression is slow, and weakness most often symmetric. Occasionally, functional spinal curvature is seen, but patients ambulate into their second or third decade, and scoliosis is an uncommon finding. This is in contrast to childhood dystrophia myotonica, which is sometimes complicated by scoliosis. Asymmetry of muscle weakness, leading to scoliosis while the patient is yet ambulatory, can occur in the childhood type of FSH, where the curve can rapidly decompensate, as well as the Becker form of muscular dystrophy, where the scoliosis is usually not found to be progressive.[78]

In DMD, paraspinal weakness is symmetric and soliosis unusual in the well-balanced patient who is still walking. However, pelvic tilt secondary to lower extremity contracture can lead to scoliosis in the ambulating Duchenne dystrophic. Asymmetric arm position can also cause secondary spinal deviation and irregularity of upper extremity placement unbalancing the torso and bending the spine.

Caution should be exercised when one attempts to straighten and stabilize the spine of a walking dystrophic patient, either surgically or with an orthosis. Such patients require torso shift for balance, and spinal rigidity (particularly at the eighth thoracic level, the nodal point for spinal axis rotation) prohibits ambulation. Oscillation of body weight necessitates alternating lateral spinal bending, providing excellent symmetric spinal exercise during ambulation, and a modest lumbar lordosis locks the lumbar and lumbosacral facets, inhibiting lateral spinal deviation with the production of spinal curvature.

Many patients with DMD develop scoliosis rapidly after they can no longer walk.[80] Thus ambulation should be prolonged as long as possible through early contracture release and bracing. Patients wheelchair confined after completion of vertebral growth stand a better chance of avoiding spinal deformity. These curves are usually rapidly progressive and convex toward the side of the dominant hand.[77] Additionally, when a patient can no longer independently turn in bed, he tends to develop a dorsal spinal curvature, convex to the side on which he lies. A variety of external spinal-containment systems have been designed to keep the pelvis level and spine erect and extended.[34,120,135] The Milwaukee brace has not proved useful in the management of DMD scoliosis because it is a dynamic orthosis depending on intact muscle strength for its proper function.

In studying 62 wheelchair-confined Duchenne dystrophic patients, Wilkins and Gibson noted that although many developed pronounced scoliosis and kyphosis those with hyperextended spines and rigid paraspinal contracture had comparatively little lateral curvature.[146] They analyzed the patterns of spinal deformity in DMD and suggested that the evolution of scoliosis may progress in two ways—one leading to progressive severe deformity, the other to early rigid spinal extension with maximum intrinsic stability and minor deformity. Wilkins and Gibson recommend special wheelchair seating, designed to keep the pelvis level and to shape and hold the spine in the upright extended position. It is known that if the pelvis is stabilized, the critical vertical load necessary to produce lateral spinal deformity must be doubled.

Alternatively, a rigid (Silastic, Orthoplast, isoprene, polyethylene, or Subortholen) torso support with a firm, level pelvic seat can be provided when wheelchair confinement becomes inevitable before the onset of spinal curvature. At this time, the spine is essentially flaccid and responds to the exoskeletal thoracopelvic distribution forces such a jacket provides. One obtains spinal alignment by fitting the thoracolumbosacral orthosis (TLSO) with the patient in cervical traction, supporting the abdomen, elevating the ribs from a contoured pelvic foundation, and (with utilization of residual neck extension strength) forcing the shoulders back, and exaggerating lumbar lordosis "locking" the lumbar and lumbrosacral facet joints, which inhibits lateral bending. With correction of abdominal ptosis, the diaphragm is allowed increased freedom of movement and vital capacity is thereby enhanced. Such an appliance must be refitted as the child grows.

Spinal fusion has been used to correct and stabilize scoliosis associated with inheritable neurologic conditions, such as familial dysautonomia, Freidreich's ataxia, spinal muscular atrophy, and Charcot-Marie-Tooth disease.[64] Spinal fusion has also been effective in treating scoliosis in childhood FSH, where weakness is sometimes less than in the other types of childhood myopathy, and prognosis for continued function and life expectancy is, as a general rule, more hopeful.[120] These patients tolerate major spinal surgery well, muscle strength permits use of the Milwaukee brace, and their scolioses are generally amenable to more traditional forms of therapy. In selected cases, spinal stabilization operations can arrest spinal deformity, thus maintaining ambulatory function. Complications are few, but pseudarthrosis is more common in such patients than in those with non-neurologic problems. Many authors,[19,53,118] Robin and Brief[110] among the first, concur in the opinion that spinal fusion is sometimes indicated for severely scoliotic, wheelchair-bound dystrophics.[108,109] Sakai and colleagues[117] reported on posterior spinal fusion for progressive spinal collapse in 10 nonambulatory DMD patients. Although the procedure was extensive and accompanied by significant blood loss, bony fusion was achieved in every case, permitting long-term sitting stability. In all patients with vital capacities of less than 40% or nonfunctional coughs, a preoperative tracheostomy was performed to minimize pulmonary complications.

Straightening a thoracic kyphosis can significantly increase the "dead space" along which air must be moved and can reduce pulmonary function by as much as 20% by restricting chest-wall compliance. In some patients, however, straightening the thoracic cage may allow more efficient movement.[45] Patients with muscular dystrophy undergoing spinal surgery require very close attention to respiratory function before, during, and after surgery. Because of their poor pulmonary reserve, surgery may cause an absolute loss of vital capacity for several weeks after the operation. This is related to overstretching of intercostal muscles on the convex side of the curve with relaxation of intercostals on the concave side, compression of the concave lung with overexpansion of the convex lung, decreased reserve in the accessory muscles of respiration, and postopera-

tive pain. The prolonged work of postoperative breathing is exhausting for these patients, and although they can often be managed with an indwelling transnasal or transtracheostomy-intratracheal tube, the use of a tank respirator is sometimes indicated.

Spinal stabilization, whether through orthotic or surgical methods, improves body image, enhances cardiorespiratory function, obviates discomfort, facilitates transfer, and frees the upper extremities from a purely supportive role for more functional use. It is a desirable and important technique in the orthopaedic rehabilitation of these patients.[9,82,112]

The following summarizes surgical management in muscular dystrophy in regard to procedure and timing:

1. *Lower extremity*
   a. "Prophylactic" (under 7 years)
      (1) Posterior tibial transfer
      (2) Tensor fasciae latae release
   b. Early (7 to 9 years)
      (1) Heel cord or tensor fasciae latae release
         (a) Quadriceps must be rated fair or better
         (b) Fit floor-reaction ankle-foot orthosis
   c. Middle (9 to 12 years)
      (1) Triple release (hip flexors–tensor fasciae latae–heel cords)
         (a) Fit knee-ankle-foot orthosis
      (2) Posterior tibial transfer
   d. Late (12$^+$ years)
      (1) Tarsal medullostomy
         (a) Posterior tibial release
         (b) Plantar fasciotomy
2. *Miscellaneous*
   a. Scapular stabilization in FSH
      (1) When functional loss requires
   b. Spinal fusion
      (1) In ambulatory FSH and Becker's where indicated
      (2) In wheelchair-bound DMD when necessary

Fractures. Fractures in patients with myopathies are incurred secondary to bone atrophy caused by lack of muscle tension related to decrease in muscle volume, as well as disuse osteoporosis. No aberrations of bone mineral metabolism are found.[65] The incidence of fracture increases with the severity of the disease. More, and more severe, fractures are seen in wheelchair patients (without remarkable trauma) than in those still ambulatory. The metaphysis of long bones are most frequently broken, and the humerus and femur are most commonly involved. There is usually minimal displacement of bone fragments and not much pain because there is little muscle spasm. Such fractures heal without complication in the expected time. The danger of restrictive procedures in children with DMD must be recognized and their fractures treated with minimal splintage (light long leg walking casts for femoral fractures, light plaster mold and sling for humeral fractures, and so on) to encourage continued ambulation for as long as possible.[127]

SUMMARY

No cure has yet been found to correct the underlying disease and arrest the relentless progression of muscular dystrophy. Nonetheless, "incurable" is not synonymous with "untreatable." A knowledge of these diseases and their differential diagnosis is important for purposes of prognosis, treatment, detection of carriers in the sex-linked varieties, and genetic counseling. Accurate diagnosis is particularly important in the case of inflammatory myopathy where a specific treatment is available. Diagnosis depends on the history and clinical examination, augmented by the electromyogram, serum muscle enzyme quantification, and muscle biopsy.

Once diagnosis is established, management should consist of supportive and symptomatic therapy, and every effort should be expended to keep the patient upright and walking for as long as possible. Progressive disability can be delayed by a variety of physiatric and orthopaedic techniques. Serial functional assessment aids in determining the stage of the disease and indicating specific therapies. Complications must be anticipated and vigorously treated. Occupational therapy is utilized to assist the patient in meeting the needs of his activities of daily living within the restrictions imposed by his disease. Physical therapy helps in augmenting strength and relieving contractures through passive stretch. Attention should be paid to pulmonary complications, cardiomyopathy, social and psychologic problems, speech difficulties, nutritional problems, dermatologic conditions, and fractures. Orthopaedic surgery, when indicated, must be aimed at realistic functional goals (standing, walking, transfer)

and enable immediate postoperative mobilization because dystrophic patients suffer rapid loss of strength when even briefly confined. Orthopaedic techniques are available for the surgical release of lower extremity contracture, the correction of foot and ankle deformity, shoulder stabilization, and so on. Bracing should be suitably staged and orthoses constructed to provide maximal support with minimal weight. Spinal deformity must be prevented, where feasible, and appropriately treated when present. After patients are wheelchair confined, their function can be enhanced through the use of a variety of special supports and appliances that encourage proper sitting posture and utilize residual muscle strength to facilitate ongoing care. The Muscular Dystrophy Association (MDA), through its nationwide network of clinics, supports a program of research and management of the muscular dystrophies and related conditions. Proper treatment of muscular dystrophy whould be multidisciplined and aggressive. Management conducted in an atmosphere of intelligent concern can minimize the frustrating aspects of these conditions while maximizing the benefits obtained through available care, thus significantly enhancing the quality of life, and perhaps even the life expectancy, of these patients.

REFERENCES

1. Aberion, G., Alba, A., Lee, M.H.M., and Solomon, M.: Pulmonary care of Duchenne type of muscular dystrophy, N.Y. State J. Med. **73:**1206, 1973.
2. Adams, M.A., and Chandler, L.S.: Effects of physical therapy program on vital capacity of patients with muscular dystrophy, Phys. Ther. **54:**494, 1974.
3. Adkins, H.V.: Improvement of breathing ability in children with respiratory paralysis, Phys. Ther. **48:**477, 1968.
4. Albright, J.A., and Brand, R.A.: The scientific basis of orthopaedics, New York, 1969, Appleton-Century-Crofts.
5. Alexander, M., Johson, E., Petty, J., and Stauch, D.: Mechanical ventilation of patients with late stage Duchenne muscular dystrophy: management in the home, Arch. Phys. Med. Rehabil. **60:**289, 1979.
6. Allen, N.R.: Hearing acuity in patient with muscular dystrophy, Dev. Med. Child Neurol. **15:**500, 1973.
7. Archibald, K.C., and Vignos, P.J., Jr.: A study of contractures in muscular dystrophy, Arch. Phys. Med. Rehabil. **40:**150, 1959.
8. Armstrong, R.M., Koenigsberger, R., Mellinger, J., and Lovelace, R.E.: Central core disease with congenital hip dislocation, Neurology **21:**369, 1971.
9. Bernhang, A.M., Rosen, H., and Leivy, D.: Internal methyl methacrylate splint, Orthop. Rev. **7:**25, 1978.
10. Bethlem, J.: Myopathies, Philadelphia, 1977, J.B. Lippincott Co.
11. Bohan, A., and Peter, J.B.: Polymyositis and dermatomyositis. Part 1, N. Engl. J. Med. **292**(7):344, 1975.

12. Bohan, A., and Peter, J.B.: Polymyositis and dermato-myositis. Part 2, N. Engl. J. Med. **292**(8):403, 1975.

13. Bonsett, C.A.: Pseudohypertrophic muscular dystrophy, Springfield, Ill., 1969, Charles C Thomas, Publisher.

14. Bonsett, C.A.: Prophylactic bracing in pseudohypertrophic muscular dystrophy, J. Indiana State Med. Assoc. **68**:181, 1975.

15. Bowker, J.H., and Halpin, P.J.: Factors determining success in reambulation of the child with progressive muscular dystrophy, Orthop. Clin. North Am. **9**:431, 1978.

16. Brooke, M.H.: A clinician's view of neuromuscular diseases, Baltimore, 1977, The Williams & Wilkins Co.

17. Buchsbaum, H.D., Martin, W.A., Turino, G.M., and Rowland, L.P.: Chronic alveolar hypoventilation due to muscular dystrophy, Neurology **18**(4):319, 1968.

18. Bunch, W.: Scapulo-thoracic fusion, Minn. Med. **56**:391, 1973.

19. Bunch, W.: Muscular dystrophy. In Hardy, J.H., editor: Spinal deformity in neurological and muscular disorders, St. Louis, 1973, The C.V. Mosby Co.

20. Burke, S.S., Grove, N.M., Houser, C.R., and Johnson, D.M.: Respiratory aspects of pseudohypertrophic muscular dystrophy, Am. J. Dis. Child. **121**:230, 1971.

21. Caughey, J.E., and Myrianthopoulos, N.C.: Dystrophia myotonica and related disorders, Springfield, Ill., 1963, Charles C Thomas, Publisher.

22. Cherry, D.B.: Transfer techniques for children with muscular dystrophy, Phys. Ther. **53**:970, 1973.

23. Chyatte, S.B., Long, C., and Vignos, P.J., Jr.: The balanced forearm orthosis in muscular dystrophy, Arch. Phys. Med. Rehabil. **46**:633, 1965.

24. Cobham, I.G., and Davis, H.S.: Anesthesia for muscular dystrophy patients, Anesth. Analg. **43**:22, 1964.

25. Curtis, B.H.: Orthopaedic management of muscular dystrophy and related disorders, AAOS: Instructional course lectures **19**:78, St. Louis, 1970, The C.V. Mosby Co.

26. Dail, C.W.: Respiratory aspects of rehabilitation in neuromuscular conditions, Arch. Phys. Med. Rehabil. **47**:655, 1965.

27. Danieli, G.A., and Angeline, C.: Duchenne carrier detection (letter), Lancet **2**:90, 1976.

28. Datey, K.K., Deshmukh, M.M., Engineer, S.D., and Dalvi, C.P.: Straight back syndrome, Br. Heart J. **26**:614, 1964.

29. De La Teur, B.J., and Biaconi, R.M.: Effect on maximal strength of submaximal exercise in Duchenne muscular dystrophy, Am. J. Phys. Med. **58**:26, 1979.

30. DeLeon, A.C., Jr., Perloff, J.K., Twigg, H., and Majd, M.: The straight back syndrome: clinical cardiovascular manifestations, Circulation **32**:193, 1965.

31. Demos, J.: Early diagnosis and treatment of rapidly developing Duchenne de Boulogne type myopathy, Am. J. Phys. Med. **50**:271, 1971.

32. Dubowitz, V.: Intellectual impairment in muscular dystrophy, Arch. Dis. Child. **40**:296, 1965.

33. Dubowitz, V.: The floppy infant. In Clinics in developmental medicine, No. 31, London, 1969, William Heinemann Medical Books Ltd. (Spastics International Medical Publications).

34. Dubowitz, V.: Prevention of deformities, Isr. J. Med. Sci. **13**:183, 1977.

35. Dubowitz, V.: Muscle disorders in childhood, Philadelphia, 1978, W. B. Saunders Co.

36. Dubowitz, V., and Brooke, M.H.: Muscle biopsy: a modern approach, Philadelphia, 1973, W.B. Saunders Co.

37. Duchenne de Boulogne, G.B.A.: Recherches sur la paralysie musculaire pseudohypertrophique, ou paralysie myosclérosique, Archives Générales de Médecine (6 ser.):11, 1868.

38. Dujovne, C.A., and Azarnoff, D.L.: Clinical complications of corticosteroid therapy: a selected review, Med. Clin. North Am. **57**(5):1331, 1973.

39. Edelstein, G.: Correlation of handedness and degree of joint contracture in bilateral muscle and joint disease, Am. J. Phys. Med. **38**:45, 1959.

40. Emery, A.E.H.: Genetic counselling in X-linked muscular dystrophy, J. Neurol. Sci. **8**:579, 1969.

41. Epstein, B.S., and Abramson, J.L.: Roentgenologic changes in the bones in cases of pseudohypertrophic muscular dystrophy, Arch. Neurol. Psychiat. **46**:868, 1941.

42. Eyring, E.J., Johnson, E.W., and Burnett, C.: Surgery in muscular dystrophy, J.A.M.A. **222**:1056, 1972.

43. Falewski de Leon, G.: Maintenance of mobility, Isr. J. Med. Sci. **13**:177, 1977.

44. Fisher, S.V., and Gullickson, G., Jr.: Energy cost of ambulation in health and disability: a literature review, Arch. Phys. Med. Rehabil. **59**:124, 1978.

45. Florence, J.M., Brooke, M.H., and Carroll, J.E.: Evaluation of the child with muscular weakness, Orthop. Clin. North Am. **9**:409, 1978.

46. Galasko, C.S.B.: Incidence of orthopedic problems in children with muscle disease, Isr. J. Med. Sci. **13**:165, 1977.

47. Galasko, C.S.B.: The difficult spine, Isr. J. Med. Sci. **13**:197, 1977.

48. Gardner-Medwin, D.: Management of muscular dystrophy, Physiotherapy **63**:46, 1977.

49. Gardner-Medwin, D.: Objectives in the management of Duchenne muscular dystrophy, Isr. J. Med. Sci. **13**:229, 1977.

50. Garrett, J.M., DuBose, T.D., Jr., Jackson, J.E., and Norman, J.R.: Esophageal and pulmonary disturbances in myotonia dystrophica, Arch. Intern. Med. **123**:26, 1969.

51. Gay, B.B., Jr., and Weems, H.S.: Roentgenologic evaluation of disorders of muscle, Semin. Roentgenol. **8**(1):25, 1973.

52. Gibson, D.A., Albisser, A.M., and Koreska, J.: Role of the wheelchair in the management of the muscular dystrophy patient, Can. Med. Assoc. J. **113**:964, 1975.

53. Gibson, D.A., Koreska, J., Robertson, D., Kahn, A., III, and Albisser, A.M.: The management of spinal deformity in Duchenne's muscular dystrophy, Orthop. Clin. North Am. **9**:437, 1978.

54. Gooch, A.D., Maranhao, V., Goldberg, H., and Mills, B.: The straight thoracic spine in cardiac diagnosis, Am. Heart J. **74**:595, 1967.

55. Gordon, E.E., and Texidor, T.A.: Problems in muscle biopsy: an experimental study, Arch. Phys. Med. Rehabil. **45**:396, 1964.

56. Green, R.E., editor: Myasthenia gravis, Philadelphia, 1969, J.B. Lippincott Co.

57. Greenberg, M., and Edmonds, J.: Chronic respiratory problems in neuromyopathic disorders, Pediatr. Clin. North Am. **21**:927, 1974.

58. Greenfield, J.G., Shy, G.M., Alvord, E.C., Jr., and Berg, L.: An atlas of muscle pathology in neuromuscular diseases, Baltimore, 1957, The Williams & Wilkins Co.

59. Gucker, T.: Muscular dystrophy, Phys. Ther. **44**:243, 1964.

60. Haas, D.C.: Treatment of polymyositis with immunosuppressive drugs, Neurology **23**:55, 1973.

61. Hall, D.S., and Vignos, P.J., Jr.: Clothing adaptations for the child with progressive muscular dystrophy, Am. J. Occup. Ther. **18**:108, 1964.

62. Harper, P.S.: Myotonic dystrophy, Philadelphia, 1979, W.B. Saunders Co.

63. Harris, S.E., and Cherry, D.B.: Childhood progressive muscular dystrophy and the role of physical therapy, Phys. Ther. **54**:4, 1974.

64. Hensinger, R.N., and MacEwen, G.D.: Spinal deformity associated with heritable neurological conditions: spinal muscular atrophy, Friedreich's ataxia, familial dysautonomia, and Charcot-Marie-Tooth disease, J. Bone Joint Surg. **58A**:13, 1976.

65. Hirotani, H., et al.: Fractures in patients with myopathies, Arch. Phys. Med. Rehabil. **60**:178, 1979.

66. Hoberman, M.: Physical medicine and rehabilitation: its value and limitations in progressive muscular dystrophy, Am. J. Phys. Med. **34**:109, 1955.

67. Houser, C.R., and Johnson, D.M.: Breathing exercises for children with pseudohypertrophic muscular dystrophy, Phys. Ther. **51**:751, 1971.

68. Hsu, J.D.: Management of foot deformity in Duchenne's pseudohypertrophic muscular dystrophy, Orthop. Clin. North Am. **7**:979, 1976.

69. Hsu, J.D., Perry, R.E., Gonzales, V., Fracalosy, C., Hash, D., and Podrasky, E.: Functional abilities of the muscle disease patient. Presented at the annual meeting of the American Academy of Orthopaedic Surgeons, San Francisco, 1975.

70. Huvos, A.G., and Pruzanski, W.: Smooth muscle involvement in primary muscle disease. I. Myotonic dystrophy, Arch. Pathol. **83**:229, 1967.

71. Inkley, S.R., Oldenburg, F.C., and Vignos, P.J., Jr.: Pulmonary function in Duchenne muscular dystrophy related to stage of disease, Am. J. Med. **56**:297, 1974.

72. Ionasescu, V., and Zellweger, H.: Duchenne muscular dystrophy in young girls, Acta Neurol. Scand. **50**:619, 1974.

73. Johnson, E.W.: Pathokinesiology of Duchenne muscular dystrophy: implications of management, Arch. Phys. Med. Rehabil. **58**:4, 1977.

74. Johnson, E.W., and Braddom, R.: Over-work weakness in facioscapulohumeral muscular dystrophy, Arch. Phys. Med Rehabil. **52**:333, 1971.

75. Johnson, E.W., and Kennedy, J.H.: Comprehensive management of Duchenne muscular dystrophy, Arch Phys. Med. Rehabil. **52**:110, 1971.

76. Johnson, E.W., Weingarden, H., and Alexander, M.: Asymmetric iliotibial band contracture following muscle biopsy: case report, Arch. Phys. Med. Rehabil. **58**:28, 1977.

77. Johnson, E.W., and Yarnell, S.K.: Hand dominance and scoliosis in Duchenne muscular dystrophy, Arch. Phys. Med. Rehabil. **57**:462, 1976.

78. Kaneda, R.R.: Becker's muscular dystrophy: orthopedic implications, J. Am. Osteopath. Assoc. **79**:332, 1980.

79. Karagan, N.: Intellectual functioning in Duchenne muscular dystrophy: a review, Psychol. Bull. **86**:250, 1979.

70. Kenrick, M.M.: Certain aspects of managing patients with muscular dystrophy, South. Med. J. **58**:996, 1965.

81. Ketenjian, A.Y.: Muscular dystrophy: diagnosis and treatment, Orthop. Clin. North Am. **9**:25, 1978.

82. Knight, G.: Paraspinal acrylic inlays in the treatment of cervical and lumbar spondylosis and other conditions, Lancet **2**:147, 1959.

83. Kornfeld, M., and Seigel, I.M.: Parental group therapy in the management of a fatal childhood disease, Health Social Work **4**:99, 1979.

84. Kottke, F.J.: The effects of limitation of activity upon the human body, J.A.M.A. **196**:10, 117, 1966.

85. Larsen, W.G.: Polymyositis dermatomyositis, Arch. Derm. **96**:724, 1976.

86. Lehmann, J.F.: Biomechanics of ankle-foot orthoses: prescription and design, Ach. Phys. Med. Rehabil. **60**:200, 1979.

87. Lewitan, A., and Nathanson, L.: The roentgen features of muscular dystrophy, Am. J. Roentgenol. **73**(2):226, 1955.

88. Ludman, H.: Dysphagia in dystrophia myotonica, J. Laryngol. **76**:234, 1962.

89. Mann, R.A., Hagy, J.L., White, V., and Liddell, O.: The initiation of gait, J. Bone Joint Surg. **61A**(2):232, 1979.

90. Marsh, G.G., and Munsat, T.L.: Evidence of early impairment of verbal intelligence in Duchenne muscular dystrophy, Arch. Dis. Child. **49**(2):118, 1974.

91. McKenzie, M.W., and Rogers, J.E.: Use of trunk supports for severely paralyzed people, Am. J. Occup. Ther. **27**:147, 1973.

92. Miller, J.: Assessment in the treatment of muscle disease, Tex. Rep. Biol. Med. **22**:871, 1964.

93. Miller, J.: Management of muscular dystrophy, AAOS: Instructional course lectures 18(J2):307, St. Louis, 1973, The C.V. Mosby Co. (reprint of J. Bone Joint Surg. **49A**(6):1205, Sept. 1967).

94. Morris, A.G., and Vignos, P.J., Jr.: A self-care program for the child with progressive muscular dystrophy, Am. J. Occup. Ther. **14**(6):301, 1960.

95. Moser, H., and Emery, A.E.H.: The manifesting carrier in Duchenne muscular dystrophy, Clin. Gen. **5**:271, 1974.

96. Mullendore, J.M., and Stoudt, R.J., Jr.: Speech patterns of muscular dystrophic individuals, J. Speech Hear. Disord. **26**:252, 1961.

97. Munsat, T.L., Baloh, R., Pearson, C.M., and Fowler, W., Jr.: Serum enzyme alterations in neuromuscular disorders, J.A.M.A. **226**(13):1536, 1973.

98. Nevins, M.A., Saan, M., Bright, M., and Lyon, L.J.: Pitfalls in interpreting serum creatine phosphokinase activity, J.A.M.A. **224**(10):1382, 1973.

99. Pearson, C.M.: Muscular dystrophy (review and recent observations), Am. J. Med. **35**(5):632, 1963.

100. Pearson, K.: The control of walking, Sci. Am. **235**(6):72, 1976.

101. Penn, A.S., Lisak, R.P., and Rowland, L.P.: Muscular dystrophy in young girls, Neurology **20**:147, 1970.

102. Perloff, J.K.: Cardiomyopathy associated with heredofamilial neuropathic diseases, Mod. Concepts Cardiovasc. Dis. **40**:23, 1971.

103. Perloff, J.K., DeLeon, A.C., Jr., and O'Dougherty, D.: The cardiomyopathy of progressive muscular dystrophy, Circulation **33**:625, 1966.

104. Radin, E.L., Simon, S.R., Rose, R.M., and Paul, L.L.: Practical biomechanics for the orthopaedic surgeon, New York, 1979, John Wiley & Sons.

105. Ramsey, P.L., and Hensinger, R.N.: Congenital dislocation of the hip associated with central core disease, J. Bone Joint Surg. **57A**:648, 1975.

106. Rayport, M.: A disposable isometric muscle biopsy clamp, J.A.M.A. **210**(8):1451, 1969.

107. Reinherz, R., and Mann, I.: Lower extremity involvement in Duchenne muscular dystrophy, J. Am. Podiatry Assoc. **67**:796, 1977.

108. Robin, G.C.: Neurological disease and scoliosis, Isr. J. Med. Sci. **9**:739, 1973.

109. Robin, G.C.: Scoliosis in Duchenne muscular dystrophy, Isr. J. Med. Sci. **13**:203, 1977.

110. Robin, G.C., and Brief, L.P.: Scoliosis in childhood muscular dystrophy, J. Bone Joint Surg. **53A**:466, 1971.

111. Robin, G.C., and Falewski de Leon, G.: Acute gastric dilatation in progressive muscular dystrophy, Lancet **2**:171, 1963.

112. Robin, G.C., Stein, H., Simein, A., and Seigel, I.M.: The effect of methacrylate cement on loading of Harrington instruments in the spine: a preliminary experimental study, Med. Biol. Eng. **12**:241, 1974.

113. Roses, M.S., Nicholson, M.T., Kircher, C.S., and Roses, A.D.: Evaluation and detection of Duchenne's and Becker's muscular dystrophy carriers by manual muscle testing, Neurology **27**:20, 1977.

114. Rowland, L.P.: Pathogenesis of muscular dystrophies, Arch. Neurol. **33**:315, 1976.

115. Roy, L., and Gibson, D.A.: Pseudohypertrophic muscular dystrophy and its surgical management: review of 30 patients, Can. J. Surg. **13**:13, 1970.

116. Sackner, M.A.: Diaphragmatic breathing exercises, J.A.M.A. **231**:295, 1975.

117. Sakai, D.N., Hsu, J.D., Bonnett, C.A., and Brown, J.C.: Stabilization of the collapsing spine in Duchenne muscular dystrophy, Clin. Orthop. **128**:256, 1977.

118. Schwentker, E.P., and Gibson, D.A.: The orthopaedic aspects of spinal muscular atrophy, J. Bone Joint Surg. **58A**:32, 1976.

119. Siegel, I.M.: Pathomechanics of stance in Duchenne muscular dystrophy, Arch. Phys. Med. Rehabil. **53**:403, 1972.

120. Siegel, I.M.: Scoliosis in muscular dystrophy, Clin. Orthop. **93**:235, 1973.

121. Siegel, I.M.: Orthopaedic correction of musculoskeletal deformity in muscular dystrophy. In Griggs, R.C., and Moxley, R.T., III, editors: Advances in neurology, Vol. 17, Treatment of neuromuscular diseases, New York, 1973, Raven Press, Publishers, p. 343.

122. Siegel, I.M.: Plastic-molded knee-ankle-foot orthoses in the treatment of Duchenne muscular dystrophy, Arch. Phys. Med. Rehabil. **56**:322, 1975.

123. Siegel, I.M.: Pulmonary problems in Duchenne muscular dystrophy, Phys. Ther. **55**:160, 1975.

124. Siegel, I.M.: Very early diagnosis of Duchene muscular dystrophy, Lancet **2**:90, 1976.

125. Siegel, I.M.: The clinical management of muscular disease, London, 1977, William Heinemann Medical Books Ltd.

126. Siegel, I.M.: Equinocavovarus in muscular dystrophy. Treatment by percutaneous tarsal medullostomy and soft tissue release, Isr. J. Med. Sci. **13**:189, 1977.

127. Siegel, I.M.: Fractures of long bones in Duchenne muscular dystrophy, J. Trauma **17**:219, 1977.

128. Siegel, I.M.: The management of muscular dystrophy: a clinical review, Muscle Nerve **1**:453, 1978.

129. Siegel, I.M., and Kornfeld, M.S.: Kinetic family drawing test for evaluating families having children with muscular dystrophy, J. Am. Phys. Ther. **60**(3):293, 1980.

130. Siegel, I.M., Miller, J.E., and Ray, R.D.: Subcutaneous lower limb tenotomy in the treatment of pseudohypertrophic muscular dystrophy, J. Bone Joint Surg. **50A**:1437, 1968.

131. Slucka, C.: The electrocardiogram in Duchenne progressive muscular dystrophy, Circulation **38**:933, 1968.

132. Smith, I., and Thomson, W.H.S.: Carrier detection in X-linked (Duchenne) muscular dystrophy: pyruvate kinase isoenzymes and creatine phosphokinase in serum and blood cells, Clin. Chim. Acta **78**:439, 1977.

133. Sockolov, R., Irwin, B., Dressendorfer, R.H., and Bernauer, E.M.: Exercise performance in 6 to 11 year old boys with Duchenne muscular dystrophy, Arch. Phys. Med. Rehabil. **58**:195, 1977.

134. Spencer, G.E.: Orthopaedic care of progressive muscular dystrophy, AAOS: Instructional course lectures **18**(J2):303, St. Louis, 1973, The C.V. Mosby Co. (reprint from J. Bone Joint Surg. **49A**(6):1201, 1967).

135. Spencer, G.E.: Orthopaedic considerations in the management of muscular dystrophy. In Ahstrom, J., editor: Recent advances in orthopaedics, Baltimore, 1973, The Williams & Wilkins Co.

136. Spencer, G.E., and Vignos, P.J., Jr.: Bracing for ambulation in childhood progressive muscular dystrophy, J. Bone Joint Surg. **44**:234, 1962.

137. Steinhauer, P.D., Mushin, D.N., and Rae-Grant, Q.: Psychological aspects of chronic illness, Pediatr. Clin. North Am. **21**:825, 1974.

138. Swaiman, K.L., and Wright, F.S.: Neuromuscular diseases of infancy and childhood, Springfield, Ill., 1970, Charles C Thomas, Publisher.

139. Taft, L.T.: The care and management of the child with muscular dystrophy, Dev. Med. Child Neurol. **15**:510, 1973.

140. Vick, N.A.: Disease of skeletal muscle: current ideas of diagnosis and management, Chicago Med. **76**(16):621, 1973.

141. Vignos, P.J.: Rehabilitation in progressive muscular dystrophy. In Licht, S.H., editor: Rehabilitation and medicine, New Haven, Conn., 1968, Elizabeth Licht, publisher.

142. Vignos, P.J.: REspiratory function and pulmonary infection in Duchenne muscular dystrophy, Isr. J. Med. Sci. **13**:207, 1977.

143. Vignos, P.J., Jr., and Archibald, K.C.: Maintenance of ambulation in childhood muscular dystrophy, J. Chronic Dis. **12**:272, 1960.

144. Vignos, P.J., Jr., and Watkins, M.P.: The effect of exercise in muscular dystrophy, J.A.M.A. **197**:843, 1966.

145. Walton, J.N., editor: Disorders of voluntary muscles, ed. 3, London, 1974, J & A Churchill Ltd.

146. Wilkins, K.E., and Gibson, D.A.: The patterns of spinal deformity in Duchenne muscular dystrophy, J. Bone Joint Surg. **58**:24, 1976.

147. Williams, E., and Nichols, P.J.R.: Expectations of the adolescent labeled as muscular dystrophy, Proc. R. Soc. Med. **68:**1, 1975.

148. Winters, J., and McLaughlin, L.A.: The diagnosis and treatment of Duchenne muscular dystrophy, South Med. J. **63:**530, 1970.

149. Worden, D.K., and Vignos, P.J., Jr: Intellectual function in childhood progressive muscular dystrophy, Pediatrics **29:**968, 1962.

150. Yates, G.: Molded plastics in bracing, Clin. Orthop. **102:**46, 1974.

151. Ziter, F.A., and Allsop, K.G.: Comprehensive treatment of childhood muscular dystrophy, Rocky Mt. Med. J. **72:**329, 1975.

152. Ziter, F.A., Allsop, K.G., and Tyler, F.H.: Assessment of muscle strength in Duchenne muscular dystrophy, Neurology **27:**981, 1977.

Chapter 2

Bone banking: current methods and suggested guidelines

GARY E. FRIEDLAENDER, M.D.
New Haven, Connecticut

HENRY J. MANKIN, M.D.
Boston, Massachusetts

Part A

Background and current methods

Since Ollier's first suggestion in 1867[53] and Inclan's implementation in 1942,[37] numerous accounts have documented the successful use of preserved bone allografts in the treatment of benign skeletal diseases.[3,10,11,31,36,67,70] More recently, renewed interest in the use of transplantable osteochondral tissues has resulted from descriptions of allograft reconstruction after limb-sparing tumor resections[34,39,48,54,55,75] and fresh articular cartilage alloimplants as resurfacing for joints partially destroyed by degenerative arthritis.[32,50]

It should be clearly noted at the outset that we fully recognize the superiority of autografts over allografts and the approach to be discussed is not meant to detract from the optimal use of autografts in skeletal reconstruction. Allografts do, however, have certain advantages in that their use obviates the need to sacrifice normal structures,

avoids potential donor-site morbidity, and overcomes inherent limitations in size, shape, and quantity of available autogenous tissues. Key to this last issue, availability, is the subject of banking, without which much of the current progress in the field could not occur. The use of massive osteochondral grafts, in particular, would not be possible without biologically safe and effective preserved allografts or without bone (or tissue) banks capable of providing appropriate material to the surgeon when urgent need arises. This chapter discusses the methods employed in banking of osteochondral allografts at our institutions (the Yale–New Haven Hospital and Massachusetts General Hospital) after a brief review of potential concerns related to the use of these tissues.

POTENTIAL DISADVANTAGES OF PRESERVED BONE AND CARTILAGE ALLOGRAFTS

Despite the advantages of availability, the clinical application of osteochondral allografts raises serious questions regarding their biologic behavior, the presence and significance of associated immunologic responses, and potential transfer of disease from donor to recipient. These questions must be addressed and attempts at possible solutions incorporated into the techniques of banking of musculoskeletal tissues.

□ Supported in part by NIH grants CA-22267 and AM-21896 and Office of Naval Research Contract N00014-77-0442. The opinions or assertions contained herein are the private ones of the authors and are not to be construed as official or reflecting the views of the U.S. Navy or the Naval Service at large.

36

Biologic potential

The most serious handicap in the evaluation of the biologic potential of bone allografts is the relative paucity of knowledge concerning biologic events associated with autografts. It is clear that both autografts and allografts provide a stimulus to new bone formation emanating from the host bed, perhaps mediated through humoral substances,[73,74] but methods for quantitating vascular invasion, resorption of old matrix, synthesis of new bone, and control mechanisms are crude, and the data obtained confusing and poorly understood.

Numerous investigators have attempted to compare the incorporation process or bone-induction properties of preserved bone allografts to autografts in animals. The studies of Carr and Hyatt,[14] Heiple and co-workers,[33] Urist,[73] and Schachar and associates[65] suggest that preserved bone allografts (or alloimplants) are biologically useful as an alternate graft material, although the incorporation rate is generally slower than that observed with fresh autografts and at times the result is unpredictable. Burchardt and Enneking[7,8] have studied freeze-dried fibular allografts in dogs and concluded that these tissues are biologically and mechanically inferior to similar autografts in the same species. A wide disparity in animal models, preservation techniques, and methods of evaluating results is sufficient to explain these differences of opinion and leaves the objective evaluation of biologic potential and its relationship to storage methods unresolved.

Despite these problematic and confusing findings in animal species, the clinical long-term success associated with transplants in humans provides a substantial argument for not only further study but for continued application and expanded use of preserved osteochondral allografts in reconstructive orthopaedic procedures. If one considers the human experience, a large body of literature attests to the use of this technique beginning with accounts of ancient civilizations and references in church records and works of art.[1] The first reliable report of a successful fresh allograft was provided by Macewen,[47] in 1881, who documented the reconstruction of a sizable humeral shaft defect in a child using bone wedges removed from bowed tibias of other children. In 1908, Lexer[45] described the use of osteochondral allografts for whole joint and hemijoint recon-

struction, and despite the crude technology available, long-term evaluation reported by Lexer[46] suggested that clinical success occurred in approximately half the cases. Inclan,[37] in 1942, Wilson,[77] in 1951, and Carr and Hyatt[14] (representing the U.S. Navy Tissue Bank), in 1955, described their approaches to the banking and clinical application of bone allografts preserved by various methods, and all were associated with encouraging results. Since then numerous reports have supported the clinical usefulness of preserved bone allografts in the treatment of a wide variety of orthopaedic disorders[10,11,67] including repair of fracture nonunions,[31] arthrodeses for cervical spondylosis,[66] and filling benign cystic defects.[70] As mentioned previously, the application of osteochondral allografts after tumor ablation[34,39,48,54,55,75] and replacement of articular cartilage defects[32,50] represent rewarding approaches that are gaining increasing popularity. Thus there is sufficient indication, though measured by the crude parameter of clinical success, that preserved bone allografts represent a satisfactory alternative to bone autografts in many benign or malignant skeletal processes and are the basis for pursuing limb-sparing reconstructive approaches in which biologic tissues are desired.

Antigenicity

Evaluation of bone and cartilage allograft immunogenicity has borrowed heavily from the evolving discipline of transplantation immunology. Therefore early reports of the degree of recipient sensitization or evidence for or against graft rejection may have more directly reflected sophistication of technology available at the time than the actual status of the host response. Past approaches applied to evaluate bone allografts in animals include histologic assessment of the graft and associated cellular infiltrate,[2,12,15,21,41] second-set skin graft rejection patterns,[6,9,15,21] changes in weight and cell populations of lymph nodes draining the site of implantation,[12,13,40] and in vitro assays of humoral,[21-23,26,42-44,58,59,64] and cell-mediated immunologic responses.[26,42,51]

Despite the many methods used and the variation in their sensitivity, there is a remarkable degree of agreement in data collected to date.[10,22] Fresh bone allografts are strongly antigenic, as would be expected of any fresh-tissue transplant, and this reaction appears detrimental to graft incorporation.[10] The process appears to be dose dependent in that small amounts of bone associated with fresh articular cartilage have been routinely well tolerated. Freezing and drying greatly diminish the antigenicity of bone, but probably not without a qualitative and quantitative effect on the efficacy of the graft.[8,41] Deep-freezing (without drying) shows little adverse effect on the biologic condition and mechanical suitability of the graft and causes a decrease in the antigenicity intermediate between that of fresh grafts and those that have been freeze dried. The reported magnitude of the antigenic response has varied, presumably related to differences in size of the graft, the animal models studied, and the assay techniques utilized.[2,6,10,21,26,33,42,64]

Most investigators have considered the cell surface antigens as the major source of osteochondral allograft antigenicity; however, recent studies have also focused attention on matrix components.[16,22,24,28,29,57,76,79] Collagen-free extracts of xenogeneic cartilage (containing purified proteoglycan subunits and link protein) have been shown to evoke humoral and cell-mediated responses in several animal models. Furthermore, recent evidence has suggested that collagen, often considered to be nonantigenic or a very weak antigen, cannot be excluded as a potential source of recipient sensitization after implantation of experimental osteochondral allografts.[17,72]

Relatively little is known about the antigenicity of osteochondral allografts in humans, but available data roughly corresponds with experience in animal models.[26,27,44,59,64] A high rate of sensitization to cell-surface transplantation antigens can be demonstrated after a fresh osetochondral allograft,[44] antibodies reactive with a panel of random lymphocytes in the postoperative serums of recipients of massive frozen ($-70°$ C) osteochondral allografts are detected in high frequency,[59] and approximately 20% of patients receiving a freeze-dried bone allograft developed donor-specific anti–HL-A antibodies.[27]

Of considerable importance to understanding the meaning of these data, however, is the fact that the clinical success or failure in each of three series just cited[27,44,59] did not correlate with the antibody titer and in no instance has a poor result been directly attributed to graft-evoked immune responses. It is still possible that immune responses may play an important role in the physiologic mechanisms of bone repair or graft incor-

poration, but these studies emphasize that the significance of bone allograft antigenicity and its demonstration by the techniques applied to date are of limited or no predictive value regarding the clinical success of the graft. Even more importantly, one must be aware that these observed responses have not been adequately defined nor have they been objectively related either to the physiologic mechanism of bone remodeling (or graft incorporation) at the cellular level or to biomechanical parameters important in the clinical success of the graft. Furthermore, the mechanism by which freezing or freeze-drying reduces bone allograft antigenicity is not entirely clear; it certainly extends beyond simple cell viability. Darcy,[19] in 1955, suggested that freeze-drying physically altered transplantation antigens and removed their capacity to function in immunologic assays. Others, however, have demonstrated that solubilized, isolated, and purified murine histocompatibility antigens retain their antigenicity during the freeze-drying process.[52,62,80] In fact, Greiff[30] has demonstrated that lymphocytes that have been subjected to the freezing and drying process may retain biologic function (including behavior in immunologic assays) after reconstitution. Sell[68] has shown that the ability to preserve cell-bound histocompatibility antigens during freezing varies considerably with the use of different cryoprotectant agents. In his studies, dimethyl sulfoxide (DMSO) not only failed to preserve antigenicity, but it actually interfered with the protective properties of polyvinylpyrrolidone (PVP)-sucrose.

The discussion above is brief and hopefully germane to the subject of bone banking. The interested reader may find a more extensive discussion of the biologic properties, clinical application, and immune responses associated with osteochondral allografts in several extensive surveys.[10,22,63,67]

Inadvertent transfer of disease

The final concern raised in the safe and effective use of preserved bone allografts relates to potential transfer of pathogens or disease from donor to recipient. This is more that a theoretical hazard, since fatal cases of rabies[35] and Creutzfeldt-Jakob disease[20] have been documented following corneal transplants from donors dying of the same rare viral disorders. Potentially fatal tumors have been inadvertently transferred with renal allografts into immunosuppressed individuals, and although the majority of these have promptly been rejected (along with the kidney) after withdrawal of immunosuppressive therapy, metastases and death have been reported.[56,78] There is evidence to support the position that allogeneic tumors, directly inoculated into healthy (or even terminally ill) individuals who are not iatrogenically immunosuppressed will not show growth or even persistence of viable tumor on subsequent biopsy.[49] Nonetheless, transfer of viral or malignant disease remains a serious concern, and the potential danger is best minimized by appropriate donor-selection criteria and tissue-banking techniques.

Bacterial disease, on the other hand, is a major problem, and there is little doubt that many pathogens can survive the rigors of freezing or even freezing and drying and retain the capacity to produce clinical infection in the recipient. This problem may be of limited significance to the kidney recipient, where the transplanted tissue is viable and suffused with blood (and antibiotics), but for the hapless individual who receives a "dead" allograft that contains viable bacteria, the problem is a very serious one. The donor tissue has no inherent barriers to proliferation and extension of the bacterial disease and even long-term high-dose intravenous antibiotics will not reach the offending colonies of microorganisms. Reported from one of our institutions is a recent series of seven patients who developed infections in their allografts and required either resection of the graft (four patients, two of whom received a second allograft) or amputation (three patients).[34] Hence many of the safeguards in the banking procedures to be described are concerned with maintenance of bacteriologic sterility of allografts during harvest, during storage in the bank, and during preparation for implantation.

TISSUE-BANKING METHODOLOGY

The development of guidelines for the banking of osteochondral grafts has recently received considerable attention from members of the Musculoskeletal Council of the American Association of Tissue Banks, and the suggestions that have evolved as a result of numerous meetings of this forum have now been published[25] and appear as Part B of this chapter. As the introduction to these guidelines clearly states, the goal of bone banking is to provide safe and biologically effective graft material, consistent with current scientific information. Thus, as our knowledge of osteochondral allograft biology, immunology, and biomechanics improves, these guidelines will require revision. Furthermore, it should be noted that these guidelines are not only preliminary but represent *minimum* standards, which may require modification for specific clinical circumstances. The committee that produced the guidelines fully recognized that the responsible physician may alter or amend the guidelines for specific purposes and also in response to the sometime rapid evolution of methodology associated with new knowledge and new approaches to reconstructive orthopaedic surgery.

As a final caveat, we would like to point out that the optimal method for bone banking is not yet known, and probably many techniques are efficacious whereas one or several may be most effective for specific clinical applications. The procedures described here are based upon techniques currently being used by us at the Yale–New Haven Hospital and Massachusetts General Hospital and seem to serve our purposes reasonably well. The background experience provided by service with the U.S. Navy Tissue Bank has been invaluable in designing this approach.[5,36,67]

Donor selection

Donor selection is the first and perhaps the most important step in acquiring safe and efficacious tissues for transplantation. This process encompasses not only the biologic parameters that make up the criteria for donor selection, but also embraces ethical considerations, medicolegal factors, and the process of public education.

If one accepts that the transplantation of human tissues to replace injured or diseased parts is feasible and desirable, the prominent ethical questions revolve around protection of an individual's freedom of choice in determining the timing, extent, conditions of use, and even recipients of anatomic donations. Balanced against these factors are the increasing needs of society to acquire such tissues for medical care, research, or teaching.[60,61] In the United States, the rights of the individual clearly prevail. The physician must exert great vigilance in protecting these rights and must in fact apply the same diligence in providing informed consent to tissue donors (or the responsible next of kin) as for other medical treatment. Regardless of the law, the role of the physician as the patient's advocate remains clear, and regardless of need, the donor's (and next of kin's) rights must be preserved.

The preceding statement, however, should not preclude the possibility that the physician may exert some influence or provide some education regarding the process of procurement and the eventual use of the graft. The relatively recent development of modern banking techniques and more widespread clinical applications of osteochondral allografts make it important that involved professionals initiate educational programs directed at the lay public as well as at medical colleagues. The need for bone and cartilage grafts and general tissue-banking methodology must be clearly described to both these groups.

It is also imperative for the successful growth of bone banking that legal mechanisms be available to expedite an individual's desire to make a donation of anatomic tissues. The Uniform Anatomic Gift Act was approved by the National Conference of Commissioners on Uniform State Laws on July 30, 1968,[18,60] with exemplary speed, and subsequently all 50 states and the District of Columbia have adopted legislation consistent with the objectives identified in this act. The act permits donation after death of any specified human body part or parts by an individual 18 years or older (ante mortem) or by the next of kin (post mortem) to a designated medical facility or professional for education, research, or transplantation purposes. The donation is facilitated by acceptance of written documentation provided by the donor or, in the absence of known prior objection of the donor, when the appropriate next of kin gives a written or recorded telephone message. In fact, the traditional ultimate authority regarding disposition of the body vested in the next of kin is modified by the Uniform Anatomic Gift Act to allow the donor's instructions to take precedence. The act also states that the time of death of the donor shall be established by the attending physician (provided that he does not participate in the actual removal or transplantation of tissues). It is further specified that any physician or person acting in good faith to carry out the anatomic gift is protected from any legal repercussions.[18]

The medicolegal aspects of the donor's rights in offering his or her body or parts can be initiated either by a properly executed donor card (which can be obtained from most medical organizations interested in transplantation, from the American Medical Association, or from the form found on the back of driver's licenses in many states), or, in the absence of a known antemortem statement, by a postmortem authorization from the next of kin. Most hospitals have developed standard forms to allow gifts to be made by the appropriate relative. Since the same form is often used to authorize removal of a variety of organs and tissues, in the interest of informed consent the particular anatomic parts to be donated should be clearly listed. Furthermore, the form should specify whether these tissues are to be used for research, teaching, or therapy, such as transplantation. Informed consent also requires that a frank discussion be held with the appropriate individual regarding the possibility of disfigurement related to bone procurement. In our personal series we have found this problem can be minimized by careful planning of surgical incisions and appropriate reconstruction of the cadaver after tissue donation (Fig. 2-1). Toward this end, it is of great benefit to discuss the need for and nature of tissue procurement with morticians so that they can understand the problems we face and we can more fully appreciate the need to minimize damage to major blood vessels in order to facilitate the embalming process.

In most communities, potential donors whose death has resulted from trauma or occurred under unknown circumstances are considered to be medical examiner's or coroner's cases. The authorities are legally required to assess the cause of death and have the right to perform autopsies or other studies as they deem necessary for that purpose. In such circumstances the medical examiner or coroner should be notified and permission requested when one wishes to obtain the donation prior to (or in some cases after) the examination. If the medical examiner grants such permission, a note should be appended to the chart so stating. We have found that most local officials are willing to cooperate in the various aspects of bone banking if the procedure and its merits are discussed.

The donor-selection and tissue-harvesting activities of each individual transplant program within a medical center or community should be coordinated so that maximum advantage can be derived from acceptable donors with minimal inconvenience to the next of kin. Cooperative approaches

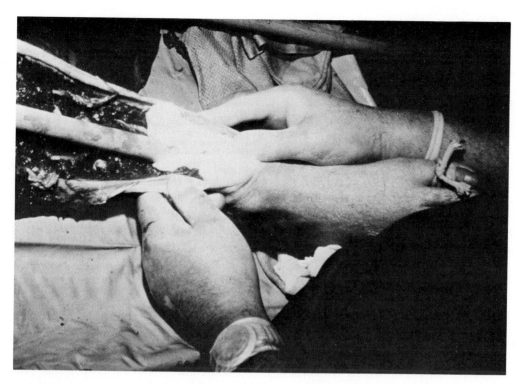

Fig. 2-1. Reconstruction of the cadaver is facilitated by insertion of wooden dowels in place of resected long bones. Plaster, sponges, or towels may also be used for this purpose.

also promote efficient use of personnel, equipment, laboratory screening tests, and educational programs. Harvesting priorities associated with each type of tissue or organ must be understood by all the involved teams and the program coordinated. Removal of viable organs, of course, takes precedence over the retrieval of musculoskeletal and other "dead" tissues in the temporal sequence of tissue procurement.

Potential sources of satisfactory tissue for transplantation include both properly screened cadavers and living donors. It is our preference to rely upon cadavers, since larger amounts of graft material may be removed and more extensive "quality-control" testing is applicable, including an autopsy, but a complete medical history, physical examination, and the laboratory studies to be outlined provide sufficient information to consider living tissue donors. Unlike viable-organ transplantation in which case only momentary warm ischemia time is tolerable, osteochondral tissues may be removed within 24 hours after death and remain biologically useful provided that the cadaver has been properly refrigerated during this

period. This estimated time constraint is based upon postmortem tissue-viability studies (the ability to culture fibroblasts in vitro) carried out at the U.S. Navy Tissue Bank[5] and merely represents a guideline. Undesirable autolysis begins immediately after death; so the shortest possible delay in procuring tissues and subjecting them to preservation techniques is recommended. In the case of fresh osteochondral allografts, implantation should be expedited within this same time frame.

As mentioned before, the single most important aspect of tissue banking is proper donor selection. The goal of the selection process is to eliminate donors with potentially transmissible disease and at the same time provide grafts that are biologically and biomechanically suited for their intended applications. Direct methods to screen potential donors or tissues for harmful diseases are limited to bacteriologic and serologic tests and therefore place great emphasis on the donor's medical history. Particular attention should be placed when one assesses the clinical evidence that suggests the presence of infection, tumor, venereal disease, metabolic bone disease, or toxic substances.

Active systemic infection, microbial contamination of tissues to be collected, or a recent history of potentially transmissible infectious disease are considered contraindications to removal of tissues for subsequent human transplantation. Past experience suggests that patients on respirators for more than 72 hours or dying within 3 days of major surgery have a high incidence of occult bacteremia and septicemia as manifest by blood and tissue cultures.[5] Similarly, patients on high-dose corticosteroids for longer than a week are believed to be more prone to have bacteremic showers and are exempted by our donor criteria. We must reemphasize that fatal slow virus diseases[20,35] and hepatitis[69] have been transmitted by means of tissue transplantation.

It is of almost equal concern in screening donors to be certain that the individual has no overt malignant disease. The inadvertent transfer and subsequent behavior of tumors associated with renal allografts have been reviewed by Wilson and Penn,[56,78] who found that tumors of donor origin could grow and metastasize in recipients (who are routinely immunosuppressed). Several of their recipients were rendered disease free by debulking the tumor (usually by removal of the kidney *and* by withdrawal of immunosuppressive therapy), but 5 of 15 patients who were known to have received tumors with their renal allografts died with (though not necessarily because of) metastatic disease. A similar experience after bone or joint transplantation is far less likely since the transplants are not vascularized and no effort is made to match tissue types or immunosuppress the patients. It should also be pointed out that others have demonstrated the inability of subcutaneous allogeneic bone tumor implants to survive, even in terminally ill cancer patients being screened for an immunotherapeutic approach.[49] Nonetheless, the authors recommend avoiding potential donors with known malignancies. Furthermore, because preservation techniques permit bone graft implantation to be delayed for long periods of time after procurement, obtaining a complete autopsy provides added assurance that inadvertent transfer of malignant disease will be minimized.

Other disorders to be considered in the assessment of potential donors include granulomatous, metabolic, nonspecific inflammatory, and toxic diseases. The theoretical transfer of venereal disease itself or conversion of serologic tests for syphilis make individuals with these diseases unacceptable donors. Similarly, the potential conversion from a negative skin test or actual transfer of disease also detracts from the suitability of donors with tuberculosis or other granulomatous diseases,[38] even after medical treatment. Metabolic bone diseases, diffuse connective tissue disorders, and serious systemic illness potentially alter important biologic and biomechanical properties of bone and thereby make potential donors with these illness less satisfactory for tissue donation. Care must be taken in the evaluation of potential donors known to have absorbed toxic substances in toxic doses such as victims of poisoning. The pharmacologic nature of the toxic substance, its affinity for specific tissues (that is, bone), and the amount of tissue to be transplanted have a bearing upon the importance of this factor. Chronic drug abuse is associated with a high and unacceptable incidence of hepatitis, and high-dose radiation to the skeleton raises concern over the possible induction of tumors in the years after exposure. Death from unknown causes, the presence of a diffuse connective tissue disease, or inflammatory disorder of unknown cause create an unacceptable lack of knowledge in the assessment of donor suitability and the evaluation of risks to the allograft recipient.

Some donor-selection criteria depend on the intended clinical use of the allograft. For example, age becomes an important factor in the selection of donors for massive segmental allografts since these bones should not contain open epiphyseal plates, which may slip during the incorporation process. Upper age limits are more difficult to establish objectively, but aging is accompanied by a physiologic osteopenia. This may compromise intrinsic structural properties but has not been found significant in providing satisfactory graft for filling benign cystic defects of bone.[4] There may actually be a biologic advantage to osteoporotic bone, since partially decalcified bone has been shown to effectively induce new bone formation.[10,73,74]

The donor-screening process should include a currently acceptable laboratory test for hepatitis[69] (such as the Australia antigen assay) and syphilis (such as the VDRL test), and in the case of cadaver donors an unrestricted autopsy is carried out *after* sterile tissue procurement. At this time there is no evidence to suggest that blood or tissues types must be matched; however, a clearer understanding of these factors will require careful retrospective analysis of graft failures. For this reason, it is suggested that blood and tissue types of donors and recipients be recorded whenever possible.

Tissue procurement

Many recommendations exist for the procurement, preservation, and storage of musculoskeletal allografts.[5,10,36] We prefer to begin with sterile tissues and remove them under aseptic conditions in an operating room.

The skin is cleansed in the standard manner used for surgical procedures. This may be facilitated by suspension of the hands or feet of the cadaver from overhead anchors, a method making possible sterile preparation of the entire required body surface. With limited facilities and personnel it is generally safer to approach tissue procurement region by region, with each area being prepped and draped in rotation, gowns and gloves changed, and additional instruments substituted as necessary. After the application of sterile drapes, the skin is cultured aerobically and blood samples are obtained by cardiac puncture for aerobic and anaerobic bacterial assessment. Past experience has shown that femoral venipuncture is associated with a high incidence of false-positive cultures. Microbiology specimens should be followed a minimum of 7 days in a standard medium (discussed later).

Attention is first directed to the upper extremities. The long bones are approached through a standard deltopectoral incision with detachment of the anterior deltoid origin. This permits easy disarticulation of the proximal humerus along with a generous margin of capsule and rotator cuff, which will expedite reconstruction when the graft is later implanted. The extended incision proceeds down the lateral aspect of the arm, between elbow flexors and extensors, to the lateral epicondyle of the humerus. Generally only one forearm bone is removed to facilitate cosmetic restoration of the cadaver for funeral purposes. If the radius is to be removed, the incision extends in a straight line toward the radial styloid, ending 2 cm proximally to the wrist so as not to be exposed at the funeral. If the ulna is to be acquired, the incision from the lateral epicondyle follows the subcutaneous border of that bone, again ending short of the wrist. Either forearm bone can be

disarticulated through this approach, as can the elbow and shoulder joints. The collateral ligaments and capsule are left as long as possible on the grafts; otherwise the entire dissection is carried subperiosteally. If the ends of the long bones are not required, segments of the shaft may be transected with a saw at any desired level.

Long bones of the lower extremity are approached subperiosteally through a longitudinal incision beginning at the anteriorsuperior spine of the ilium and then directed over the greater trochanter and down the thigh laterally to the knee (Fig. 2-2). The incision is swung midanteriorly at the level of the patellar tendon and then carried directly over the crest of the tibia to the ankle joint. The entire femur, tibia, and fibula may be removed through this incision and disarticulated (leaving capsule and ligaments attached), or any portion of these bones or joints may be acquired (Fig. 2-3). As previously mentioned, efforts are made to avoid injury to major blood vessels to facilitate the embalming process and promote cooperation with morticians.

Additional separate incisions can be used for removal of virtually any bone in the body (with patella, ribs, and metatarsals being other common choices) if the need exists. The iliac wing or entire hemipelvis may be removed by extension of the incision from anterior to posterior along the crest. If the bowel is perforated, all tissue procurement ceases at that point. In fact, each bone should be separately wrapped in a towel as it is procured, to prevent cross-contamination of specimens inadvertently infected at the time of tissue procurement.

After removal of tissues, each graft may be cut into any desired size or shape in anticipation of specific surgical applications in the future, including anterior cervical fusions (wafers or plugs), filling of benign cystic defects (small fragments), repair of nonunions (plates or strips), and segmental replacements (as appropriate).

As each tissue is removed, bacterologic cultures are obtained. The only method capable of attesting to the sterility of the entire graft would be cultures made from the entire specimen. Since this is obviously impractical, an estimate of sterility is obtained by a touch culture (surface swab) or by removal and culture of a small portion of the graft (from the medullary canal or cortical surface). We prefer the latter method. If a portion of the cortical surface is removed, it should be taken from

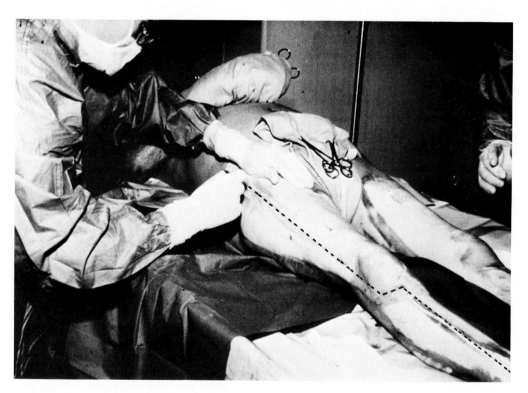

Fig. 2-2. Long bones of the lower extremity are approached through a longitudinal lateral thigh incision that is curved anteriorly at the level of the patellar tendon and follows the crest of the tibia to the ankle.

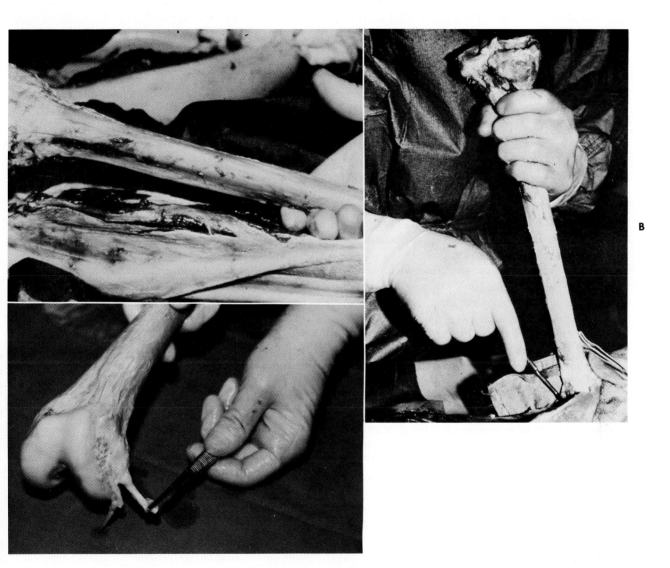

Fig. 2-3. Entire tibia, or any other long bone, may be removed by subperiosteal dissection, **A,** followed by transection at the desired level or disarticulation, **B.** Ligaments, tendons, and capsular structures that may be of value for reconstruction of the joint are retained with the allograft, **C.**

a bony prominence so as not to compromise the structural integrity of the graft. Individual specimen cultures in the context of the medical history, blood cultures, and other specimen cultures represent a reasonable survey of the bacterologic status of the bone. If blood cultures are positive, one must assume that sepsis was present and all bone is infected with the same organism, even if individual specimens are negative. Similarly, if a significant portion of specimens from a single donor reveal contamination with the same organism or organisms, the remainder of grafts are presumed to contain that organism. We have arbitrarily chosen contamination of 25% of specimens by identical bacteria to indicate ubiquitous infection, even if blood and other fluid cultures are negative, and would not consider this bone sterile.

To further complicate matters of assessing the bacteriologic status of a graft, one must keep in mind that "sterility" is a somewhat arbitrary definition. The clinical significance of contamination reflects a combination of factors, including the number of organisms present, the virulence of specific microorganisms, the nature of the recipient bed and host-defense capabilities, and the intrinsic adverse circumstances of implanting a nonviable foreign body.[71] Conservatism must be exercised after each of these facets of the problem is taken into account, since an infected allograft is a substantial threat to preserving a reconstructed limb.[34]

We rely upon the standard approach used by our bacteriology laboratories to screen for aerobic and anaerobic microbial and fungal contamination, except that these cultures are observed for 7 days. Thioglycollate broth with Filde's enrichment is the medium currently employed. An alternate approach (or for identification of microorganisms found during screening in thioglycollate broth) is dispersion of the specimen in trypticase soy broth and plating onto various growth media such as blood agar, deoxycholate, colistin–nalidixic acid (CNA) agar, anaerobic blood agar with neomycin, and enriched thioglycollate broth, if not already done. The U.S. Navy Tissue Bank has used a medium containing equal amounts of thioglycollate and trypticase soy broths and then observed these cultures for 20 days.[5]

In addition to the specimen cultures, blood, skin (touched with a swab), each fluid that comes into contact with the graft during the tissue procurement (such as glycerol), and any additional available body fluids (urine, pleural fluid) are also cultured in a routine manner.

Detection of tissue contamination with viruses remains an unsolved problem. There are currently no practical screening tests for pathogenic viruses; so we rely upon the medical history and postmortem evaluation for guidance. An exception is the Australia antigen (hepatitis B surface antigen) assay for hepatitis B viruses.

Antibiotics are not routinely used during the tissue-procurement process. They make interpretation of graft cultures taken at the time of implantation difficult and may preclude use of particular grafts in patients sensitive to these drugs. If antibiotics are used during the procurement process, specimen cultures must be obtained before exposure.

Tissue preservation

Numerous methods have been proposed for the preservation of bone, but freezing or freeze-drying are the most widely utilized approaches. A detailed discussion of alternate methods and presumed merits of each has been prepared by Burwell.[10] Freeze-drying of bone was introduced by the U.S. Navy Tissue Bank and described in detail elsewhere,[5,36] and the method of preparing "AAA" chemosterilized, antigen-extracted, autodigested alloimplants has been published by Urist.[74] We have relied upon deep-freezing to −70° C for long-term storage. This is based on the fact that bone does not freeze at conventional freezer temperatures (−10° C) and that colder temperatures are required to retard autolysis.[10,36] Empiric success with this method is also a factor in our decision, since there is an absence of objective knowledge relating freezing temperatures to biologic properties known to be significant for bone graft function and only anecdotal information correlating temperatures with absolute "shelf life."[10,77] There is no question, however, that clinical success has been achieved with bone frozen to −20° C[10,55] as well as −170° C.[3]

It should be pointed out that virtually all efforts to preserve bone for transplantation result in loss of cell viability, but not necessarily biologic potential as a graft.[10] The articular surface, on the other hand, must contain viable chondrocytes to maintain the specilized hyaline matrix. Nonviable articular cartilage in our experience is replaced by fibrocartilage, and this has a limited capacity for weight-bearing joint function over time. Previous animal experiments by one of us (H.J.M.)[48,65] form the basis for current efforts to maintain chondrocyte viability during the freezing process. After their acquisition, articular surfaces of each graft are immersed in a 10% solution of sterile glycerol for 30 or more minutes, and after refrigeration for 18 hours, specimens are then frozen to −70° C. This appears to result in approximately 40% chondrocyte viability when grafts are quickly thawed. The percentage of chondrocytes required to maintain a functional articular matrix is unknown. The use of other cryoprotectant agents (such as dimethyl sulfoxide), various concentrations of such agents, and different freezing and thawing conditions are being explored.

Storage

After bacteriologic testing and, when appropriate, exposure of articular surfaces to a cryoprotectant agent, specimens are placed in a sterile polyethylene bag (Fig. 2-4). They are then wrapped in a double layer of sterile towels, fastened with freezer tape, and appropriately labeled. A second outer polyethylene bag is optional. Specimens treated with glycerol are placed in a refrigerator (at 4° C) overnight or for 18 hours to allow for more complete penetration of the cryoprotectant into the cartilage, and, as a final step, all specimens are placed in a −70° C freezer equipped with a temperature monitor/recorder and alarm system. Grafts remain frozen until required for clinical application. At this low temperature, autolysis is considerably retarded and storage for several years appears possible. As mentioned previously, there have been no objective measurements of "shelf life" related to variously preserved osteochondral allografts, but past clinical success would attest to the usefulness of tissues stored at −70° C for at least 2 years. No evidence is currently available to establish a time limit for the long-term storage of allografts by the technique described here.

X-ray films of segmental or osteochondral grafts are made in two standard planes prior to freezing of the grafts (Fig. 2-5). One can easily judge magnification by the use of a known fixed focal distance or by applying a standard reference object to the outside of the package (taking care to place this at the same distance from the film as the bone). A coin taped to the package serves this purpose. Accurate sizing of specimens used to reconstruct articular surfaces appears to be of considerable importance in minimizing late degenerative joint disease caused by instability and joint incongruity.

For the purposes of quality control, approximately 5% of specimens are recultured every 6 months. This can be satisfied by routine cultures taken at the time of clinical application.

Distribution and use

Most tissues are used within the local geographic region in which they are acquired, and this is certainly the case with our banks. When transfer from one institution to another is necessary, storage temperatures must be maintained during transit, and the integrity of the storage "container" must be protected.

Tissues remain frozen until the time of surgery. At that point they are thawed in a warm physiologic solution (such as Ringer's lactate). Antibiotics may be added to this fluid provided that bacteriologic cultures are obtained before emersion of the graft; the antibiotic solution should not be one to which the recipient is hypersensitive, nor should the antibiotic be toxic to chondrocytes. Penicillin, polymyxin, or bacitracin appear to be tolerated by cartilage.

Descriptions of the surgical procedure (allograft implantation) have appeared elsewhere.[34,39,48,54,55,75]

Record keeping

It is imperative that accurate and complete record keeping be maintained so that responsible clinical evaluation can occur and the graft recipient will be protected in the event that other tissues removed from the same donor should prove unsatisfactory. We follow the recommendations outlined by the American Association of Tissue Banks *Guidelines for the Banking of Musculoskeletal Tissues*[25] (see p. 52). Records should clearly identify the graft donor (including name, hospital unit number, age, and sex), circumstances surrounding death, past medical history, and a summary of laboratory, bacteriologic, and autopsy results. Similar data should be recorded for the recipient of the graft as well as a description of the specific graft implanted, the nature of the operative procedure, graft culture results from the time of surgery, any adverse reactions related to the allo-

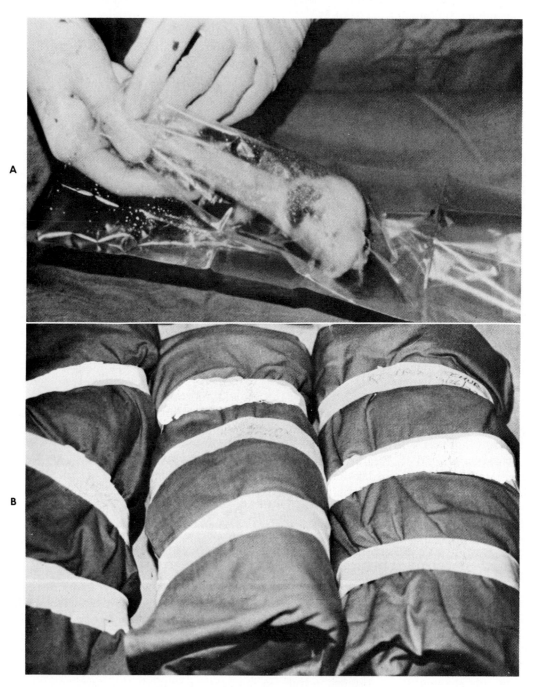

Fig. 2-4. After removal from the donor, obtaining of bacteriologic cultures, and soaking of articular surfaces in cryoprotectant agent, each graft is inserted into a sterile polyethylene bag, **A,** and then wrapped in a double layer of towels and labeled, **B.** The graft is first refrigerated for 18 hours if cartilage preservation is desired; otherwise it is placed directly into the freezer (at $-70°$ C).

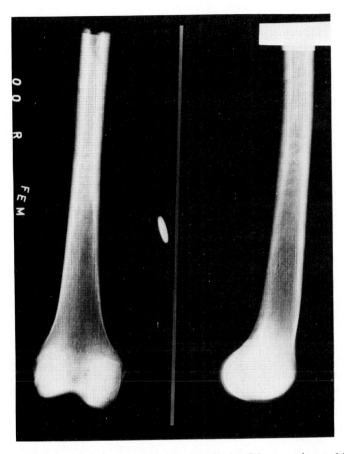

Fig. 2-5. Roentgenograms of each specimen are obtained in two planes. Magnification can be controlled by use of a standard distance from the x-ray source to the graft and between the graft and film or by inclusion of a standard reference marker at the level of the graft, such as the nickel, shown in the middle of this illustration.

graft, and an estimate of clinical progress at follow-up. The physician or physicians responsible for graft procurement and transplantation should be identified, and methods used for banking are detailed for future reference.

SUMMARY

There is considerable evidence to support the clinical usefulness of preserved osteochondral allografts in reconstructive orthopaedic surgery. Responsible methods for banking these tissues are required to provide biologically useful and predictable grafts that are free of potentially significant pathogenic agents or transmissible disease.

Although much remains unknown concerning the biology, immunology, and biomechanics of fresh and preserved osteochondral allografts and undoubtedly the best method or methods for banking these tissues have not been identified, the approach outlined here (and in the AATB *Guidelines*) reflects our interpretation of the present state of the art. We fully recognize the possibility that alternative approaches may meet special needs of other investigators and, in fact, expect our approach to change as additional knowledge becomes available and as clinical applications expand.

REFERENCES TO PART A

1. Bick, E.M.: Source book of orthopaedics, New York, 1968, Hafner Publishing Co.
2. Bonfiglio, M., Jeter, W.S., and Smith, C.L.: The immune concept: its relation to bone transplantation, Ann. N.Y. Acad. Sci. **59**:417, 1955.
3. Boyne, P.J.: Review of the literature on cryopreservation of bone, Cryobiology **4**:341, 1968.
4. Bright, R.W.: Personal communication, 1976, Gainesville, Fla.
5. Bright, R.W., Friedlaender, G.E., and Sell, K.W.: Current concepts: tissue banking: the United States Navy Tissue Bank, Milit. Med. **142**(7):503, 1977.

6. Brooks, D.B., Heiple, K.G., Herndon, C.H., and Powell, A.E.: Immunological factors in homogenous bone transplantation. IV. The effect of various methods of preparation and irradiation on antigenicity, J. Bone Joint Surg. **45A:**1617, 1963.

7. Burchardt, H., and Enneking, W.F.: Transplantation of bone, Surg. Clin. North Am. **58:**403, 1978.

8. Burchardt, H., Jones, H., Glowczewskie, F., Rudner, C., and Enneking, W.F.: Freeze-dried allogeneic segmental cortical-bone grafts in dogs, J. Bone Joint Surg. **60A:**1082, 1978.

9. Burwell, R.G.: Studies in the transplantation of bone. V. The capacity of fresh and treated homografts of bone to evoke transplantation immunity, J. Bone Joint Surg. **45B:**386, 1963.

10. Burwell, R.G.: The fate of bone grafts. In Apley, A.G., editor: Recent advances in orthopaedics, Baltimore, 1969, The Williams & Wilkins Co., p. 115.

11. Burwell, R.G.: The fate of freeze-dried bone allografts, Transplant. Proc. **8**(suppl. 1):95, 1976.

12. Burwell, R.G., and Gowland, G.: Studies in the transplantation of bone. III. The immune responses of lymph nodes draining components of fresh homologous cancellous bone and homologous bone treated by different methods, J. Bone Joint Surg. **44B:**131, 1962.

13. Burwell, R.G., Gowland, G., and Dexter, F.: Studies in the transplantion of bone. VI. Further observations concerning the antigenicity of homologous cortical and cancellous bone, J. Bone Joint Surg. **45B:**597, 1963.

14. Carr, C.R., and Hyatt, G.W.: Clinical evaluation of freeze-dried bone grafts, J. Bone Joint Surg. **37A:**549, 1955.

15. Chalmers, J.: Transplantation immunity in bone grafting, J. Bone Joint Surg. **41B:**160, 1959.

16. Chrisman, O.D., Fessel, J.M., and Southwick, W.O.: Experimental production of synovitis and marginal articular exostoses in the knee joint of dogs, Yale J. Biol. Med. **37:**409, 1964.

17. Cracchiolo, A., III, Michaeli, D., Goldberg, L.S., and Fudenberg, H.H.: The occurrence of antibodies to collagen in synovial fluids, Clin. Immunol. Immunopathol. **3:**567, 1975.

18. Curran, W.J.: The Uniform Anatomical Gift Act, N. Engl. J. Med. **280:**36, 1969.

19. Darcy, D.A.: Reaction of rabbits to frozen homografts, Pathol. Bacteriol. **70:**143, 1955.

20. Duffy, P., Wolf, J., Collins, G., DeVoe, A.G., Streeten, B., and Cowen, D.: Possible person-to-person transmission of Creutzfeldt-Jakob disease, N. Engl. J. Med. **290:**692, 1974.

21. Elves, M.W.: Humoral immune response to allografts of bone, Int. Arch. Allergy Appl. Immunol. **47:**708, 1974.

22. Elves, M.W.: Newer knowledge of the immunology of bone and cartilage, Clin. Orthop. **120:**232, 1976.

23. Elves, M.W., and Ford, C.H.J.: A study of the humoral immunce response to osteoarticular allografts in the sheep, Clin. Exp. Immunol. **17:**497, 1974.

24. Friedlaender, G.E., Ladenbauer-Bellis, I., and Chrisman, O.D.: Cartilage matrix components as antigenic agents in an osteoarthritis model, Trans. Orthop. Res. Soc. **5:**170, 1980.

25. Friedlaender, G.E., and Mankin, H.J.: Guidelines for the banking of musculoskeletal tissues, Am. Assoc. Tissue Banks Newsletter **4**(suppl.):30, 1980.

26. Friedlaender, G.E., Strong, D.M., and Sell, K.W.: Studies on the antigenicity of bone. I. Freeze-dried and deep-frozen bone allografts in rabbits, J. Bone Joint Surg. **58A:**854, 1976.

27. Friedlaender, G.E., Strong, D.M., and Sell, K.W.: Donor graft specific anti–HL-A antibodies following freeze-dried bone allografts, Trans. Orthop. Res. Soc. **2:**87, 1977.

28. George, R.C., and Chrisman, O.D.: The role of cartilage polysaccharides in osteoarthritis, Clin. Orthop. **57:**259, 1968.

29. Glant, T., Hadas, E., and Nagy, M.: Cell-mediated and humoral immune responses to cartilage antigenic components, Scand. J. Immunol. **9:**29, 1979.

30. Greiff, D., and Milson, T.J.: Functional activities of isolated lymphocytes following drying by sublimation of ice *in vacuo*. I. Rosette formation, stimulation by plant lectins (mitogens) and the mixed lymphocyte reaction, Cryobiology **17:**319, 1980.

31. Gresham, R.B.: The freeze-dried cortical bone homograft: a roentgenographic and histologic evaluation, Clin. Orthop. **37:**194, 1964.

32. Gross, A.E., Langer, F., Houpt, J., Pritzker, K., and Friedlaender, G.E.: Allotransplantation of partial joints in the treatment of osteoarthritis of the knee, Transplant. Proc. **8**(suppl. 1):129, 1976.

33. Heiple, K.G., Chase, S.W., and Herndon, C.H.: A comparative study of the healing process following different types of bone transplantation, J. Bone Joint Surg. **45A:**1593, 1963.

34. Hiki, V., and Mankin, H.J.: Radical resection and allograft replacement in the treatment of bone tumors, J. Jpn. Orthop. Assoc. **54:**475, 1980.

35. Houff, S.A., Burton, R.C., Wilson, R.W., et al.: Human-to-human transmission of rabies virus by corneal transplant, N. Engl. J. Med. **300:**603, 1979.

36. Hyatt, G.W., and Butler, M.C.: Bone grafting. The procurement, storage, and clinical use of bone homografts. In American Association of Orthopaedic Surgeons: Instructional course lectures, **14:**343, Ann Arbor, Mich., 1957, J.W. Edwards Co.

37. Inclan, A.: Use of preserved bone graft in orthopaedic surgery, J. Bone Joint Surg. **24:**81, 1942.

38. James, J.I.P.: Tuberculosis transmitted by banked bone, J. Bone Joint Surg. **35B:**578, 1953.

39. Koskinen, E.V., Salenius, P., and Alho, A.: Allogeneic transplantation in low-grade malignant bone tumors, Acta Orthop. Scand. **50:**129, 1979.

40. Kossowska-Paul, B.: Studies on the regional lymph node blastic reaction evoked by allogeneic grafts of fresh and preserved bone tissue, Bull. Acad. Polon. Sci. **14:**651, 1966.

41. Kruez, F.P., Hyatt, G.W., Turner, T.C., and Bassett, A.L.: The preservation and clinical use of freeze-dried bone, J. Bone Joint Surg. **33A:**863, 1951.

42. Langer, F., Czitrom, A., Pritzker, K.P., and Gross, A.E.: The immunogenicity of fresh and frozen allogeneic bone, J. Bone Joint Surg. **57A:**216, 1975.

43. Lee, E.H., Langer, F., Halloran, P. Gross, A.E., and Ziv. I.: The effect of major and minor histocompatibility differences on bone transplant healing in inbred mice, Trans. Orthop. Res. Soc. **4:**60, 1979.

44. Lee, E.H., Langer, F., Halloran, P., Gross, A.E., and Ziv, I.: The immunology of osteochondral and massive allografts, Trans. Orthop. Res. Soc. **4:**61, 1979.

45. Lexer, E.: Die Verwendung der freien Knochenplastik nebst Versuchen über Gelenkversteifung und Gelenktransplantation, Arch. Klin. Chir. **86:**939, 1908.

46. Lexer, E.: Joint transplantation and arthroplasty, Surg. Gynecol. Obstet **40:**782, 1925.

47. Macewen, W.: Observations concerning transplantation of bone. Illustrated by a case of inter-human osseous transplantation, whereby over two-thirds of the shaft of a humerus was restored, Proc. R. Soc. Lond. **32:**232, 1881.

48. Mankin, H.J., Fogelson, F.S., Trasher, A.Z., and Jaffer, F.: Massive resection and allograft transplantation in the treatment of malignant bone tumors, N. Engl. J. Med. **294:**1247, 1976.

49. Marsh, B., Flynn, L., and Enneking, W: Immunologic aspects of osteosarcoma and their application to therapy: a preliminary report, J. Bone Joint Surg. **54A:**1367, 1972.

50. Meyers, M.H., and Chatterjee, S.N.: Osteochondral transplantation, Surg. Clin. North Am. **58:**429, 1978.

51. Musculo, D.L., Kawai, S., and Ray, R.D.: Cellular and humoral immune response analysis of bone-allografted rats, J. Bone Joint Surg. **58A:**826, 1976.

52. Nimelstein, S.H., Hotti, A.R., and Holman, H.R.: Transformation of a histocompatibility immunogen into a tolerogen, J. Exp. Med. **128:**723, 1973.

53. Ollier, L.: Traité expérimental et clinique de la régénération des os, Paris, 1867, Victor Masson et Fils.

54. Ottolenghi, C.E.: Massive osteo and osteo-articular bone grafts: technic and results of 62 cases, Clin. Orthop. **87:**156, 1972.

55. Parrish, F.F.: Allograft replacement of all or part of the end of a long bone following excision of a tumor: report of twenty-one cases, J. Bone Joint Surg. **55A:**1, 1973.

56. Penn, I.: The incidence of malignancies in transplant recipients, Transplant. Proc. **7(2):**323, 1975.

57. Poole, A.R., Reiner, A., Choi, H., and Rosenberg, L.C.: Immunological studies of proteoglycan subunit from bovine and human cartilages, Trans. Orthop. Res. Soc. **4:**55, 1979.

58. Rodrigo, J.J.: Distal rat femur allografts: a surgical model for the induction of humoral cytotoxic antibodies, Trans. Orthop. Res. Soc. **2:**265, 1977.

59. Rodrigo, J.J., Fuller, T.C., and Mankin, H.J.: Cytotoxic HL-A antibodies in patient with bone and cartilage allografts, Trans. Orthop. Res. Soc. **1:**131, 1976.

60. Sadler, A.M., Jr., Sadler, B.L., Stason, E.B., and Stickel, D.L.: Transplantation—a case for consent, N. Engl. J. Med. **280:**862, 1969.

61. Sadler, B.L., and Sadler, A.M., Jr.: Providing cadaver organs: three legal alternatives, Hastings Center Studies **1:**14, 1973.

62. Sagi, S., Turianskyj, F.H., and Gyenes, L.: Immunogenicity of soluble murine histocompatibility antigens, Immunol. Commun. **3:**85, 1974.

63. Schachar, N.S., Friedlaender, G.E., and Mankin, H.J.: Bone transplantation. In Slavin, S., ed. Organ transplantation: present state, future goals, Amsterdam, Elsevier/North-Holland Biomedical Press B.V. (In press.)

64. Schachar, N.S., Fuller, T.C., Wadsworth, P.L., Henry, W.B., and Mankin, H.J.: A feline model for the study of frozen osteoarticular allografts. II. Development of lymphocytotoxic antibodies in allograft recipients, Trans. Orthop. Res. Soc. **3:**131, 1978.

65. Schachar, N.S., Henry, W.B., Wadsworth, P.L., Castronovo, F.P., Jr., and Mankin, H.J.: A feline model for the study of frozen osteoarticular allografts. I. Quantitative assessment of cartilage viability and bone healing, Trans. Orthop. Res. Soc. **3:**130, 1978.

66. Schneider, J.R., and Bright, R.W.: Anterior cervical fusion using preserved bone allografts, Transplant. Proc. **8(suppl. 1):**73, 1976.

67. Sell, K.W., and Friedlaender, G.E., editors: Tissue banking for transplantation, New York, 1976, Grune & Stratton, Inc.

68. Sell, K.W., Friedlaender, G.E., and Strong, D.M.: Immunogenicity and freeze-drying, Cryoimmunology **17:**187, 1976.

69. Shutkin, N.M.: Homologous-serum hepatitis following use of refrigerated bone-bank bone: report of a case, J. Bone Joint Surg. **36A:**160, 1954.

70. Spence, K.F., Sell, K.W., and Brown, R.H.: Solitary bone cyst: treatment with freeze-dried cancellous bone allograft, J. Bone Joint Surg. **51A:**87, 1969.

71. Tomford, W.W., Starkweather, R.J., and Goldman, M.H.: A study of the clinical incidence of infection in the use of banked allograft bone, J. Bone Joint Surg. **63A:**244, 1981.

72. Trentham, D.E., Townes, A.S., Kang, A.H., and David, J.R.: Humoral and cellular sensitivity to collagen in type II collagen induced arthritis in rats, J. Clin. Invest. **61:**89, 1978.

73. Urist, M.R.: Practical applications of basic research on bone graft physiology. In AAOS: Instructional Course Lectures, **25:**1, St. Louis, 1976, The C.V. Mosby Co.

74. Urist, M.R., Mikulski, A., and Boyd, S.D.: A chemosterilized antigen-extracted autodigested alloimplant for bone banks, Arch. Surg. **110:**416, 1975.

75. Volkov, M.V., and Imamaliyev, A.S.: Use of allogenous articular bone implants as substitutes for autotransplants in adult patients, Clin. Orthop. **114:**192, 1976.

76. Weislander, J., and Heinegard, D.: Immunochemical analysis of cartilage proteoglycans: antigenic determinants of substructures, Biochem. J. **179:**35, 1979.

77. Wilson, P.D.: Follow-up study of the use of refrigerated homogenous bone transplants in orthopaedic operations, J. Bone Joint Surg. **33A:**307, 1951.

78. Wilson, R.E., and Penn, I: Fate of tumors transplanted with a renal allograft, Transplant. Proc. **7(2):**327, 1975.

79. Yablon, I.G., Brandt, K.D., and DeLellis, R.A.: The antigenic determinants of articular cartilage: their role in the homograft rejection, Trans. Orthop. Res. Soc. **2:**90, 1977.

80. Yamane, K., and Nathenson, S.G.: Biochemical similarity of papain-solubilized H-2d alloantigens from tumor cells and from normal cells, Biochemistry **9:**4743, 1970.

Part B

Guidelines for banking of musculoskeletal tissues

MISSION AND GOALS

Based upon substantial past clinical experience, it is clear that allografts (or alloimplants) of musculoskeletal tissues are a reasonable alternative to fresh autografts or synthetic implants in properly selected cases. There is no question that the biologic properties of fresh autografts are optimal and represent the standard against which alternative materials are to be compared (with the recognition that aspects of fresh autograft biologic properties are not as yet completely defined). The potential disadvantages of fresh autografts, particularly in terms of donor morbidity and limitations in size, shape, and quantity of available tissue diminish the potential applicability of the material and suggest that increased quantities of musculoskeletal allografts will be required in the future (even before additional knowledge concerning graft biologic properties can be accumulated). It is important that methods for donor selection, tissue procurement and processing, storage, quality control, distribution, and record keeping be identified so as to ensure the availability of safe and efficacious musculoskeletal allografts that remain biologically predictable within the period of their intended use. These guidelines must protect the graft recipient to the extent current scientific knowledge can practically allow, but at the same time must acknowledge that guidelines that are "premature, overdrawn, or overzealously applied . . . can become impediments to product development and, as such, impediments to health care."[1]

The following guidelines represent suggestions for the banking of musculoskeletal allografts. It is expected these guidelines will change as knowledge of fresh and preserved bone graft biologic properties progress and as applications of allografts continue to evolve. It is also recognized that each graft donor and graft recipient may present individual considerations that make portions of these guidelines inappropriate, too restrictive, or

not sufficiently defined. The banking of musculoskeletal tissues other than nonviable but biologically useful osteochondral grafts may also require different approaches. Deviations from the proposed guidelines should, however, be consistent with the spirit of methodology set forth, that is, to provide safe and efficacious allografts. One should clearly note that the guidelines listed below for banking procedures for musculoskeletal tissue may have limited applicability to other tissues or organ systems and, similarly, guidelines for selection, procurement, preservation, or storage of other tissues may have little or no application to bone, cartilage, or other musculoskeletal tissues.

ORGANIZATIONAL CONSIDERATIONS
General

The nature and purpose of the banking facility should be clearly established, whether it is a stand-alone operation or part of an institutional complex. It should have a functional identity with a professional staff and a commitment to maintain and preserve records and operation procedures for future reference and historical continuity.

Facilities and equipment

The facilities should include all equipment necessary to perform the tasks required. Where possible, they should be separate from other facilities and activities and security maintained.

Personnel qualifications

The tissue-banking procedures should be under the supervision of a currently licensed medical or osteopathic physician, dentist, or oral surgeon, or an individual whose past training clearly indicates competence in the application and evaluation of all procedures involved in the safe banking of effective tissues. Other personnel involved in the bank must be trained and judge competent by the tissue bank supervisor for those procedures he or she performs.

Operational procedures

All aspects of donor selection, procurement, processing, storage, quality control, distribution and record keeping should be recorded in an *operational manual*, which should be reviewed periodically and revised as required.

☐ Revised and reprinted with permission from the American Association of Tissue Banks Newsletter **4**(suppl.):30, 1980.

Records

Accurate record keeping is required and must be available to the transplant surgeon. At a minimum, records should include the following:

1. *Donor information*
   a. Donor identification, age, sex, and social security number
   b. Description of the specimen and radiograph(s) where indicated
   c. Cause of death if cadaver donor
   d. Significant past medical history
   e. Blood and tissue types if known
   f. Identification of methods used for procurement, processing, and storage of the graft, including mention of any antibiotics employed
   g. Summary of laboratory, culture, and autopsy records
   h. Results of quality control
   i. Place where tissue was procured and individual responsible
2. *Recipient information*
   a. Recipient identification, age, sex, address, and social security number
   b. Transplant surgeon identification and address
   c. Application for which graft used, date, and location of procedure
   d. Any adverse reactions attributed to graft
   In addition, it is desirable to record the following if known:
   e. Recipient blood and tissue types
   f. Report of graft culture obtained at time of graft use
   g. Any deviations from recommended directions for reconstitution of grafts or from suggestions for their handling
   h. An estimate of clinical graft success

Quality control

Each bank is urged to develop or participate in methods to evaluate those biologic functions for which grafts are employed. A periodic survey of the bacteriologic status of grafts should also be undertaken. This should include reculture of at least 5% of randomly selected representative samples every 6 months (with more specimens cultured more frequently if contamination problems are suspected or demonstrated) and methods to evaluate the effectiveness of storage containers before the clinical use of the allografts.

ACQUISITION OF TISSUES
General and ethicolegal considerations

General. Acceptable sources of musculoskeletal tissue allografts include cadavers, particularly if an autopsy is performed, and living donors, such as at the time of amputation or reconstructive surgery, provided that sufficient clinical information and laboratory tests are available. The primary goals of donor selection are the elimination of potentially harmful transmissible disease and providing tissues that biologically and biomechanically behave satisfactorily for their intended use.

Consent. Appropriate permission must be obtained for tissue donation, either ante mortem from the donor or post mortem from the next of kin. Practices commonly accepted for other medical consent procedures should be followed for tissue donation, including notification or approval of the medical examiner or coroner when appropriate.

Selection criteria

Age. Age alone does not preclude an individual as appropriate for tissue donation; however, age may be a significant factor in terms of intended clinical applications.

Time lag. Tissue should be harvested and subjected to a satisfactory preservation method within 12 hours after death if the cadaver remains in the room temperature environment or within 24 hours if the cadaver is placed in a refrigerator at 4° C ($\pm$4° C) shortly after death. Tissues obtained from living donors should be placed in a closed container or package immediately, refrigerated within 4 hours, and subjected to a satisfactory preservation method within 24 hours after procurement.

Medical history. A review of the past medical history (preferably the written record, but a reliable verbal source may be used) and a review of medical records pertaining to the circumstances of death in the case of a cadaver donor must be accomplished before the clinical application of tissue allografts. Potential donors should be rejected if the medical history includes the following:

1. Active systemic infection
2. Active infection involving tissue to be procured
3. Active or past history of a slow virus disease
4. Malignancy with a propensity to metastasize to tissues being collected

5. History or existence of active hepatitis, or unexplained jaundice
6. Diffuse connective tissue disease, metabolic bone disease, or other serious systemic disorders of unknown cause
7. Death from unknown causes
8. Chronic parenteral drug abuse
9. Heavy irradiation to area of tissue being collected
10. Toxic substances that may be transferred in toxic doses

Laboratory tests. The following tests should be obtained from cadaver and living donors:

1. Australia antigen or other test commonly acceptable for detection of hepatitis
2. VDRL or other test commonly acceptable for detection of syphilis

Blood typing and tissue typing are recommended whenever possible (to further evaluate the clinical significance of these factors), though no attempt to match donor and recipient is required and no specific blood or tissue types are known to play a significant role in donor selection.

Autopsy. An autopsy is desirable, especially when the medical history appears to be incomplete.

It must be emphasized that many considerations regarding donor selection are influenced by, if not dependent on, intended allograft use. Under unusual circumstances, it may also be acceptable to obtain tissues from donors normally excluded provided that the nature of the deviation from the usual and its potential consequences are properly explained to and apparently understood and accepted by the graft recipient.

Tissue procurement and processing

Whenever possible, tissue should be removed by the use of sterile techniques consistent with standard operating room practices. One must understand that aseptic technique does not necessarily preclude the need for additional tissue sterilization. Allografts procured by use of nonsterile techniques may be suitable for transplantation if a satisfactory method of sterilization can be employed. (See Sterilization in the next column.)

Media. If used, the media should be sterile and have the same physiologic pH as the tissue.

Antibiotics. If used, the cultures should be obtained prior to exposure of tissues to antibiotics, and the antibiotics used should be clearly identified to the allograft surgeon.

Cultures. All potential grafts should be cultured for bacteria and fungi at least once prior to final packaging. Either touch cultures (swabs) or specimen cultures (a portion of the graft) should be followed aerobically and anaerobically for a minimum of 7 days by use of commonly acceptable bacteriologic medium and techniques. Blood cultures should be obtained from cadaver donors and handled in a similar fashion to the tissue cultures. The advisability of obtaining blood cultures from living donors depends on individual circumstances, and the need should be determined by the bank for each case.

Sterilization. When sterilization of tissues is required, the method chosen must be effective, without unacceptable risk of potential hazard to the recipient and not cause biologic or biomechanical alterations sufficient to impair graft function with respect to its intended use. Methods of surface decontamination are acceptable only when surface contamination is the only bacteriologic concern.

Reconstruction of cadaver. After tissue procurement appropriate reconstruction of the cadaver is recommended.

TISSUE PRESERVATION AND STORAGE

General. The most acceptable methods for allograft preservation and storage appear to vary with the type of tissue and its intended clinical application.

Deep-freezing and freeze-drying. Although the optimal methods are not yet defined, the preferred methods for long-term preservation and storage of nonviable but biologically useful osteochondral allografts are deep-freezing to $-15°$ C or colder or freeze-drying to a residual moisture of 2% to 5%.

Refrigeration. Short-term preservation of allografts may be accomplished by storage at 4° C ($\pm 4°$ C) for periods up to 48 hours after tissue procurement.

Storage containers. Storage containers must be sterile, nontoxic, and freezable and must maintain a vapor barrier beyond that time that tissues will be stored. Appropriate plastics or glass are recommended.

DISTRIBUTION

1. Safe and effective distribution of tissues requires maintenance of storage temperatures

during transit and a mode of transportation that will not jeopardize the integrity of the storage container.

2. Grafts should be accompanied by directions for reconstitution and use. A frozen graft should be thawed and kept refrigerated at 4° C (±4° C) for no longer than 24 hours before use. A freeze-dried graft should be reconstituted at 4° C (±4° C) for an appropriate length of time (up to 24 hours, depending on the size of the graft) and should be used within 24 hours of complete reconstitution.

3. The donor information outlined in Organizational Considerations (Records) and Acquisition of Tissues (Selection Criteria) must be made available to the transplant surgeon.

4. The importance of culturing the graft at the time of clinical application should be stressed to the transplant surgeon.

5. The importance of obtaining informed consent from the graft recipient should be stressed to the transplant surgeon.

6. The recipient information outlined in Organizational Considerations (Records—Recipient Information) should be completed by the transplant surgeon or his or her designate.

REFERENCE TO PART B
1. Meyers, H.M., Jr.: Standards for tissue banks and transplantation, Trans. Proc. **8**(2, suppl. 1):253, June 1976.

Chapter 3

Neurofibromatosis in childhood

ALVIN H. CRAWFORD, M.D.
Cincinnati, Ohio

Neurofibromatosis is a disease that may manifest itself as abnormalities of the skin, nervous tissue, bones, and soft tissues and is often hereditary. It is believed to be a hamartomatous disorder of neural crest derivation. It was first described by von Recklinghausen in 1882 in an article entitled "Fibrome der Haut."[77] Even though the name "von Recklinghausen's disease" is assigned to neurofibromatosis because of his monograph, he gives credit to Tilesius von Tilenau for the first adequate description of fibroma molluscum in 1793.

R.W. Smith,[69] better known for his work on reverse Colles' fractures, published a remarkable volume in 1849 in which he reported in great detail two cases of generalized neurofibromatosis with necropsy and made pathologic observations.

In 1956, the clinical spectrum of neurofibromatosis in adults was elucidated by Crowe and associates.[19] Its manifestations in children have been reviewed by Suzuki and associates[72] in 1963 and Chao[15] in 1959 and comprehensively described by Fienman and Yakovac[25] in 1970. Allibone and associates[3] found that neurofibromatosis was frequently associated with skeletal anomalies. Later, Brooks and Lehman[13] presented a comprehensive classification of skeletal changes in neurofibromatosis, which included scoliosis, abnormalities of growth on individual bones, and irregularities of the outlines of bones. More recently, Fisher and Vuzevski[26] provided electron microscopic evidence of collagenous fibrils arising from interdigitating extensions of the basement membranes of Schwann cells in neurofibromatosis to connect the mesenchymal and neurectodermal elements of the disease.

Except for the papers of Moore,[54] Miller and associates,[53] and McCarroll,[47] most of the information regarding osseous manifestations of neurofibromatosis has appeared in the radiologic literature. Reports in the orthopaedic literature have dealt with specific entities, such as scoliosis,[14] pseudarthrosis of the tibia, paraplegia, hemihypertrophy, or neoplasia.

At the Alfred I. duPont Institute a study was made of all patients with the diagnosis of neurofibromatosis. Eighty-two have been conclusively diagnosed. Criteria for diagnosis required at least two of the most commonly found entities: multiple café-au-lait spots, abnormal family history, or definitive biopsy or characteristic bony lesions (such as pseudarthrosis tibiae, characteristic hemihypertrophy, or short, sharply angulated spinal curvature). All our patients were under 12 years of age at the time of diagnosis. These 82 patients comprise the largest group of children with neurofibromatosis ever reported from one institution.

Of the patients, 72 were white, 10 black with 46 females and 34 males. The presenting complaints (Table 3-1) represent a myriad of entities and are heavily weighted toward spinal deformity. This finding could possibly be prejudicious, since the Alfred I. duPont Institute is known for its treatment of scoliosis patients.

GENETICS

In 1918, neurofibromatosis was first noted by Preiser and Davenport[61] to be autosomal dominant. It is now considered to be an autosomal dominant trait with variable penetrance and a very high rate of genetic mutation. It has been documented to have a frequency of one patient

Table 3-1. Presenting complaints

Curved spine	43
1 noted to coincident to intravenous pyelogram	
1 preoperative excision to intrathoracic ganglioneurofibroma	
Limb-length discrepancy	12
Abnormal neurologic defects	6
1 proprioceptive defect	
1 neuromuscular clubfoot	
Family study	6
Pseudarthrosis tibiae	6
3 tibial fractures	
1 pseudarthrosis	
1 bowing (prepseudarthrosis)	
Pain	
2 hip (1 pathologic fracture)	
1 knee	
Café-au-lait spots	3
Foot swelling	1
Facial enlargement	1
Digital enlargement	1
Visual problem	1
Foot turning in	1

per 2500 to 3000 births. Spontaneous mutations may explain why an abnormal familial history can be obtained in less than one half the families with involved members. A family history was obtained in 32 of our 82 patients (40%).

FINDINGS
Cutaneous lesions

The café-au-lait type of pigmentation is a characteristic lesion of neurofibromatosis. This pigmentation is tan, macular, and melanotic in origin and is located in and around the basal layer of the epidermis. Café-au-lait spots were present in 74 of our 82 patients (90%). The presence of a café-au-lait spot may be normal. McCarroll[47] routinely examined nursing students and found that 20% had café-au-lait spots without associated anomalies. Crowe and associates[19] concluded that an adult patient who has more than six café-au-lait spots measuring 1.5 cm or more in diameter must be presumed to have neurofibromatosis. Whitehouse[80] evaluated 365 children under the age of five and stated that two or less café-au-lait spots occur in only 0.75% of normal children and that five spots with a diameter of at least 0.5 cm should be considered diagnostic of neurofibromatosis until proved otherwise. Most of our patients who did not have café-au-lait spots initially developed them at a later age. Those patients presenting with only a few spots as children showed an increase in number with increasing age. The café-au-lait spots of neurofibromatosis have smooth edges (coast of California) as contrasted by the jagged edges seen in fibrous dysplasia (coast of Maine).

Nodules

Ten of our patients (12%) had cutaneous nodules (fibroma molluscum). They were all adolescents. These lesions are manifestations of longstanding or adult disease and do not occur with any frequency in childhood.[35] The soft tumors may grow under, be flush with, or be raised above the level of the skin. Although they are usually the color of normal skin, early lesions may be violaceous. Ormsby and Montgomery[58] interpreted these tumors as true neurofibromas arising from peripheral nerves and their supporting structures, but this conclusion has not been proved. Stout[71] considered these tumors to be simple proliferations of fibrous tissue.

Nevus

Five patients (6%) presented with nevi, including one patient with "nevus lateralis," which can be described as dark brown pigmented skin over one half the abdominal wall, with the change occurring along the midline. Other patients presented with large nevi that covered broad areas of skin and were occasionally quite tender. This tenderness was observed in two patients, one who was unable to tolerate a brace because of the presence of the sensitive lesion and the other who had difficulty wearing a scoliosis jacket. This skin type may also have decreased sensation, thus allowing sores to develop under a brace or cast without the patient's knowledge.

Elephantiasis

Frequently large soft tissue masses are seen in neurofibromatosis. These masses have been termed "pachydermatocele," or "elephantiasis neuromatosa." They are characterized by a rough, raised verrucous or villous type of skin hypertrophy presenting an unmistakable appearance. Although more frequently occurring in adult life, we encountered nine patients (10%) with varying degrees of involvement (Fig. 3-1). Weiss[78] has described this finding to be characteristic of neurofibromatosis. There may be dysplasia of the underlying bone.[37]

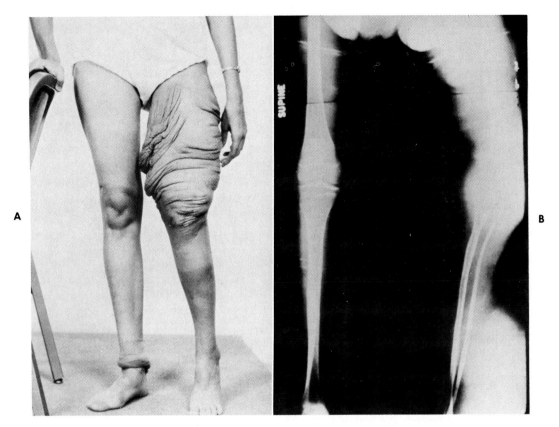

Fig. 3-1. Clinical and radiographic appearance of elephantiasis neuromatosa. **A,** Teenager with elephantiasis involving only the left thigh. There is thickening and overgrowth of the skin as well as of the limb. Note the scars around the knee after attempted distal femoral and proximal tibial epiphyseal arrest. **B,** Anteroposterior roentgenogram of both lower extremities showing normal-appearing bone on the *right* and the dysplastic narrow, elongated bone on the *left*. Soft-tissue shadows partially obliterate the femor on the *left*.

SKELETAL MANIFESTATIONS
Spinal deformities

 Scoliosis is the most common osseous defect associated with neurofibromatosis. Gould[29] and Weiss[78] were the first to point out the high incidence of scoliosis that varies in severity from mild nonprogressive forms to severe scoliosis.[27]

Miller[52] described the course of neurofibromatosis as a kyphoscoliosis with a site of predilection in the lower dorsal area, which may be noticed in early childhood. A characteristic feature is the sharp angulation at the apex of the gibbus. Scott[67] evaluated the spinal deformities in 81 patients and found no evidence of any pattern of scoliosis in neurofibromatosis. He noted that the severity of some of the curves resembled congenital scoliosis. Veliskakis and associates[76] noted that in 43 of 55 patients a characteristic short curve composed of five or fewer segments with sharp apical wedging and rotation in the lower thoracic area prevailed. The wedging was occasionally so severe it was mistaken for a hemivertebra, They believed that the tendency of this curve to progress rapidly warranted early spine fusion of the involved segments to prevent progression. Our study revealed the short-segmented sharply angulated curvature to be the anteroposterior x-ray presentation of a kyphoscoliosis.

The consensus is that there are probably two patterns of scoliosis with neurofibromatosis, that

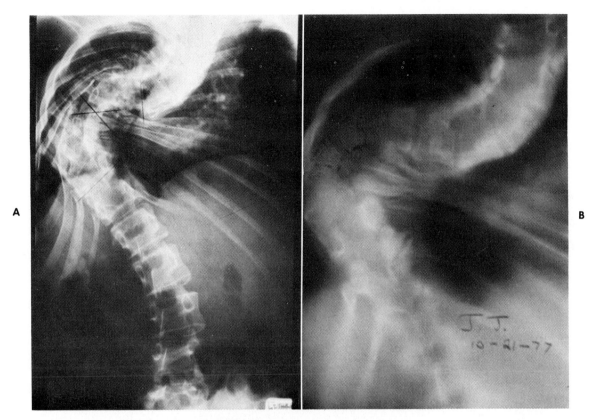

Fig. 3-2. Dysplastic neurofibromatotic curvature with short-segmented, sharply angulated "kinky" spinal deformity: plain film and tomography. **A,** AP roentgenogram of a child with spinal deformity associated with neurofibromatosis. There is scalloping of the vertebral margins, gross rotation of the apical vertebrae, relative appearance of a paraspinous mass, and penciling of the ribs in the concavity. **B,** Plain polytomography reveals widening of the spinal canal in the upper thoracic region inferring dural ectasia. There appears to be a 180-degree vertebral body rotation between the upper thoracic vertebra and the apical vertebrae. Note the proximity of the apical vertebrae to the ribs. (**A** and **B,** Courtesy Dr. Michael Schafer, Chicago, Ill.)

is, the characteristic short-segmented dysplastic sharply angulated curve and curves resembling idiopathic scoliosis.[7,14,43,46,64] The dysplastic curvature is characterized by severe wedging of the apical vertebral bodies, strong rotation of apical vertebrae, scalloping of vertebral bodies, spindling or transverse processes, foraminal enlargement, and penciling of the apical ribs (Fig. 3-2).

Fifty of our patients (60%) presented with scoliosis. Only eight had the characteristic neurofibromatosis curve, and the remainder had curves indistinguishable from the idopathic type. The x-ray characteristics and response to treatment in these curves were similar to those of patients without neurofibromatosis (Fig. 3-3).

Forty-five of our 50 patients with spinal deformities were females, that is, 90%. Seven were detected because of our ongoing family study to determine the genetic aspects of scoliosis.[18] The finding of neurofibromatosis in the family study reconfirms the genetic aspect. Although a scoliosis family history was obtained in only 23 of our 82 patients (28%), this figure agrees with Crowe's data of less than 50% having an abnormal family history. This finding also reiterates the high rate of genetic spontaneous mutation described by Fienman and Yakovac.

Thirty-six patients underwent posterior spinal fusion, and of these, nine had reexploration for possible pseudarthrosis, of which five were found

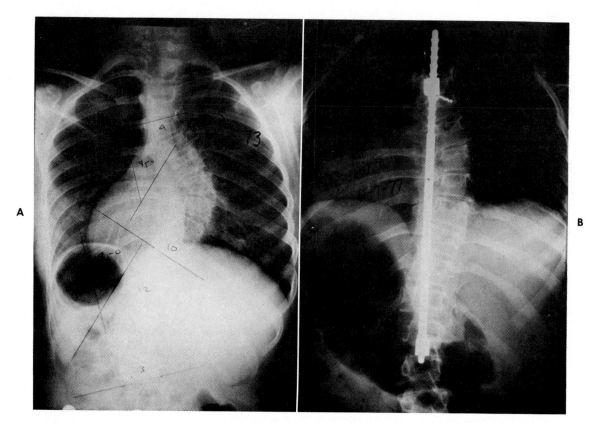

Fig. 3-3. Idiopathic spinal deformity in a patient with neurofibromatosis. **A,** Right dorsal T4-T10 spinal deformity with compensatory lumbar curve in 14-year-old female with neurofibromatosis. (Her 17-year-old brother had severe kyphosis requiring surgery.) There is no evidence of scalloping of vertebral margins or paraspinal masses. **B,** Four-year follow-up showing maintenance of correction and solid fusion.

to have defects in the fusion mass (a 17% pseud-arthrosis rate). One other patient is known to have a pseudarthrosis but has not been explored. This percentage is much higher then that for the idiopathic curves treated during the same period of time.

Kyphoscoliosis

The severe kyphoscoliosis seen in neurofibro-matosis is distinguished by the predominance of kyphosis over the scoliosis with acute angulation being a typical sign. The vertebral bodies frequently are so deformed and attenuated at the apex that it may be impossible to identify them on routine roentgenograms. Curtis and others[20] believed that the kyphosis contributed more to the production of paraplegia than did the scoliosis. This view is supported by the biomechanical studies of Breig,[10] which showed that flexion of the spine caused elongation of the spinal canal and deformation of the spinal cord. Pathologically increased spinal flexion as by a kyphotic deformity leads to excessive axial tension in the cord parenchyma and may result in neurologic impairment.

Of the 50 patients, four presented with more kyphosis than scoliosis. One patient 6 years of age underwent a posterior spinal fusion of T4 to T12 and an attempted anterior spinal fusion for progressive kyphosis, but it could not be carried out because of pronounced local invasion of the soft tissue with neurofibromatosis material. The kyphosis has been temporarily stabilized with external support. The other three patients underwent attempts at obtaining surgical stabilization with varying success. Recently Winter and others[81] have reported a 64% incidence of pseudarthrosis in patients with dysplastic scoliosis with kyphosis of more than 50 degrees.

Spondylolisthesis

McCarroll noted spondylolisthesis in four of his patients. Only one of our patients was noted to have spondylolisthesis even though lateral x-ray films of the lumbar spine were taken on all (a lower incidence than in the general population).

Intrathoracic meningocele

In 1933, Pohl[60] reported the first case of an intrathoracic meningocele associated with neurofibromatosis. Roentgenographically with myelogra-phy, a soft-tissue mass is seen protruding from the spinal canal into the posterior mediastinum. Structural defects in the pedicles, enlargements of the intervertebral foramina, and abnormalities of the vertebral bodies may accompany the mass. An intrathoracic meningocele is relatively rare, and less than 50 cases are reported in the literature.[38,44,65] No case was noted in our series.

Disorders of bone growth

Disorders of bone growth are quite frequently associated with changes in the soft tissue overlying the bony deformity.[9,13,24,28,57,74] The changes in the soft tissue are usually those of hemangioma-tosis, lymphangiomatosis, elephantiasis, or occasionally beaded plexiform neuromas. The zones of overgrowth in bone and soft tissue are usually unilateral involving the lower extremity or the head and neck.[37,44] Sir Arthur Treves, a British surgeon is renown for his kind assistance to Joseph Carey Merrick (called "John" Merrick in the movie). Merrick was afflicted by neurofibromatosis with a profound disorder of facial bone growth, and he traveled with freak shows as the "Elephant Man." The diffuse hypertrophy of an extremity may first command the attention of the orthopaedic surgeon (Fig. 3-4). Eleven of our patients presented with limb-length discrepancy, of which four had associated elephantoid changes. Increased blood supply of the hemangiomatous and lymphangiomatous elements in the soft-tissue masses offers the most plausible explanation for the overgrowth in length. Two of these subsequently developed retroperitoneal sarcoma.

Congenital bowing and pseudarthrosis

The relationship of pseudarthrosis of the tibia to neurofibromatosis was first described by Ducroquet[21] in 1937. Of his 11 patients with tibial pseudarthrosis, nine had manifestations of neurofibromatosis. The bowing of the tibia in neurofibromatosis is characteristically anterolateral and is usually evident within the first years of life. The single bone most commonly affected by neurofibromatosis is the tibia.[4,5,22,32,48,49,55] Other affected bones have been reported, such as the ulna,[17] fibula, femur, clavicle,[2,43,56] radius,[62] and humerus.

Pseudarthrosis has also been reported as familial.[79] Only one pseudarthrosis has been reported in a patient beyond 11 years of age.[6] This was

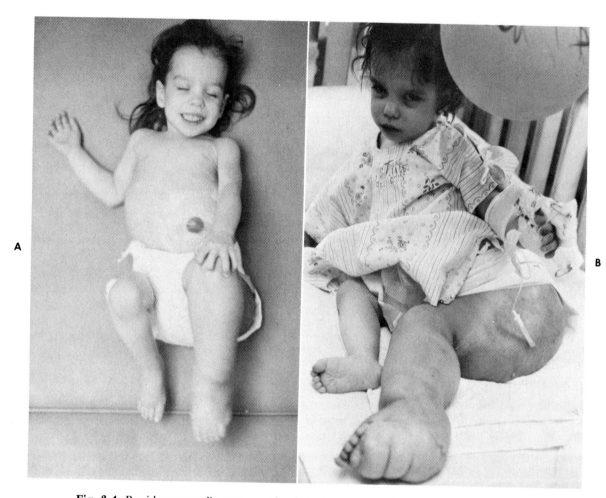

Fig. 3-4. Rapid monomelic overgrowth of the lower extremity in a young child. **A,** At 2 years of age this child underwent a ureterosigmoidostomy because of ureteral blockade from retroperitoneal ganglioneuroma. There is significant overgrowth of the left lower extremity. **B,** Two years later, the limb has increased in size by a factor of three. The limb was longer and weighed more than the rest of the child. She was totally immobilized because of it and required a hip disarticulation.

caused by a fracture in a 41-year-old male. The cause of pseudarthrosis is questionable. Except for the case report of Green and Rudo[30] in which the histologic studies showed neurofibromatotic tissue growing in the pseudarthrosis segment, studies have failed to show neurofibromatotic tissue at the pseudarthrotic site. Aegerter[1] believed that the basic lesion was in the surrounding soft tissue with secondary bony involvement. He speculated that if all the tumor tissue were removed, normal callous tissue would still form. Briner and Yunis[12] examined by electron microscopy the soft tissue removed from three patients with pseudarthrosis tibiae and found fibroblasts rather than Schwann cells or perineural cells. This finding differed from true neurofibromatosis and neurilemomas, in which both Schwann cells and fibroblasts are found, as well as occasional unmyelinated axons.

Pseudarthrosis poses a difficult orthopaedic problem in management. Many surgical procedures to improve alignment and internally stabilize the bone fragments have been described. Few satisfy the basic requirements of stability of fixation and promotion of osteogenesis.[8,50,75] The widely used methods include the massive onlay graft,[33] dual autogenous onlay,[39] trough with chip graft[31] delayed autogenous onlay,[39] bypass,[23] fragmentation, and turn-around.[70] Charnley[16] used an intramedullary nail for better fixation. Langenskiöld devised a procedure for stabilizing the ankle.[41] Lloyd-Roberts and Shaw[45] suggested prefracture grafting of the kyphotic tibia as a means of preventing pseudarthrosis. Lavine and others[42] and Brighton and others[11] recently reported the application of an electric current to a pseudarthrosis defect.

Eight patients presented with angular deformities of the tibias under 2 years of age. These included five frank tibial fractures, one pseudarthrosis, and two with anterolateral bowing (prepseudarthrosis). The treatment of seven of these patients has been reported by Rathgeb and others.[63] Attempts were made to classify the radiographic appearance of the lesion and prognosticate response to treatment.

Seventeen surgical procedures were performed, including onlay grafting, multiple osteotomies, plate fixation, and three below-knee amputations and the application of electrical current in two. The four radiologic types of pseudarthrosis tibiae in these cases are as follows.

Type I. Anterolateral bow with a normal medullary canal. These patient have the best prognosis, can usually be followed without bracing, and may never have a fracture.

Type II. Anterolateral bowing with narrowed sclerotic medullary canal—"high risk." These patients inevitably have a fracture. Although two patients healed after several procedures, the shortening and deformity were unacceptable and amputation was necessary. These patients should be protected from the time the diagnosis is made and prepared for surgical intervention, possibly prophylactically.

Type III. Anterolateral bow with cystic lesion. These patient should have a graft because of their tendency to early fracture with the resulting dire consequences.

Type IV. Anterolateral bow with fracture, cyst, or frank pseudarthrosis. These patients have the worst possible prognosis. All aspects of the patient must be considered in the eagerness to achieve union. The number of operations and length of hospitalization must be carefully considered in terms of whether the psychologic costs are a fair price to pay for the anticipated result. Amputation should be considered early in the course of treatment. Some of the happiest patients have had amputations, particularly those who had experienced several operations requiring prolonged confinement. Observation of children with similar problems often helps the psychologic effect on the patient and the family (Fig. 3-5).

Erosive defects of bone from contiguous neurogenic tumors

Erosive defects are considered by some authors as the most characteristic bone changes in neurofibromatosis.[13,24,27,28] Nøgaard[57] described these erosions as a pit or cave in the bone. There were seven cases of erosive defects in the series ranging from gross enlargement of the vertebral neural foramina to extrinsic cystic lesions of the tibia and femur (Fig. 3-6).

Bone cyst

One of the most unusual anomalies and possibly the most controversial skeletal abnormality is the cystic lesion.[37] The problem arises as to whether or not the lesion is an intrinsic cyst, one resulting from pressure erosion from an adjacent peripheral nerve with (1) neurofibromatotic involvement, (2) secondary overgrowth of the peri-

Text continued on p. 68.

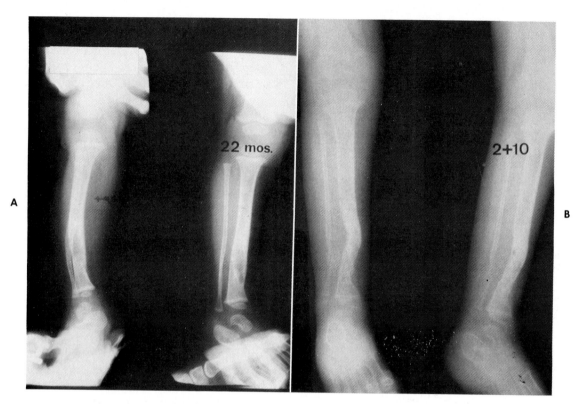

Fig. 3-5. Example of presentation and successive operative procedures on a child with neurofibromatosis and type IV pseudarthrosis tibiae. The amount of time, emotional commitment, and psychologic deterioration of the child should cause one to consider other options with the type IV pseudarthrosis tibiae lesion. **A,** At 22 months of age the child was brought in by the parents after they noticed a limp for several months. There is a healing fracture with cystic response. **B,** Two years 10 months at time of removal of cast after third known fracture. There is a frank oligotrophic pseudarthrosis of the fibula. **C,** Three years 9 months. The fracture was considered to be completely healed. He was allowed to walk with external support. The fibular pseudarthrosis appears segmental. **D,** Five years 8 months after immobilization over a prolonged period. It was considered that the union was solid enough to allow weight-bearing without support. The area of union was sclerotic with no medullary canal. **E,** Five years 9 months. One month after independent weight-bearing, the fracture occurred just below the area of sclerosis in the medullary canal. **F,** Six years 7 months. After 11 months of immobilization with no evidence of union, onlay bone grafting was carried out with an intramedullary stabilization rod.

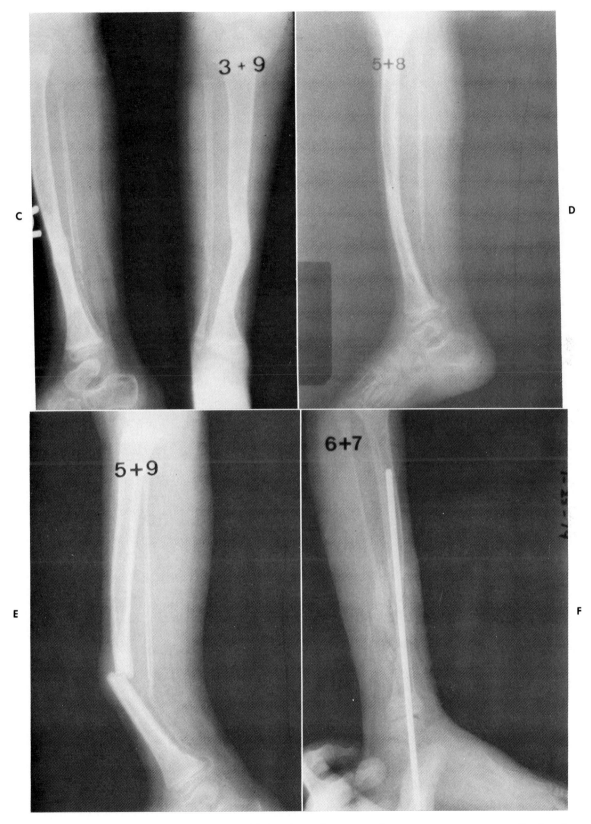

Fig. 3-5, cont'd. For legend see opposite page.   *Continued.*

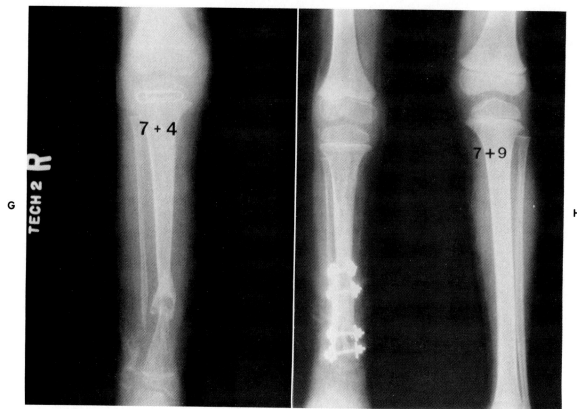

Fig. 3-5, cont'd. G, Seven years 4 months. Nine months after bone grafting, there is no evidence of union, even though the graft appeared to unite to the proximal fragment. **H,** Seven years 9 months. Several months after onlay plates with rigid fixation, there is still no bony union. The child is only 7 years 9 months old; the limb is 3 inches short with virtually no foot or ankle motion.

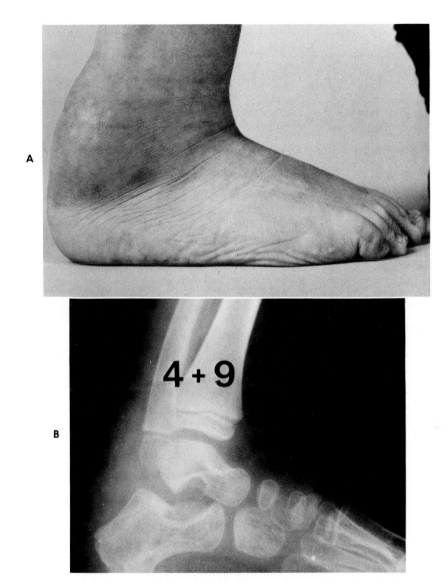

Fig. 3-6. Neurofibromatous mass in the subtalar joint. **A,** This young child was noted to have a mass over the posterolateral aspect of his right foot and ankle. A biopsy revealed the mass to be neurofibromatous tissure in the subtalar joint. **B,** Lateral x-ray studies of the foot show the characteristic erosive defect in the subtalar joint. The sclerotic margins infer that the lesion has been present for a long time. Wavy thickened trabeculas of the anterior aspect of the os calcis are characteristic of bony changes in neurofibromatosis.

osteum, and (3) cyst formation in response to the extrinsic neurofibromas, or a cyst resulting from direct invasion of the periosteum by a plexiform neuroma and infiltration of the cortex and haversian canals by neurofibromatous tissue.

Only one patient, 10 years of age, in our series had a true bone cyst. She also had a hemangioma of the palm, a mass on her left arm, and café-au-lait spots on her abdomen, arms, and legs. The cyst in the proximal femur was reported as a simple bone cyst, but the mass on the arm was found to be a neurofibroma. The cyst recurred at 12 years of age and responded to curettage and grafting. She was examined 18 years later and noted to have more numerous café-au-lait spots and subcutaneous nodules. We believe that this lesion does not represent the cystic lesion of neu-

rofibromatosis, but only that of a simple cyst of the femur that occurred in a patient with neurofibromatosis.

Subperiosteal bone proliferation

Among the protean manifestations of multiple neurofibromatosis is the occurrence of the subperiosteal bone proliferation as described by Brooks and Lehman.[13] Two cases were described in their original report; others[29,34,35,40,47,59,66] have reported similar lesions.

We have noted a total of five such lesions in our series, three of which have been previously reported.[59] One of these, a male patient noted to have a scoliosis and bony overgrowth of the left tibia with a subperiosteal cortical cyst, underwent a spinal fusion and was scheduled for a tibial epi-

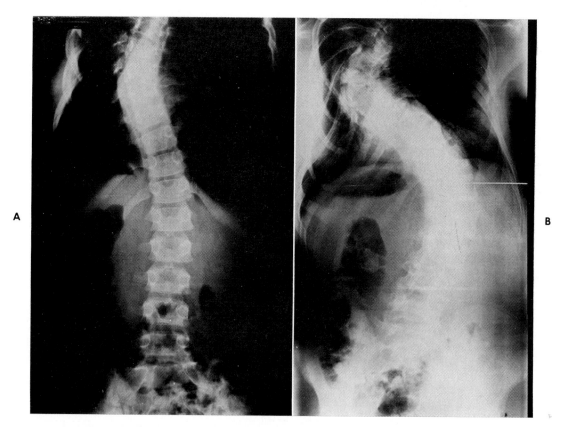

Fig. 3-7. Progressive neurofibromatotic spinal deformity with neurofibrosarcoma presenting as a pseudarthrosis. **A,** Initial presentation of moderate left thoracic spinal deformity. **B,** Two years after initial evaluation there has been noticeable progression of the spinal deformity giving it the kinky short-segmented, sharply angulated appearance of the neurofibromatous spinal deformity.

physiodesis; however, he never returned for follow-up. Another patient was first seen because of enlargement of the right tibia and fibula, café-au-lait spots, and verrucous skin hypertrophy. He was treated at 8 years of age with an epiphysiodesis of the right tibia and fibula. He subsequently developed Charcot changes of the right ankle. The other three patients had similar conditions and were reported in an earlier article.[59]

All five of these patients had elephantoid overgrowth of soft tissue and pachydermatocele formation. All had overgrowth of the bone that had cystic subperiosteal involvement.

Neoplasia

Any study of a large series of patients diagnosed as having neurofibromatosis will reveal soft-tissue neoplasms.[36,51,68] Most are of neurogenic origin and are either central or peripheral in location. The existence of other neurologic hamartomatous lesions in neurofibromatosis is uncommon but not rare. Also the tendency for these lesions to undergo malignant change has been cited by others[51,71] (Fig. 3-7).

Thirteen of our 82 patients were noted to have neoplastic lesions. These included benign lesions that presented in a malignant fashion, that is, a retroperitoneal mass, a dumbbell tumor extending into the spinal canal and brachial plexus with neurologic compromise, and lesions that recurred after initial excision with overgrowth into vital areas that prevented repeat excision and threatened life (Table 3-2).

Although all the benign tumors represented

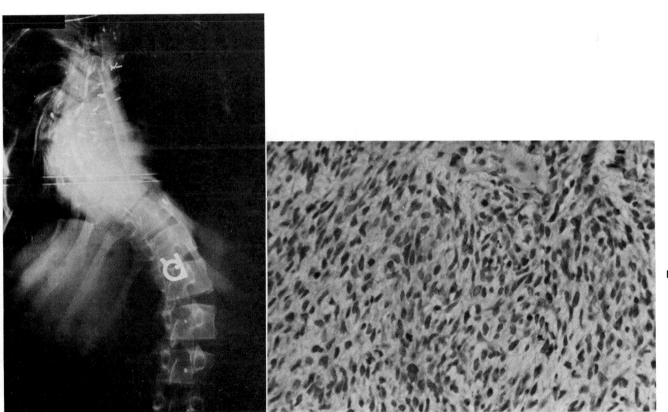

Fig. 3-7, cont'd. There has been commissural rib and chest cage deformity. **C,** After a normal myelogram, a stabilization procedure was carried out with an anterior fibular short-strut graft and a posterior in situ fusion. **D,** Because of pain and motion of the fusion mass, an exploration for pseudarthrosis was carried out. The tissue at pseudarthrosis was grossly abnormal and histologic findings showed characteristics of neurofibrosarcoma. (**A** to **D,** Courtesy Dr. James C. Drennan, Newington Children's Hospital, Newington, Conn.)

Table 3-2. Neoplasms

Patient	Unit number	Lesion	Sequelae
P.K.	11321	Fibrosarcoma	Retroperitoneal mass compressing abdominal contents, leading to anorexia and death
D.P.	11398	Neurofibrosarcoma	Sarcomatous changes in original neurofibromas of cervical area with subsequent involvement of spinal cord, clivus, and brain, leading to death
J.O.	13565	Acoustic neuroma	Neurofibromatous involvement of acoustic nerve, olfactory groove, optic atrophy extension of spinal cord, leading to death
L.S.	7537	Neurogenic sarcoma	Metastatic neurosarcoma to brain with headaches and clonic seizure, leading to death
P.C.	18085	Retrobulbar glioma	Loss of right optic nerve
F.P.	10158	Thalamic glioma	Ptosis of both eyes with subsequent brain involvement, requiring ventriculoperitoneal shunt, followed by abdominal laparotomy and death
M.B.B.	24776	Mediastinal neuroblastoma	Exploratory thoracotomy, radiation therapy, and posterior spinal fusion
W.C.	15883	GR III astrocytoma T10-L1	Paraplegia
K.M.	19104	Ganglioneuroblastoma picked up as mediastinal mass on roentgenogram	Anterior and posterior spinal fusion
C.W.	8907	Retroperitoneal neurofibroma	Palpable abdominal masses with abnormal function
R.S.	10299	Retroperitoneal neurofibroma	Dumbbell extension of retroperitoneal tumor into thorax and abdomen
E.B.	9447	Sarcomas of paravertebral (neck) soft tissue	Excisional biopsy and irradiation
P.N.	19242	Sarcomatous degeneration of mediastinal mass	Maintenance in external support after unsuccessful attempts at anterior and posterior spinal stabilization

neural elements, they could not be considered benign because of the functional impairment of the central nervous system at the target organs. Not only was the target organ intrinsically impaired, but also attempts at resection of the lesion usually resulted in further neurologic loss.

DISCUSSION

The cutaneous manifestation of neurofibromatosis was demonstrated in our series in that café-au-lait spots were present in 74 of the 82 patients. The series reconfirmed the observation that only a few café-au-lait spots may be present (five lesions of greater than 0.5 cm) in children, but they may increase in number and size with age.[80] Several of the patients who had abnormal biopsy results did not have café-au-lait spots at the time of their initial examination but subsequently developed multiple skin lesions in later years. Only those children over 12 years of age demonstrated the cutaneous nodules (fibroma molluscum) of neurofibromatosis. One patient who had no evidence of lesions on initial presentation revealed multiple fibroma molluscum all over her body at follow-up 18 years later.

We agree with Biot and others[7] that spinal deformities in neurofibromatosis are divided into two groups. The first and most serious deformities complicating neurofibromatosis include severe dysplasia of the vertebral bodies, posterior arches, and spinal canal and are usually found in the thoracic area with a scoliosis, kyphosis, or kyphoscoliosis. They may appear in early infancy and continue to increase after puberty. They may develop neurologic problems including paraplegia. The second group develop scoliotic deformities that are in appearance identical to idopathic scoliosis. These curves have the same prognosis and evolution as idopathic curves have, except that they have a higher risk of pseudarthrosis after fusion and possibly a greater risk of progression with or without corrective treatment. However, during the evolutionary period some had a tendency to take on dysplastic characteristics that were more characteristic of the first group. Of the 50 patients who presented with curvatures, only eight had the characteristic neurofibromatotic curve, that is, the low thoracodorsal curve with the appearance of dysplasia. The remainder had a condition like idiopathic scoliosis associated with neurofibromatosis.

No patients in our series had paraplegia resulting from a kyphosis associated with a progressive deformity. An attempt in one patient for anterior and posterior spinal stabilization failed. In this patient, the kyphotic deformity has been temporarily stabilized by bracing, but the possibility of progression and paraplegia is real. Twelve of our patients appear to be well controlled in spinal braces. McCarroll[47] noted spondylolisthesis in four of his 33 cases of vertebral involvement. The incidence of spondylolisthesis in our series is only one of 50 with adequate roentgenograms and is statistically not so great as the incidence of spondylolisthesis in our patients with idiopathic scoliosis.

The most impressive disorders of bone growth included patients who had coexistent pachydermatocele or elephantoid skin characteristics. Two of the patients with a combination of bony overgrowth and elephantoid skin changes subsequently developed retroperitoneal sarcomas. The one patient not having skin changes associated with bony overgrowth underwent progressive enlargement of her right mandible. After 16 plastic surgical procedures, she is quite disfigured and has asymmetric growth in her mandible.

The relationship of pseudarthrosis or congenital anterolateral bowing of the tibia to neurofibromatosis cannot be overemphasized. Usually the patients have the condition under 2 years of age with no other evidence of neurofibromatosis at that time. One patient had undergone eight procedures before she was a teen-ager and did not manifest café-au-lait spots until 8 years of age. She subsequently developed multiple café-au-lait spots and fibroma molluscum. Because of the considerable shortening and disfigurement of the leg, despite union after the eighth procedure, she

elected to have an amputation. She subsequently presented with a neck mass diagnosed as neurofibrosarcoma by biopsy.

The four types of lesions we have described and their recommended form of treatment are self-explanatory. Although the association of the pseudarthrosis tibiae to neurofibromatosis is not 100%, we believe that the patterned type of pseudarthrotic lesions, that is, anterolateral bowing whether associated with neurofibromatosis or not, requires the same treatment. Strong emphasis must again be placed on the type IV lesion. I believe that amputation should be considered very early because of the tendency of this lesion to resist all methods of obtaining a union. We have noted that patients with the type IV lesion who have undergone Boyd-Syme type of amputations (retaining the os calcis and weight-bearing skin) primarily and placed in a prosthesis have accomplished synostosis of the defect. This same lesion has been known to resist multiple attempts at synostosis by bone grafting.

It was noted that all five of our patients who showed manifestations of subperiosteal bone proliferation had elephantoid overgrowth of the soft tissue. These patients also presented with subperiosteal hematomas but ran a very progressive and malignant course, despite aspiration, tamponading, and further attempts to control bleeding. They all ran a relentless course of bony enlargement that was refractive to epiphyseal arrest. It was further noted that two of these patients developed Charcot-like changes in the joints of the affected extremities.

The incidence of neoplasia was quite high in our young population. Most series report a 5% incidence. Of our 15 cases of neoplasia in 82 patients, that is, 18%, there were only two frankly malignant lesions, but the other lesions involving compromise of the neuraxis led to death in three of our patients. They were considered malignant because of their inaccessibility or their compromise to structures essential to the maintenance of life. At least three other patients from our series now being treated at other institutions have subsequently developed neoplastic lesions.

Organic manifestations of neurofibromatosis previously reported in children, such as sexual precocity and retarded sexual development, malignant hypertension secondary to renal artery stenosis and diffuse small vessel changes,[73] and mental retardation, were not statistically analyzed in our series. Our data did reveal a very definite trend toward mental retardation, with all patients being somewhat slow in comprehension. Some had delayed speech and motor development when compared to their peers. There were not enough of our patients with intelligence tests available to arrive at a definite conclusion. We do believe that the incidence of retarded development was greater in these patients.

CONCLUSIONS

We have reviewed 82 patients conclusively diagnosed with neurofibromatosis, who presented to the Alfred I. duPont Institute under 12 years of age. The following observations were made:

1. The most common presenting complaint was that of spinal deformities (60%).
2. The scoliosis appeared to be divided into two categories:
   a. Those associated with neurofibromatosis in which there were dysplastic vertebral bodies, progressive deformity with scoliosis and kyphosis, and a tendency toward pseudarthrosis after spinal fusion.
   b. Those associated with neurofibromatosis that present as a idiopathic scoliosis and have the same prognosis.
3. The presence of café-au-lait spots was the most consistent finding (90%), and the numbers and size tended to increase with age.
4. The verrucous skin hypertrophy or elephantoid or pachydermatocele formation appeared as ominous sign in that not only did patients with severe bony overgrowth show this manifestation, but also on occasion patients who had this manifestation developed sarcomatous changes.
5. The pseudarthrosis tibiae could be classified into four distant types with corresponding treatment programs.
6. The incidence of neoplasia far exceeded that of the average population, and some lesions that were not considered frankly malignant, resulted in catastrophic consequences because of their anatomic locations.

REFERENCES

1. Aegerter, E.: The possible relationship of neurofibromatosis, congenital pseudarthrosis and fibrous dysplasia, J. Bone Joint Surg. **32A**(3):618-626, 1950.
2. Alldred, A.J.: Congenital pseudarthrosis of the clavicle, J. Bone Joint Surg. **45B**:312, 1963.
3. Allibone, E.C., Illingworth, R.S., and Wright, T.: Neurofibromatosis (von Recklinghausen's disease) of the vertebral column, Arch. Dis. Child. **35**:153-158, 1960.
4. Andersen, K.: Congenital pseudarthrosis of the leg, J. Bone Joint Surg. **58A**(5):657-662, 1976.
5. Barber, C.G.: Congenital bowing and pseudarthrosis of the lower leg: manifestations of von Recklinghausen's neurofibromatosis, Surg. Gynecol. Obstet. **69**:618-626, 1939.
6. Berk, L., and Mankin, H.J.: Spontaneous pseudarthrosis of the tibia occurring in a patient with neurofibromatosis: report of a case in a man forty-one years old, J. Bone Joint Surg. **46A**(3):619-624, April 1964.
7. Biot, B., et al: Les lésions vertébrales de la neurofibromatose, Rev. Chir. Orthop. **60**:607-621, 1974.
8. Boyd, H.B., and Sage, F.P.: Congenital pseudarthrosis of the tibia, J. Bone Joint Surg. **40A**:1245-1270, 1958.
9. Brasfield, R.D., and Das Gupta, T.K.: Von Recklinghausen's disease: a clinicopathological study, Ann. Surg. **175**(1):86-103, Jan. 1972.
10. Breig, A.: Biomechanics of the central nervous system: some basic normal and pathological phenomena concerning spine, discs, and cord, Stockholm, 1960, Almquist & Wiksell, Printers & Publishers.
11. Brighton, C.T., Friedenberg, Z.B., Zemsky, L.M., and Pollis, P.R.: Direct-current stimulation of non-union and congenital pseudarthrosis: exploration of its clinical application, J. Bone Joint Surg. **57A**(3):368, 1975.
12. Briner, J., and Yunis, E.: Ultrastructure of congenital pseudarthrosis of the tibia, Arch. Pathol. **95**:97-99, Feb. 1973.
13. Brooks, B., and Lehman, E.P.: The bone changes in Recklinghausen's neurofibromatosis, Surg. Gynecol. Obstet. **38**:587-595, 1924.
14. Chaglassian, J.H., Riseborough, E.J., and Hall, J.L.: Neurofibromatous scoliosis: natural history and results of treatment in thirty-seven cases, J. Bone Joint Surg. **58A**(5):695-702, 1976.
15. Chao, D.H.: Congenital neurocutaneous syndromes in childhood. I. Neurofibromatosis, J. Pediat. **55**:189, 1959.
16. Charnley, J.: Congenital pseudarthrosis of the tibia treated by the intramedullary nail, J. Bone Joint Surg. **38A**:238-290, 1956.
17. Cobb, N.: Neurofibromatosis and pseudarthrosis of the ulna: a case report, J. Bone Joint Surg. **50B**(1):146-149, Feb. 1968.
18. Cowell, H.R., Hall, J.N., and MacEwen, G.D.: Genetic aspects of idiopathic scoliosis: a Nicholas Andry Award essay, 1970, Clin. Orthop. **86**:121-131, July-August 1972.
19. Crowe, F.W., Schull, W.J., and Neel, J.U.: A clinical pathological and genetic study of multiple neurofibromatosis, Springfield, Ill., 1956, Charles C Thomas, Publisher.
20. Curtis, B.H., et al.: Neurofibromatosis with paraplegia: report of eight cases, J. Bone Joint Surg. **51A**(5):843-860, 1969.
21. Ducroquet, R.L.: À propos des pseudarthroses et inflexions congénitales du tibia, Mem. Acad. Chir. **63**:863-868, 1937.
22. Dunn, A.W.: Case of overgrowth of leg and anterolateral bowing of tibia in neurofibromatosis, Am. J. Orthop. **7**:120-123, Sept.-Dec. 1965.
23. Eyre-Brook, A.L., Baily, R.A.J., and Price, C.H.G.: Infantile pseudarthrosis of the tibia, J. Bone Joint Surg. **51B**:604, 1969.

24. Fairbank, H.A.T.: Neurofibromatosis: atlas of general affections of the skeleton, J. Bone Joint Surg. **32B**(2):266-270, May 1950.

25. Fienman, N.L., and Yakovac, W.C.: Neurofibromatosis in childhood, J. Pediat. **76**(3):339-346, 1970.

26. Fisher, E.R., and Vuzevski, V.D.: Cytogenesis of schwannoma (neurilemoma), neurofibroma, dermatofibroma and dermatofibrosarcoma as revealed by electron microscopy, Am. J. Clin. Pathol. **49**:141-154, 1968.

27. Friedman, M.M.: Neurofibromatosis of bone, Am. J. Roentgenol. **51**:623-630, 1944.

28. Goel, M.K.: Osseous lesions in neurofibromatosis. (Unpublished data.)

29. Gould, E.P.: The bone changes occurring in von Recklinghausen's disease, Q. J. Med. **XI**:221, 1918.

30. Green, W.T., and Rudo, N.: Pseudarthrosis and neurofibromatosis, Arch. Surg. **46**:639-651, 1943.

31. Hallock, H.: The use of multiple small bone transplants in the treatment of pseudarthrosis of the tibia of congenital origin or following osteotomy for the correction of congenital deformity, J. Bone Joint Surg. **20A**:648, 1938.

32. Harding, K.: Congenital anterior bowing of the tibia: the significance of the different types in relations to pseudarthrosis, Ann. R. Coll. Surg. Engl. **51**:17-30, 1972.

33. Henderson, M.S.: Congenital pseudarthrosis of the tibia, J. Bone Joint Surg. **10**:483, 1928.

34. Hensley, C.D.: The rapid development of a "subperiosteal bone cyst" in multiple neurofibromatosis, J. Bone Joint Surg. **35A**:197, 1953.

35. Holt, J.F., and Wright, E.M.: The radiologic features of neurofibromatosis, Radiology **51**:647, 1948.

36. Hosol, K.: Multiple neurofibromatosis (von Recklinghausen's disease) with special reference to malignant transformation, Arch. Surg. **22**:258-281, Feb. 1931.

37. Hunt, J.C., and Pugh, D.G.: Skeletal lesions in neurofibromatosis, Radiology **76**(1):1-19, 1961.

38. Kessel, A.W.L.: Intrathoracic meningocele, spinal deformity and multiple neurofibromatosis, J. Bone Joint Surg. **33B**:87-98, Feb. 1951.

39. Kite, J.H.: Congenital pseudarthrosis of tibia, fibula: report of 15 cases, South. Med. J. **34**:1021, 1941.

40. Kullman, L., and Wouters, H.W.: Neurofibromatosis, gigantism, and subperiosteal hematoma: report of two children with extensive subperiosteal bone formation, J. Bone Joint Surg. **54B**(1):130-138, 1972.

41. Langenskiöld, A.: Pseudarthrosis of the fibula and progressive valgus deformity of the ankle in children: treatment by fusion of the distal tibial and fibular metaphyses: review of three cases, J. Bone Joint Surg. **49A**(3):436-470, 1967.

42. Lavine, L.S., Lustrin, I., Shamos, M.H., Rinaldi, R.A., and Liboff, A.R.: Electric enhancement of bone healing, Science **175**:118, 1972.

43. Laws, J.W., and Pallis, C.: Spinal deformities in neurofibromatosis, J. Bone Joint Surg. **45B**:674-682, Nov. 1963.

44. Levine, D.B.: Spondylolisthesis, neurofibromatosis, and thoracic meningocele: a case report, J. Bone Joint Surg. **52A**(2):403, 1970.

45. Lloyd-Roberts, G.C., and Shaw, N.E.: The prevention of pseudarthrosis in congenital kyphosis of the tibia, J. Bone Joint Surg. **51B**:100-105, 1969.

46. Loop, J.W., Akeson, W.H., and Clawson, D.K.: Acquired thoracic abnormalities in neurofibromatosis, Am. J. Roentgenol. **93**:416-424, 1965.

47. McCarroll, H.R.: Clinical manifestations of congenital neurofibromatosis, J. Bone Joint Surg. **32A**(3):601-617, 1950.

48. McFarland, B.: Pseudarthrosis of the tibia in childhood, J. Bone Joint Surg. **33B**:36-46, 1951.

49. McKeller, C.C.: Congenital pseudarthrosis of the tibia: treatment by tibial lengthening and corrective osteotomy seven years after successful bone graft: a case report, J. Bone Joint Surg. **55A**(1):193-196, 1973.

50. Masserman, R.L., Peterson, H.A., and Bianco, A.: Congenital pseudarthrosis of the tibia: a review of the literature and 52 cases from the Mayo Clinic, Clin. Orthop. Related Res. **99**:140-145, March-April 1974.

51. Merten, D.F., Gooding, C.A., Newton, T.H., and Malamud, N.: Meningiomas of childhood and adolescence, J. Pediat. **84**(5):696-700, 1974.

52. Miller, A.: Neurofibromatosis with reference to skeletal changes, compression myelitis, and malignant degeneration, Arch. Surg. **32**:109, 1936.

53. Miller, D.S., et al.: Orthopaedic manifestations in neurofibromatosis, Q. Bull. Northwestern U. Med. School **31**:245-252, 1957.

54. Moore, B.H.: Some orthopaedic relationships of neurofibromatosis, J. Bone Joint Surg. **23**(1):109-140, 1943.

55. Moore, J.R.: Congenital pseudarthrosis of the tibia. AAOS Instructional course lectures. **14**:222-237, Ann Arbor, Mich., 1957, J.W. Edwards, Publishers.

56. Moore, J.R.: Delayed autogenous bone graft in the treatment of congenital pseudarthrosis, J. Bone Joint Surg. **31**:23, 1949.

57. Nøgaard, F.: Osseous changes in Recklinghausen neurofibromatosis, Acta Radiol. **18**:460-470, 1937.

58. Ormsby, O.S., and Montgomery, H.: Disease of the skin, ed. 8, Philadelphia, 1954, Lea & Febiger.

59. Pitt, M., Mosher, J.F., and Edeiken, J.: Abnormal periosteum and bone in neurofibromatosis, Radiology **103**:143-146, April 1972.

60. Pohl, R.: Meningocele im Brustraum unter dem Bilde eines intrathorakalen Rundschattens, Röntgen-Praxis **5**:747-749, Oct. 1933.

61. Preiser, S.A., and Davenport, C.B.: Multiple neurofibromatosis, Am. J. Med. Sci., n.s. **Clvi**:507, 1918.

62. Rankin, E.: Neurofibromatosis in the radius of a nine year old. (Personal communication, 1975.)

63. Rathgeb, J.M., Ramsey, P.L., and Cowell, H.R.: Congenital kyphoscoliosis of the tibia, Clin. Orthop. **103**:178-190, 1974.

64. Robin, G.C.: Scoliosis and neurological disease, Isr. J. Med. Sci. **9**:578-586, May 1973.

65. Sammons, B.P., and Thomas, D.F.: Extensive lumbar meningocele associated with neurofibromatosis, Am. J. Roentgenol. **81**:1021-1025, 1959.

66. Sane, S., Yunis, E., and Greer, R.: Subperiosteal or cortical cyst and intramedullary neurofibromatosis: uncommon manifestations of neurofibromatosis: a case report, J. Bone Joint Surg. **53A**(6):1194-1200, 1971.

67. Scott, J.C.: Scoliosis and neurofibromatosis, J. Bone Joint Surg. **47B**(2):240-246, May 1965.

68. Sheklakov, N.D.: A case of neurofibromatosis with 9, 242 tumors, Vestn. Venereol. Dermatol. **3:**51-52, May-June 1950.

69. Smith, R.W.: A treatise on the pathology, diagnosis and treatment of neuroma, Dublin, 1849, Hodges & Smith.

70. Sofield, H.A., and Millar, E.A.: Fragmentation, realignment and intramedullary rod fixation of deformities of the long bones in children: a ten-year appraisal, J. Bone Joint Surg. **41A:**1371, 1959.

71. Stout, A.P.: Tumors of the peripheral nervous system. In Atlas of tumor pathology, Section 2, Fascicle 6, Washington, D.C., 1949, Armed Forces Institute of Pathology.

72. Suzuki, M., Tamura, E., Kamoshita, S., and Saito, M.: Clinical observations of phacomatosis in infancy and childhood. I. von Recklinghausen's disease, Paediat. Univ. Tokyo **9:**23, 1963.

73. Tilford, D.L., and Kelsch, R.C.: Renal artery stenosis in childhood neurofibromatosis, Am. J. Dis. Child. **126:**665-668, Nov. 1973.

74. Tucker, J.T., and Carpenter, E.B.: Localized neurofibromatosis with associated overgrowth of an extremity, J. Bone Joint Surg. **33A**(1):103-106, 1951.

75. Van Nes, C.P.: Congenital pseudarthrosis of the leg, J. Bone Joint Surg. **48A:**1467-1483, 1966.

76. Veliskakis, K.P., et al.: Neurofibromatosis and scoliosis: significance of the short angular spinal curve, J. Bone Joint Surg. **52A**(4):833, 1970.

77. von Recklinghausen, F.D.: Ueber die multiplen Fibrome der Haut und ihre Beziehung zu den multiplen Neuromen, Berlin, 1882, Hirschwald.

78. Weiss, R.A.: A curvature of the spine in von Recklinghausen's disease, von Recklinghausen's disease in a Negro, Arch. Dermatol. Syph. **iii:**144-151, 1921.

79. Wellwood, J.M., Bulmer, J.H., and Graff, D.J.C.: Congenital defects of the tibia in siblings with neurofibromatosis, J. Bone Joint Surg. **53B**(2):314-318, 1971.

80. Whitehouse, D.: Diagnosis value of the café-au-lait spot in children, Arch. Dis. Child. **41:**316-319, 1966.

81. Winter, R.B., Moe, J.H., Bradford, D.S. et al.: Spine deformity in neurofibromatosis, J. Bone Joint Surg. **61A**(5):677-694, July 1979.

Chapter 4

Treatment of Legg-Calvé-Perthes disease

G. DEAN MacEWEN, M.D.
Wilmington, Delaware

The concept of treatment of Legg-Calvé-Perthes disease can be basically divided into two categories: (1) early treatment and (2) reconstructive treatment.

1. The early treatment program is for the patient still in the early stages of the disease process, whose symptoms have been present for only a short period of time, with little or no deformity of the cartilage of the femoral head.
2. The reconstructive stage is present when the patient with a significant deformity of the femoral head has already been into the disease process, with or without treatment, for a considerable length of time, but the Perthes disease process still has not run its full course.

EARLY TREATMENT

It has been previously recognized that some patients do not require treatment. The early treatment program basically aims (1) to obtain and maintain an essentially normal range of motion and (2) to contain the femoral head deeply within the acetabulum. Historically, non–containment treatment methods have been either by bedrest, which has been impractical except for a maximum of a few weeks to regain motion, or by so-called ischial non–weight-bearing braces, which have not demonstrated the ability to reduce the weight-bearing across the hip joint or to maintain the femoral head deeply within the acetabulum.

Obtaining motion

It is important to obtain and maintain essentially a full range of motion in Perthes' disease. This is best done with a period of bedrest and traction that will gradually carry the hip out into full abduction (Fig. 4-1). An adductor tenotomy is rarely indicated. Internal rotation is the most difficult to recover, and occasionally an internal rotator strap applied to the thigh is useful. If full abduction is difficult to obtain, the application of a set of Petrie casts, held in moderate abduction for a few days and then given gradually increasing abduction at several day intervals, usually relieves the problem. If this technique is used, it is advisable to defer weight-bearing until the desired abduction is obtained.

Techniques to refine this method with abduction and weight-bearing, such as Tachdjian's caliper, have been difficult to control and maintain. The Snyder sling (Fig. 4-2, *A*) and the Forte harness have not produced containment and have not been successful in most patients because they tend to walk on the leg, or at least kneel and produce the same pressure on the femoral head. The methods of containment that have been most satisfactory have been the Petrie (Fig. 4-2, *B*) cast and abduction/internal rotation braces. The Petrie cast, which maintains abduction and moderate internal rotation, holds the head deeply within the acetabulum. This method produces a very loose and relaxed joint, but it is difficult to apply, difficult to maintain, and has an associated risk of stiffness of the knees with secondary degenerative changes. The last is probably more theoretical than realistic if the cast is changed every 2 to 2½ months. The Petrie cast method is very helpful in the early part of the treatment program. If there is any tendency for stiffness, the casts may be used for a 6-week period only. The abduction method has been refined into different bracing techniques such as the Toronto brace (Fig. 4-2 *C*), the Newing-

75

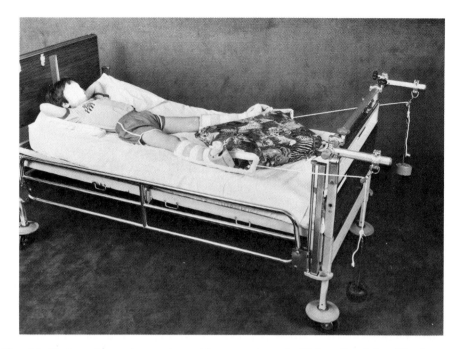

Fig. 4-1. Patient shown in traction with approximately 10 kg of weight. The legs are gradually abducted, and a bolster assists the maintenance of this position.

A

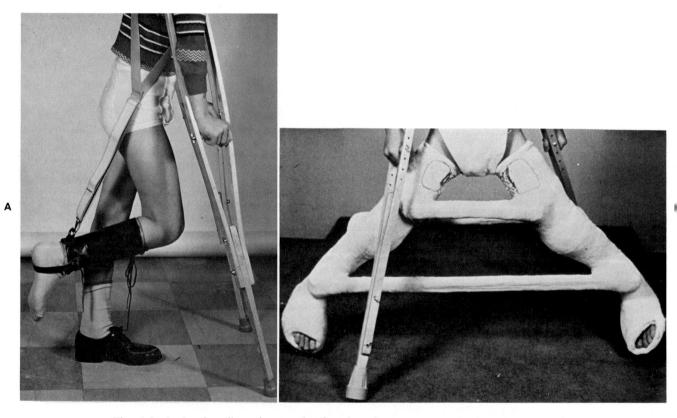

Fig. 4-2. A, Snyder sling elevates the foot but does not prevent pressure across the knee. This technique does not promote containment; therefore it is of little use in the treatment of Perthes' disease. **B,** Petrie casts hold the femoral heads deeply within the acetabuli and stimulate increased motion of the hip joints. **C,** Toronto brace maintains centering of the femoral heads. **D,** Abduction brace of Dr. John Roberts consists of leather lacers and metal crossbars and provides for abduction and internal rotation. **E,** Atlanta brace controls only abduction, is satisfactory for most patients, and only slightly inhibits the patient's activities.

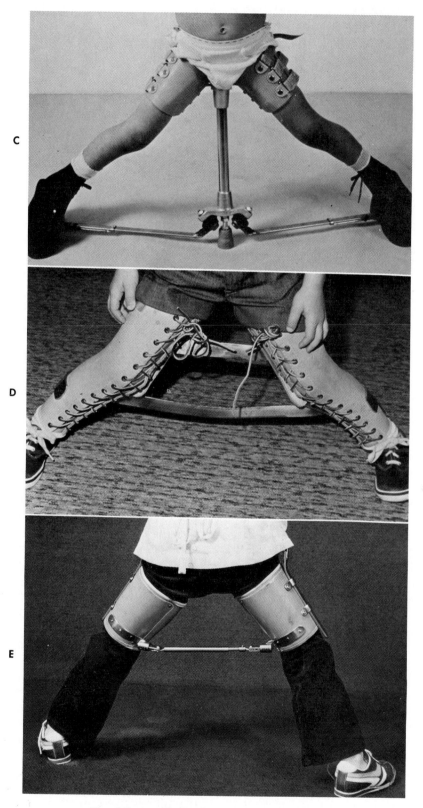

Fig. 4-2, cont'd. For legend see opposite page.

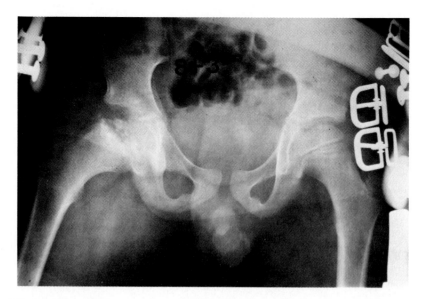

Fig. 4-3. Standing anteroposterior roentgenograph taken with patient in the brace. A slightly greater degree of abduction than shown here is desired so that the lateral portion of the epiphyseal line reaches the outer corner of the acetabulum.

ton brace, the Craig splint from California, and the technique by Dr. John Roberts with an abduction/internal rotation position of leather lacers and metal bars (Fig. 4-2, *D*). These modifications have allowed an easier fitting and have permitted the patient to be removed from the device for daily range-of-motion exercise. The most recent extension of this treatment has been the Atlanta brace (Fig. 4-2, *E*), which controls only abduction and not rotation. It would appear that internal rotation may be desirable in a small group of patients, but most patients only require abduction that can be well controlled in the Atlanta brace.

It is important to obtain a standing radiograph in any device that is used in order to show that adequate coverage has been obtained (Fig. 4-3). Ideally, the lateral portion of the epiphyseal line should advance to the corner of the acetabulum so that extrusion of the lateral portion of the head cannot occur. Another important concept is that the patient should be removed from the brace at each outpatient visit to determine that a full range of motion has been maintained. Ferguson stated, and we agree, that if a patient has a full range of motion, probably very little if anything has gone wrong within the hip joint. In summary, treatment of the acute phase is that of obtaining and maintaining a full range of motion and maintaining a concentric reduction by abduction methods, with control of rotation rarely being needed.

Discontinuation of treatment program

The classical treatment has been to continue the program until the subchondral bone plate of the femoral epiphysis has reconstituted itself on the anteroposterior and lateral radiologic views. Our experience, at the time of review by Kamhi and in a subsequential review by Westin, showed that the treatment could be discontinued well before this time. It would appear that once the dense or sclerotic bone has disappeared from the head and there is a good range of motion and the head is relatively round (Fig. 4-4), the patient can then resume weight-bearing in the neutral position. These changes in the femoral head usually occur approximately 12 to 14 months after the onset of the condition. Therefore it makes the nonoperative treatment of the acute phase very important since, on the average, it requires 6 months to evaluate the full extent of the involvement. If an additional 6 to 8 months is all that is needed to complete the nonoperative treatment, the time difference between the operative and nonoperative phases is essentially nil. We therefore believe

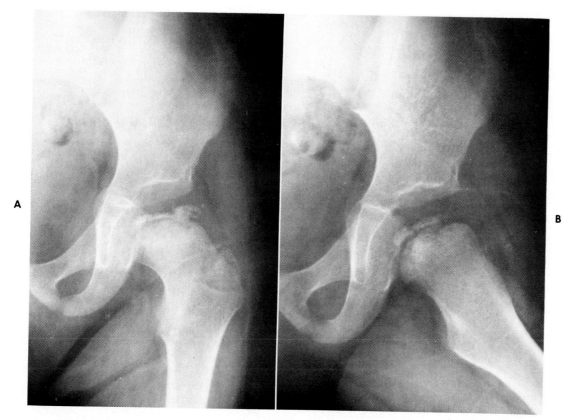

Fig. 4-4. A, Anteroposterior and, **B,** frog-leg views showing that the dense bone has disappeared and the femoral head is relatively round. Weight-bearing can be resumed at this stage.

that most children, seen early and treated adequately during the active phase of the condition, can be well treated by nonoperative methods.

SURGERY
Early containment

In the early treatment of Perthes' disease, surgery can be thought of as an alternative to bracing, and thereby the choice of the treatment program is often determined by the psychologic and social implications. Some patients and families cannot tolerate the concept of bracing and will do better with surgical intervention. The surgical considerations include varus femoral osteotomy or pelvic osteotomy. Note, however, that surgical treatment has a tendency to reduce the motion in the hip. If there is any residual stiffness after the initial traction or other conservative regimen, one should be hesitant to enter a surgical program because of greater risk of increasing the severity of the stiffness. This is more of a problem with pel-

vic osteotomy, which increases the pressure on the femoral head.

Femoral osteotomy. The angle of the femoral neck should be brought down approximately 20 degrees (Fig. 4-5) and should *never* approximate 90 degrees. At times, the normal neck-shaft angle can be reconstituted, but one should not reduce the angle to a severe pathologic degree. Internal fixation is desirable and is best done with a device that will not necessitate great force to insert. I prefer a version of the Coventry or Richards screw technique. It also is important that the internal fixation device not enter the greater trochanteric apophysis because of the risk of producing a premature closure and a secondary valgus. This may produce a valgus position of the neck that was greater than the original angle, a most undesirable position.

Pelvic osteotomy. Containment can also be obtained by an osteotomy of the pelvis of the Salter type (Fig. 4-6). This appears to be technically

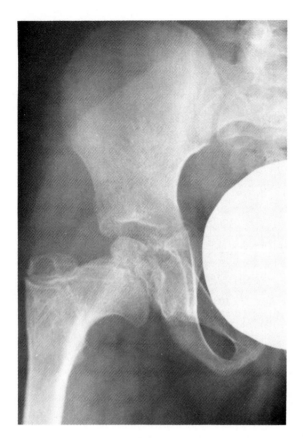

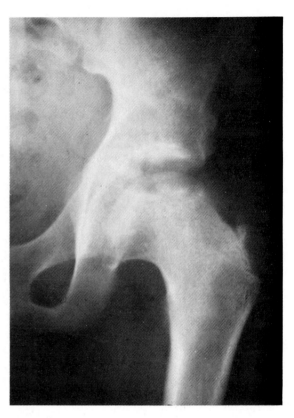

Fig. 4-5. Ten months after varus osteotomy. Note the neck shaft angle has only been reduced to approximately 115 degrees.

Fig. 4-6. One year after Salter osteotomy showing good containment of the femoral head and only mild residual deformity.

more difficult than a femoral osteotomy for many surgeons. It is most important that an arthrogram be done prior to this procedure to determine whether the head is essentially round (Fig. 4-7) because with any amount of deformity there is a risk of producing further crushing of the femoral head.

In summary then, whether to operate above or below the acetabulum is to some degree dependent on the experience of the surgeon and whether he is more at ease doing a femoral or pelvic osteotomy. However, if there is any tendency toward restriction in motion, there is a greater risk of stiffness after a pelvic osteotomy. Therefore any tendency to stiffness results in a contraindication to the pelvic osteotomy of Salter. If there is an associated shortening of the extremity, consideration should favor the pelvic procedure to lengthen the limb to some degree, once the other prerequisites have been met.

Treatment in reconstructive stage

Treatment is late when a femoral head is already deformed. Then the question is, can the femoral head be successfully reduced inside the acetabulum and maintained for an adequate period of time to produce a concentric alignment. In most patients, even with major deformity, the acetabulum has relatively little deformity or is deformed to a much lesser degree than the femoral head is. If the head is not centered, there is the possiblity of hinge abduction (Fig. 4-8) where the corner of the femoral head impinges against the corner of the acetabulum and produces a distraction in the lower portion of the head from the acetabulum. A pooling of the dye can also be seen if an arthrogram is done at this stage. If the head cannot be concentrically reduced, it is usually better to discontinue treatment rather than to perform additional surgery. Exceptions to this are when the patient has a painful hip or where the

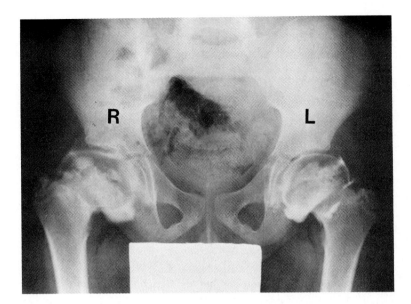

Fig. 4-7. An example of a patient with bilateral Perthes' disease undergoing arthrography. The right side already shows advanced deformity of the femoral head and acetabulum, which is a relative contraindication to the previously described surgical procedures. On the left the femoral head is spheric, an indication that could allow for surgical consideration.

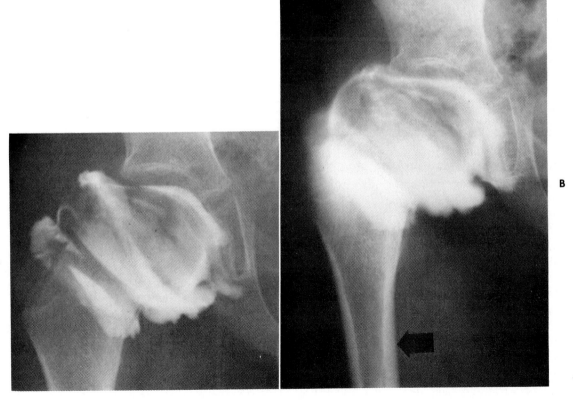

Fig. 4-8. Arthrogram in neutral, **A,** and in stressed, **B,** abduction. This shows hinging of the deformed femoral head on the corner of the acetabulum with pooling of the dye medially, which is a contraindication to abduction treatment unless this can be corrected.

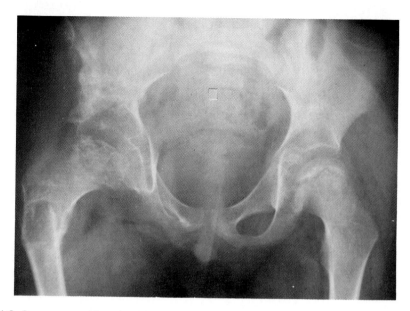

Fig. 4-9. Seven-year-old patient 6 months after a combined Salter and varus osteotomy. A fair result is anticipated because the femoral head is deep within the acetabulum and the epiphyseal line appears to be open.

hip will not abduct beyond a few degrees in the extended position. In these rare circumstances a partial excision of the femoral head may be considered.

After a period of traction, if the head successfully centers itself, a varus osteotomy or a combination of a varus osteotomy plus an acetabuloplasty (Fig. 4-9) can be carried out. If the epiphyseal line remains open, an excellent result can be anticipated. If the same procedure is carried out and the epiphyseal line closes, a poor alignment will result. If it appears that the epiphyseal line will close prematurely, this should downgrade any consideration for reconstructive surgery because there will be a poor result with or without the surgery.

Arrest of the greater trochanter may be considered when there has been premature closure of the physeal line. This must be accomplished before a patient is 8 years of age to be practical. In most patients with Legg-Calvé-Perthes disease, a final diagnosis of physeal closure is usually not made until after this age; therefore this procedure is rarely indicated for children with Perthes' disease.

The question of possible containment is a major consideration in the reconstructive phase. Is there value in treatment of a large femoral head where the medial portion of the femoral head is in contact with the medial acetabulum? It appears in this group of patients that there is enough contact between the femoral head and acetabulum to produce a normally full weight-bearing surface (Fig. 4-10). Producing a varus neck angle or an acetabular deformity will only *change* the area of weight-bearing and not actually *increase* it. The concept of Chiari should not be considered in this type of patient, since there is such a large surface area of contact already present. It is our belief that there is essentially no indication for the Chiari procedure in Perthes' disease in the child or adolescent.

In the occasional patient where the lateral portion of the femoral head is extruded from the acetabulum and cannot be reduced inside the acetabulum and where no abduction is present, one can consider resection of the lateral portion of the femoral head (Fig. 4-10). This procedure, a cheilotomy, is rarely indicated. When indicated, the surgical procedure must be deferred until reconstruction of the femoral head proceeds to such a degree that further extrusion and deformity will not reoccur after the surgery. This usually means that the process should be followed for 2 or more years before cheilotomy is performed.

Always remember that in the natural history of Perthes' disease even a severely involved femoral

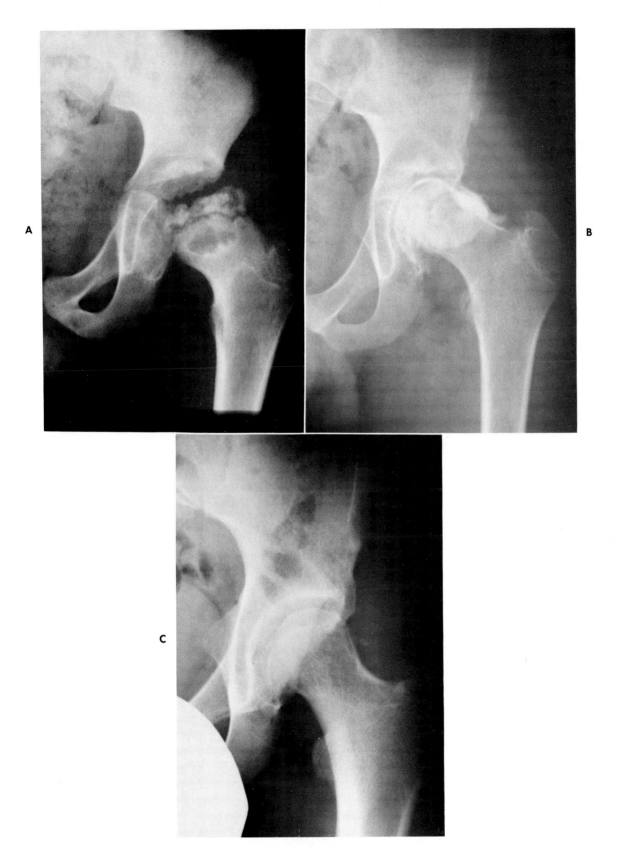

Fig. 4-10. A, Ten-year-old patient with extrusion of the lateral portion of the femoral head completely limiting abduction. **B,** Arthrogram 3 months after cheilotomy showing the removal of the obstruction that limited abduction. **C,** Five years later there has been remodeling with retention of a good range of motion.

head may not cause significant symptoms for 20 to 30 years. Therefore it is important not to produce any secondary changes that may shorten this interval. Containment at this stage can, at best, produce remodeling of the hip that is already deformed. Reconstructive surgery or containment must *not* be done in the face of a fixed deformity.

SUMMARY

It seems that early, energetic treatment with containment of the femoral head and preservation of the range of motion are the methods of choice for the patient in the early stages of the problem. Most patients with early involvement can be treated with the conservative method. This can be concluded within approximately 12 to 14 months, when the sclerotic and dense bone has disappeared and an adequate range of motion has been maintained. Reconstructive procedures are rarely indicated. They must be entered with great caution because of the risk of shortening the symptom-free interval, which presently is about 20 or 30 years, before reconstructive treatment is necessary.

REFERENCES

1. Ayer, A.: Subtrochanteric osteotomy in the treatment of Perthes' disease, J. Bone Joint Surg. **47B**:489, Aug. 1965.
2. Bobechko, W.P., McLaurin, C.A., and Motloch, W.M.: Toronto orthosis for Legg-Perthes disease, Artif. Limbs **12**:36, 1968.
3. Canale, S.T., D'Anca, A.F., Cotler, J.M., and Snedden, H.E.: Innominate osteotomy in Legg-Calvé-Perthes disease, J. Bone Joint Surg. **54A**:25, Jan. 1972.
4. Chuinard, E.G.: Femoral osteotomy in treatment of Legg-Calvé-Perthes syndrome, Orthop. Rev. **8**:113, March 1979.
5. Cotler, J.M.: Surgery in Legg-Calvé-Perthes syndrome, AAOS: Instructional course lectures **25**:135, St. Louis, 1976, The C.V. Mosby Co.
6. Curtis, B.H., Gunther, S.F., Gossling, H.R., and Siegfried, W.P.: Treatment for Legg-Perthes disease with the Newington ambulation-abduction brace, J. Bone Joint Surg. **56A**:1135, Sept. 1974.
7. Dickens, D.L.V., and Menelaus, M.D.: The assessment of prognosis in Perthes' disease, J. Bone Joint Surg. **60B**(2):189, May 1978.
8. Eaton, G.O.: Long-term results of treatment in coxa plana, J. Bone Joint Surg. **49A**:1031, Sept. 1967.
9. Ferguson, A.B., and Howorth, M.B.: Coxa plana and related conditions at the hip, J. Bone Joint Surg. **16**:781, 1934.
10. Goff, C.W.: Legg-Calvé-Perthes syndrome and related osteochondroses of youth, Springfield, Ill., 1954, Charles C Thomas, Publisher.
11. Harrison, M.H.M., and Turner, M.H.: Containment splintage for Perthes' disease of the hip, J. Bone Joint Surg. **56B**:199, Feb. 1974.
12. Kamhi, E., and MacEwen, G.D.: Treatment of Legg-Calvé-Perthes disease: prognostic value of Catterall classification, J. Bone Joint Surg. **57A**:651, July 1975.
13. Katz, J.F.: Non-operative therapy in Legg-Calvé-Perthes disease, Orthop. Rev. **8**:69, March 1979.
14. Lloyd-Roberts, G.C., Catterall, A., and Salamon, P.B.: A controlled study of the indications for and the results of femoral osteotomy in Perthes' disease, J. Bone Joint Surg. **58B**:31, Feb. 1976.
15. Lloyd-Roberts, G.C., and Ratliff, A.H.C.: Perthes' disease. In Hip disorders in children, London, 1978, Butterworth & Co. (Publishers).
16. MacEwen, G.D., and Ramsey, P.: The hip. In Lovell, W.W., and Winter, R.B., editors: Pediatric orthopaedics, Philadelphia, 1978, J.B. Lippincott Co.
17. Thompson, G.H., and Westin, G.W.: Legg-Calvé-Perthes disease: results of discontinuing treatment in the early reossification phase, Clin. Orthop. **139**:70, March-April 1979.

Chapter 5

Biotrigonometric analysis and practical applications of osteotomies of tibia in children

S. TERRY CANALE, M.D.
Memphis, Tennessee

MARION C. HARPER, M.D.
Columbia, Missouri

As noted by Gordon, Paul of Aegena was first credited with performing an osteotomy in a long bone.[20] In 1838, Mayer[18] coined the term "osteotomy" for a tibial resection for an angulation deformity. Since that time, various shapes and designs of osteotomies have been popularized; most variations were introduced prior to 1900, before skeletal fixation, to provide stability at the osteotomy site.[20] Today in orthopaedics, osteotomies are commonplace; however, the techniques and methods have been "handed down" from one generation to the next with very little standardization. The purpose of this paper is to present objective, mathematically proved guidelines for osteotomy and to describe some of the more common osteotomy techniques in the lower extremity in children. This information will, we hope, help orthopaedic surgeons avoid some of the pitfalls learned the hard way.

BIOMECHANICAL ANALYSIS

Much of what we know of the exact science of osteotomies has been learned through empiricism. Questions such as, What is the result in length gained or lost in straightening an angulated bone? or What is the optimal site to perform an osteotomy? have never been objectively answered. An exception to this is Milch's work in 1947[20]; a description of his pelvic osteotomy and review of other osteotomies in 1965[19] is still considered a classic.

Although a search of the orthopaedic literature reveals numerous types and designs of osteotomies, with general guidelines and recommendations based on empiricism,[1,4,7,11,12,14,15,20,21,24,26] little engineering or mathematical documentation is available. Using biomechanical techniques and trigonometric functions, four basic questions will be answered objectively. All computations were theoretical and apply only to acutely angulated deformities, though the following inferences can be made concerning deformities secondary to bowing.

Is there any gain in length when an angulated bone is corrected, and can this be calculated?

If there is a "crooked" bone, such as the tibia, and if this is straightened, disregarding the type of osteotomy (opening or closing wedge), empirically the answer should be that there is a gain in length. This can be proved objectively. The model and equation is given in Fig. 5-1. When one solves for *HD* (length gained) it is apparent that if the type of osteotomy is not considered there is an obvious gain in effective length when an angulated bone is straightened. A practical example of an

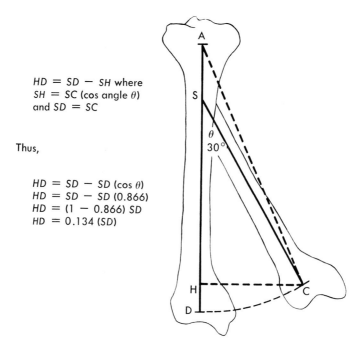

$HD = SD - SH$ where
$SH = SC$ (cos angle θ)
and $SD = SC$

Thus,

$HD = SD - SD$ (cos θ)
$HD = SD - SD$ (0.866)
$HD = (1 - 0.866)$ SD
$HD = 0.134$ (SD)

Fig. 5-1. Model and equation to prove a gain in length if an angulated bone is straightened, regardless of the type of osteotomy. *S*, Maximum point of 30-degree angulation (θ); *SC*, angulated bone, corrected to *SD*; thus *HD*, absolute gain in length from osteotomy.

osteotomy to correct a 30-degree angulation deformity using the equation in Fig. 5-1 to determine the gain in length follows:

Tibia: 15 inches long with 30-degree angulation deformity; 3 inches below the knee (12 inches)
HD: Gained length
SD: 13 inches

HD   = 0.134 (SD)
HD   = 0.134 (12 inches
Gained length = 1.6 inches

What is the best level to perform an osteotomy?

Corrective dome osteotomy performed at the site of angulation (*S*) (Fig. 5-1) with angulation of the distal segment through the angle (θ) will shift the mechanical axis back to its normal position, restore the effective length, and restore the angular relationship of the two articular surfaces to normal. The optimum location, as seen in Fig. 5-1, is at the site of the maximum angulation; however, clinically quite often the maximum angulation site is to be avoided. If so, then what is the next best site to perform an osteotomy? If the os-

teotomy is performed at a level proximal or distal to the maximum angulation, a compensatory osteotomy needs to be performed. From Fig. 5-2, it is apparent that as the osteotomy site is moved distally, increasingly greater angles of correction are necessary to correct the deformity, and there is greater loss in restored length. This loss of length is real and can be computed independently of the type of osteotomy performed (opening or closing wedge). On the other hand, as one moves proximally (Fig. 5-3), less angle of correction is necessary and less loss in restored length occurs. What was known empirically can be proved objectively: osteotomy proximal to the area of maximum angulation requires fewer degrees for correction to the midline than does an osteotomy distal to the maximum site of angulation.

Proof of the principle stated above, and illustrated diagrammatically in Figs. 5-2 and 5-3 is obtained when one solves for the appropriate corrective angle ($\emptyset$) for any proximal or distal site and thus for the effective length of the angulated segment (*L*) and the amount of length regained. An example using this technique is given in Tables 5-1 and 5-2 for a 30-degree angulation deformity occurring 8 cm below the knee in a tibia

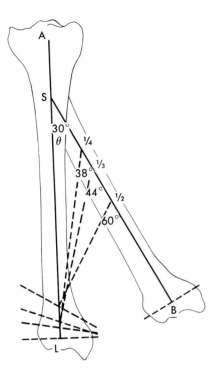

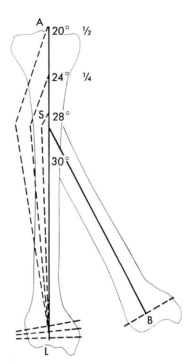

Fig. 5-2. Model illustrating 30-degree angulation deformity and computing compensatory osteotomies moving progressively distal to realign the tibia. At one fourth the distance from the maximum angulation (*S*), a 38-degree wedge osteotomy is necessary to correct a 30-degree angulation deformity. At a point one half the distance from *S*, a 60-degree compensatory osteotomy is necessary to correct a 30-degree angulation deformity. Also note that as the osteotomy is performed more distally, the absolute gain in length, *L*, progressively diminishes.

Fig. 5-3. Same model as in Fig. 5-2 but with compensatory osteotomies being performed proximal to maximum angulation of 30 degrees, *S*. At one fourth the distance proximal to *S*, it takes only a 24-degree wedge to correct to the midline, and at one half the distance, it only takes a 20-degree wedge to correct to the midline. Notice that when one moves more proximally from the site of maximum angulation, there is a loss of anticipated gain in length, but not so much as when an osteotomy is performed in the same location distal to the maximum angulation site.

measuring 38 cm. It can be seen that a closing or opening wedge done either 1 cm proximally (Table 5-1) or distally (Table 5-2) from the site of angulation will result in a significant gain in effective length. Although *K* is the distance from the site of angulation to the site of corrective osteotomy and *B* is the length of angulated segment, the detailed proofs of the equations are beyond the scope of this paper. However, in general, it can be stated that (1) the maximum length that can be gained is by an opening wedge osteotomy near the point of maximum angulation; (2) less wedge (fewer degrees) is needed and less loss of restored length occurs as the osteotomy site is moved proximal to the site of maximum angulation; and (3) conversely, more wedge (more degrees) is necessary and more loss of restored length occurs as

one moves distal to the maximum angulation to perform the osteotomy.

Knowing the diameter of the bone and the angle of correction (degrees of the osteotomy), how can the base of the wedge be determined practically?

This is illustrated in Fig. 5-4. The angle of the osteotomy is usually calculated preoperatively, but how is the length (*w*) along the cortex determined? The simplest method, requiring virtually no mathematics, is given in Fig. 5-5. Since the angle is known preoperatively, various diameters can be drawn. At surgery, one determines the diameter by placing a guide wire across the bone and measuring for the diameter. The vertical line of the appropriate diameter can then be mea-

Table 5-1. Equations and examples for solving amount of restored lengths in relationship to level of osteotomy (proximal): number of degrees of either opening or closing wedge and amount of regained length

$$\emptyset = \arctan \frac{B \sin \theta}{K + B \cos \theta}$$

$$L = K \cos \emptyset + \frac{K \sin \emptyset}{\sin (\theta - \emptyset)} \cos(\theta - \emptyset)$$

Proximal site (cm)	Type	Corrective wedge angle (degrees)	Height regained (cm)
1	Open	29.1	4.99
	Closing	29.1	2.77
2	Open	28.2	4.84
	Closing	28.2	2.69
3	Open	27.4	4.73
	Closing	27.4	2.65
4	Open	26.6	4.57
	Closing	26.6	2.57
5	Open	25.8	4.42
	Closing	25.8	2.47
6	Open	25.1	4.26
	Closing	25.1	2.39
7	Open	24.5	4.16
	Closing	24.5	2.34

Table 5-2. Equations and examples for solving amount of restored length in relationship to level of osteotomy (distal): number of degrees of either opening or closing wedge and amount of regained length

$$\emptyset = \theta + \arcsin \frac{K}{B} \sin \theta$$

$$L = K \cos \theta + \frac{K \sin \theta}{\sin (\emptyset - \theta)} \cos (\emptyset - \theta)$$

Distal site (cm)	Type	Corrective wedge angle (degrees)	Height regained (cm)
1	Open	31.0	5.15
	Closing	31.0	2.75
2	Open	32.0	4.99
	Closing	32.0	2.48
3	Open	33.2	4.91
	Closing	33.2	2.30
4	Open	34.4	4.78
	Closing	34.4	2.09
5	Open	35.7	4.69
	Closing	35.7	1.80
6	Open	37.2	4.54
	Closing	37.2	1.51
7	Open	38.8	4.42
	Closing	38.8	1.21
8	Open	40.5	4.29
	Closing	40.5	0.88
9	Open	42.4	4.16
	Closing	42.4	0.51
10	Open	44.5	4.02
	Closing	44.5	0.09

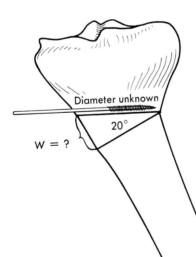

Fig. 5-4. Illustration at surgery of measuring with a guide pin the diameter of bone at the planned site of osteotomy to later aid in determining the amount of wedge, *W*, to be removed.

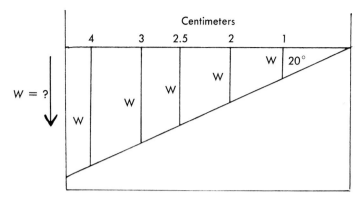

Fig. 5-5. Method used to determine length of wedge, *W*, to be removed when one knows preoperatively the desired angle (20 degrees) and determines the diameter at surgery.

sured with the ruler and the length of the base of the osteotomy determined.[25]

Another method utilizing biotrigonometry is given in Fig. 5-6; however, the tangent of the angle must be determined, and without the use of tangent tables this has very little practical application. One application it does have is to test the empiric approximation used in regard to high tibial osteotomy that for every degree of correction needed, 1 mm of wedge should be taken (1 mm = 1 degree of correction needed).[1,6] To test this hypothesis, diameters of 5 and 6 cm were used and a hypothetical 25-degree angle was chosen for the osteotomy.

$$W = \text{Diameter} \times \text{Tangent of } 25°$$

$W = 6 \text{ cm} \times 0.4663$	$W = 5 \text{ cm} \times 0.4663$
$W = 27.6 \text{ mm}$	$W = 23.3 \text{ mm}$

From the above equations, one can see that 27.6 and 23.3 mm closely approximate 25 degrees. Thus the "1 mm equals 1 degree" formula is reasonably accurate for performing a high tibial osteotomy only when one deals with a tibia approximately 5 to 6 cm in diameter. However, applying the same equation to a bone of smaller diameter, such as one with a 4 cm diameter, produces a different result:

$$W = \text{Diameter} \times \text{Tangent of } \emptyset$$
$$W = 4 \text{ cm} \times \text{Tangent of } 25°$$
$$W = 4 \text{ cm} \times 0.4663$$
$$W = 18.5 \text{ mm}$$

One can see that 18.5 mm does not approximate 25 degrees and, in fact, is in error by almost

$$W \text{ (wedge)} = D \text{ (diameter)} \times \text{Tangent}$$

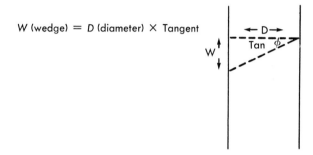

Fig. 5-6. Biotrigonometric method of determining length of wedge, *W*, to be removed in closing wedge or opened in opening-wedge osteotomy. The tangent of the desired angle and the diameter must be known.

40% (6.6 mm difference); thus the formula of "1 mm = 1 degree of correction needed" is applicable only in a bone with a diameter of approximately 5 to 6 cm and is generally not of value in a child, and since the adult proximal tibia 2 cm below the knee is 8 to 10 cm, it is also not useful in adults.

Because it is not practical to ask the orthopaedic surgeon to use tangent tables, a simplified formula has been devised for determination of the wedge *(W)* when the angles are from 5 to 45 degrees. Although this simplified formula has a 10% to 15% margin of error, it is practical and clinically useful.

$$W = \text{Diameter} \times 0.02 \times \text{Angle}$$

The accuracy of this formula is compared with trigonometric proof by use of the tangent and a comparison of both equations when one solves for the wedge *(W)*.

W = Diameter × Tangent $\emptyset$ = W = Diameter × 0.02 × Angle

W = 4 cm × Tangent of 25° =	W = 4 cm × 0.02 × 25°
W = 4 × 0.4663	W = 4 × 0.50
W = 1.85 cm	W = 2.0 cm

When one performs a closing wedge osteotomy, how much absolute shortening occurs by taking the wedge itself?

When one considers a corrective angulation osteotomy in terms of an opening or closing wedge technique, the effect of the wedge on restoration of length is often given prime consideration. One should remember, however, that significant length will be restored when the angulated bone is moved to the midline. Using a biotrigonometric model (Fig. 5-7), one can see that an opening or closing wedge osteotomy would change the abso-

$$\text{Tan } \phi = \frac{W}{D}$$

$$\text{Tan } \phi = \frac{w}{D/_2}$$

$$\text{Tan } \phi = \frac{D}{2w}$$

$$2w = D \tan \phi$$

$$2w = \frac{DW}{D}$$

$$2w = \frac{D}{W}$$

$$w = \frac{W}{2}$$

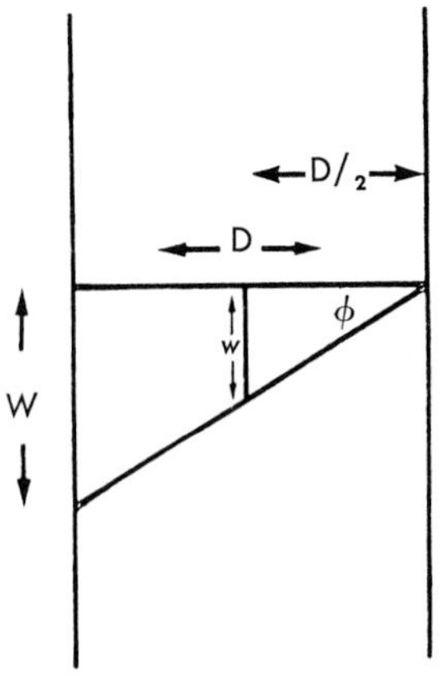

Fig. 5-7. Model showing that in a closing or opening wedge osteotomy the absolute amount of loss or gain from the wedge itself is the length of the center line, *w*, and also the formula proving the center line, *w*, to be equal to one half the base of the wedge, *W*.

lute length of the bone at the "center line" by the length of *w*. From the equation in Fig. 5-7, it can be proved that the length of the center line *(w)* is one half the base of the osteotomy *(W)*. Thus the absolute amount of length lost or gained by a closing or opening wedge osteotomy is one half the base of the osteotomy wedge.

OSTEOTOMIES OF TIBIAS IN CHILDREN

Varus, valgus, and anterior and posterior angulation, as well as internal and external rotation of the tibia, can occur with or without leg-length inequality. It is beyond the scope of this treatise to discuss the problems of leg-length inequality, and the osteotomies described are for either angulation or rotational deformities. Angulation in the tibia can contribute to significant deformities in the knee and ankle (genu varum, valgum, recurvatum, and so on), and often a tibial osteotomy can be useful in correcting joint malalignment.

The largest group of deformities of the tibia occurs secondary to normal physiologic growth. The normal pattern is one of varus of the tibia through the first 18 months of life (physiologic bowing). From about 18 months to 3 years of age, a valgus deformity predominates. These physiologic angulations correct themselves without treatment, and only rarely is operative treatment indicated.[9,21,22]

Deformity and differential diagnosis

The deformity in the tibia can occur secondary to congenital anomalies, either of an isolated bone, such as in fibula hemimelia, or of multiple bones, such as in achondroplasia or multiple epiphyseal dysplasia. Not all children of short stature with angulated tibias need osteotomies; some can be managed successfully with a period of bracing (Fig. 5-8).

Metabolic abnormalities such as rickets and scurvy can cause angulation deformities of the tibia and should be considered in the differential diagnosis. In general, the young child with the usual type of vitamin D–deficient rickets can be treated with vitamin D, calcium, phosphorus, and bracing. Ultimately a straight extremity can be expected and an osteotomy avoided. Contrary to this, angulation deformities in older children caused by vitamin D–resistant rickets or rickets secondary to renal abnormalities, regardless of treatment with newer drugs such as 1,25-dihydrocholecalciferol, frequently will need an osteotomy. One word of caution: avoid medical treatment at the time of osteotomy (discontinue high levels of vitamin D derivative, calcium, and phosphorus for 3 weeks before and after osteotomy) to avoid the possibility that, while the patient is immobilized, hypercalcemia with extraosseous calcification, such as renal calculi, may develop.[8]

Angulation deformities can occur secondary to developmental abnormalities such as in Blount's disease. Not all children with Blount's disease need osteotomies. If seen and treated with long-leg ambulatory braces at an early age, the process can, in some cases, be reversed and osteotomy avoided (Fig. 5-9). Osteotomy of the tibia, if not controlled by bracing, should be performed early to avoid the late deformities at the tibial epiphysis seen in Blount's disease. However, osteotomies should be delayed until at least 3 years of age or older so that the diagnosis of Blount's disease versus that of physiologic bowing of the tibia can be determined by roentgenogram.[2,16]

Angulation deformities of the tibia after fracture or secondary to epiphyseal growth arrest, either in the proximal or distal tibia, can occur. Osteotomy alone or in conjunction with a bony bridge resection of the proximal or supramalleolar area of the tibia can be performed.[5,15]

Indications

Indications for osteotomies of the proximal tibia include (1) significant angulation deformity, (2) progressive angulation deformity uncontrolled by bracing, (3) knee or ankle malalignment, (4) angulation deformity causing ligamentous laxity of the knee joint, and (5) rarely pain.

Defining a significant angulation deformity is particularly difficult. Clinically, when one is standing straight, the knees should touch, as should the medial malleoli of the ankle. In an older child, when there is more than 6 cm between the medial malleoli with the knees touching, a clinically significant valgus deformity is present. When there

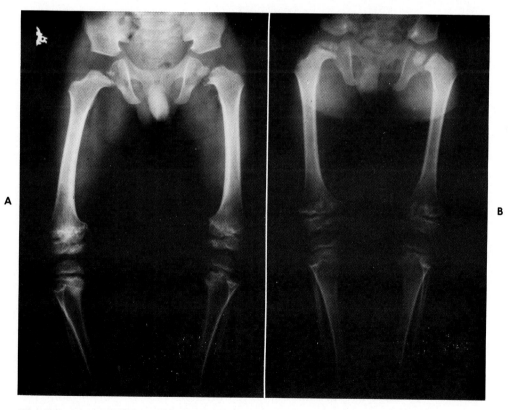

Fig. 5-8. A, Roentgenograms of 6-year-old male with spondyloepiphyseal dysplasia and resultant genu varum. **B,** Roentgenogram after 1 year in long leg-corrective braces for genu varum with good result. Coxa vara still persists in right hip.

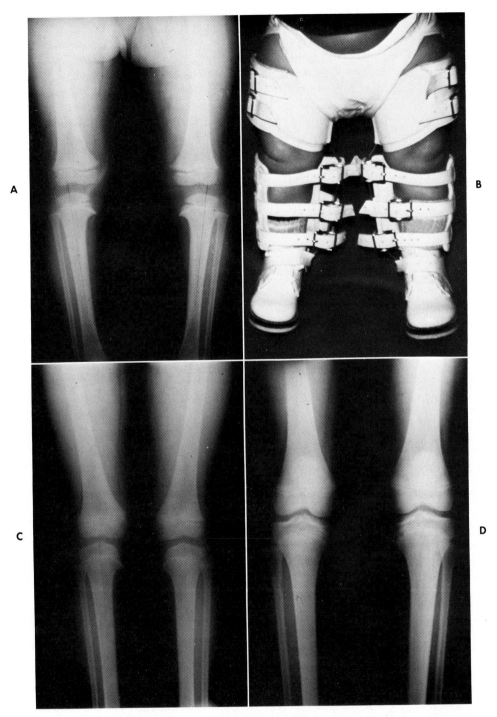

Fig. 5-9. A, Roentgenogram of a child with varus deformity of the tibia secondary to Blount's disease. **B,** Ambulatory "bowleg" braces utilized early in the course of the disease by this child for 18 months. **C,** Roentgenogram 2 years later showing adequate correction. **D,** Roentgenograms of same child 9 years later with permanent correction.

is more than 4 cm between the knees with the ankles touching, a significant varus deformity is present. If either of the situations occurs in the child, further investigation with the use of standing leg-length roentgenograms is in order. With standing leg-length roentgenograms, the tibiofemoral angle (the angle formed by the inclination of the tibia to the femur) should measure, according to Blount,[28] 5 to 9 degrees of valgus in females and 4 to 7 degrees of valgus in males. This difference occurs because of the broader pelvis in females. There should be no degrees of varus angulation in either males or females. When contemplating either conservative or operative treatment, the surgeon should subtract the normal valgus angulation for boys (4 to 7 degrees) and girls (5 to 9 degrees) from the pathologic valgus deformity and add it to the pathologic varus deformity. It is our opinion that absolute valgus deformities of between 9 and 14 degrees and absolute varus deformities of 0 to 5 degrees should be treated, either conservatively by bracing or by operation.

Another difficult question to answer is whether to perform a proximal tibial osteotomy or a supracondylar osteotomy of the femur. In general, if the knee joint is parallel to the floor on a standing roentgenogram and there is significant angular deformity, a proximal tibial osteotomy should be performed. On the other hand, if there is a significant angular deformity of the knee joint in relationship to the parallelism of the floor, a supracondylar osteotomy of the femur should be considered.[12] One exception is a Langenskiöld type V or VI Blount's disease with significant angulation of the epiphysis itself (Fig. 15-19).

Indications for supramalleolar osteotomy are generally for growth arrest secondary to trauma or, rarely, secondary to osteochondromas causing angular deformities at the ankle. Lloyd-Roberts,[17] believing the talus to be externally rotated in the ankle in clubfeet, occasionally uses an internal rotation supramalleolar osteotomy. Although experience with this procedure is limited, it would appear that when the deformity is in the foot, compensatory supramalleolar osteotomy will only rarely be indicated and further correction of the foot itself may be needed.

Techniques

Frequently, when one is performing an osteotomy, complementary procedures may be neces-

sary. Two of the more common are epiphysiodesis and reconstruction of ligamentous laxity about the knee. Blount's axiom of trying to avoid an epiphysiodesis of an already shortened extremity is a good one,[3] but occasionally this may be necessary. Considerable planning and preoperative evaluation should be carried out before large ligamentous reconstruction procedures are performed. One should remember that it is considered "bad form" to drill or burr large holes through a child's or adolescent's growth plate.

When one is performing an osteotomy of the tibia, two supplementary procedures are useful: (1) excision of a small portion of the fibula rather than a simple division of the bone, which allows for potentially maximum correction of the tibial osteotomy, and (2) an anterolateral fasciotomy, a simple procedure that can be performed quickly and usually through the already present incision and that may avoid neurovascular sequelae.

Some form of skeletal fixation should be used to avoid immediate loss of correction. Percutaneous pins incorporated in plaster have the advantage of avoiding a second operation such as has to be performed to remove plates or staples. Occasionally, when multiple osteotomies on the ipsilateral or contralateral extremity are performed, the Roger-Anderson apparatus is useful to align and secure an osteotomy while another is being carried out. Once completed, all the pins can be incorporated in the plaster and the Roger-Anderson device removed (Fig. 5-10).

All the osteotomies described can be performed in the proximal or supramalleolar area of the tibia. The closing wedge osteotomy (Fig. 5-11) is recommended because of its inherent stability. Absolute length lost is only one half the base of the wedge. A segment of the fibula should be excised. A power saw is useful in performing the tibial closing wedge osteotomy, but protection posteriorly is mandatory. Two, or preferably three, pins placed parallel and ultimately incorporated in plaster are recommended.

The opening wedge osteotomy (Fig. 5-12) has the advantage of gaining absolute length of about one half the base of the wedge. Its disadvantage is the lack of stability (Fig. 5-13). The segment taken from the fibula can be used as a wedge and placed in the osteotomy site in its most stable position (Fig. 5-14). Pins and plaster will add to the stability of the osteotomy. The "broomstick" or "dome-shaped" osteotomy (Fig. 5-15) has the advantage

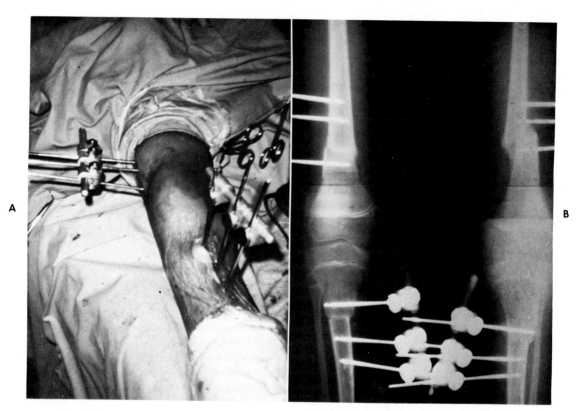

Fig. 5-10. A, Roger Anderson apparatus used to stabilize and align supracondylar osteotomy and subsequent tibial osteotomy. **B,** Roentgenograms of multiple osteotomies held firmly by Roger Anderson apparatus before application of pins and plaster.

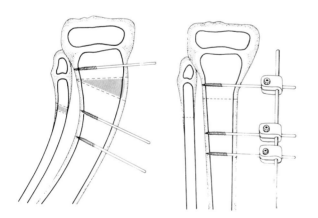

Fig. 5-11. Illustration of closing-wedge osteotomy. At the termination of the procedure, the pins should be parallel and ultimately incorporated in plaster.

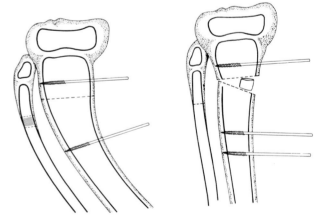

Fig. 5-12. Illustration of opening-wedge osteotomy using segment of the fibula. The fibular wedge should be cut in a desired manner to give the most inherent stability.

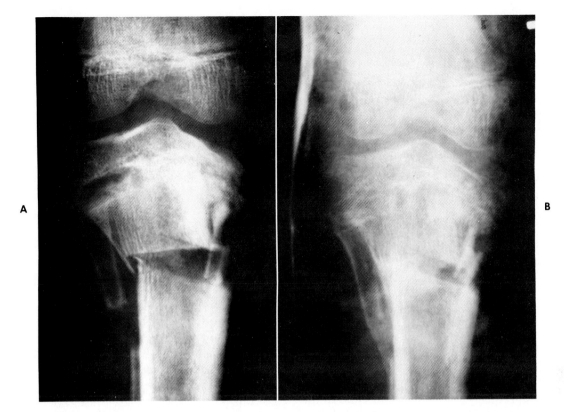

Fig. 5-13. A, Roentgenograms of opening-wedge osteotomy using fibula graft set "on end" without skeletal fixation. **B,** Shortly after the procedure the graft slipped, with subsequent loss of correction.

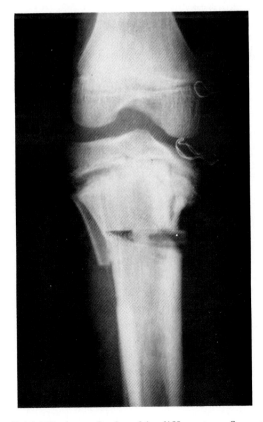

Fig. 5-14. Fibula graft placed in different configuration with more inherent stability.

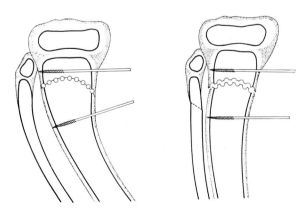

Fig. 5-15. Illustration of dome-shaped or "broomstick" osteotomy, primarily utilized for inherent stability and ease of correction.

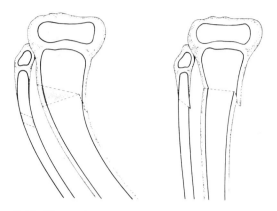

Fig. 5-16. Illustration of closing-wedge osteotomy utilizing medial hinge for inherent stability.

of being a partial opening wedge osteotomy with some inherent stability. Because of the difficulty of constructing the dome with the power saw, multiple drill holes are preferred. The osteotomy is completed when the holes are connected with an osteotome.

Occasionally, when skeletal fixation is to be avoided, as after infection or in the hemophiliac, a hinge osteotomy (Fig. 5-16) is preferable. This provides inherent stability. The hinge portion of the osteotomy can be "notched" and then "greensticked" for more stability. The medial hinge osteotomy gives good stability against loss of correction for varus and valgus. However, if anteroposterior stability is sought, a small ledge or hinge should also be constructed, preferably posteriorly.

When a rotational osteotomy is used (Fig. 5-17), one must remember that the tibia should be considered as a circle with a circumference of 360 degrees and that a rotational osteotomy of 45 degrees requires, in reality, very little rotation. Skeletal pins placed at the desired angle of degree and then rotated until parallel are also useful when the amount of rotation is determined.

The epiphyseal plus metaphyseal osteotomy is a recent and controversial innovation (Fig. 5-18). Its usefulness is in epiphyseal growth arrest or in older children with Blount's disease whose medial epiphysis is sloped approximately 90 degrees and fused or partially fused (Langenskiöld type V and VI) (Fig. 5-19). There are, in reality, two deformities: one in the angulated epiphysis and the other in the varus deformity of the shaft. To correct only the varus of the shaft is to invite early recurrence of the deformity and later degenerative changes in the knee joint. Siffert[24] of New York

and Ingram[12] of the Campbell Clinic believe that, although the long-term results of this double osteotomy are unknown, it may be indicated in a small number of older children with severe Langenskiöld type V or VI Blount's disease. Epiphyseal osteotomy, which seemingly violates all axioms concerning epiphyseal involvement, is performed through the epiphyseal line, which is fused and is carried into the knee joint. The epiphysis is then elevated, especially posteriorly, to parallel the lateral portion of the knee joint. A fibular graft is placed in the created opening wedge. The osteotomy and graft are secured with pin fixation. A second closing wedge osteotomy is performed in the metaphysis for correction of the varus deformity (Fig. 5-20).

Quite often, to avoid recurrence of a deformity, a bony bridge resection in conjunction with a tibial osteotomy can be performed (Fig. 5-21). We believe that both Bright[5] and Langenskiöld[15] would agree that when there is significant angulation deformity, simply resecting the bony bridge will not correct the already present deformity and that an osteotomy also needs to be performed. This, indeed, may be fortuitous because through the osteotomy site a central bridge, previously believed not to be resectable, can be resected. A guide pin is placed parallel and close to the open epiphyseal plate. An osteotomy is performed parallel to the level of the pin and near the open epiphyseal line. A lamina spreader is used to open the osteotomy site. The tip or beginning of the bony bridge is seen as an area of white, sclerotic bone, as compared to the reddish, cancellous bone. With the use of a power dental burr, the entire sclerotic bridge is resected, and the defect is filled with either autogenous fat, Silastic, or silicone material. A section of fibula is used in the opening wedge osteotomy. Parallel pins are then incorporated in plaster (Fig. 5-22).

Guidelines for tibial osteotomies

1. Correct static deformities to neutral. Progressive deformities need to be significantly overcorrected for fear of recurrence.
2. Overcorrect more into the valgus position; overcorrect less into the varus position. Foot and ankle mechanics tolerate very little varus alignment.
3. Reduce the incidence of loss of immediate correction by using skeletal fixation.
4. Determine the proper site of osteotomy (tibia

Text continued on p. 101.

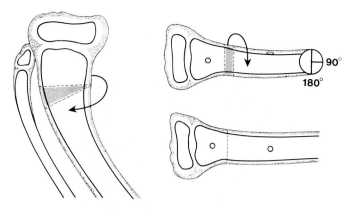

Fig. 5-17. Illustration of a closing-wedge derotation osteotomy. In performing a rotatory osteotomy one should consider the bone as a circumference of 360 degrees, and for a 45-degree osteotomy very little rotation is necessary. Pins set at the correct degree of rotation and then brought parallel are helpful.

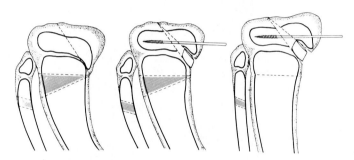

Fig. 5-18. Illustration of epiphyseal and metaphyseal osteotomy. Epiphyseal osteotomy is performed through the closed or nearly closed growth plate and carried into the joint. This osteotomy is elevated with the aid of a fibula graft. A second closing-wedge osteotomy is performed for the varus deformity of the shaft, and both osteotomies are secured in pins and plaster.

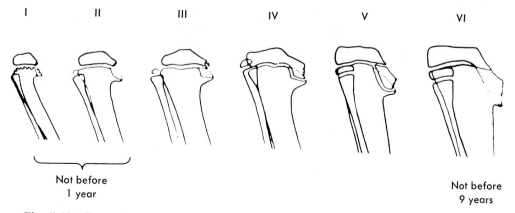

Fig. 5-19. Illustration of Langenskiöld's six stages of Blount's disease. In types V and VI, which occur in older children, the epiphysis is sloped 90 degrees and fused or about to fuse.

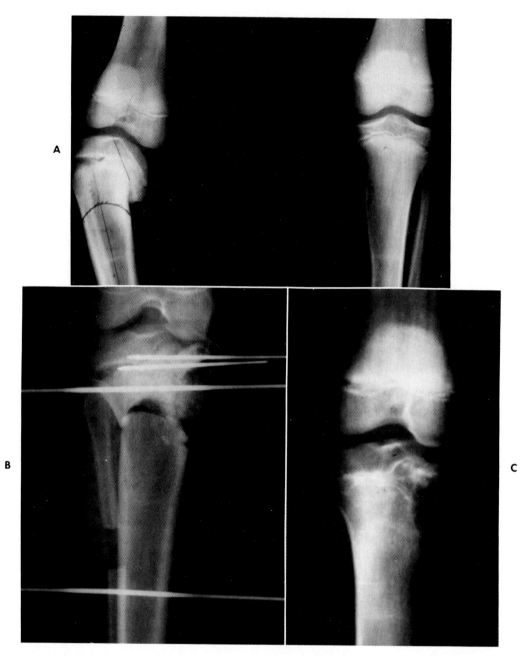

Fig. 5-20. A, Preoperative roentgenogram of a child with type VI Blount's disease of the right tibia with a closed epiphysis and sloped at 90 degrees. A significant varus deformity of the shaft is also present. **B,** Roentgenogram of epiphyseal and metaphyseal osteotomy with fibula graft, all secured with pins. **C,** Roentgenograms at short-term follow-up showing good correction of knee joint and a straight extremity. (Courtesy Alvin J. Ingram, M.D. Memphis, Tenn.)

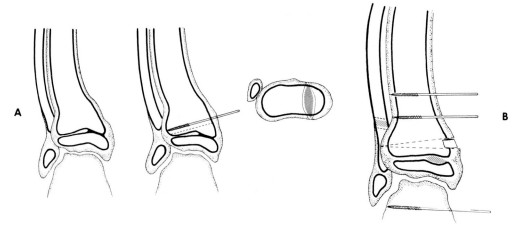

Fig. 5-21. A, Illustration of bony bridge resection and supramalleolar osteotomy. Guide pin is placed parallel to open epiphyseal plate. The osteotomy is performed adjacent and parallel to the guide pin, and the sclerotic bony bridge is visualized. **B,** Illustration of resection of bony bridge; opening-wedge osteotomy utilizing fibula graft and skeletal-pin fixation.

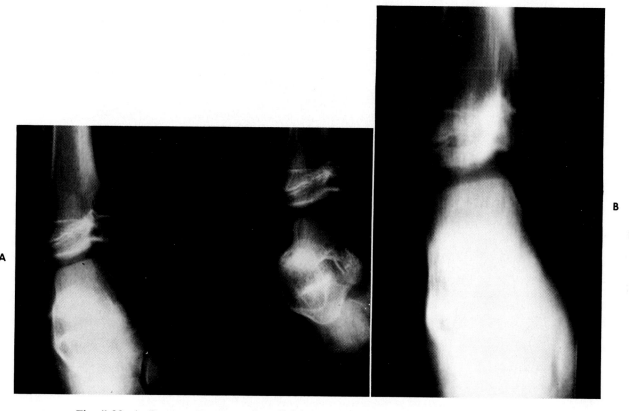

Fig. 5-22. A, Roentgenograms of medial bony bridge with varus deformity secondary to trauma. **B,** Tomogram taken to localize the bony bridge.

Continued.

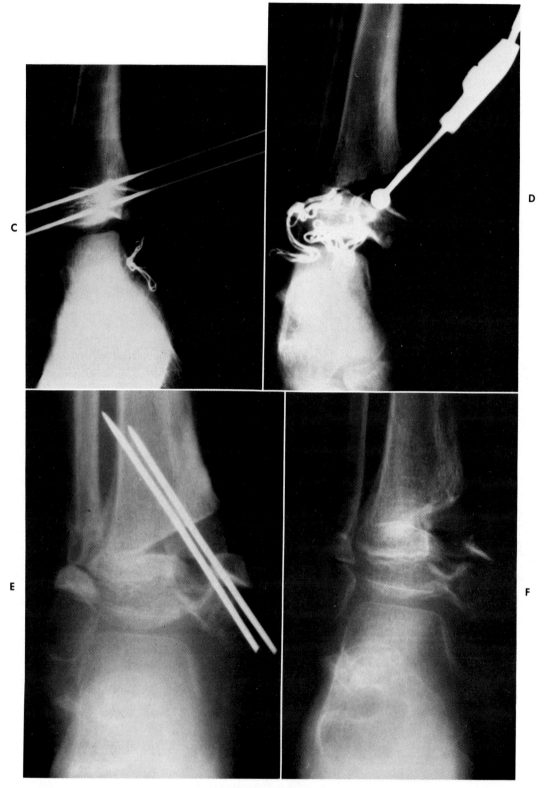

Fig. 5-22, cont'd. C, Roentgenogram of guide pins placed parallel to open epiphyseal plate. **D,** Osteotomy was performed parallel and adjacent to proximal pin. Osteotomy was opened with a lamina spreader and a power dental burr utilized to excise the sclerotic bony bridge. The defect was filled with autogenous fat. **E,** Roentgenograms of pins and plaster used to hold opening-wedge osteotomy. **F,** Roentgenograms of same patient as a short-term follow-up showing correction of the deformity and a defect at the bony bridge site.

versus supracondylar) by utilizing a standing roentgenogram and noting the parallelism of the articular surface to the floor.

5. Reduce the incidence of neurovascular sequelae by performing an anterolateral fasciotomy.

Complications

Nonunions or malunions rarely occur; the most frequent and catastrophic complications are neurovascular. These can include peroneal nerve palsy, anterior compartment syndrome, or stretching or kinking of the proximal vasculature as described by Steel.[27] It is important to differentiate between these three entities so that proper treatment can be instituted immediately. With peroneal nerve palsy, there is no pain on passive plantar flexion of the toes. In an ischemic syndrome secondary to stretching or kinking of the proximal artery, there is immediate postoperative onset of pain with plantar flexion of the toes. This occurs as early as 1 to 3 hours after surgery. Contrary to this, in an anterior compartment syndrome the pathologic process takes longer to develop. At 8 to 10 hours after surgery, there is diffuse swelling about the foot and extreme pain on passive motion of the toes. In each of these entities, all the dressings should be removed completely. If an anterior compartment syndrome is suspected, the patient should be prepared for extensive fasciotomy. If a peroneal nerve palsy or arterial compromise is suspected, the extremity should be returned to its original position before osteotomy. Remember that an angulated, functional lower extremity is superior to a straight but functionless lower extremity. Furthermore, if there is any suggestion of vascular damage, an arteriogram should be performed immediately and appropriate peripheral vascular consultation sought.

REFERENCES

1. Bauer, G.C.H., Insall, J., and Koshino, T.: Tibial osteotomy in gonarthrosis, J. Bone Joint Surg. **51A**:1545-1563, Dec. 1969.
2. Blount, W.P.: Tibia vara (osteochondrosis deformans tibiae). In Adams, J.P., editor: Current practice in orthopaedic surgery, vol. 3, St. Louis, 1966, The C.V. Mosby Co.
3. Blount, W.P.: Unequal leg length, AAOS: Instructional course lectures, **17**:218-254, St. Louis, 1960, The C.V. Mosby Co.
4. Brackett, E.G.: A study of the different approaches to the hip-joint, with special reference to the operations for curved trochanteric osteotomy and for arthrodesis, Boston Med. Surg. J. **166**:235-242, 1912.
5. Bright, R.W.: Operative correction of partial epiphyseal plate closure by osseous bridge resection and silicone rubber implant, J. Bone Joint Surg. **56A**:655-664, June 1974.
6. Coventry, M.B.: Osteotomy about the knee for degenerative and rheumatoid arthritis: indications, operative technique and results, J. Bone Joint Surg. **55A**:23-47, Jan. 1973.
7. Coventry, M.B.: Osteotomy of the upper portion of the tibia for degenerative arthritis of the knee: a preliminary report, J. Bone Joint Surg. **47A**:984-990, July 1965.
8. Edmonson, A.S., and Crenshaw, A.H., editors: Campbell's operative orthopaedics, ed. 6, St. Louis, 1980, The C.V. Mosby Co.
9. Engel, G.M., and Staheli, L.T.: The natural history of torsion and other factors influencing gait in childhood, Clin. Orthop. **99**:12-17, March-April 1974.
10. Evans, F.G.: Mechanical properties of bone, Springfield, Ill., 1973, Charles C Thomas, Publisher.
11. Harris, W.R., and Kostuik, J.P.: High tibial osteotomy for osteo-arthritis of the knee, J. Bone Joint Surg. **52A**:330-336, March 1970.
12. Ingram, A. J.: Personal communication, Memphis, Tenn., 1980.
13. Insall, J., Shoji, H., and Mayer, V.: High tibial osteotomy, J. Bone Joint Surg. **56A**:1397-1405, Oct. 1974.
14. Jackson, J.P., Waugh, W., and Green, J.P.: High tibial osteotomy for osteoarthritis of the knee, J. Bone Joint Surg. **51B**:88-94, Feb. 1969.
15. Langenskiöld, A.: An operation for partial closure of an epiphysial plate in children, and its experimental basis, J. Bone Joint Surg. **57B**:325, 1975.
16. Langenskiöld, A., and Riska, E.B.: Tibia vara (osteochondrosis deformans tibiae), J. Bone Joint Surg. **46A**:1405-1420, Oct. 1964.
17. Lloyd-Roberts, G.C., Swann, M., and Catterall, A.: Medial rotation osteotomy for severe residual deformity in clubfoot, J. Bone Joint Surg. **56B**:37-43, Feb. 1974.
18. Mayer, A.: Historische and statistische Notizen. Die von Dr. Mayer verrichtete Osteotomien, Deutsche Klinik von Göschen **8**:119, 1856. Cited in Milch, H.: Osteotomy of the long bones, Springfield, Ill., 1947, Charles C Thomas, Publisher.
19. Milch, H.: Osteotomy at the upper end of the femur, Baltimore, 1965, The Williams & Wilkins Co.
20. Milch, H.: Osteotomy of the long bones, Springfield, Ill., 1947, Charles C Thomas, Publisher.
21. Morley, A.J.M.: Knock knee in children, Br. Med. J. **11**:976, 1957.
22. Salenius, P., and Vankka, E.: Development of the tibiofemoral angle in children, J. Bone Joint Surg. **57A**:259-261, March 1975.
23. Shoji, H., and Insall, J.: High tibial osteotomy for osteoarthritis of the knee with valgus deformity, J. Bone Joint Surg. **55A**:963, July 1973.
24. Siffert, R.: Personal communication, New York, 1980.
25. Slocum, D.B., Larson, R.E., James, S.L., and Grenier, R.: High tibial osteotomy, Clin. Orthop. **104**:239-243, 1974.
26. Sorrell, E.: Ostéotomie "en chevron," Paris Med. **95**:569, 1935.
27. Steel, H.H., Sandrow, R.E., and Sullivan, P.D.: Complications of tibial osteotomy in children for genu varum or valgum, J. Bone Joint Surg. **53A**:1629-1635, Dec. 1971.
28. Zuege, R.C., Kempken, T.G., and Blount, W.P.: Epiphyseal stapling for angular deformity of the knee, J. Bone Joint Surg. **61A**:320-329, April 1979.

TRAUMA

Chapter 6

Management of multiply injured patients

TAYLOR K. SMITH, M.D.
Houston, Texas

LORRAINE J. DAY, M.D.
San Francisco, California

SIGVARD T. HANSEN, Jr., M.D.
Seattle, Washington

RENNER M. JOHNSTON, M.D.
Denver, Colorado

The challenge to improve the survival of multiply injured patients has presented orthopaedic surgeons with the need to develop and utilize methods of care that will complement and assist in the overall management of these patients.

Initially the orthopaedist's role in the care of the severely injured patients is of secondary importance. However, frequently a critically ill patient will survive to be left with a musculoskeletal problem that should, and could, have been better managed with judicious and sometimes aggressive early treatment. For this reason we cannot emphasize enough how important it is for the orthopaedist to be involved early in the decision-making regarding these patients. The orthopaedist's care should not increase the patient's problems but should be directed toward providing the earliest mobility with the least morbidity.

ORTHOPAEDIC SURGEON'S ROLE IN TRAUMA TEAM

In most trauma centers the overall direction of care of the multiply injured patient is managed by the general surgeon. Other specialty surgeons consult on the case, but the overall direction of care, management of systemic problems, and coordination of surgical procedures is handled by the general surgical trauma service. In other medical centers the captain of the team or the service responsible for the coordination of activities will be the speciality managing the most serious aspect of the case. A patient with a severe head injury and multiple extremity fractures may be on the neurosurgical service with the orthopaedic service consulting until the neurologic problem is resolved or stabilized. Regardless of which method of organization is preferred, it is important that the team responsible be established before the patient arrives. The other services involved must understand and accept the chain of command. Without a well-organized trauma service plan the patient may suffer from errors of omission, indecision, or conflicting treatments. Communication between services and between house officers and staff must be frequent and easy to obtain.

The nonphysician members of the trauma team must also be aware of the chain of command for each patient so that the treatment plan can be carried out efficiently.

105

TIMING AND STAGING OF ORTHOPAEDIC SURGICAL PROCEDURES IN CARE OF MULTIPLY INJURED PATIENT

A recent trauma victim whose vital signs are stabilized is usually, at that time, in the best condition for aggressive surgical management of his orthopaedic problems, even if prolonged anesthesia and moderate blood replacement should result from this definitive treatment. The advantages of early operative stabilization of axial and long bone fractures greatly outweigh the disadvantages of deferral of definitive fracture surgery.

If by immediately stabilizing the patient's spinal and extremity fractures one can avoid traction and the patient can be allowed to sit or stand, many of the well-known complications of trauma can be avoided. The benefits of early mobilization on pulmonary function, nutrition, and mental status in the early postinjury period are well established. The mobile patient can be easily evaluated by physicians and nurses, can be moved with less difficulty and pain, and can undergo diagnostic and therapeutic procedures that are not available to the immobilized patient in traction or in cumbersome casts.

The fact that a patient has a fracture that can be internally fixed is not in and of itself a reason for operative fixation of fractures. Surgical intervention should not be contemplated unless the benefits outweigh the disadvantages of additional trauma to an already traumatized patient. For example, it makes little sense to operatively fix a closed supracondylar femur fracture immediately in a multiply injured patient who will be treated in traction anyway for a central fracture dislocation of the acetabulum on the same side. On the other hand, the patient who has several broken ribs and a contused lung, in addition to an open humeral shaft fracture on the same side, might well benefit from immediate compression plating of the humerus, with the wound being left open for delayed primary closure at a later date. This would decrease the patient's discomfort and need for narcotics, enable him to better cooperate with pulmonary therapy, and allow him to gain the use of his arm and hand early to assist with his own care. If the type of fixation selected would not provide rigid immobilization, or the fracture could not be reapproximated with any semblance of strength, then surgical fixation would be contraindicated because the patient would still require external fixation and would have limited use of the extremity.

Early operative fixation of fractures in the multiply injured patient should therefore be encouraged when it enhances patient care and should be discouraged if it does not. In a short period of time the patient will be in a rather severe catabolic state, will be requiring multiple medicines including narcotics, and may become septic or may have major pulmonary problems with acute respiratory distress syndrome, fat emboli, pulmonary emboli, or lung contusions. Therefore he will be a greater surgical risk a few days after surgery.

If two or more areas need operative attention, sufficient manpower should be available to operate simultaneously at several sites. This should decrease anesthesia time and the amount of blood loss.

PHYSIOLOGIC EFFECTS OF TRAUMA

Immediately after severe injury, a whole series of physiologic changes occur in the patient. Collapse or failure of any one of the major defense mechanisms or organ systems has a profoundly deleterious effect on all the others; therefore it is of the utmost importance to anticipate such adverse responses and to ensure that the patient does not develop problems in these areas.

Blood loss must be evaluated and treated adequately. The tendency, however, is to overload the patient with crystalloid and blood products and so adequate steps to monitor fluid replacement must be instituted. The measurement of central venous pressure by a CVP line has been shown to be quite inaccurate and misleading. The use of a Swan-Ganz catheter to monitor the patient's status and his response to treatment has, on the other hand, proved to be very useful in the management of the multiply injured patient.

Pulmonary insufficiency may develop acutely from direct lung contusion or from the adult respiratory distress syndrome. It may develop later because of pulmonary emboli, fat emboli, or sepsis. Usually several days elapse before severe pulmonary compromise occurs. This is one of the reasons we advocate early aggressive surgical management of long bone and spine fractures. The mobilization gained contributes to the care of the patient. If respiratory distress does develop, it may prevent definitive care of orthopaedic problems for quite some time.

Lastly, the role of sepsis in the development of posttraumatic pulmonary insufficiency must be emphasized. It has been shown that the clinical event most often associated with fatal posttraumatic pulmonary insufficiency is sepsis. Although we do not know all the mechanisms causing adult respiratory distress syndrome, we can greatly decrease the incidence by avoiding sepsis. Strict sterile care of indwelling urinary and intravenous catheters, endotracheal tubes, and wound dressings will help prevent sepsis, as will the judicious use of antibiotics, both prophylactically and therapeutically.

One of the responses of the body to acute stress in trauma is the outpouring of antidiuretic hormone (ADH) by the hypothalamus. ADH acts on the distal tubules of the kidneys to permit the reabsorption of water into the vascular system. This has the effect of raising the blood volume and thus acts as a vasopressor. ADH also causes the retention of sodium by blocking the excretion of sodium ions and sodium bicarbonate in urine, sweat, saliva, and the small bowel. The retention of water by the effect of ADH may, in the period after fluid resuscitation for severe trauma, cause a fluid overload. The effect of excess fluids on an already compromised lung is obvious.

NUTRITION

A severely traumatized patient has caloric and protein needs far in excess of the actively working uninjured person. In fact, the multiply injured patient lying quietly in bed in traction in the immediate postinjury period requires calories and protein in phenomenal amounts. A healthy active orthopaedic resident may need 2500 calories per day, but a patient with several long-bone fractures and abdominal injuries may be utilizing 5000 to 6000 calories per day. Of the three somatic sources of energy, glycogen, fat, and protein, the protein stores are the most useful. Glycogen stored mainly in the liver is quickly depleted, often within 12 hours. Fat, though frequently present in considerable amounts, often cannot be broken down and utilized in stress situations. Protein is thus catabolized in the body's attempt to provide calories for the excess demands placed on it by the stress of trauma. There are no stores of protein in the body. Even in health every molecule of protein is serving a vital function. Consequently, catabolism of body protein during trauma results in depletion of somatic protein in the form of skeletal muscle, and visceral protein in the form of albumin, lymphocytes, and other blood components. This results in decreased muscle mass and strength, and inhibition of wound healing and immunocompetence. Therefore it is important for the orthopaedist to anticipate the profound protein catabolism that can occur in the multiply injured patient. Early in the course of treatment, he should institute calorie and protein replacement. A dose of 3000 ml of 5% dextrose (average maintenance quantity) provides only 600 calories per day, much less than the actual need of most trauma victims.

There are two routes for the administration of nutritional substrates. The enteric route includes supplemental oral feedings, a nasogastric tube or gastrostomy or enterostomy feeding tube. The patient being held "nothing by mouth" for an ileus or frequent trips to the operating room rarely will be able to obtain his needed protein and calories by this regimen. Parenteral hyperalimentation may then be necessary. The introduction of hyperosmolar solutions in large amounts in peripheral veins is not feasible. Intravenous hyperalimentation has become possible with the use of central venous lines for the introduction of solutions containing large quantities of glucose, essential amino acids, vitamins, and trace elements.

The orthopaedist caring for the multiply injured patient should thus anticipate the massive protein and caloric needs of these patients and make provision early for adequate replacement.

ANESTHESIA IN MULTIPLY INJURED PATIENT

For the trauma team to function efficiently, the activities and problems faced by other members of the team must be appreciated. The anesthesiologist taking care of the traumatized patient is responsible for many more things than just keeping the patient asleep. In addition to maintaining anesthesia they replace blood and fluid loss and they maintain a proper pH balance and physiologic temperatures. Each of these areas is discussed briefly.

The choice of anesthesia of course is a crucial one and must be done by the anesthesiologist who is experienced in these techniques. Trauma victims are almost always better off with a general anesthetic rather than a spinal or a regional block because their vital functions can be controlled more easily and they will not develop major problems with vasodilatation. If a patient has eaten recently, a spinal or regional block may be necessary. Most patients with head injuries are hypertensive until the end stage of head injury or they are suffering serious blood losses. If a patient is unconscious from a head injury, the anesthesiologist will often use only a muscle relaxant and oxygen for anesthesia. Levels of unconsciousness and evidence of lateralizing signs can be monitored during general anesthesia, and in most cases the patient with a closed head injury can tolerate anesthesia without problems. Ketamine may be used in situations requiring a mild degree of anesthesia. It can be injected intramuscularly and will produce profound analgesia while the patient is awake. Therefore it is useful in such areas as burn débridement or fracture reductions that do not require a significant degree of relaxation. It is also the agent of choice for many patients who are conscious but hypotensive. One of the serious disadvantages of ketamine is the extreme apprehension that patients experience after the anesthetic; some may even develop postanesthetic hallucinations.

The anesthesiologist should also be carefully monitoring the patient's temperature. The multiply injured patient is frequently exposed to a cool operating room environment, may have large surface areas exposed to room air or cool irrigation solutions, and may be receiving large amounts of cool intravenous fluids. As the patient's blood cools, his platelet activity is greatly decreased; therefore a bleeding diathesis may be created inadvertently when the patient's temperature is allowed to drop below normal levels. If the patient's temperature is low and he is rewarmed, there is a very great danger that significant acidosis will develop. If the blood pH level falls below 7.15, an abrupt loss of consciousness associated with respiratory inadequacy may develop. Correction of the acidosis quite often will give a dramatic reversal in the clinical picture; therefore it is quite important to monitor the pH during the rewarming of trauma victims. The third problem with hypothermia in the traumatized patient is the increase in myocardial irritability associated with a drop in temperature.

The functions of the anesthesiologist in the management of the multiply injured patient are crucial, and the orthopaedist can, with knowledge of these functions, assist the anesthesiologist in the management in his part of the team efforts.

FRACTURES OF SPINE

Patients with significant injuries should be presumed to have a fracture of the spine until proved otherwise. Transportation and movement of the patient for diagnostic procedures should be very carefully carried out until a fractured spine has been ruled out. The complete physical examination of the multiply injured patient should, of course, include palpation of the spine from the base of the skull to the coccyx. Log-rolling the patient to one side with inspection of the posterior aspects of the body and palpation of the spine should be carried out once a cervical spine injury has been ruled out. A complete neurologic evaluation is often difficult to perform because of the patient's depressed sensorium or lack of cooperation. However, follow-up neurologic examinations at frequent intervals should be included in the management of any multiply injured patient. A patient with neck pain or significant injury to the head or face should have an adequate cross-table lateral and an anteroposterior cervical spine x-ray examination carried out before any manipulation. This is particularly true if there is facial trauma that may require intubation or a tracheostomy.

If it has been determined that the patient has a spinal cord injury or instability of the spine, stabilization of that area during transportation and treatment of his other problems should be a high-priority objective. Rigid collars can be used for patients having hyperflexion or hyperextension injures that are not grossly unstable or are not associated with neurologic problems. If, however, there is a significant disruption of the alignment of the cervical spine or a facet joint dislocation, the patient should be placed in skull traction. One of the most satisfactory types of skull traction equipment to be found in the emergency room is the Gardner-Wells tongs. We prefer, however, to apply a halo in the emergency room because this device allows one to place the head in the desired position during traction or to utilize the halo vest. All sizes of halos should be available in the emergency room, and the orthopaedic team should be well versed in their application. Once stabilization of the spine by traction has been accomplished, transporting the patient for diagnosis and treatment is made easier and safer than if it were not done. Traction can and should be maintained while the patient is on the operating room table receiving treatment for his other injuries. The patient can convalesce in a regular bed, with traction being maintained through the halo.

We prefer not to use the horizontal or circular electric turning frames with patients having unstable spine injuries. It has been shown that the prone position on the horizontal turning frame considerably restricts the patient's pulmonary function and significant degrees of displacement of cervical spine fractures can occur during the turning of a patient with an unstable spine fracture. The circular electric turning frame likewise does not prevent axial loading of the spine. In fact, when the patient is turned upright on this frame, he may bear up to 90% of his body weight through his feet. For the nursing of patients with unstable spines or with neurologic injuries secondary to spinal fractures, we prefer that the patient be placed in a regular bed with frequent turning and positioning with pillows. Halo vests may be applied in the emergency room shortly after the patient is admitted so that rigid stability of the spine can be obtained.

There are two indications for early operative intervention in spinal fractures associated with other multiple injuries: instability and neurologic compromise as a result of displacement. Those patients who have gross instability of their spine or neurologic compromise that could be improved by surgical realignment of the spine deserve early operative intervention. If a unilateral facet dislocation can be reduced with manipulation under anesthesia, the stability of the patient's spine is usually quite good and he can be managed in a halo vest without difficulty. If there is a bilateral facet dislocation, we prefer early operative reduction and fusion because these patients often will undergo subluxation and their hyperflexion deformity will recur even though the facets have been reduced earlier by traction. In multiply injured patients this can be done as part of the initial treatment plan. The stability gained would allow early mobilization.

High thoracic spine injuries are best maintained by a halo also, but midthoracic and low thoracic spine injuries may require stabilization with Harrington rods or other forms of internal fixation. One should carefully evaluate the status of the aorta and the possible presence of a hemothorax in patients who have sustained thoracic spine fractures. Hemothorax frequently develops postoper-

atively after stabilization of the thoracic spine fracture because the reduction allows the hematoma that is developing in the fracture site to evacuate into the negative pressure of the pleural space. Cardiac contusion associated with fractures of the sternum or the thoracic spine must also be ruled out. If Harrington rods are used in the thoracic area, the distal hooks should be staggered at different levels to avoid encroachment on the canal by more than one hook at any one level. Thoracolumbar and lumbar spine fractures can be managed also either by early operative intervention or by traction. In most cases, an unstable thoracolumbar spine fracture will be best handled with early reduction and stabilization followed by the application of a Taylor-Knight brace. In patients who have burns or other contraindications for surgery, halo femoral or halo tibial traction can be utilized. It is quite possible to reduce and maintain reduction of a thoracolumbar fracture through the use of halo femoral traction, but this requires immobilization of the patient and brings with it many potential complications.

In summary, the treatment of unstable spine fractures or spine fractures associated with neurologic injuries in the multiply injured patient should be aggressive, and early reduction and stabilization should be achieved. The goal is to facilitate the overall care of the patient and to prevent further injuries to the spine during the recovery period.

PELVIC FRACTURES

Quite often the patient with multiple injuries has a pelvic fracture. This possibility should be anticipated, and all patients with multiple injuries should have an anteroposterior film of the pelvis included in their diagnostic x-ray workup. Pelvic fractures are often associated with damage to the genitourinary and visceral structures, blood loss, and pelvic instability and deformity resulting from the fracture.

All patients with pelvic fractures, especially those with diastasis of the symphysis pubis or fractures though pubic rami, should be considered to have injuries to the urethra or bladder until proved otherwise. The physical examination should include a rectal examination to determine whether the prostate is floating and is higher than its normal position. The urethral meatus should be inspected to determine whether blood is present. If there is possibility of a urethral injury, a urethral catheter should not be passed until a urethrogram has been performed. Twenty milliliters of Renographin injected into the urethral meatus, followed by a roentgenogram, will determine the status of the urethra. If the urethra is partially or completely torn, no attempt should be made to pass a urethral catheter until a urologic consultation has been obtained. A suprapubic catheter or needle aspiration can be used to evacuate the bladder. Once a catheter has been placed in the bladder, a cystogram, followed by an intravenous pyelogram, should be part of the workup on all multiply injured patients with pelvic trauma.

Blood loss from pelvic fractures can be considerable. An attempt should be made to stabilize the pelvic fracture as early as possible, and movement of the patient should be limited. The torn pelvic veins risk being opened up every time the patient is turned or manipulated, and so this should be avoided. If at all possible, a laparotomy, especially an opening into the retroperitoneal space, should be avoided to eliminate possible additional hemorrhage from loss of the tamponade effect. A g suit, or MAST suit, can be utilized in patients who are bleeding significantly from their pelvic fractures. This is easily applied and can quickly stabilize the pelvis and decrease the amount of blood loss into the retroperitoneal area. In cases of suspected pelvic injury or massive blood loss from lower extremity injury, the patients can be placed directly onto the opened suit before they are lifted onto the emergency stretcher, and the suit can be inflated during transportation. This method also serves to stabilize long-bone fractures in the lower extremities. The only absolute contraindication is pulmonary edema from fluid overload. The suit must be used with caution in patients with impaired pulmonary function because there is a decrease in vital capacity from increased intra-abdominal pressure. The suit must be decompressed with care, and the patient's hypovolemia must be corrected before decompression.

Another method of reducing and stabilizing a pelvic fracture early is the application of a pelvic external fixator device. These external skeletal fixation devices are available now in most trauma centers and can be applied to the unstable pelvic fractures in any one of several configurations. This quickly provides stability to the pelvic fracture and cuts down considerably on the blood loss. Use of the external fixator for pelvic fractures can eliminate the long-term traction previously required for many unstable pelvic fractures.

A final method is the immediate application of a spica cast with the incorporation of distal femoral pins. This method is an effective alternative if special equipment or skills are not present.

EXTREMITY FRACTURES

The treatment of extremity fractures in the multiply injured patient is, of necessity, sometimes different from the treatment of patients with isolated extremity fractures. The goals of fracture treatment in patients with polytrauma are different also in that lifesaving measures and the measures to produce mobility take precedence over some of the basic conservative concepts that we still believe are appropriate in the treatment of isolated fractures. Cast immobilization, traction, and external skeletal fixation are all mainstays of treatment that can and should be utilized if they will benefit the patient and not interfere with his total treatment plan. Early internal fixation of fractures can and should be used if it will benefit the overall care of the patient. This is true even of open fractures that can be internally fixed if the wound is debrided early and adequately. In this case, the wound is always left open for delayed primary closure. It appears that the incidence of infection is no greater than in the open wound not internally fixed. Rigid internal fixation of intra-articular fractures is commonly performed early because the "golden" period for operative correction is short. This allows early motion at joints and a decrease in the morbidity caused by malunions and joint contractures.

In lower extremity fractures, intramedullary fixation will most often be biomechanically superior and technically less demanding on the surgeon and the patient than other methods are. We prefer blind intramedullary nailing of lower extremity long-bone fractures and occasionally humeral shaft fractures. Most types of intramedullary devices should be available, and the surgeon should have the option to choose the device he believes most appropriate. Rather than prolong the operative time in fractures that are difficult to reduce closed, we prefer a limited open reduction. If a few screws or circlage wires can improve the stability and reduction, they should be used. The goal, of course, is to stabilize the long-bone fractures so that the total care of the patient is enhanced. Any operative wound under tension, or with tissue viability possibly compromised, should be left open for later delayed primary closure. Wire sutures can be laid in place to be twisted down later on the ward, if necessary.

For lower extremity fractures, early weight-bearing can be allowed with intramedullary rods but not with plate fixation. Upper extremity fractures, on the other hand, are usually fixed by the use of plates because motion, not weight-bearing, is the prime early goal. Unless reduction can be obtained and held, however, open reduction and internal fixation should not be attempted. If comminution or instability are too great, often open reduction and internal fixation can be supplemented with external fixation of a functional nature, such as a cast brace or a walking spica or the newer plastic functional braces for the upper extremity.

External skeletal fixation is receiving a new wave of popularity; however, one must be aware of the increased risk of nonunion if the external fixator is left in place too long. The pin tracks are also a source of infection in multiply injured patients who are often suppressed immunologically. Traction, with all of its shortcomings, is still frequently used in managing the skeletally injured patient. There are instances however when perhaps more aggressive fixation forms should be used. A humeral fracture, for instance, in a patient with a flail chest or other pulmonary or abdominal problems is very difficult to manage in skeletal traction or with the use of a Velpeau bandage. These forms of treatment may severely compromise the treatment of the patient's pulmonary and abdominal problems, and, in this case, open reduction and internal fixation of the humeral shaft fracture shortly after the time of injury would greatly facilitate the overall care of the patient. The patient with a head injury who is thrashing about is very difficult to manage in traction. In this case, blind intramedullary nailing or external fixation would be preferable. Time and again we see patients with head injuries who recover and are left with severe malunions because of the problems associated with management of these patients in traction.

Multiply injured patients with burns and skeletal injuries are unique because fractures must be cared for within 12 to 16 hours after injury if early internal fixation is to be used. After the patients are septic, surgery on the skeletal system can be quite hazardous. Skeletal traction or external fixation, even through an area of a third-degree burn, will give excellent immobilization and maintenance of reduction and the liability of open reduction with internal fixation is avoided. Patients with burns make multiple trips to the operating room for débridement and grafting, and if the patient's fractures can be managed with internal or external fixation rather than traction, their care is greatly facilitated.

SUMMARY

The care that the orthopaedic surgeon provides the multiply injured patient must be carefully coordinated with other members of the trauma team. That care should be rendered aggressively and early if it will facilitate the patient's mobilization and benefit the overall management of the patient's multiple system problems.

Chapter 7

External skeletal fixation

Part A

Introduction to external skeletal fixation

FRED BEHRENS, M.D., F.R.C.S.(C)
St. Paul, Minnesota

External fixators have been employed sporadically for more than a century.[11,16,18] Unsuitable metals, inappropriate designs, and a high rate of complications, however, created a bad reputation for these devices[8,13,23] and limited their use to a small number of hardy enthusiasts. The few published series have made contradictory recommendations and have therefore not promoted the development of a consistent approach. Despite a sudden surge in the popularity of external fixators in the early 1970s, this situation has remained largely unchanged.

Based on the experience with external fixators in four North American centers over the past 7 years, we have made a conscientious effort to (1) go beyond the description of individual, serendipitous cases, (2) formulate general concepts that remain valid in different clinical situations and do not depend on the use of a particular device, and (3) show that for the achievement of optimal results, external fixation must be an integral part of a well thought-out treatment plan, which may include repeated bone grafting, various soft-tissue procedures, and the concomitant or sequential use of other methods of immobilization.

□ Supported by Grant 8263 from the Medical Education and Reseach Foundation, St. Paul–Ramsey Hospital, St. Paul, Minnesota.

HISTORICAL PERSPECTIVES

To our knowledge, external fixation was used for the first time by Malgaigne[18] in 1853. Discouraged by the conservative management of displaced patellar fractures, he suggested a system of metal "claws" that if percutaneously applied would approximate the displaced fragments and hold them in place until the fracture was healed. In 1897, Parkhill[21] from Denver reported a "100 percent success rate" in nine tibial fractures using his own device. A few years later Lambotte[16] developed a fixator that has become the precursor for many modern designs. In those days external fixators were mainly used for the immobilization of unstable closed fractures. Because they prevented shortening and loss of reduction, they appeared superior to plaster-of-paris casts without carrying the feared complications typical for internal fixation.

In the early 1930s, Cuendet[9], Anderson[3], and Hoffmann[11] made major advances in the design of external fixators when they first introduced such features as transfixion pins, adjustable connecting rods, and universal joints (Fig. 7-1). Only with the beginning of World War II did it become clear that external fixation could greatly improve the management of open fractures and facilitate the transport of the wounded.[4,12] Unfortunately, indiscriminate use of these devices by men with little training in the method led to a high rate of

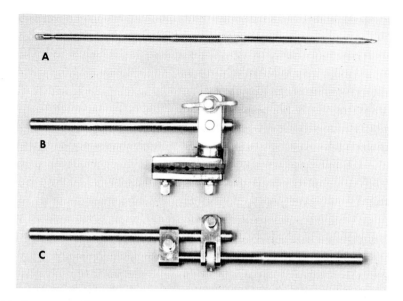

Fig. 7-1. Important fixator components developed during the 1930s. **A,** Transfixion pin. **B,** Universal joint. **C,** Adjustable connecting rod. (Copyright Dr. F. Behrens.)

component failures, nonunions, and osteomyelitis secondary to pin-tract infections.[8,23] Consequently the surgeon general severely limited the use of all external fixators in 1943.

After World War II, the design of external fixators was advanced by many people who tried to adapt them to different purposes. A careful mechanical analysis of the Hoffmann device by Adrey, Vidal, and Rabishong[1] and their suggestion for a more rigid configuration—the "quadrilateral frame" (Fig. 7-6, *B*)—in 1969 led to improved clinical results and a rapidly increasing popularity of these devices. Earlier Wagner[27] had developed a simple and effective leg-lengthening apparatus (Fig. 7-2), and modifications of Charnley's compression clamp[7] ultimately led to such devices as the ASIF "tubular" fixator (Fig. 7-5, *B*). Probably the most interesting search, however, went on in Russia where, in an attempt to equal the precision of internal fixation, a number of surgeons developed highly adjustable ring fixators.[26]

Until recently, external fixators were almost exclusively designed and used for the management of extremity lesions. Over the past 10 years, mechanical investigations and clinical experience have shown that a number of devices can successfully stabilize injuries to the pelvic ring (Fig. 7-3), particularly when the sacroiliac joints are not com-

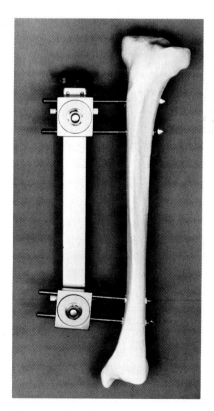

Fig. 7-2. Wagner's leg-lengthening apparatus. (Copyright Dr. F. Behrens.)

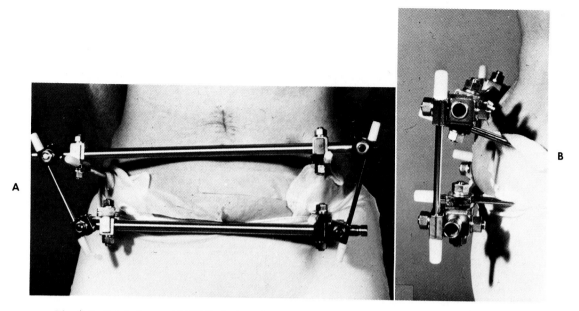

Fig. 7-3. Pelvic frame (ASIF "tubular" fixator). **A,** Frontal view. **B,** Lateral view. (Copyright Dr. F. Behrens.)

pletely disrupted.[24] This has decreased the hospital stay for lesser lesions and will greatly facilitate the management of open pelvic injuries.

CLASSIFICATION OF EXTERNAL FIXATORS

As a guide to the functional capabilities of the many fixators that are presently on the market, I suggest the following classification:

Pin fixators. The strong bone-holding pins are directly connected to the longitudinal rods and form a principle structural component of the fixator frame (Fig. 7-4). These fixators are best subclassified according to their adjustability.

Simple pin fixators. Each bone-holding pin (over an independent joint) is directly connected to a longitudinal rod. Within the plane of pin insertion each pin can be placed at the most desirable angle to the bone. But once two pins are inserted into each main bony fragment, angular and rotational adjustments are severely limited. Depending on such features as joint design and hinged connectors, the adjustability of different simple pin fixators can vary considerably (Fig. 7-5).

EXAMPLES: Roger Anderson, Denham, ASIF "tubular" fixator.

Modular pin fixators. The bone-holding pins inserted into each main fragment must be parallel to each other. They are all held by the same

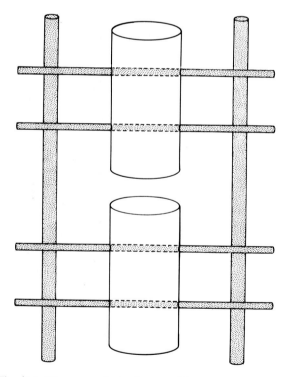

Fig. 7-4. Diagram of pin fixator. The pins form a crucial part of the fixator structure. (Copyright Dr. F. Behrens.)

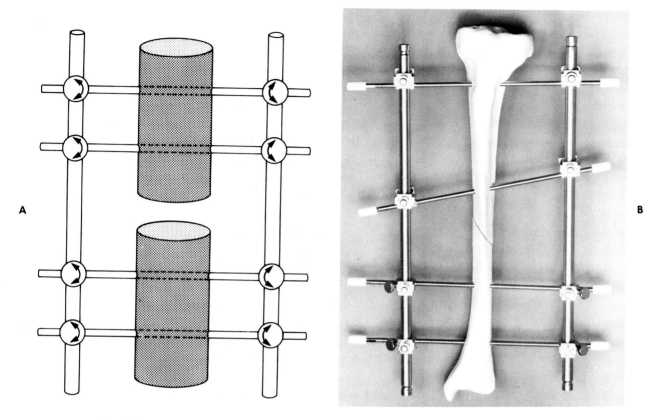

Fig. 7-5. A, Diagram of a simple pin fixator. Each pin is connected over an adjustable clamp. **B,** Example: ASIF "tubular" fixator (type 2 frame). (Copyright Dr. F. Behrens.)

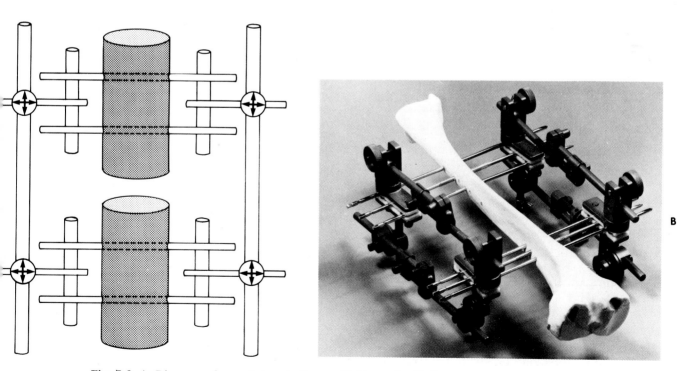

Fig. 7-6. A, Diagram of a modular pin fixator. **B,** Example: Hoffman apparatus (quadrilateral frame). (Copyright Dr. F. Behrens.)

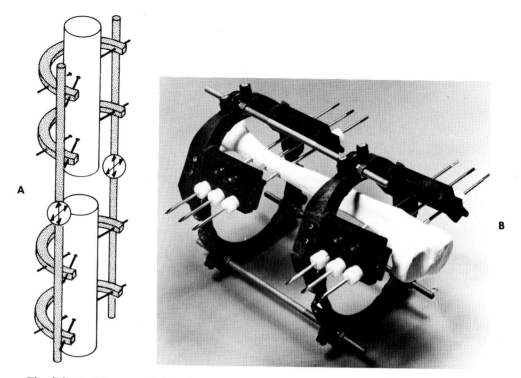

Fig. 7-7. A, Diagram of ring fixator. The pins are not a necessary part of the frame. **B,** Example: Kronner circular compression frame. (Copyright Dr. F. Behrens.)

clamp, which, over a universal joint, is connected to the longitudinal rod. These fixators provide considerably less freedom with respect to pin insertion but, provided that all joints are loosened simultaneously, allow for universal adjustments (Fig. 7-6).

EXAMPLES: Hoffmann, ICLH.

Ring fixators. The structure of the fixator frame is formed by circular elements (rings, partial rings) and longitudinal rods. The bone-holding pins have the sole purpose of connecting the bony fragments to the frame (Fig. 7-7). Some Russian fixators use Kirschner wires rather than heavy Steinmann pins.

EXAMPLES: Volkov-Oganesian, Kronner circular compression frame.

None of these fixators is "perfect." Lack of adjustability is an obvious weakness of the simple pin fixators, which, however, give excellent wound access and are economically more attractive than the complex modular and ring devices.

Since presently less than 10% of all fixators used in North America are of ring design, the clinical examples are limited to pin fixators.

INDICATIONS FOR EXTERNAL FIXATION
Advantages of external fixation

Regardless of specific design features, external fixators have certain advantages over other methods of skeletal immobilization:
1. Free wound access
2. Stabilization of bony fragments at a distance from the lesion
3. Motion of adjacent joints
4. Patient mobility
5. Adjustability

External fixators therefore can not only facilitate the initial management of complex musculoskeletal lesions, but also often allow for an accelerated rehabilitation of the injured patient.

Primary indications

There is presently a certain consensus[14,20,25] that in the treatment of these lesions external fixation is superior to other methods.

Open fractures. As a guide for management and for easier comparison of results, open fractures have been divided into three categories of increasing severity, mainly in accordance with the

[Handwritten annotations at top of page:]
1° Indications
① Type 2 & 3 Open Frs
② Skeletal Infection
③ Limb lengthening

extent of the soft-tissue injury. Unfortunately, the various classifications[6,10,15] are rather vague, differ considerably, and do not account appropriately for the characteristics of the bony lesion.

Type 1: A bony fragment from within has pierced the skin and made a small laceration (1 to 2 cm). There is minimal soft-tissue damage.

Type 2: A larger skin laceration is present, generally caused by an outside object. There is a moderate amount of soft-tissue damage.

Type 3: This is the most severe injury, with massive destruction of muscle tissue. It may include avulsion of soft-tissue flaps, crush injuries, and nerve and vascular lesions.

The treatment of a type 1 injury is similar to that of a corresponding closed fracture. The use of a fixator is unlikely to shorten the healing process or improve the ultimate outcome. For type 2 and 3 fractures, however, external fixation will provide early stabilization of the fracture fragments and allow simultaneously free access to the wound for débridement and reconstructive procedures. This is particularly important in complex injuries (crush, avulsion, concomitant vascular lesions) where the full extent of the tissue necrosis may not become immediately apparent.

Skeletal infections. Included in this category are acute and chronic osteomyelitis, infected pseudarthrosis, chronic joint infections, and salvage procedures in connection with infected implants. External fixation is ideally suited to allow for meticulous wound care over protracted time periods while maintaining the rigid immobilization necessary for bone consolidation.

Limb lengthening. External fixators are frequently used for the distraction of overlapping fracture fragments and elective leg-lengthening procedures. It appears, however, that the specially modified devices, such as the leg-lengthening apparatus designed by Wagner,[27] are generally better suited to this specific task (Fig. 7-3). However, these distraction devices are rarely versatile enough for the optimal management of fresh fractures or infected nonunions. Concepts and techniques pertaining to limb lengthening have recently been reviewed and are outside the scope of this course.[2,27]

Secondary indications

Secondary indications include lesions that could be well treated by other methods of immobilization.

Patients with multiple injuries: External fixators have become increasingly important in the management of multiply injured patients. These devices are frequently the only safe means to avoid skeletal traction and its deleterious pulmonary and cutaneous side effects.[22] Joint mobility is easily maintained and ambulation accelerated.

Fractures complicated by burns or other skin conditions: These present similar problems as open fractures.[5]

Closed fractures with severe comminution: These lesions invariably shorten when managed in a cast or brace. Open reduction and internal fixation often leave many devascularized fragments and precipitate late complications such as refractures.

Arthrodesis, osteotomies

"Ligamentotaxis": This is a general term for the concept that periarticular or intra-articular fractures can be kept in proper alignment if the joint is distracted temporarily. It is particularly useful for comminuted fractures of the distal radius.

Soft-tissue reconstruction: External fixators have largely replaced the cumbersome casts that were traditionally used for the immobilization of cross-leg pedicle flaps.

The basic concepts of fixator application for secondary indications differ little from those pertinent to open fractures and infected bony lesions.

Whenever a "new" treatment modality gains popularity, there is a tendency to overestimate its capabilities and, often to the detriment of the patient, apply it in areas where more "traditional methods" give better results or are considerably less hazardous. External fixators are no exception. In many situations they are inferior to cast immobilization, skeletal traction, internal fixation, or amputation.[14] Indications for their use will continue to change with time, depending on technical improvements, advances with other methods, and the surgeon's experience.

INTEGRATED TREATMENT PLAN

It is essential to realize that external fixation is only one of the many tools crucial in the optimal management of open fractures and skeletal infections. Thorough knowledge of the modern techniques of soft-tissue coverage[17,19] and bone grafting[28] is of equal importance. For this reason we shall initially review these three "elements of successful care" separately:

1. Immobilization by external fixation (Parts B and C).
2. Soft-tissue coverage (Part D).
3. Bone grafting (Part 5).

In later sections we shall apply these concepts to injuries encountered in different body regions (Parts F to H).

REFERENCES TO PART A

1. Adrey, J.: Le fixateur externe d'Hoffmann couplé en cadre, Paris, 1970, Editions Gead.
2. Amstutz, H.C., and Sakai, D.N., editors: Symposium on equalization of leg length, Clin. Orthop. **136:**2-142, 1978.
3. Anderson, R.: An automatic method of treatment of fractures of the tibia and the fibula, Surg. Gynecol. Obstet. **58:**639-646, 1934.
4. Bradford, C.H., and Wilson, P.D.: Mechanical skeletal fixation in war surgery: report of 61 cases, Surg. Gynecol. Obstet. **75:**468-476, 1942.
5. Brooker, A.F.: The use of external fixation in the treatment of burn patients with fractures. In Brooker, A.F., and Edwards, C., editors: The current state of the art, Baltimore, 1979, The Williams & Wilkins Co.
6. Cauchoix, J., Duparc, J., Boulez, P.: Traitement des fractures ouvertes de jambe, Mém. Acad. Chir. **83:**811, 1957.
7. Charnley, J.: Positive pressure in arthrodesis of the knee joint, J. Bone Joint Surg. **30B:**478-486, 1948.
8. Coates, J.B., and Cleveland, M., editors: Orthopaedic surgery in the Mediterranean theater of operations, Washington, D.C., 1957, Office of the Surgeon General, Department of the Army.
9. Cuendet, S.: Procédé de réduction des fractures de la diaphyse des deux os de l'avant-bras à l'aide de l'appareil à broches jumeliées, Livre jubilaire Albin Lambotte, Bruxelles, 1936, Vromant.
10. Gustilo, R.B., and Anderson, J.T.: Prevention of infection in the treatment of 1,025 open fractures of long bones, J. Bone Joint Surg. **58A:**453-458, 1976.
11. Hoffmann, R.: Rotules à os pour la réduction dirigée, non sanglante, des fractures (ostéotaxis), Helv. Med. Acta **6:**844-850, 1938.
12. Hoffmann, R.: Closed osteosynthesis with special reference to war surgery, Acta Chir. Scand. **86:**235-266, 1942.
13. Johnson, H.F., and Stovall, S.L.: External fixation of fractures, J. Bone Joint Surg. **32A:**466-467, 1950.
14. Karlström, G., and Olerud, S.: Fractures of the tibial shaft: a critical evaluation of treatment alternatives, Clin. Orthop. **105:**82-115, 1974.
15. Karlström, G., and Olerud, S.: Percutaneous pin fixation of open tibial fractures: Double frame anchorage using the Vidal-Adrey method, J. Bone Joint Surg. **57A:**915-924, 1975.
16. Lambotte, A.: L'intervention opératoire dans les fractures, Bruxelles, 1907, Lamartin.
17. McGraw, J.B.: Selection of alternative local flaps in the leg and foot, Clin. Plast. Surg. **6:**277-246, 1979.
18. Malgaigne, J.G.: Considérations cliniques sur les fractures de la rotule et leur traitement par les griffes, J. des Connaissances Méd. Pratiques **16:**9-12, 1853-1854.
19. Mathes, S.J., and Alpert, B.S.: Advances in muscle and musculocutaneous flaps, Clin. Plast. Surg. **7:**15-26, 1980.
20. Müller, M.E., Allgöwer, M., and Willenegger, H.: Manual of internal fixation, ed. 2, New York, 1979, Springer-Verlag New York Inc.
21. Parkhill, C.: Further observations regarding the use of the bone clamp in ununited fractures, fractures with malunion and recent fractures with a tendency to displacement, Am. Surg. Assoc. Trans. **15:**251-256, 1897.
22. Riska, E.B., von Bonsdorff, H., Hakkinen, S., et al.: Primary open fixation of long bone fractures in patients with multiple injuries, J. Trauma **17:**111, 1977.
23. Siris, I.: External pin transfixion of fractures, Ann. Surg. **120:**911-942, 1944.
24. Slätis, P., and Karaharju, E.: External fixation of the pelvic girdle with a trapezoid compression frame, Injury **7:**531-536, 1975.
25. Vidal, J., Buscayret, C.H., Connes, H., Paran, M., and Allieu, Y.: Traitement des fractures ouvertes de jambe par le fixateur externe en double cadre, Rev. Chir. Orthop. **62:**433-448, 1976.
26. Volkov, M.V., and Oganesian, O.V.: Restoration of function in the knee and elbow with a hinge-distractor apparatus, J. Bone Joint Surg. **57A:**591-600, 1975.
27. Wagner, H.: Technik und Indication der operative Verkürzung und Verlängerung von Ober-und Unterschenkel, Orthopäde **1:**59-74, 1972.
28. Weber, B.G., and Čech, O.: Pseudarthrosis: pathophysiology, biomechanics, therapy, results, New York, 1976, Grune & Stratton, Inc.

SUGGESTED READINGS

Brooker, A.F., and Edwards, C.: External fixation: the current state of the art, Baltimore, 1979, The Williams & Wilkins Co.

Mears, D.C.: Percutaneous pin fixation. In Materials and orthopaedic surgery, Baltimore, 1979, The Williams & Wilkins Co.

Part B

Basic concepts

FRED BEHRENS, M.D., F.R.C.S.(C)
St. Paul, Minnesota

Success in the treatment of an injury that is managed with the help of an external fixator depends on the following:

1. Characteristics of patient and his injury (*clinical*)
2. Structural soundness of fixator frame (*mechanical*)

☐ Supported by Grant 8263 from the Medical Education and Research Foundation, St. Paul–Ramsey Hospital, St. Paul, Minnesota.

3. Placement of *bone-holding pins,* which become a crucial part of both patient and fixator frame
4. *Miscellaneous* considerations such as timing and accessory procedures

THE PINS
Design and function

Transfixion pins. These are either smooth or have a centrally threaded section. They pierce the whole limb and two bony cortices. They provide for increased rigidity in the plane of insertion (Fig. 7-8, *A*).

Half pins. Half pins can be smooth or partially threaded. They only have one skin-entry point but pierce both bony cortices (Fig. 7-8, *B*). Threaded pins are preferred in cancellous and osteoporotic bone.

Diameter

Assuming constant material properties, the diameter of a pin determines directly its strength and its holding power in bone. To prevent serious weakening of the bone, a pin should be thinner than one third of the bone's diameter for which it is used. Diameters of 4.5 mm and larger appear ideal for pelvis, femur, and tibia, particularly if weight-bearing is intended. For the bones of the upper extremity, pin diameters of 4 mm and less are more appropriate.

Selection

Optimal pin design and diameter for a particular situation depend, on local anatomy, extent and location of the wound, fracture pattern, and desired rigidity of the fixator frame, among other factors.

CLINICAL CONSIDERATIONS

Clinical aspects that influence the application of a fixator include the patient, number and characteristics of the injuries, and regional anatomy.

Patient. An old and weak patient who has difficulties with a cumbersome cast can on occasion manage with an external fixator because it is

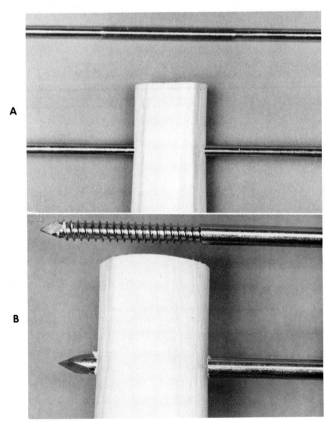

Fig. 7-8. Smooth and threaded pins. **A,** Transfixion pins. **B,** Half pins. (Copyright Dr. F. Behrens.)

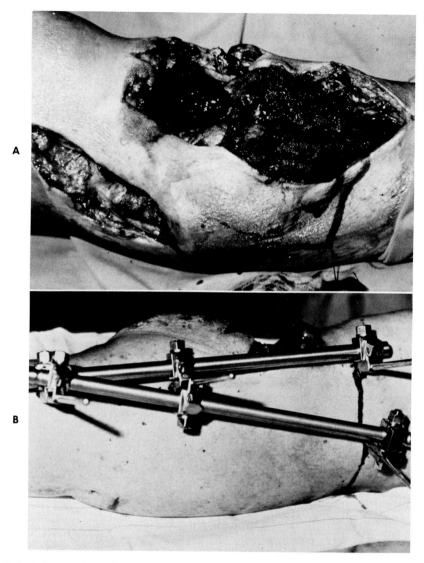

Fig. 7-9. A fixator is "tailored" to an injury. **A,** Severe lateral bone and soft-tissue dis-, ruption. **B,** Application of fixator to medial side. No interference with subsequent procedures (see p. 159). (Copyright Dr. F. Behrens.)

lighter and does not immobilize adjacent joints. The same holds true for the trauma victim with multiple injuries.

Because the patient will be responsible for the care of pins and fixator, he should be cooperative and reliable.

Injury. Ideally, the fixator frame should be "tailored" to the injury. Although under extreme circumstances the pins can be inserted directly through the injured area, we prefer to place them proximally and distally through healthy tissue. The longitudinal bars should not obstruct wound access (Fig. 7-9).

Regional anatomy. Only a thorough knowledge of the local anatomy will prevent iatrogenic damage. Neurovascular structures are particularly at risk in areas where they have a fixed relationship to the underlying bone, such as the superficial

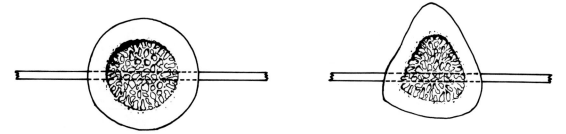

Fig. 7-10. For optimal contact, pins must be inserted through widest bone diameter. (Copyright Dr. F. Behrens.)

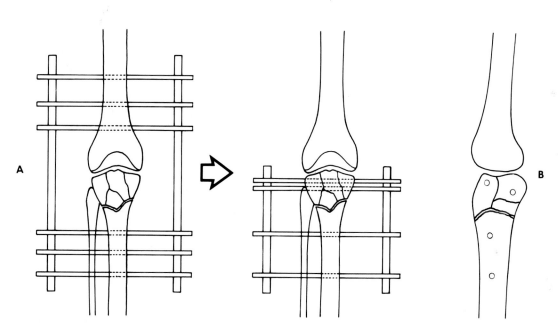

Fig. 7-11. A, Periarticular and undisplaced intra-articular fractures. Precise subchondral pin placement, **B,** preserves joint motion. (Copyright Dr. F. Behrens.)

femoral vessels in the adductor canal[3] at the junction of the middle and distal third of the femur. When there is doubt about the safety of percutaneous pin insertion, the bone should be exposed operatively and the pins placed under direct vision. This is often necessary in the upper extremity and the pelvis.

The shape of a bone and its strength directly influence the direction and location of pin insertion (Fig. 7-10).

If a lesion lies close to a joint, better immobilization of the fracture area may be obtained if the pins are placed into the adjacent bone (Fig. 7-11, *A*). Unfortunately, this will invariably lead to a loss of joint motion. Frequently, this can be prevented through precise pin placement into the

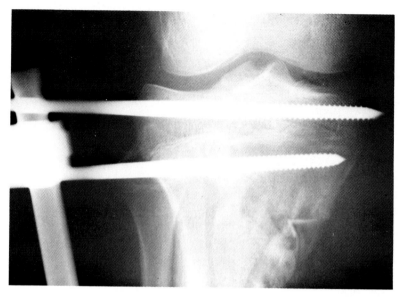

Fig. 7-12. Pin placement near epiphyseal plate. (Copyright Dr. F. Behrens.)

subchondral bone parallel to the joint surfaces (Fig. 7-11, *B*). This is best done under image intensification.

For the management of injuries close to an epiphyseal plate, parallel pins can be inserted through the epiphysis as long as the growth cartilage is not injured (Fig. 7-12).

MECHANICAL CONSIDERATIONS

Mechanical conditions at the fracture site are determined by the fracture configuration, the size and position of the inserted pins, the geometry of the fixator frame that is being built around the pins, and the forces that are acting on the injured area.

Fracture

A severely comminuted fracture or one involving bone loss is considerably more difficult to immobilize than a fracture that has transverse components. In the latter situation, improved rigidity can be achieved when compression is applied across the fracture area, whereas the rigidity of an unstable fracture is only improved when one inserts more pins, inserts them in different planes, and constructs a stronger frame. If a severely comminuted tibia is accompanied by an intact fibula, only a half frame may be needed because the fibula can replace one of the longitudinal rods.

In simple oblique fractures apposition of the fracture fragments can be improved by insertion of a lag screw perpendicular to the fracture plane. If this is done, care must be taken that the fixator frame is rigid enough to neutralize all external forces.

Pins

We have seen in the previous section that the insertion site of pins is in part determined by clinical considerations. Because pins form an important structural component of pin fixators, they also have a direct effect on the ultimate rigidity of the frame structure.

Pin anchorage in bone can be improved by a number of different methods or combinations thereof: thicker pins, replacement of smooth by threaded pins, increasing the number of pins per fragment, and bringing the protruding pin ends closer together (Fig. 7-13).

Apart from anchoring the fixator frame in bone, pins have to resist axial bending and torsional forces at the fracture site. Torsional forces are well controlled by most fixators. Resistance to axial loads is directly determined by the number of pins per fragment and the pin strength (diameter, material properties). Transfixion pins, irrespective of the number of pins per fragment, are about 10 times more effective in preventing displacement of the fracture fragments in the plane of insertion than in the plane perpendicular to it.[2]

Displacement of fracture fragments in a plane

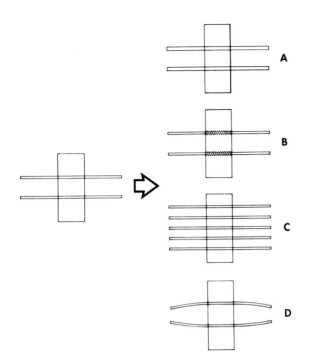

Fig. 7-13. Methods to improve pin anchorage in bone. **A,** Thicker pins. **B,** Threaded pins. **C,** More pins. **D,** Compressing two adjacent pins. (Copyright Dr. F. Behrens.)

Table 7-1. Methods to decrease motion between fracture fragments

1. Thicker pins
2. Increase in number of pins per fragment
3. Greater pin separation in each main fragment
4. Placement of pins closer to fracture site
5. Stronger longitudinal rods
6. Decreasing distance between bone and longitudinal rods
7. Adding half or full frame perpendicular to main pin plane, or using higher order frame

perpendicular to the pin-insertion plane can be diminished by use of methods 1 to 4 in Table 7-1.

Further improvement in fracture immobilization is largely dependent on the configuration of the fixator frame (Table 7-1, methods 5 to 7).

Frame configuration

Although the optimal frame designs differ somewhat for each brand of external fixator, it is useful to classify common basic configurations according to their rigidity. Based on mechanical evaluations, Hierholzer[5] has suggested such a classification for ASIF "tubular" frames. This classification has been recently expanded and adapted to accommodate most presently used fixators,[1] as follows.

Classification of fixator frames (Fig. 7-14)

Type 1 frame: Half pins are inserted in one or more planes and are connected by one or

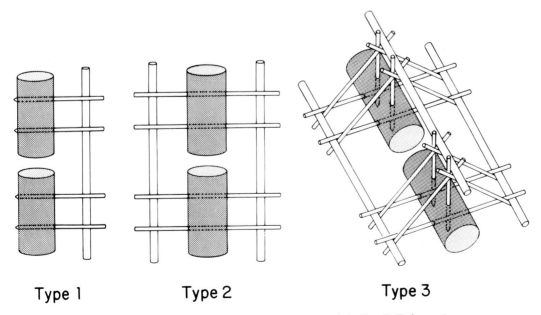

Type 1   Type 2   Type 3

Fig. 7-14. Basic frame configurations. (Copyright Dr. F. Behrens.)

more tubular rods. These are the least rigid configurations. They are particularly indicated in the upper extremity because the use of half pins makes injury to neurovascular structures less likely. If employed in the lower extremity, pins of large diameters and strong longitudinal bars should be used.

Type 2 frame: Transfixion pins are inserted into one plane and stabilized by one or more rods on each side. Since the work of Adrey, Vidal, and Rabishong these have become the "basic frames" and represent presently about 70% of all tibial frame configurations.

Type 3 frame: A combination of transfixion and half pins is inserted in different planes and connected by three or more rods. These, the most rigid frames, are only indicated in the management of skeletal infections when one is dealing with a heavy patient or a severely comminuted fracture with small main fragments.

Although more rigid, the higher orders of frames are frequently rather cumbersome for the patient and, as a large number of pins is used, present a higher risk of pin-tract infection and injury to vital structures. Most importantly, they obstruct wound access.

Forces applying at fracture site

Forces that must be considered are those generated by muscles that span the fracture area, gravity (particularly in the supine patient), and ground reaction forces during walking.

MISCELLANEOUS CONSIDERATIONS

Timing. Because immobilization facilitates bone and soft-tissue healing and decreases the likelihood of an infection,[4] the fixator should be applied as early as possible. When this presents problems (lack of proper equipment, lack of familiarity with device, lack of help, lack of time, and uncertainties about the optimal frame), the limb should be temporarily immobilized by traditional methods.

Combination of methods. On occasion, it is advantageous to combine external skeletal fixation with one of the traditional methods, such as the use of a short leg cast applied over the fixator in an ambulating patient with peroneal nerve palsy, or the use of a polypropylene ankle-foot orthosis in the same situation. Though being least desirable, traction and external fixation are at times

used simultaneously as in an open tibial fracture and an ipsilateral acetabular injury that is held optimally reduced by skeletal traction and does not lend itself to internal fixation. If a complex fracture has diaphyseal and intraarticular components, internal fixation of the articular lesion and external fixator for the diaphyseal fracture may be ideal.

Secondary procedures. Early in the treatment period and before an external fixator is applied, the need, nature, and extent of secondary procedures have to be carefully evaluated. Pins placed too close to the fracture site expose a later bone graft directly to a potentially contaminated area. This increases the chance of infection.

Changes in treatment methods. External fixators are most useful during the initial treatment phase of severe injuries, until appropriate soft-tissue coverage has been obtained. In the later phases it is often desirable to change the rigidity of the frame or to change to a different method of immobilization.

The rigidity of unstable fractures that have started to consolidate can be improved through the compression of the fracture site. Some authors believe that this simultaneously accelerates fracture healing.[6] In other situations, the initially used frame may appear to be too rigid and a reduction in pin rigidity, the number of pins, or the number of longitudinal bars may be desirable.

After the initial period of treatment, we do not hestiate to remove an external fixator and, for example, complete the treatment course in a patellar tendon–bearing cast or brace. Impending nonunions or insufficient soft-tissue coverage of an injured area by a split-thickness skin graft should be spotted early, and the appropriate procedure (see Part E of this chapter) should be carried out without delay.

REFERENCES TO PART B

1. Behrens, F.: The "tubular system"—an ASIF external fixator. In Mears, D.C.: External skeletal fixation, Baltimore, 1981, The Williams & Wilkins Co.
2. Chao, E.Y.S., Briggs, B.T., and McCoy, M.T.: Theoretical and experimental analyses of Hoffmann-Vidal external fixation system. In Brooker, A.F., and Edwards, C.: External fixation: the current state of the art, Baltimore, 1979, The Williams & Wilkins Co.
3. Connes, H.: Hoffmann's external anchorage: techniques, indications, and results, Paris, 1977, Editions Gead.
4. Friedrich, B., and Klane, P.: Mechanical stability and posttraumatic osteitis: an experimental evaluation of the relation between infection of bone and internal fixation, Injury **9:**23, 1977.

5. Hierholzer, G., Kleining, R., Hörster, G., and Zemenides, P.: External fixator: classification and indications, Arch. Orthop. Traumat. Surg. **92:**175-182, 1978.
6. Vidal, J., Buscayret, C.H., Connes, H., Paran, M., and Allieu, Y.: Traitement des fractures ouvertes de jambe par le fixateur externe en double cadre, Rev. Chir. Orthop. **62:**433-448, 1976.

Part C

External fixator application

FRED BEHRENS, M.D., F.R.C.S.(C)
St. Paul, Minnesota
RICHARD E. JONES III, M.D.
Dallas, Texas
DAVID A. FISCHER, M.D.
Minneapolis, Minnesota

PLANNING

As any other operative procedure, the mounting of an external fixator can only be successful if it has been carefully planned. This encompasses all the clinical, mechanical, and miscellaneous considerations discussed in Parts A and B. Before an external fixator is actually applied, the following five points must be checked:

1. *Indications.* Taking all considerations into account: Is external fixation the optimal method? Should the external fixator be used alone or in conjunction with other means of immobilization?
2. *Timing.* Should the external fixator be applied during the initial débridement or during a later visit to the operating room?
3. *Long-range plan.* How does an externally stabilized injury affect the management of other lesions? What kind of secondary procedures will be necessary and when?
4. *Frame design*
   a. Pin placement. How are optimal pin purchase in bone, needs for wound care, and mechanical requirements best realized?
   b. Optimal frame. Similar considerations as for pin placement. Often it is more instructive to draw possible frame configurations on a piece of paper or build them

preoperatively. This furthermore assures that all necessary equipment is available.

5. *Equipment check*

Unless unusual circumstances prevail, we apply the external fixator under general or regional anesthesia after formal preparing and draping of the injured region (Fig. 7-15). All fixator components and necessary instrumentation are sterilized.

Exact pin placement is facilitated if (1) the proximal and distal joints lie within the operating field, (2) pertinent skeletal landmarks are carefully identified by palpation, (3) probe pins or Kirschner wires are used, and (4) an image intensifier is employed. Although these methods can provide excellent orientation in a limited area, they are generally not reliable enough to determine correct angular and rotatory alignment. For

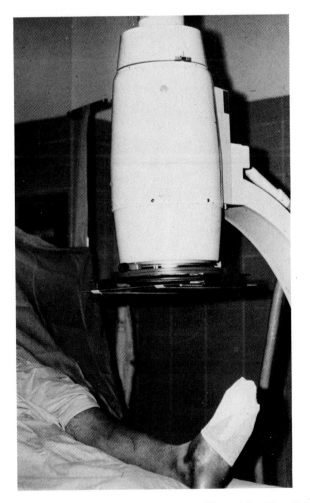

Fig. 7-15. Operating room setup. (Copyright Dr. F. Behrens.)

☐ Supported by Grant 8263 from the Medical Education and Research Foundation, St. Paul–Ramsey Hospital, St. Paul, Minnesota.

this purpose, radiographs in two planes on long cassettes must be obtained.

As there are principle differences in the mounting of single and modular pin fixators, we shall go through the main steps of application for both types. We have chosen, as an example of a simple fixator, the ASIF "tubular" fixator,[1] and as an example of the modular fixator, the Hoffmann apparatus.[2,3]

In our experience the placement of "self-drilling" pins into diaphyseal bone is imprecise, time consuming, cumbersome, and frequently complicated by the development of heat necrosis. If the necessary instrumentation is not provided by the manufacturer, we predrill, preferably with power, before pin insertion. For cortical bone, we recommend a drill bit 0.2 to 0.4 mm smaller than the pin diameter. In cancellous bone, the drill bit can be 1 to 1.5 mm smaller than the pin diameter. Drill guides that protect soft tissues are most desirable.

APPLICATION OF A SIMPLE PIN FIXATOR (ASIF "TUBULAR" FIXATOR)[1]
Components and instrumentation (Fig. 7-16)

Pins. The traditional pin designs come in two sizes. The pins, the appropriate drill bits, and drill sleeves are correlated in Table 7-2.

Clamps. Two basic designs are available:
Standard clamps: Pins and rods are held at a fixed angle of 90 degrees.
Simple, adjustable clamps: These allow for any desired angle between pin and rod.

Tubular rods. The connecting bars come in various lengths from 10 to 45 cm and are of tubular construction.

Adjusting devices. Hinged connectors allow for angular correction of up to 18 degrees in one plane.

Compression devices facilitate compression or distraction between two parts of the fixator frame and are removable.

Instrumentation (Fig. 7-17)
Power drill
Drill guides
Hand drill
Wrenches

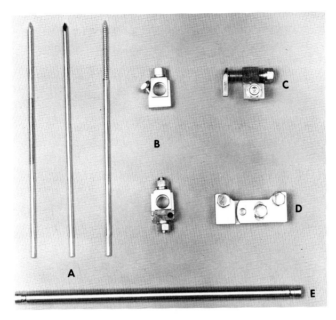

Fig. 7-16. ASIF "tubular" fixator components. *A*, Pins; *B*, standard clamp, single adjustable clamp; *C*, compression device; *D*, hinged connector; *E*, tubular rod. (Copyright Dr. F. Behrens.)

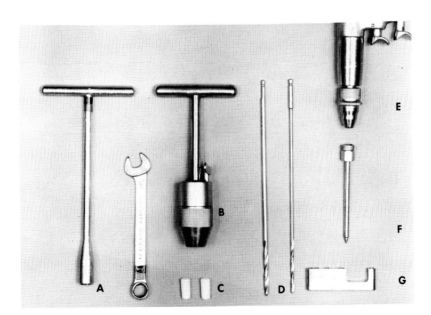

Fig. 7-17. ASIF "tubular" fixator instrumentation. *A*, Wrenches; *B*, hand drill; *C*, pin caps; *D*, drill bits; *E*, power drill; *F*, drill sleeve and trochar; *G*, drill guide. (Copyright Dr. F. Behrens.)

Steps of application

Before the first pin is inserted, a preliminary reduction of the fracture is obtained. The frame is then mounted in four well-defined steps, as follows.

Step 1: Insertion of one pin into each main fragment. Unless unusual circumstances prevail, pins are not inserted closer than 3 cm to the joint line.

1. Skin incision.
2. Drill sleeve with trochar is advanced down to bone.
3. Drilling of bone with appropriate drill bit (Table 7-2) generally parallel to the joint line (Fig. 7-18, *A*) by use of a power drill.
4. Insertion of pin with hand drill (Fig. 7-18, *B*).
5. Same procedure in opposite main fragment (Fig. 7-18, *C*).

Table 7-2. Correlation of pins and drill bits

Instruments	For cancellous bone (mm)	For cortical bone (mm)
Drill bits	3.5	4.5
Pins		
Smooth	5.0	4.5
Threaded	5.0*	4.5†

*Threaded near tip (Schanz screws).
†Centrally threaded.

Step 2: Reduction of fracture

1. Application of standard clamps to both ends of one pin and of adjustable clamps to the ends of the other pin; connection of the two pins with longitudinal rods (all clamps necessary for completion of the frame must be lined up on the respective longitudinal rods before they are connected to the initial pins) (Fig. 7-19, *A*).
2. Manual reduction of fragments is generally initiated by slight distraction of the fracture fragments.
3. The four clamps are tightened as soon as optimal apposition and alignment have been achieved. Particular attention must be paid to rotational alignment because malrotation is most difficult to adjust at a later time (Fig. 7-19, *B*).

APPLICATION OF A "SIMPLE" EXTERNAL FIXATOR

Step 1: Insertion of one pin into each main fragment

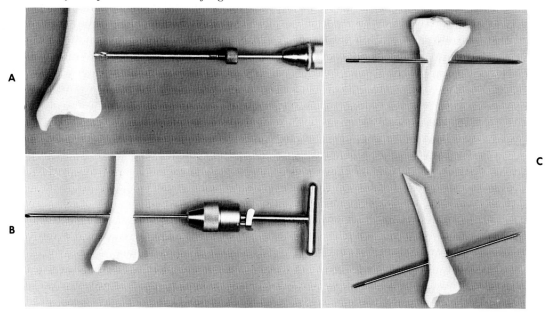

Fig. 7-18. A, Predrilling with power drill. **B,** Pin insertion with hand drill. **C,** One pin in each fragment. (Copyright Dr. F. Behrens.)

Step 2: Reduction

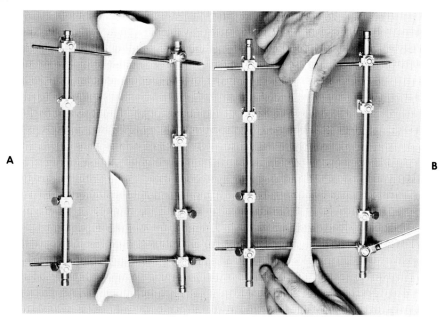

Fig. 7-19. A, Connection of longitudinal rods. **B,** Manual reduction and tightening of clamps as soon as fragments are properly aligned. (Copyright Dr. F. Behrens.)

Step 3: Insertion of remaining pins. The drill sleeves are inserted through drill guides or directly through the clamps, and the remainder of the pins are placed. Parallel pin insertion is not necessary but tends to make later adjustments easier (Fig. 7-20).

Step 4: Adjustments. Adjustments, when necessary, are possible in the following planes and axes:

1. In the *transverse plane,* one makes adjustments by loosening the adjustable clamps and then changing the alignment of the respective fragment in the desired direction (Fig. 7-21, *A*).
2. Angular adjustments of up to 18 degrees are possible in the *sagittal plane* by use of the hinged connector. If more massive malalignments have to be corrected, one pin in one fragment has to be removed and replaced after proper alignment has been obtained (Fig. 7-21, *B*).
3. If substantial *rotational* realignment is necessary, pin removal and reinsertion in the correct position is inevitable (Fig. 7-21, *C*).
4. Axial adjustments are carried out by use of the removable compression devices (Fig. 7-21, *D*).

Step 3: Insertion of remaining pins

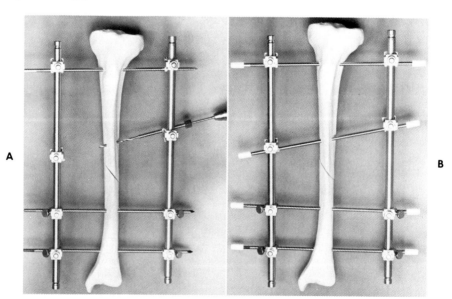

Fig. 7-20. A, Parallel or oblique insertion of remaining pins. **B,** Complete frame. (Copyright Dr. F. Behrens.)

Step 4: Adjustments

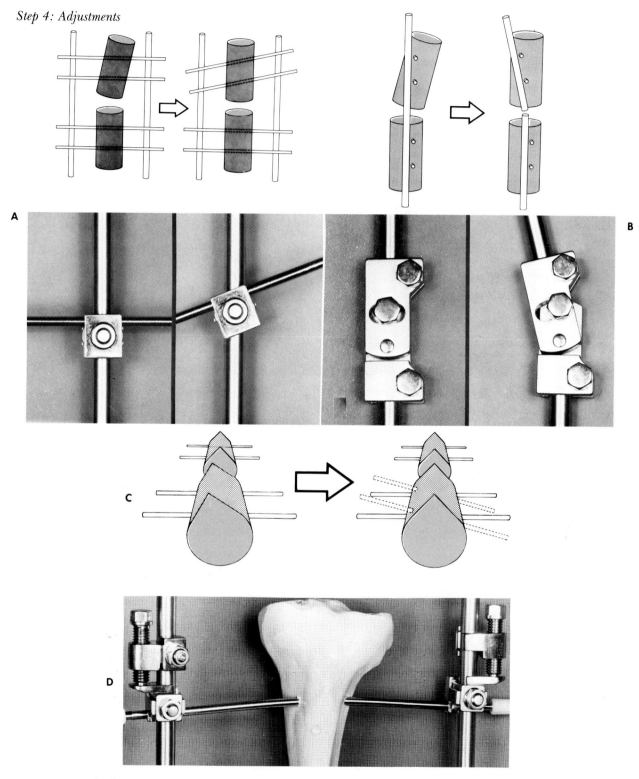

Fig. 7-21. A, Transverse plane: adjustable clamps. **B,** Sagittal plane up to 18 degrees: hinged connectors. **C,** Longitudinal axis: rotation. Pins in one fragment must be removed and reinserted after correction. **D,** Longitudinal axis: compression and distraction. Removable compression device. (Copyright Dr. F. Behrens.)

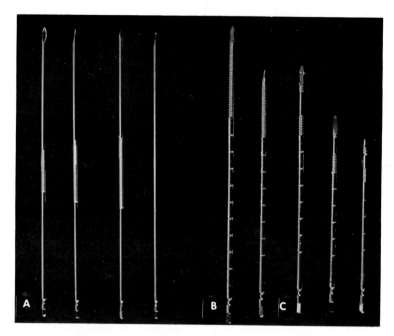

Fig. 7-22. A, Transfixing pins. **B,** Continuous-thread half pins. **C,** Split-thread half pins designed for cortical bone.

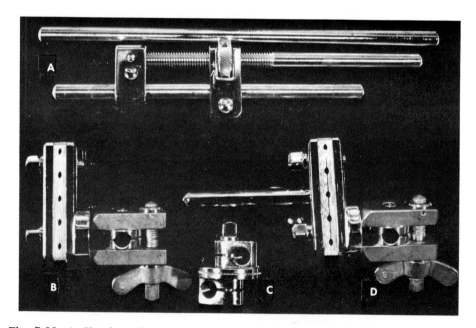

Fig. 7-23. *A,* Simple and compression-distraction rod; *B,* simple ball joint clamp; *C,* articulated coupling; *D,* universal pin clamp (ball joint) with rod. (From Fisher, D.A.: The Hoffmann external fixator: technique of application. In Brooker, A.F., and Edwards, C.C., editors: External fixation: the current state of the art, Baltimore, 1979, The Williams & Wilkins Co.)

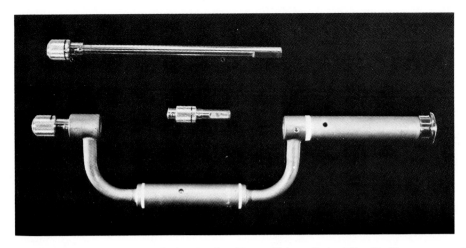

Fig. 7-24. Brace with assorted pin chucks. (From Fisher, D.A.: The Hoffman external fixator: technique of application. In Brooker, A.F., and Edwards, C.C., editors: External fixation: the current state of the art, Baltimore, 1979, The Williams & Wilkins Co.)

APPLICATION OF A MODULAR PIN FIXATOR (HOFFMANN APPARATUS)[2]
Components and instrumentation

Pins (Fig. 7-22). Transfixing pins of 4 mm diameter are available either with or without a centrally threaded portion. Recommended half pins are 4 mm in diameter with a continuously threaded tip or a split thread designed for cortical bone. All pins are designed to be self-drilling, self-tapping; however, predrilling is encouraged.

Clamps and connecting rods (Fig. 7-23). All pins in each group must be parallel to each other to be accommodated in the pin clamps. The pin clamps (universal ball joints) will hold up to five pins each. Depending on the type of external frame to be applied, a clamp with or without a short connecting post is used.

Connecting rods are 8 mm bars of either a simple type used on frames in either a neutralization or distraction mounting, or compression-distraction rods for the application of controlled compression or distraction.

An articulated coupling is an universal joint used to attach connecting rods to the bars of the pin clamps.

Drill brace (Fig. 7-24). The drill brace and either the regular or extended chuck are used for the manual insertion of all pins.

Pin guide (Fig. 7-25). Pins in each group are parallel. The extended guide assures parallel insertion and can be sprung open slightly to allow passage of the threaded portion of the transfixing pins.

T wrench. The wrench is used for final secure tightening of the components after application of the frame and reduction of the fracture.

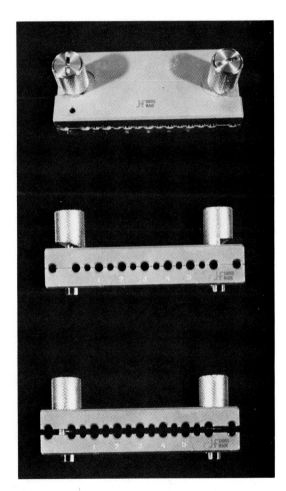

Fig. 7-25. Extended pin guide that may be opened slightly to allow passage of threaded portions of transfixing pins. (From Fisher, D.A.: The Hoffmann external fixator: technique of application. In Brooker, A.F., and Edwards, C.C., editors: External fixation: the current state of the art, Baltimore, 1979, The Williams & Wilkins Co.)

Steps of application

In the case of a modular pin fixator, adjustments in alignment are made after insertion of all pins and partial application of the external frame. Restoration of the length before pin insertion is necessary to avoid soft-tissue tethering over the pins, which will occur if the pins are placed through a shortened limb that is then suddenly restored to proper length.

The standard Vidal-Hoffmann frame is applied in three steps, as follows.

Step 1: Insertion of pin groups and partial application of frame. The insertion of transfixing pins is shown in Fig. 7-26. Using the guide after free-handing the insertion of the first pin in each group, one inserts the pins manually through the largest diameter of the bone. When more than two pins in a set are used, the proximal and distal pins of each group are inserted first, to assure ad-

APPLICATION OF A "MODULAR" EXTERNAL FIXATOR

Step 1: Pin insertion and partial application of frame

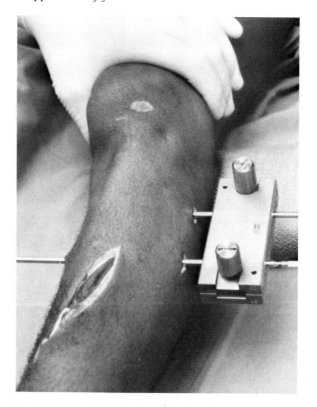

Fig. 7-26. Manual insertion of pins through extended guide. Note generous skin incisions. (From Fisher, D.A.: The Hoffmann external fixator: technique of application. In Brooker, A.F., and Edwards, C.C., editors: External fixation: the current state of the art, Baltimore, 1979, The Williams & Wilkins Co.)

equate location of all pins in the bone (Fig. 7-27). Generous skin incisions are made at both the entrance and exit sites of each pin. Pins are placed in the proximal and distal fragments. It is not necessary to place the proximal and distal groups of pins parallel to each other.

A pin clamp (universal ball joint) is applied to each set of pins (in this case, a pin clamp with a post) (Fig. 7-28). The clamp is securely tightened to the pins by use of the T wrench. Two connecting rods are placed in the ball joints but not tightened.

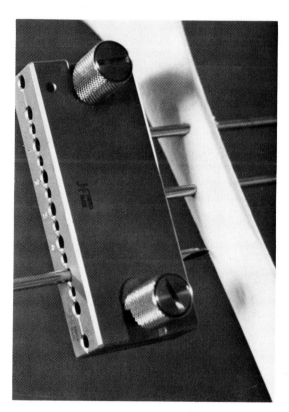

Fig. 7-27. Pins must be parallel. If neighboring pins are inserted first and are not in optimum location, the insertion of further pins may be either impossible or undesirable. (From Fisher, D.A.: The Hoffmann external fixator: technique of application. In Brooker, A.F., and Edwards, C.C., editors: External fixation: the current state of the art, Baltimore, 1979, The Williams & Wilkins Co.)

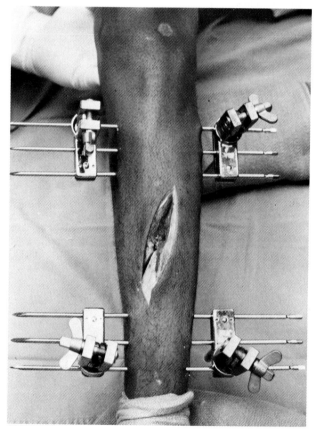

Fig. 7-28. Insertion of proximal and distal groups of pins completed. Ball joints with rods securely attached to each pin set.

Step 2: Reduction of fracture. The fracture is reduced manually and the universal joints are tightened to maintain reduction (Fig. 7-29). If the reduction is satisfactory, the universal joints are securely tightened by use of the T wrench.

Step 3: Completion of frame and adjustments of components. The Vidal-Hoffmann frame is completed by attachment of two more connecting rods to the bars on the pin holders by use of the articulated couplings. Final tightening of all components completes the frame application (Fig. 7-30).

After the frame has been tightened, only adjustments in compression or distraction are possible. Changes in displacement, rotation, and angulation must be done with the universal joints loosened.

The relationship of the pins to the universal joints is rigid with the frame tightened and attempts to correct angulation by adjustment of the lengths of the connecting rods without loosening of the universal joints will result in deformation of the pins and frame with little change in the angulation of the fracture (Fig. 7-31).

Step 2: Reduction

Step 3: Completion and adjustments

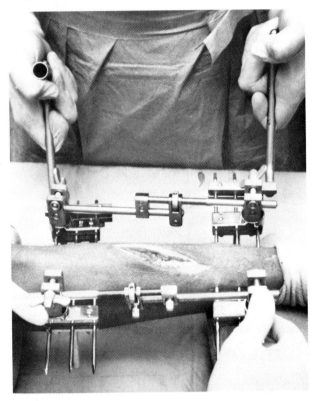

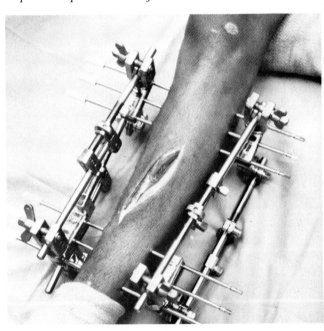

Fig. 7-30. Completed Vidal-Hoffmann frame.

Fig. 7-29. Two connecting rods have been loosely attached to the ball joints. The fracture is manually aligned and the ball joints are tightened. (From Fisher, D.A.: The Hoffmann external fixator: technique of application. In Brooker, A.F., and Edwards, C.C., editors: External fixation: the current state of the art, Baltimore, 1979, The Williams & Wilkins Co.)

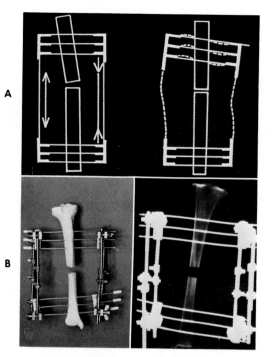

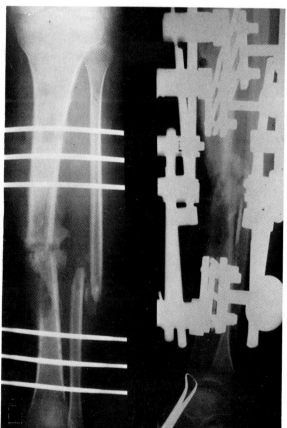

Fig. 7-31. A, Diagram of pin and frame deformation that will occur if an attempt is made to correct angulation by mechanically changing lengths of connecting rods after the frame is tightened. **B,** Observed deformation on model and roentgenogram. (From Fisher, D.A.: The Hoffmann external fixator: technique of application. In Brooker, A.F., and Edwards, C.C., editors: External fixation: the current state of the art, Baltimore, 1979, The Williams & Wilkins Co.)

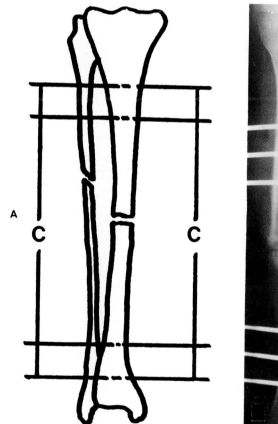

Fig. 7-32. A, Compression mode, *C.* **B,** Compression mode: hypertrophic nonunion. Note gentle bowing of transfixing pins.

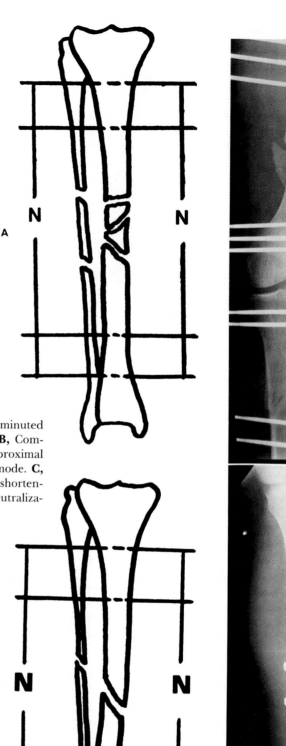

Fig. 7-33. A, Neutralization mode, *N*. Comminuted fracture. Compression will cause shortening. **B,** Comminuted fractures of the distal femur and proximal tibia are both maintained in a neutralization mode. **C,** Neutralization mode. Compression will cause shortening on displacement. **D,** Spiral fracture in neutralization mode.

All frames are mounted in one of the three modes: compression (Fig. 7-32), neutralization (Fig. 7-33), or distraction (Fig. 7-34). In the acute period, mechanical compression of a fracture is not possible when the frame is acting in either the neutralization or distraction mode because displacement or shortening will occur. During the phase of bone consolidation, light compression is possible and is recommended.

In the case of fractures amenable to early compression (primarily transverse fractures), compression by the fixator will add to the stability of the reduction. Do not overcompress. Permanent pin deformation can result easily when the mechanical advantage of the external bars is misused. The fracture should be compressed only until a gentle bowing is noted in the pins.

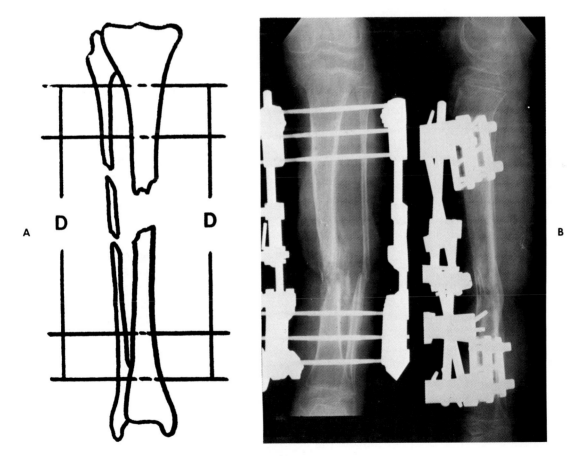

Fig. 7-34. A, Distraction mode, *D.* **B,** Bone loss with subsequent cancellous bone grafting of defect. Distraction mode. Defect is bridged, and at this time light compression is applied.

MAINTAINING A FIXATOR FRAME

After frame application, attention to detail in the management of the frame and injury may make the difference between a happy patient and surgeon and failure.

Soft tissue and adjacent uninvolved joint

The immediate postinjury and post–frame application period is characterized by soft-tissue pain and swelling. Inasmuch as the fracture is stabilized, the patients are comfortable as long as the soft tissue is rested also. During this time, which may last from a few days to a few weeks, the soft tissues are supported with soft dressings (Fig. 7-35). This applies to both the tissues directly injured and, in the case of the leg, the dependent posterior soft tissues.

The frame can be suspended directly from the fracture bed. This is comfortable for the patient and distributes the weight of the leg evenly through the frame. A simple modification of the frame will facilitate immobilization of the foot and ankle in a neutral position (Fig. 7-36) for patient comfort and to prevent an early equinus contracture.

After the initial swelling has subsided, the soft-tissue support may be removed. The footrest, however, is continued until the patient has regained strong active dorsiflexion.

During the period between resolution of the postinjury swelling and pain and until the patient is completely capable of maintaining a range-of-motion and exercise program independently, regular motion and exercise programs are performed under the direct supervision of the physical therapist and nursing staff (Fig. 7-37).

Pin care

Because of motion of muscle over the pins, a rather unremarkable serous drainage is observed wherever pins penetrate muscle. For this reason, drainage around pins in the thigh and lateral leg is always greater than around pins placed into the anteromedial tibia where the bone is subcutaneous. In the first few days after pin insertion, the drainage is a mixture of blood and serous fluid and may be substantial. During this period pin care may be necessary two or three times a day and gauze dressings are applied to absorb the fluid.

The important aspect of regular pin care is to thoroughly cleanse the pin-skin interface so that no accumulation of drainage occurs. Although cleansing may be necessary only on a daily basis after the first few days, all the serous and blood crusting must be completely removed (Fig. 7-38).

Skin tension on a pin must be avoided. This may happen simply as the swelling subsides. Skin tension is painful initially and local necrosis of the skin about the pin predisposes to infection.

Regular pin care is a patient responsibility and the patient is taught early how to care for the pins and to report the development of a tender pin site to the nursing or physician staff.

Normally a pin secure in bone with free drainage will not become infected.

However, the most frequent complication of external fixation is pin-tract infection. How do you handle an infected pin?

1. Check to be sure there is no skin tension around the pin. The skin may be infiltrated with local anesthetic and the tented skin incised generously.
2. Increase the frequency of the cleansings.
3. Temporarily decrease the activity of the patient to minimize muscle activity over the pin.
4. If the infection does not respond to this, the pin is most likely loose. The pin clamp is loosened, and the pin is lightly shaken by hand. If the pin is loose or this maneuver painful, the pin must be removed. Pin loosening with subsequent infection most commonly occurs as a result of two conditions:
   a. Excessive heat generation during pin insertion resulting in thermal necrosis of bone.
   b. Incorrect location of the pin, usually too anterior in the tibial shaft where the length of pin–to–bone contact is short because of the triangular shape of the tibia. Pin insertion through such dense cortical bone also generates excessive heat.
5. Systemic antibiotics may be useful in controlling localized cellulitis but will not be definitive if the pin is loose. Local antibacterial compounds containing iodine may be used routinely at the pin site. However, with long-term use many patients will develop a localized sensitivity to the iodine, which will appear as a tender reddened pin site. This will be noted at every pin site and clears rapidly when the iodine-containing compounds are discontinued.

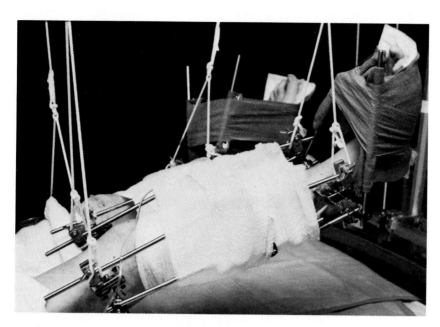

Fig. 7-35. Elevation and soft-tissue support in the immediate postinjury period.

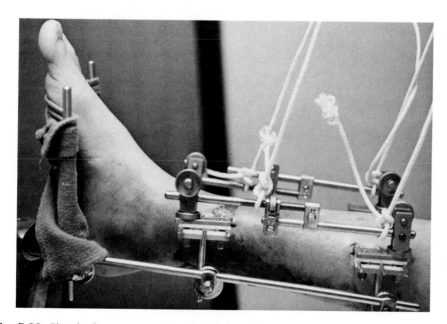

Fig. 7-36. Simple frame extension allows foot support. Frame may be suspended directly from overhead frame. (From Kryschyshen, P.L., and Fischer, D.A.: Am. J. Nurs. **80**(2):256, Feb. 1980.)

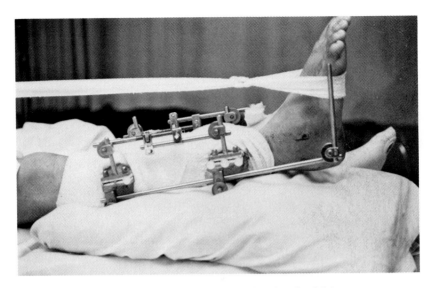

Fig. 7-37. Active mobilization of uninvolved joints.

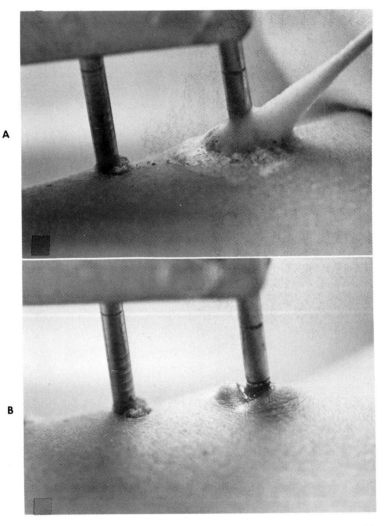

Fig. 7-38. A, By use of cotton applicators and hydrogen peroxide, the pin-skin interface is thoroughly cleansed. **B,** Pin has been cleansed. It may be left open to the air, or a porous local antibacterial may be applied.

Secondary bone and soft-tissue procedures performed in a frame

If possible, the initial placement of the pins and frame should be such as to interfere as little as possible with subsequent procedures. Extremities stabilized in fixators can be treated with a Whirlpool regularly for soft-tissue care. This also keeps the frames clean. A large surgical adhesive drape can be used to isolate the frame at the time of major secondary procedures.

REFERENCES TO PART C

1. Behrens, F.: The "tubular system"—an ASIF external fixator. In Mears, D.C., editor: External skeletal fixation, Baltimore, 1981, The Williams & Wilkins Co.
2. Fischer, D.A.: The Hoffmann external fixator: technique of application. In Brooker, A.F., and Edwards, C.C.: External fixation: the current state of the art, Baltimore, 1979, The Williams & Wilkins Co.

Part D

Soft-tissue coverage

RICHARD E. JONES III, M.D.
Dallas, Texas

Complex open fractures are complicated by a high rate of osteomyelitis, nonunion, and delayed union. These injuries result from high-energy forces, which cause significant comminution, displacement, and extensive soft-tissue damage with associated skin loss, all of which complicate treatment regimens. The principles of care of open fractures[2] rightly emphasize that management of the soft-tissue wound is of primary concern. The concept of the open fracture wound,[4] which involves the skin, fascia, muscle, periosteum, and bone, is the key to the understanding of wound healing in these complex injuries. In the complex open fracture there is a lag phase during which restoration of the viable soft-tissue envelope must be accomplished before hard-tissue healing can begin.[3] Although methods of treatment for complex open fractures such as debridement and healing by secondary granulation tissue or skin grafting over such tissue may provide satisfactory early results, this mode of therapy frequently yields unstable soft-tissue cover. The skin is adherent to bone, particularly in the pretibial area, and this is susceptible to recurrent trauma and breakdown. Additionally, when such methods fail, the serious problem of exposed, dead cortical bone, exposed tendinous or neurovascular structures, and diminished blood supply to adjacent tissues all severely compromise the treatment outcome.

METHODS

The treatment options available for soft-tissue coverage of open fractures with severe soft-tissue damage include débridement and stimulation of secondary granulation tissue, relaxing incisions, local rotational flaps, split-thickness skin graft, local muscle or myocutaneous flaps, cross-leg pedicle flaps, and distant free flaps.

Split-thickness skin grafts can be applied to a bone that has granulation tissue. Cortical bone, denuded of its periosteum as a result of extensive comminution, will not accept a free skin graft. In the best of circumstances, successful split-thickness skin-graft cover provides an unstable scar, adherent to bone and vulnerable to breakdown when exposed to direct trauma.

Rotational flaps can occasionally be used, but again, because of the local effects of trauma, the skin is frequently damaged. Additionally, in the leg the skin is relatively avascular overlying the medial aspect of the tibia, further compromising skin viability.

Local myoplasty or myocutaneous flaps offer the best solution at this time to soft-tissue coverage to type III tibial open fracture wounds (Table 7-3). External skeletal stabilization[5] is clearly indicated for these high-energy fractures to decrease dead space and provide ready access for wound care. Further, extensive additional periosteal stripping is avoided if internal fixation is not used. The early provision of a viable soft-tissue envelope about the fracture site encourages and accelerates bone healing by providing a favorable mes-

Table 7-3. Myoplasty/myocutaneous coverage

Site of soft-tissue defect	Soft tissue transposed
Tibia–proximal third	Gastrocnemius, medial soleus
Tibia–proximal/middle junction	Gastrocnemius, soleus
Tibia–middle third	Gastrocnemius, soleus
Tibia–middle/distal junction	Soleus
	Flexor digitorum longus
Tibia–distal third	Flexor digitorum longus
	Peroneus; distal soleus

enchymal milieu.[9] Transposition of local muscle flaps accomplishes early coverage of exposed bone, tendons, or joint, or neurovascular structures while introducing a viable soft-tissue envelope to the area of the fracture. This promotes healing, combats infection, and can provide an excellent vascular bed for a split-thickness skin graft. The open fracture is converted to a closed fracture and a live wound is created and maintained to enhance and hasten the healing of both the soft and hard tissues.

SURGICAL ANATOMY

A review of the surgical anatomy and surgical technique for utilization of gastrocnemius and soleus muscles in providing coverage of the upper and middle third of the tibia is presented here.

Particularly in the distal portion of the leg, the skin receives its blood supply from segmental vessels that penetrate from the underlying muscle fascia.[7] This anatomic pattern provides the basic for myocutaneous flaps. If the skin is already traumatized by severe injury, loss of an entire skin flap is an all too frequent complication of careless blunt dissection through the skin and fascia plane.

The gastrocnemius muscle is covered by deep fascia that separates it medially from the saphenous vein. Proximally the sural nerve (white line of Henry) passes between the two heads of the gastrocnemius, piercing the deep fascia in the midline to accompany the short saphenous vein. The two heads of the gastrocnemius remain separate until their tendinous insertion distally. The vascular supply is independent to each head and the vascular hila are constantly located at the level of the tibial tubercle.

Deep to the gastrocnemius is the soleus muscle, which rises from the proximal aspect of the fibula and the middle third of the posteromedial border of the tibia. Proximally the gastrocnemius and soleus are separated by a fascial layer, and distally the aponeuroses of the two muscles merge to form the Achilles tendon. The blood supply to the soleus is segmental and based upon the popliteal, the peroneal, and posterior tibial arteries. A distinct fascia separates the soleus from the underlying neurovascular bundle and deeper muscles of the posterior compartment, and this fascia protects the bundle during dissection.

SURGICAL TECHNIQUES
Soleus myoplasty flap

A long, vertical, medial incision (Fig. 7-39) is made from the level of the tibial tubercle to the distal third of the tibia and situated between the posterior medial border of the tibia and the ten-

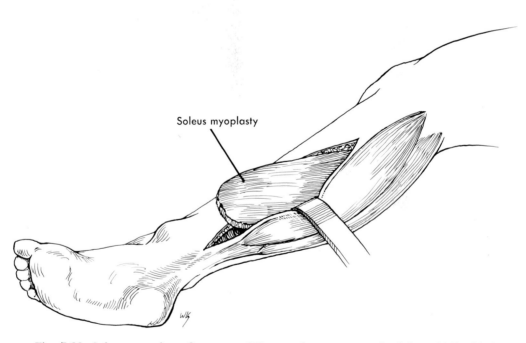

Soleus myoplasty

Fig. 7-39. Soleus myoplasty for a type III open fracture wound of the middle third tibia.

docalcaneus.[1] In the distal segment of the wound the deep fascia is incised and the tendocalcaneus is identified. To avoid confusion with the gastrocnemius, dissection is continued proximally to identify the plantaris tendon and the medial head of the gastrocnemius superficial to the soleus. The muscle fibers are sharply separated from the deep surface of the Achilles tendon and the gastrocnemius muscle is retracted laterally. The distal pedicles from the posterior tibial artery are identified and ligated, and the muscle is mobilized from distal to proximal after sharp detachment of the fibers from the Achilles tendon, approximately 3 cm distal to the most distal muscle fibers. Stay sutures should be placed in the lower end of the muscle and the dissection continued proximally, defining the anterior border of the muscle. Stay sutures should also be placed at the gastrocnemius-skin interface to prevent separation and

damage to the skin vasculature. When sufficient muscle is mobilized, the muscle is rotated forward to cover the defect. The muscle is then sutured into the freshened skin edges, and hemostasis is accomplished. The donor skin defect can usually be closed primarily and a meshed split-thickness skin graft[6] can be immediately applied to the muscle (Fig. 7-40).

Gastrocnemius myoplasty flap

The medial gastrocnemius may be transposed as a muscle or a musculocutaneous unit to cover the middle or the upper third of the tibia. A medial longitudinal incision is made along the posterior border of the tibia from the tibial condyle to the distal third of the leg. The gastrocnemius is identified and separated from the soleus muscle in the raphe between the medial and lateral heads. It is also identified and divided from distal

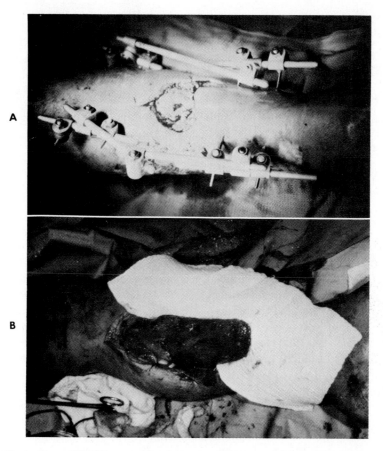

Fig. 7-40. A, Type III tibia open fracture wound with large soft-tissue defect stabilized by external fixation. **B,** Soleus muscle detached from tendocalcaneus and mobilized.

Continued.

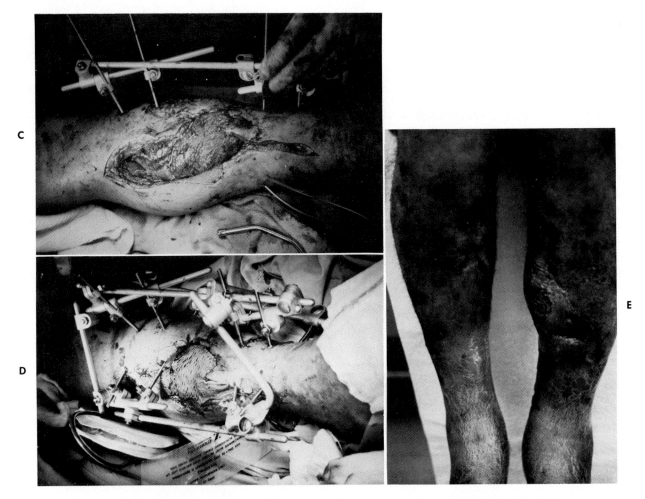

Fig. 7-40, cont'd. C, Soleus muscle transposed anteriorly to cover soft-tissue defect. **D,** Soleus myoplasty with meshed split-thickness skin graft immediately applied and external fixation converted to biplane to enhance stability. **E,** Appearance of leg at time of fracture union 13 weeks after myoplasty and 14 weeks after injury.

to proximal. Fibers are also separated from the Achilles tendon, and this requires a sharp resection. The muscle is elevated to the level of the tibial condyles where the arc of rotation is generally adequate for anterior tibial coverage. If a greater arc of rotation is necessary, the unit can be elevated. The primary vascular trunk that enters the muscle at the level of the tibial tubercle should be protected. Additionally, the muscle can be tunneled under the skin to enable more lateral cover. However, this is not recommended because the skin tunnel may be devascularized or compression from the skin bridge may occur.

The lateral head of the gastrocnemius can be elevated in a similar manner with a lateral, vertical

incision. In elevating the lateral head, one needs to take caution in the proximal area of the dissection to identify and protect the peroneal nerve.

If the donor defect cannot be primarily closed, skin grafting should be performed. The muscle can be grafted with meshed split-thickness skin immediately, or skin may be taken at the time of operation and delayed split coverage of the muscle can be performed.

Either medial or lateral gastrocnemius can be taken as a musculocutaneous unit.[8] Because the compound myocutaneous gastrocnemius flap is as simple to do as a gastrocnemius local muscle flap, the myocutaneous flap is preferred in most situations. Both the medial and the lateral head of the

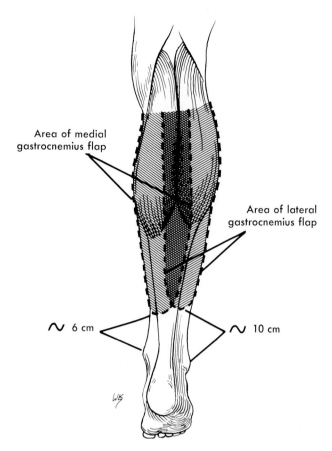

Area of medial
gastrocnemius flap

Area of lateral
gastrocnemius flap

∿ 6 cm   ∿ 10 cm

Fig. 7-41. Cutaneous borders of gastrocnemius myocutaneous flap, posterior view.

gastrocnemius directly supply all the overlying skin. Additionally the skin distal to each head of the gastrocnemius can be carried on this musculocutaneous unit to a distance approximately equal to the width of each head (Fig. 7-41). McGraw has specifically defined the medial gastrocnemius myocutaneous flap as supplying an area of skin distal to the muscle that extends to the midline posteriorly to a point some 6 cm proximal to the medial malleolus, distally and anteriorly extending downward from the anterior border of the muscle (Fig. 7-42). The lateral gastrocnemius myocutaneous flap will carry a skin area with the medial margin in the midline posteriorly, with the anterior margin overlapping the fibula and extending distally to a point some 10 cm above the lateral malleolus. It is important to note that the lateral myocutaneous gastrocnemius flap does not include the skin over the anterior compartment, proximally and distally, which is supplied by the peroneal artery (Fig. 7-43).

The surgical technique of elevation of either medial or lateral gastrocnemius myocutaneous flap is similar (Fig. 7-44). The muscle is outlined as are the anterior, posterior, and distal borders of the skin flap (Fig. 7-45, *A* to *C*). The distal segment of skin is elevated with the deep fascia leaving a bared Achilles tendon (Fig. 7-45, *D*). It is important to include the fascia because the viability of the flap depends on the extensive arcades penetrating to the skin from the fascia. Care is taken to avoid injury to either the sural nerve or the saphenous nerve or vein. The gastrocnemius must then be isolated from the soleus muscle and stay sutures are placed in the skin and muscle-fascial margins to maintain continuity of the unit. The two heads of the gastrocnemius are sharply separated, and the sural nerve must be protected at this juncture. The vascular pedicle is located at the level of the tibial tubercle and of course must be protected. The flap is then rotated into place and sutured into the freshened skin edges. The

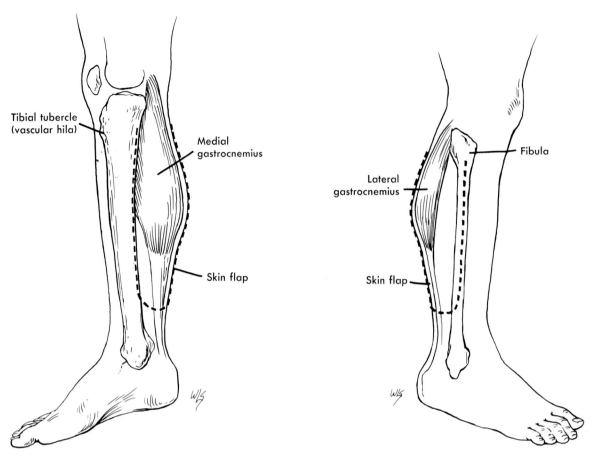

Fig. 7-42. Cutaneous border of gastrocnemius myocutaneous flap, medial view.

Fig. 7-43. Cutaneous border of gastrocnemius myocutaneous flap, lateral view.

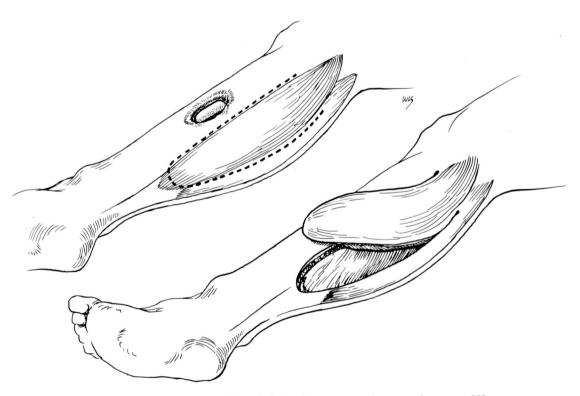

Fig. 7-44. Myocutaneous flap of medial head gastrocnemius covering type III open fracture wound of middle third of tibia .

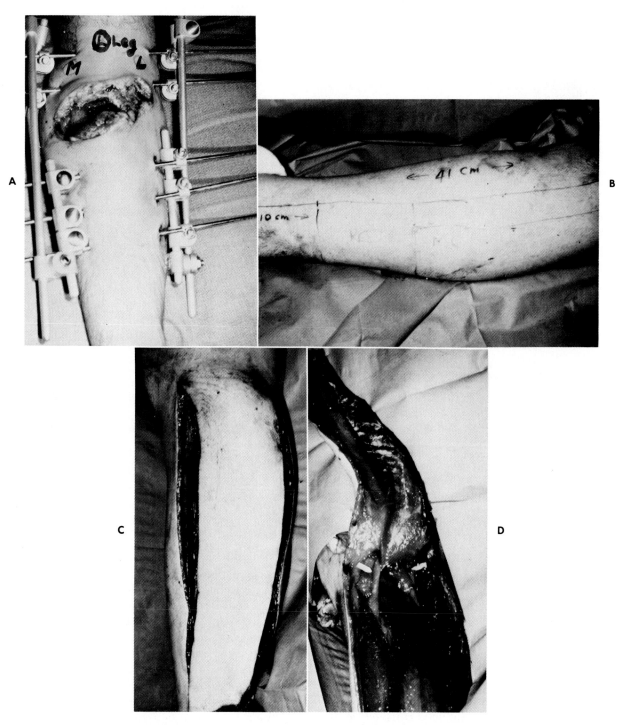

Fig. 7-45. A, Appearance of soft-tissue defect 6 days after injury and débridement of type III proximal tibia open fracture wound. **B,** Cutaneous borders of lateral gastrocnemius myocutaneous flap outlined. **C,** Flap incision as outlined in **B. D,** Composite lateral gastrocnemius flap elevated. Note top marker on lateral gastrocnemius vascular hilum and bottom marker on medial gastrocnemius vascular pedicle.

Continued.

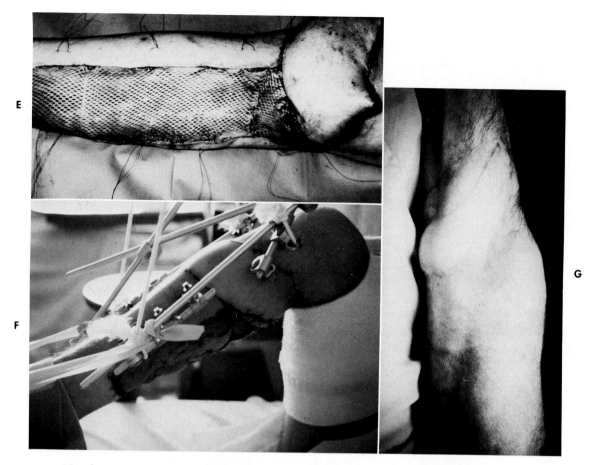

Fig. 7-45, cont'd. E, Composite flap sutured in place over soft-tissue defect with meshed split-thickness skin graft over donor area. **F,** Appearance of leg 2 weeks after soft-tissue coverage. Note external fixation and knee mobility. **G,** Appearance of leg at time of fracture union 12 weeks after myocutaneous coverage and 13 weeks after injury.

donor defect is covered with meshed split-thickness skin graft (Fig. 7-45, *E*).

The medial gastrocnemius myocutaneous flap can resurface the entire middle and upper pretibial areas and will reach as much as 15 cm proximal to the knee joint either anteriorly or posteriorly. The lateral flap does not have the same excursion but can readily cover proximal and anterior defects with upward mobility only some 10 cm above the knee joint (Fig. 7-45, *F* and *G*).

The fluorescein test should be performed intraoperatively to assure viability of the transposed skin. Fluorescein (5 to 10 mg/kg) is injected intravenously. Fifteen minutes later, under Wood's lamp, ultraviolet fluorescence of the skin indicates the areas of viable skin. Dark-skinned patients should receive the upper-range dose levels. The test can be repeated every 8 to 12 hours.

Distant flaps

Cross-leg pedicle flaps should be moved with muscle as well as skin (Fig. 7-46). The muscle creates a good vascular envelope around the fracture. Cross-leg flaps are particularly useful when the myocutaneous territories of the posterior leg have been violated or severely damaged by the initial trauma. External skeletal fixation of the limb permits complete mobility of the joints above and below the pedicled cross-leg flap.

Distant free flaps, particularly composite grafts, are useful when there is segmental loss of bone. These must be performed with microvascular anastomosis. The provision of viable bone with intact periosteum, muscular feeding vessels, and overlying skin has proved to be a significant advance in the treatment of complex open wounds (Fig. 7-47).

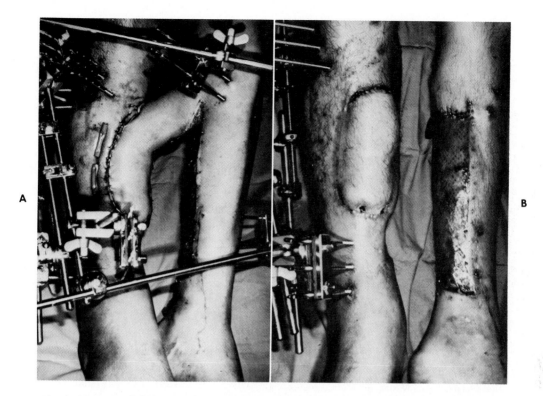

Fig. 7-46. A, Pedicled, cross-leg, medial gastrocnemius myocutaneous flap for coverage of type III open fracture wound. **B,** Flap in place at time of pedicle severance.

Fig. 7-47. Appearance of arm in a 10-year-old youth 4 months after iliac wing composite free flap for segmental defect of radius after type III shotgun open fracture wound.

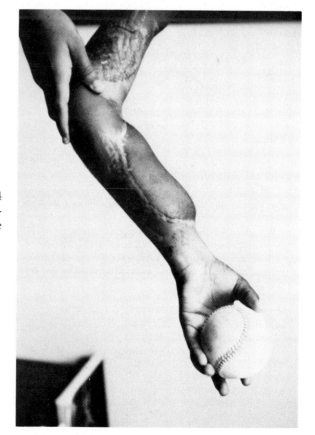

SUMMARY

Soft-tissue coverage of major defects in the lower extremity can readily be performed by the orthopedic surgeon. If there is a cooperative spirit between the orthopedic surgical specialist and a plastic surgical specialist, consultation should be encouraged. Early assessment of the open fracture wound should have a goal of creating and maintaining a live wound with conversion to a closed wound by soft-tissue coverage procedures as early as possible. Aggressive provision of soft-tissue coverage can be readily combined with stable external skeletal fixation to vastly improve the outcome of complex open fractures.

REFERENCES TO PART D

1. Ger, R.: The management of open fracture of the tibia with skin loss, J. Trauma **10:**112-212, 1970.
2. Gregory, C.F.: Open fractures. In Rockwood, C., and Green, D., editors: Fractures, Philadelphia, 1975, J.B. Lippincott Co.
3. Holden, C.E.: The role of blood supply to soft tissue in the healing of diaphyseal fractures, J. Bone Joint Surg. **54A:**993-1000, 1972.
4. Jones, R.E., and Cierny, G.C.: Management of complex open tibial fractures with external skeletal fixation and early myoplasty or myocutaneous coverage, Can. J. Surg. **23:**242-244, May 1980.
5. Karlström, G., and Olerud, S.: Percutaneous pin fixation of open tibial fractures, J. Bone Joint Surg. **57A:**915-924, 1975.
6. Kojima, T., Kohno, T., and Ito, T.: Muscle flap with simultaneous mesh skin graft for skin defects of the lower leg, J. Trauma **19:**724-729, 1979.
7. McCraw, J.B., and Dibbell, D.G.: Experimental definition of independent myocutaneous vascular territories, Plast. Reconstr. Surg. **60:**212-220, 1977.
8. McCraw, J.B., et al.: The versatile gastrocnemius myocutaneous flap, Plast. Reconstr. Surg. **62:**15, 1978.
9. Rosenthal, R.E., et al.: Non-union in open tibial fractures: analysis of reasons for failure of treatment, J. Bone Joint Surg. **59A:**244-248, 1977.

ADDITIONAL READINGS

Barfred, T., and Rumert, T.: Myoplasty for covering exposed bone or joint on the lower leg, Acta Orthop. Scand. **44:**532-538, 1973.
Daniel, R.K., and Kerrigan, C.L.: Skin flaps: anatomical and hemodynamic approach, Clin. Plast. Surg. **6:**181-200, 1979.
Ger, R.: The technique of muscle transposition in the operative treatment of traumatic and ulcerative lesions of the leg, J. Trauma **11:**502-510, 1971.
Mathes, S.J., and Nahai, F.: Clinical atlas of muscle and musculocutaneous flaps, St. Louis, 1979, The C.V. Mosby Co.
McCraw, J.B.: Selection of alternative local flaps in the leg and foot, Clin. Plast. Surg. **6:**227, 1979.
Pers, M., and Medgyesi, S.: Pedicle muscle flaps and their applications in the surgery of repair, Br. J. Plast. Surg. **26:**313-321, 1973.
Townsend, P.L.G.: An inferiorly based soleus muscle flap, Br. J. Plast. Surg. **31:**210-213, 1978.

Part E

Bone grafting: general principles and use in open fractures

FRED BEHRENS, M.D., F.R.C.S.(C)
St. Paul, Minnesota

BASIC APPROACH TO OPEN FRACTURES

After a patient has been admitted with an open fracture, which is by definition always contaminated, it is the surgeon's foremost task to *obtain and preserve a clean wound.* This is usually achieved by the following:

1. Radical débridement of dead tissue
2. Dressing the wound open with gauze soaked in antiseptic solutions
3. Systemic antibiotics

If because of improper identification of dead tissue this process is repeated too often, secondary colonization of the wound with resistant organisms will often ensue. Inserting bone graft, which consists of partially dead tissue, into such a contaminated bed and closing the soft tissues over it will invariably lead to suppuration and loss of the graft.

Frequently the need for bone grafting becomes apparent early in the treatment period. If this is the case, we prefer to carry out the soft-tissue and bony reconstruction during the initial hospitalization. The sequence of interventions is generally:

1. Application of an external fixator to gain stability of the wound, facilitate débridement, and promote soft-tissue and bone healing.
2. Soft-tissue coverage of the exposed bone ends.
3. Placement of the bone graft.

On occasion, a nonunion will develop during the latter part of the treatment course. As soon as this is apparent and once other treatment options as rigid internal fixation have been considered, the nonunion site should be grafted in order not to protract the healing process unnecessarily.

SOURCES OF BONE GRAFTS

Allografts are rarely used in posttraumatic reconstruction. In the injured patient two principle sources of bone graft are available (Fig. 7-48).

□ Supported by Grant 8263 from the Medical Education and Research Foundation, St. Paul–Ramsey Hospital, St. Paul, Minnesota.

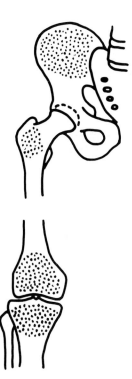

Fig. 7-48. Main sources of graft bone: iliac crests and metaphyses of long bones.

Iliac crests. Although more graft material generally can be obtained from the posterior crests, the anterior parts are generally better accessible when one is working on an extremity.

Metaphyses. The metaphyses of all long bones are ideal to obtain cancellous material, particularly the greater trochanter, the proximal tibia, and the distal femur. They contain large amounts of bone and frequently lie in the operating field.

TYPES OF BONE GRAFTS

Graft bone may be obtained in different shapes and consistencies.

Cancellous chips and strips. This type has the best osteogenic potential, frequently contains live osteoblasts, and only on rare occasions acts as a foreign body in the graft bed.

Corticocancellous strips. These are harvested from the iliac crest (Fig. 7-49) as about 2 mm thick slivers that consist of cancellous bone sandwiched between two cortical strips, contributed by the inner and outer iliac tables (Fig. 7-50).

Cortical struts. Cortical struts are generally whole or longitudinally cut fibulas. They were popular in the past for their mechanical properties but have been largely replaced by metal implents, external fixators, and free vascularized bone grafts. Their osteogenic properties are unsatisfactory.

Vascularized bone grafts. On rare occasions, medial transposition of the ipsilateral fibula on its vascular pedicle has been used for the management of segmental tibial defects.

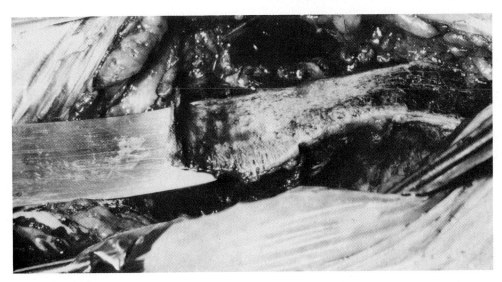

Fig. 7-49. Harvesting of corticocancellous strips from anterior iliac crest. (Copyright Dr. F. Behrens.)

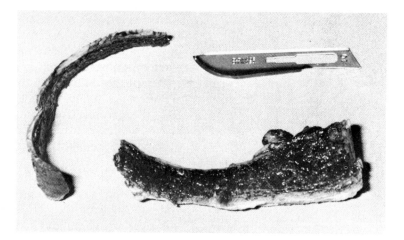

Fig. 7-50. Corticocancellous strips: 3 to 5 cm long, 1 to 2 mm thick. (Copyright Dr. F. Behrens.)

Free vascularized bone grafts have been pioneered by Östrup and co-workers[2] and Taylor and co-workers[4] and represent a major advance in the grafting of large bony defects. The donor bone is isolated on its vascular pedicle and can then be transferred to the recipient site anywhere in the body where the vessels can be reattached by microsurgical technique.

The following sources and transfers have been described[3]:

Free vascularized bone grafts. Sources include fibula, ribs, and iliac crests. Only the bone with some of the surrounding soft tissue is transferred.

Free osteocutaneous flaps. These contain bone, the overlying skin, and subcutaneous tissue and are transferred in connection with a rib or iliac crest.

Free osteocutaneous neurovascular flaps. Such flaps contain in addition to bone the sensory supply to the transferred skin. The bony base can be a rib or an iliac crest.

INDICATIONS FOR VARIOUS BONE-GRAFTING PROCEDURES
Nonunions

Established nonunions. *Hypertrophic* nonunions can be successfully treated by rigid fixation (internal or external) or by bone grafting alone. In the treatment of *hypotrophic* nonunions, the combination of bone grafting and rigid fixation has been most successful.

Among the various recommended grafting procedures for the treatment of established nonunions, the creation of osteoperiosteal flaps in-

volving two thirds of the bone's circumference is preferred.[1] Cancellous strips are then laid between these flaps and the cortical bone (Fig. 7-51).

Prospective nonunions. We have found that certain fracture characteristics frequently predict the development of nonunions. They (Fig. 7-52) include the following:
1. Fractures with comminuted and displaced butterfly fragments
2. Partial or complete cortical bone loss
3. Severely displaced fractures with extensive soft-tissue stripping

We believe that much time can be saved if prophylactic bone grafting is carried out during the initial admission. The following techniques have been successful:
1. *Metaphyseal fractures.* Cancellous chips and strips.
2. *Diaphyseal fractures.* Elevation of periosteal flaps about 3 cm proximal and distal to the fracture site and placement of long overlapping cancellous strips.

Bony defects

Partial-thickness metaphyseal and diaphyseal defects. These pose similar technical problems as prospective nonunions and are treated according to the same guidelines.

Full-thickness metaphyseal defects. Such defects rarely exceed 5 cm in length. Shortening may be a part of the reconstructive procedure but should not exceed 1.5 cm in the lower extremity. When the central part of the defect is filled with

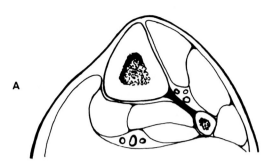

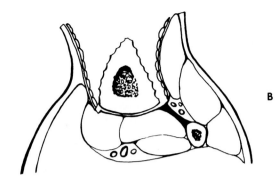

Fig. 7-51. Osteoperiosteal bone graft. **A,** Tibial cross-section. **B,** Elevation of osteoperiosteal flaps from medial and lateral tibial surfaces. Transsection of periosteum at posteromedial and posterolateral corners to make room for cancellous bone graft. **C,** Closure after insertion of cancellous strips between osteoperiosteal flaps and tibial cortices.

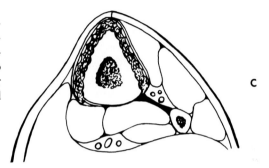

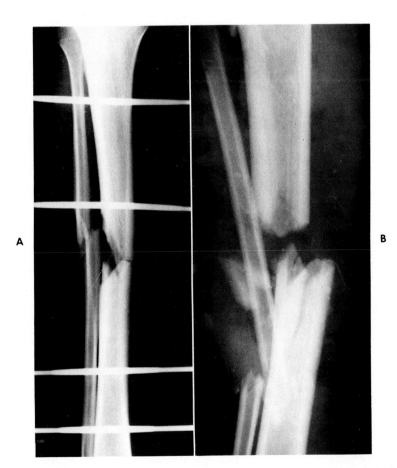

Fig. 7-52. Prospective nonunions. **A,** Partial bone loss. **B,** Large soft-tissue lesion, circumferential periosteal stripping. (Copyright Dr. F. Behrens.)

cancellous chips and the peripheral confines are maintained with corticocancellous strips, consolidation ensues generally without difficulty and maintains the original shape of the bone.

Full-thickness cortical defects

Upper extremity. In the humerus, considerable shortening can be accepted without significant loss of function. If the defect involves the radius and ulna, length is often maintained by use of internal fixation in the form of a plate because external fixators tend to be too cumbersome. Gaps are filled with cancellous grafting material, which may have to be applied repeatedly.[5]

Lower extremity. For defects between 2 and 5 cm Weber and Cěch[6] has proposed corticocancellous pegs stabilized in compression and covered with cancellous chips or corticocancellous strips. Defects exceeding 5 cm in length have in the past been treated with a combination of free fibular struts and cancellous grafts. If the fibula is intact, large tibial defects can be bridged in a 2-step procedure (Fig. 7-53). Initially a proximal and distal tibiofibular synostosis is created, and the remaining gap is subsequently filled with cancellous graft.[6,7]

Large combined segmental defects of tibia and fibula, particularly when they are accompanied by neurovascular lesions, are often best managed with an amputation in the elderly. If the appropriate facilities are available, however, a free vascularized bone graft or composite flap should be considered in the younger patient.[3]

REFERENCES TO PART E

1. Forbes, D.B.: Subcortical iliac bone grafts in fractures of the tibia, J. Bone Joint Surg. **43B:**672-679, 1961.
2. Östrup, L.T., and Fredrickson, J.M.: Distant transfer of a free living bone graft by microvascular anastomosis: an experimental study, Plast. Reconstr. Surg. **55:**563, 1975.
3. Serafin, D., and Buncke, H.J., editors: Microsurgical composite tissue, St. Louis, 1979, The C.V. Mosby Co.
4. Taylor, G.I., Miller, G.D., and Ham, F.: The free vascularized bone graft: a clinical extension of microvascular techniques, Plast. Reconstr. Surg. **55:**533, 1975.
5. Vidal, J., Buscayret, C.H., Connes, H., Paran, M., and Allieu, Y.: Traitement des fractures ouvertes de jambe par le fixateur externe en double cadre, Rev. Chir. Orthop. **62:**433-448, 1976.
6. Weber, B.G., and Cěch, O.: Pseudarthrosis: pathophysiology, biomechanics, therapy results, New York, 1976, Grune & Stratton, Inc.
7. Weinberg, H., Roth, V.G., Robin, G.C., and Floman, Y.: Early fibular bypass procedures (tibiofibular synostosis) for massive bone loss in war injuries, J. Trauma **19:**177-181, 1979.

Part F

External fixation in open fractures

TIBIA

FRED BEHRENS, M.D., F.R.C.S.(C)
St. Paul, Minnesota

Presently about 70% of all external fixators are used in the management of open tibial fractures. Other indications include infected nonunions, severely comminuted closed fracture of diaphysis and metaphyses, and typically unstable fractures 5 to 12 cm proximal to the ankle joint.

ANATOMIC AND CLINICAL CONSIDERATIONS

When compared with other long bones, the tibia is unique because less than two thirds of its circumference is covered by a well-vascularized muscle envelope. Thus injuries of only moderate severity can lead to massive skin avulsions and the development of large soft-tissue flaps of doubtful

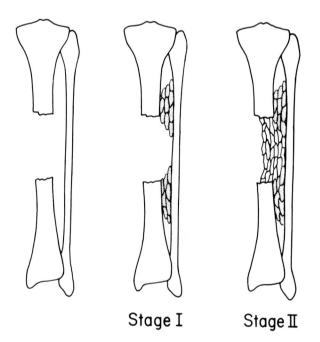

Stage I   Stage II

Fig. 7-53. Bridging of segmental tibial loss. *Stage I,* Creation of tibiofibular synostosis; *stage II,* augmentation of bone mass through second grafting procedure.

□ Supported by Grant 8263 from the Medical Education and Research Foundation, St. Paul–Ramsey Hospital, St. Paul, Minnesota.

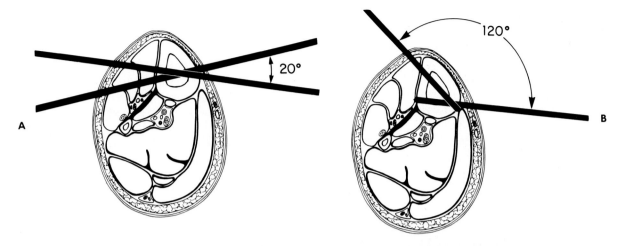

Fig. 7-54. Extreme angles of pin insertion. **A,** Transfixion pins. **B,** Half pins. (Copyright Dr. F. Behrens.)

viability. Bone ends maybe circumferentially denuded of periosteum for a distance of several centimeters. It is therefore not surprising that most bone grafts and secondary soft-tissue procedures are carried out in this region. Early assessment of the healing potential of the injured tissues is paramount as it will influence pin placement and optimal fixator frame, as well as the nature and sequence of secondary procedures.

In its proximal part, the tibia is triangular in shape. Pin purchase in bone is therefore optimal if the insertion site lies close to the posterior cortex. The anteromedial surface of the tibia is ideal for pin insertion because the close adherence of the skin to the bone reduces motion between the two tissues and therefore pin drainage.

Presently most tibial frames are of type 2 design, which is characterized by the insertion of multiple pins into the proximal fourth and distal fourth of the tibia. Unfortunately, the use of *transfixion pins* limits the angle of pin insertion severely (Fig. 7-54) and predisposes to a number of disturbing complications:

Anterior compartment syndrome. Although only recently described in the French literature,[6] this complication appears to be not uncommon, particularly when the lateral soft tissues are depressed during pin insertion. Experimentally the same workers have shown that the insertion of two transfixion pins into the proximal one third of the tibia will lead to an average increase in anterior compartment pressure of 15 mm Hg.[5]

Injury to anterior tibial artery. In the distal two fifths of the tibia, this vessel lies in contact with

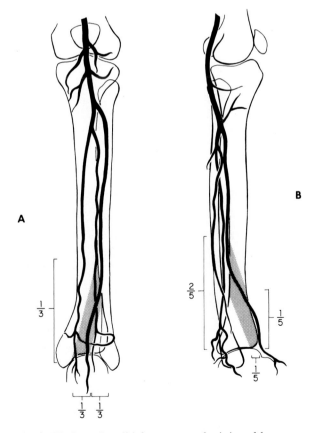

Fig. 7-55. Anterior tibial artery can be injured by transfixion or half pins in distal one third of tibia. **A,** Frontal view. **B,** Lateral view. (Copyright Dr. F. Behrens.)

the bone. It courses from a posterolateral position to lie midway between the two malleoli where it crosses the ankle joint (Fig. 7-55). Although injuries by transfixion pins have been proved angiographically, half pins could possibly have a similar effect.[6]

Injury to posterior tibial neurovascular bundle. These structures lie close to the posterior border of the tibia and are easily injured when a pin slips suddenly posteriorly during insertion. Because the disruption of one neurovascular bundle

may occur in severe leg injuries, iatrogenic interruption of the remaining arterial blood supply can be disastrous.[7]

Transfixion of anterior and lateral musculotendinous units. Transfixion of these structures will not only decrease ankle excursion while the pins are in place but often lead to residual ankle stiffness as well.[2] Regardless of the pins used, early splinting followed by active range-of-motion exercises is paramount in the prevention of this complication (Fig. 7-56).

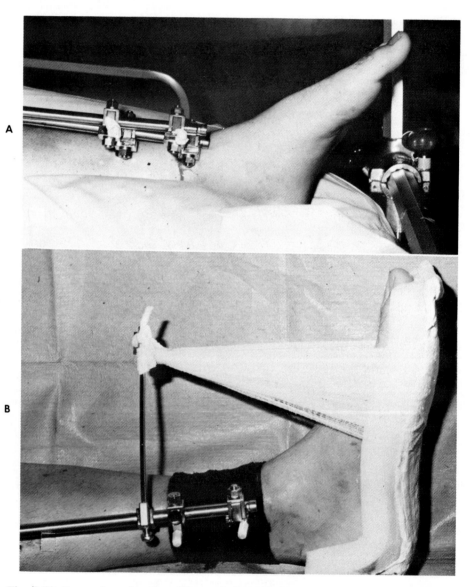

Fig. 7-56. Prevention of ankle stiffness. **A,** In a supine patient, gravitational forces pull foot in equinus. **B,** Until patient regains active ankle motion, splinting at 5 degrees of dorsiflexion is optimal. (Copyright Dr. F. Behrens.)

APPLICATION OF FIXATOR

Pin placement. Many of the severely comminuted proximal tibial fractures, even when they have intra-articular extensions, show a surprisingly well preserved articular alignment. We have found repeatedly that pin insertion into the subchondral tibial bone provides good purchase and stabilizes a rather tenuous situation. Closeness to a moving joint, however, tends to increase pin drainage. Meticulous pin care is therefore mandatory.

The tibial diaphysis provides excellent purchase for the pins, whereas pin placement near the ankle joint is made rather difficult by the many important surrounding structures.

Frame designs

Type 2 frames. Type 2 frames, mainly in the form of the Vidal-Hoffmann configuration, are presently most popular. This design was proposed in the late 1960s by Vidal and co-workers,[7] who believed that the unilateral frame with one connecting rod, as used by Hoffmann, was not rigid enough to provide adequate stability for the management of severe open fractures, particularly when they were accompanied by bone loss or extensive comminution. Despite the increased rigidity of type 2 frames, it is well to remember that they are about three times less stiff in anteroposterior than in lateral bending.[1] Type 2 frames can be left in place for up to 8 months or longer with only a minimal increase in pin-tract problems.[4,7] Full weight-bearing, however, is advisable only with caution.

Type 1 frames. Burny[2] and Jorgensen[3] have accumulated a vast experience with unilateral Hoffmann frames, which they use mainly in uncomplicated—often closed—tibial fractures. It is their contention that many of the delayed unions seen with type 2 frames are caused by the excessive rigidity of these frames. They generally keep their

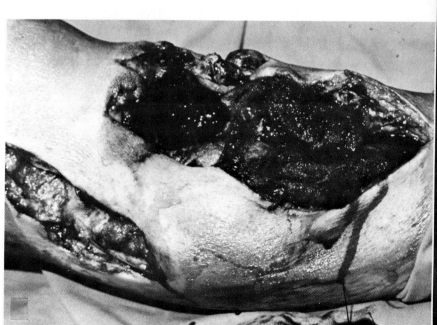
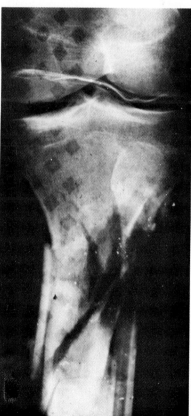

Fig. 7-57. A, Massive lateral soft-tissue and bone loss after gunshot wound. **B,** Radiographic appearance. Immobilization of injured area through medially applied external fixator. (See Fig. 7-9, *B*.) (Copyright Dr. F. Behrens.)

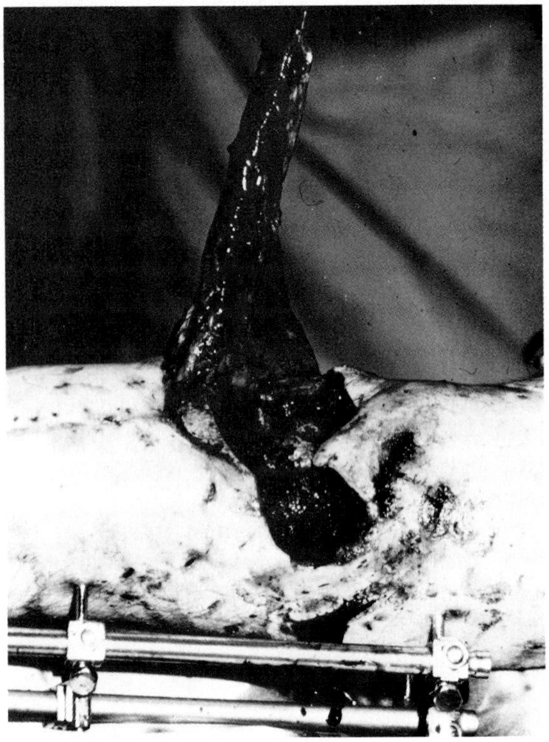

Fig. 7-58. Consolidation of soft-tissue defect with lateral gastrocnemius muscle pedicle flap and split-thickness skin graft. (Copyright Dr. F. Behrens.)

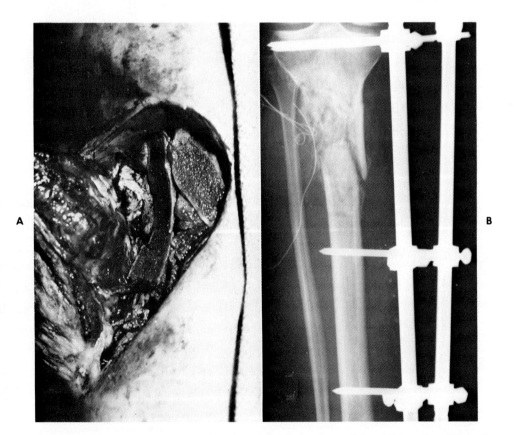

Fig. 7-59 A, One month later, medial elevation of muscle pedicle and bone grafting of residual skeletal defect. **B,** Radiographic appearance. (Copyright Dr. F. Behrens.)

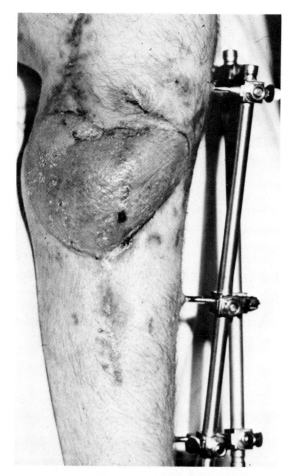

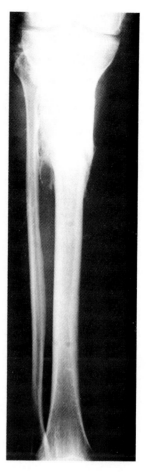

Fig. 7-60. Frontal view of tibia before removal of external fixator 5 months after the injury. (Copyright Dr. F. Behrens.)

Fig. 7-61. Final result. (Copyright Dr. F. Behrens.)

patients nonweight-bearing for 8 weeks, or until early consolidation is seen.

Disturbed by the detrimental potential of transfixion pins, we have recently adapted the ASIF "tubular" fixator to unilateral use and have found it rigid enough for the management of even the most severe bony lesions. Its adaptability to individual injury patterns has been surprising. In uncomplicated situations full weight-bearing has been possible 2 to 4 weeks after the injury (Figs. 7-57 to 7-61).

OTHER METHODS OF IMMOBILIZATION

To prevent nonunions in oblique fractures of the midtibial and distal tibial diaphysis, some authors advocate "limited open reduction" and internal fixation with a lag screw, followed by neutralization of the fracture site with an external fixator.[2] When we have a stable tibial fracture that

shows little indication to consolidate, we remove the fixator and have the patient fully bear weight in a below-knee cast or brace as soon as the soft tissues are healed and all projected secondary procedures have been carried out.

We generally manage nonunions with osteo-periosteal elevation and a bone graft or rigid internal fixation, depending on the location, nature of the nonunion, and the needs of the patient. Often a number of these auxiliary methods have to be used sequentially.

REFERENCES TO PART F—TIBIA

1. Briggs, B.T., Cabanela, M.E., Chao, E.Y.S., et al.: External fixators: biomechanical and clinical analysis of the Hoffmann, Roger Anderson, Kronner, and Volkov-Oganesian fixators (scientific exhibit), San Francisco, 1979, American Academy of Orthopaedic Surgeons.
2. Burny, F.: Elastic external fixation of tibial fractures: study of 1421 cases. In Brooker, A.F., and Edwards, C.: External fixation: The current state of the art, Baltimore, 1979, The Williams & Wilkins Co.

3. Jorgensen, T.E.: Measurements of stability of crural fractures with Hoffmann osteotaxis. 3. The uncomplicated terminal phase of healing of crural fractures, Acta Orthop. Scand. **43**:264-279, 1972.

4. Karlström, G., and Olerud, S.: Percutaneous pin fixation of open tibial fractures: double frame anchorage using the Vidal-Adrey method, J. Bone Joint Surg. **57A**:915-924, 1975.

5. Raimbeau, G., Toulemonde, J.L., Albaret, P., and Pillet, J.: L'artère tibiale antérieure: intérêt de l'artériographie de profil, Anat. Clin. **1**:325-329, 1979.

6. Raimbeau, G., Chevalier, J.M., and Raguin, J.: Les risques vasculaires du fixateur en cadre à la jambe, Rev. Chir. Orthop. **65**(suppl. II):77-82, 1979.

7. Vidal, J., Buscayret, C.H., Connes, H., et al.: Traitement des fractures ouvertes de jambe par le fixateur externe en double cadre, Rev. Chir. Orthop. **62**:433-448, 1976.

FEMUR

DANA C. MEARS, M.D.
Pittsburgh, Pennsylvania

The application of external skeletal fixation to various femoral problems is indicated less frequently than would be the case with comparable problems arising in the tibia or in the forearm. The indications include open fractures, especially those accompanied by soft-tissue or osseous loss, and excessive foreshortening with segmental bone loss, with or without a nonunion. It may be employed as a rapid means to stabilize a complicated femoral fracture associated with other complicated fractures involving the pelvis, acetabulum, or ipsilateral tibia. It may provide rapid stabilization to accompany a neurovascular repair. It may be extended across the knee joint to stabilize a ligamentous insult accompanied by a femoral fracture. It may also be employed for stabilization in the presence of an infected nonunion. This topic is discussed in Part G (p. 176). The indications are limited in view of anatomic factors and the availability of alternative methods of stabilization.

ANATOMY

A thorough knowledge of the anatomic considerations of the femur is essential to permit a surgeon to undertake the application of external fixation to the femur with safety. The proximity of the groin and urogenital organs limits access to the proximal part of the femur, and the hip joint produces a similar limitation. The sciatic nerve, its branches, and the femoral vessels inhibit ready access to the femur, particularly the proximal half. The capsule of the knee joint impedes access to the distal end of the bone, and the large anterior and posterior muscle groups with the allied subcutaneous fat thwart ready access to the diaphyseal portions of the bone. Impalement of the middle portion of the quadriceps by transfixing pins is extremely likely to provoke substantial contracture of the quadriceps muscle with associated stiffness of the knee joint.

AVAILABLE FRAMES

Three principal configurations of frame have merit for application to the femur. All these possess large components with considerable structural integrity, which is absolutely essential in view of the mechanical forces imposed upon the frame and the fracture fragments. For the management of certain diaphyseal fractures as from a shotgun blast, or of a malunion with overriding, the application of the Wagner apparatus is most satisfactory. It is of adequate strength and is preferred by the patients in view of its streamlined configuration and limited bulk. For those fractures that

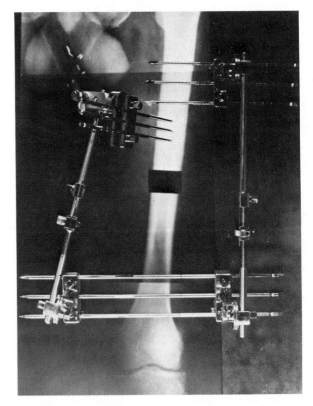

Fig. 7-62. A composite photograph illustrates the conventional femoral frame with proximal half pins and distal transfixing pins.

show considerable comminution or extension across the hip or knee joint, a more complex and structurally sound frame is essential. An appropriate model can be constructed by application of the Hoffmann or AO tubular components. These modified frames involve mediolateral transfixing pins through the distal femoral shaft or distal metaphysis. In the midshaft region transfixing pins can be inserted in the oblique axis from anteromedial to posterolateral. This technique is particularly useful for application with the Hoffmann device. For those fractures that progress in a more proximal direction, the proximal fixation is obtained by the application of multiple clusters of threaded half pins, which are inserted from a lateral and an anterior direction (Fig. 7-62). The quadriceps muscle is only impaled when this is absolutely essential or when arthrodesis of the knee is anticipated.

For the erection of the frame the pins require insertion under carefully controlled technique. Image intensification may be helpful, particularly with the use of a Wagner frame. When there is any doubt about the location of the femur and of the adjacent neurovascular structures, incisions should be made directly down to the bone so that the pins are inserted under direct visualization. Alternatively, probe pins may be inserted to identify the bone before insertion of the half pins. When the frame is erected, a distance of at least an inch between the frame and the cutaneous surface is essential so that impingement of the skin upon the frame does not occur. This problem is frequently encountered in the femur in view of the very supple nature of the skin and of its mobility when the patient rolls over in bed.

If the fracture is complicated by an ipsilateral acetabular or proximal femoral fracture, the

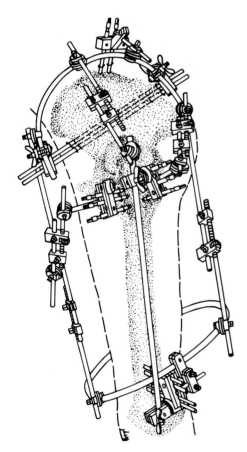

Fig. 7-63. Schematic diagram of a complex frame for application to proximal femur or central acetabulum. It employs transfixing iliac and femoral pins as well as half pins inserted in iliac crest and greater trochanter.

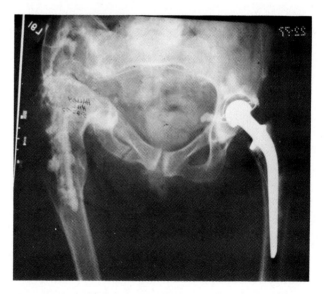

Fig. 7-64. Roentgenogram of an infected pseudarthrosis of the hip with widespread chronic osteomyelitis secondary to a failed total hip joint replacement in which external fixation was employed to achieve immobilization at the time of fusion.

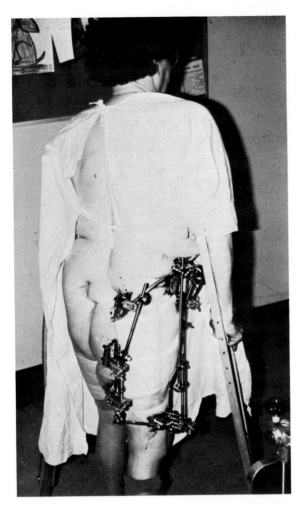

Fig. 7-65. Patient whose roentgenogram is shown in Fig. 7-64 as she walks a few days after surgery.

frame may be extended to the ipsilateral ilium (Figs. 7-63 to 7-65). Transfixing pins can be inserted in the ilium by resort to a special drill guide. Alternatively, anterior and posterior threaded half pins may be inserted into the ilium by direct exposure of the bone in the region of the anteroinferior and posteroinferior parts of the spine.

LIMITATIONS AND PITFALLS

After the application of the frame, physical therapy including quadriceps and hamstring exercises and active flexion of the knee should be undertaken within a few days. A rigorous regimen of pin-tract care is essential. This should include the use of hydrogen peroxide applied with cotton-tip swabs. As soon as excessive drainage from a pin track is evident, a local release procedure and débridement should be performed to lessen the likelihood of an established pin-track infection with osteomyelitis. With the likelihood for complaints about hygiene and social activities, as well as liabilities for pin-track infection, the surgeon should consider alternative methods. In many instances double-onlay plates may be employed for the immobilization of a comminuted or segmental fracture or for an infected nonunion with absolute loss of bone. In other situations a cast brace or intramedullary rod may provide a suitable technique of immobilization.

PELVIS

DANA C. MEARS, M.D.
Pittsburgh, Pennsylvania

External fixation is a very satisfactory method for controlling the unstable pelvic-ring fracture. Particularly in the acute setting where a patient undergoes an emergency laparotomy as part of his management, the application of external skeletal fixation currently possesses great advantages. It can be employed for the stabilization of an open or infected pelvic-ring fracture or for a comminuted central acetabular fracture. Various complex frames can be employed to stabilize the most complicated pelvic, central acetabular, and femoral-shaft fractures.

The aims of the treatment include early control of hemorrhage associated with a fracture, alleviation of pain at the fracture site, and early mobilization of the patient to facilitate respiratory care, nursing care, and rapid discharge from the hospital.

DESIGNS OF PELVIC FRAMES

The most widely employed design is the anterior frame that bridges from the anterosuperior or anteroinferior crest to the contralateral side. Perhaps the best known design is that provided by Slatis in which three half pins are inserted into either anterosuperior spine. This frame can be rapidly applied. It helps greatly in the early control of hemorrhage so that it should be considered before emergency laparotomy. At that time the frame can be erected in an inferior fashion so that it does not interfere with the approach to the abdomen. The frame can be repositioned at the conclusion of the laparotomy. This design is simple

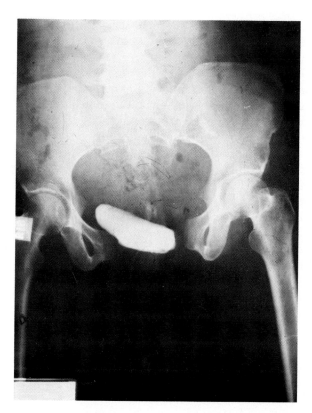

Fig. 7-66. Roentgenogram of a typical unstable pelvic-ring fracture with a wide diastasis of the symphysis and left sacroiliac dislocation. Contrast medium is observed in the intact bladder.

and provides good alleviation of discomfort. It is of inadequate stability, however, for the management of a truly unstable pelvic-ring fracture (Fig. 7-66). In this situation the frame should be augmented by the application of three supplementary half pins into either anteroinferior spine, which are inserted with an angulation of about 40 degrees with respect to the pins in the anterosuperior spine. By erection of a Vidal type of frame around these pins, a frame of adequate stability is provided so that a patient may undertake immediate bed-to-chair transfers and be discharged from the hospital without the risk of late loss of reduction. On certain occasions, particularly in the presence of substantial posterior skin loss, a posterior frame may be preferred. The pins are inserted in the region of the posterosuperior to posteroinferior areas of the spine. Although the frame is rigid and substantially less cumbersome than the anterior frame, it requires a special type of bed. The modification in the bed may include the application of two pediatric mattresses with a

gap between them or the use of an ancillary foam pad of about 6 inches in thickness. A hole is cut into the pad to provide an appropriate site for the frame.

In certain situations a more complex frame may be applicable. The frame may employ transfixing iliac pins, which is particularly desirable if transfixation should be extended to the distal femur. Such complex frames are employed for the immobilization of an unstable pelvic ring combined with a central acetabular or proximal femoral fracture, or both. These frames require special expertise and apparatus and should not be used unless the surgeon has obtained appropriate training.

ANATOMY

For the insertion of pins into the highly irregular pelvis, only an open approach down to bone should be employed. The upper half of a Smith-Petersen incision is preferred for the insertion of the anterior pins. The incision is extended along the anterior crest of the ilium distal to the anteroinferior part of the spine. The origin of the sartorius and the direct head of the rectus femoris may be sharply incised. A subperiosteal plane on the inner and outer walls of the pelvis is developed. Appropriate retractors are inserted so that the pins may be applied with direct visualization of all the related portions of bone. In view of the enormous hazards, if neurovascular structures or intra-abdominal viscera are impaled, the open technique is strongly recommended. Because of rotational anomalies and other malalignments that frequently accompany the unstable pelvic-ring fractures, the surgeon's ability to insert the pins through a stab wound is greatly compromised. Three pins are usually inserted in the anteroinferior and anterosuperior part of the spine, respectively. The most anterior portion of the iliac crest also is a suitable site. The more posterior aspect of the crest of the bone rapidly diminishes in thickness so that the pins do not provide good fixation. After insertion of the pins the wounds are closed loosely. Since most of the fractures are accompanied by widening of the pelvic ring, the cutaneous incisions should be made somewhat medial to the mobile hemipelvis. After the reduction of the fracture the cutaneous incision is positioned more accurately with the underlying bone so that the skin is less likely to be tented around the fixation pins.

The posterosuperior and posteroinferior parts of the spine may be approached by a longitudinal incision directly over the bone. The soft tissues, including a small amount of the origin of gluteus maximus, may be sharply reflected. The pins are inserted directly into bone.

ERECTION OF FRAME

For erection of a Hoffmann type of frame (Figs. 7-67 to 7-69), ball joints are applied to each of the four clusters of half pins. A smooth rod is used to connect the adjacent ipsilateral ball joints. By the use of articulation couplings, two smooth rods may be attached to each of the primary rods, which extend away from the body surface. In this way a frame may be erected a long way from the abdominal wall. Particularly in the obese patient this technique is essential to avoid excessive im-

pingement of the abdominal skin on the external frame. Once the two half frames are erected, the pelvis may be corrected in terms of rotational displacement diastasis. For the correction of apparent leg-length discrepancy, when a hemipelvis has migrated in a superior direction, some other technique is essential. We prefer to place the patient on a fracture table for undertaking the procedure. The shorter extremity is distracted with the fracture table until appropriate distal migration is restored (Fig. 7-70). Then the external frame is erected as previously described. Such distal migration should be undertaken within the first week after the injury. Afterwards the early fracture healing greatly interferes with an attempt to obtain adequate correction.

The frame may be erected by the use of adjustable slider bars or long straight rods. The former

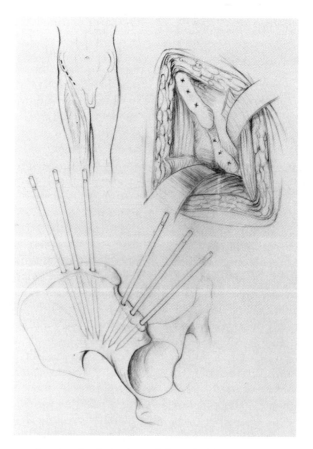

Fig. 7-67. Diagram of stages for insertion of threaded half pins into the anterior superior and inferior areas of the spine for application of an anterior frame to the pelvic ring. *Upper left,* Site of the pin incision; *upper right,* after exposure of the bone sites for insertion of the pins; *bottom,* two clusters of threaded half pins.

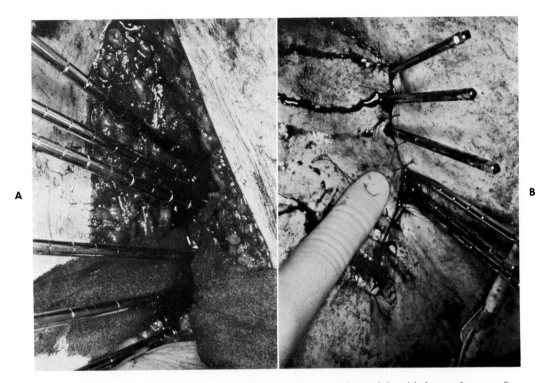

Fig. 7-68. Insertion of threaded half pins into the anterior pelvis with loose closure of the skin.

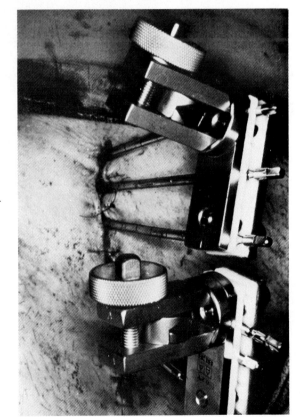

Fig. 7-69. Ball joints attached to the two clusters of half pins.

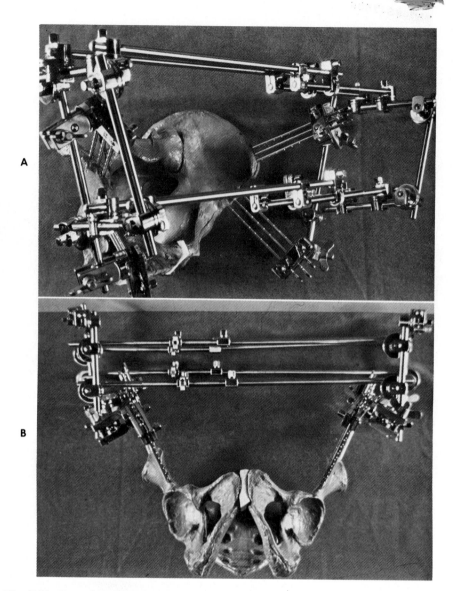

Fig. 7-70. Two views of the modified frame employed for external fixation of an unstable pelvic-ring fracture are shown. The two clusters of pins are inserted with an angulation of about 40 degrees of one cluster with respect to the other.

permits more complex postoperative adjustments, whereas the latter is lighter in weight. Usually the latter is adequate for the typical unstable pelvis fracture.

MOBILIZATION OF THE PATIENT

If other injuries permit, the patient is encouraged to transfer to a chair the day after surgery (Fig. 7-71). This maneuver greatly facilitates his respiratory care and restoration of spontaneous activity of the bowel and bladder. The patient is instructed in the conventional method of routine pin care. As soon as he can transfer himself to a chair and a bedside commode, he is permitted to be discharged from the hospital. Generally he is readmitted a minimum of 6 weeks after injury for removal of the device. In the presence of a true dislocation of the sacroiliac joint the frame is

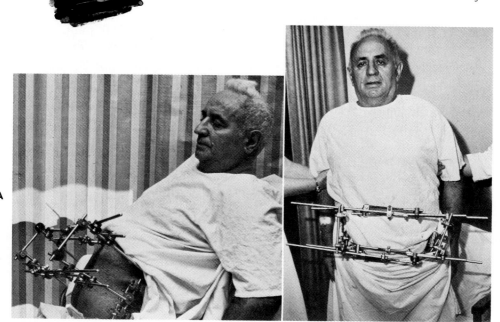

Fig. 7-71. Short obese man, 52 years old, who sustained an unstable pelvic-ring fracture with a complete rupture of the bladder and had primary repair of the bladder with external fixation.

maintained for a period of 8 to 10 weeks. It is removed in the hospital under ketamine anesthesia. Subsequently the patient is permitted to undertake weight-bearing with support to tolerance.

LIMITATIONS OF TECHNIQUE

The patient does show limited hip flexion to about 90 degrees. The absolute amount of hip flexion depends on the location of the pins and of the anterior frame itself. At the present time a patient with a totally unstable pelvic-ring fracture is not permitted to walk for at least the first 3 or 4 weeks after the injury. Otherwise, late loss of fixation might occur. Although the technique is useful for the stabilization of a conventional pelvic-ring fracture, it is not applicable for the severely comminuted ilium that arises by direct force such as a shotgun blast or more conventionally a fall from a great height. Such fractures require conservative methods or internal fixation. In the presence of an associated acetabular fracture with displacement and comminution, we prefer to undertake open reduction and internal fixation of the acetabular fracture followed immediately by external fixation of the pelvic ring. This remains a highly complicated problem where further improvements in the technique remain to be made.

UPPER EXTREMITY
RICHARD E. JONES III, M.D.
Dallas, Texas

High-energy trauma and open fracture wounds are less common in the upper extremity than in the lower extremity. Nonetheless, the indications for the use of external fixation in the upper extremity are the same as those for the lower extremity. Type III or type IIIA open fracture wounds, significant comminution of bone, segmental loss of bone, and comminuted osteochondral fractures not amenable to internal stabilization are the situations where external fixation is likely to prove most valuable in patient management. Additionally, patients with thermal injuries alone or when combined with fractures may also require external fixation. Prevention of soft-tissue contracture in patients with thermal injuries by use of percutaneous skeletal pins and external anchoring frames or dynamic splints can be performed.

The anatomy of the upper extremity dictates the placement of fixation pins. Because of the high likelihood of muscle impalement or damage to the closely applied neurovascular structures, transfixation can rarely be used in the upper extremity. Rather, half-pin configurations predominate as methods of frame anchorage. Furthermore, if a direct subcutaneous margin of bone is not available for pin fixation, an incision should be made to identify intermuscular planes and protect vital neurovascular structures. Luckily, the demands placed upon the injured upper extremity usually do not exceed the stability of half-pin anchoring frames. If additional stability is required, biplane half-pin configurations can be used.

HUMERUS

Pin placement in the scapula, if required, is best accomplished through the spine or the acromion (Fig. 7-72). In the proximal humerus the greater tuberosity is the ideal pin-placement site. Pins placed more distal than 6 cm from the acromion may endanger the axillary nerve. Pins can be placed directly posterior, through the triceps in the distal quarter of the humerus. Burny and co-workers[1] have reported on external skeletal fixation of 62 humeral shaft fractures, many of which had pins inserted through the triceps. Occasionally, elbow mobilization may be compromised by triceps impalement. Pins may also be placed laterally in the humeral diaphysis or in the lateral epicondyle (Fig. 7-73). An incision should be made to identify and protect any vital structures, particularly the radial nerve, and direct dissection to bone will identify a safe pin site.

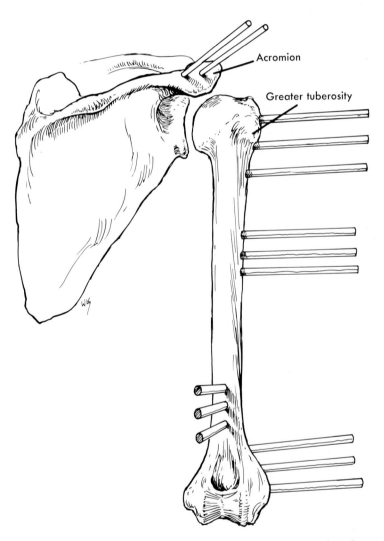

Fig. 7-72. Scapula and humerus pin-insertion sites, posterior view.

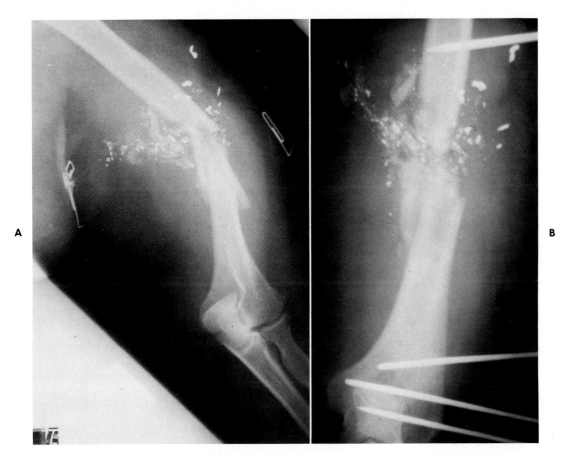

Fig. 7-73. A, Gunshot wound fracture of humerus. **B,** Gunshot wound fracture of humerus reduced with external fixation.

ELBOW

High-energy trauma causing disorganization of the elbow can be managed by olecranon-pin overhead traction, but external fixation, allowing mobilization of the entire patient, is preferable. Placement of pins in the distal third of the humerus and in the proximal third of the ulna can accomplish fixation with the limb in a functional position.

FOREARM

Again, in the forearm the major indications for external skeletal fixation are high-energy open fractures, fracture dislocations, and comminuted fractures of the distal third of the forearm. The method of insertion of the forearm pins should be based on half-frame configurations (Fig. 7-74). Since half-pin configurations are safer than transfixation, subcutaneous borders of bone can be directly penetrated with threaded pins (Fig. 7-75). Musculotendinous or neurovascular impalement can be prevented by a short skin incision for direct insertion into bone. Particularly in the distal third of the radius, the superficial sensory radial nerve should be protected. If both the radius and the ulna are fractured and percutaneous transfixation is contemplated, the forearm should be placed in full supination to maintain a wide interosseous space. Independent frames in both the radius and ulna will enable the limb to maintain rotation during the fracture-healing process.

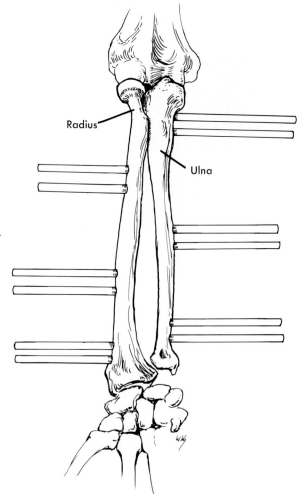

Fig. 7-74. Forearm pin-insertion sites.

DISTAL RADIUS FRACTURES

The severely comminuted fracture of the distal radius, unstable Colles' fractures, and comminuted intra-articular fractures are all prone to settling and loss of length. External fixation is readily applied. Biplane configurations help achieve more stability and control of the fracture. Tendons again should be identified and retracted. Placement of pins at the base of the second metacarpal is best performed with the thumb in wide abduction, and the extensor tendons and hood should of course be spared (Fig. 7-76). Forearm and hand percutaneous pins should be in the range of 2 to 2.3 mm in diameter.

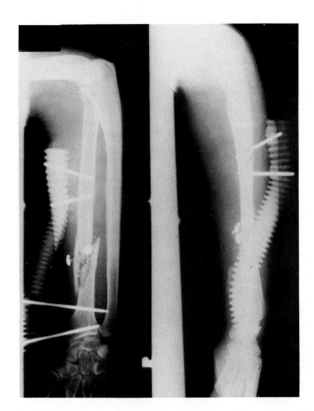

Fig. 7-75. Gunshot wound fracture of radius managed with external skeletal fixation.

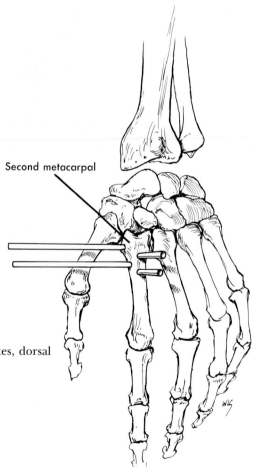

Second metacarpal

Fig. 7-76. Second metacarpal pin-insertion sites, dorsal view.

The excellent clinical experience in treatment of comminuted fractures of the distal radius by external fixation reported by Cooney and co-workers[2] and by Grana and Kopta[3] must be compared with Green's[4] report on pins and plaster treatment. The external fixation method has the advantage of being more readily adjustable than pins in plaster (Fig. 7-77). The external fixation device should be left in place for approximately 6 to 8 weeks. Mobilization of the hand and forearm is possible and helps prevent any secondary contractures.

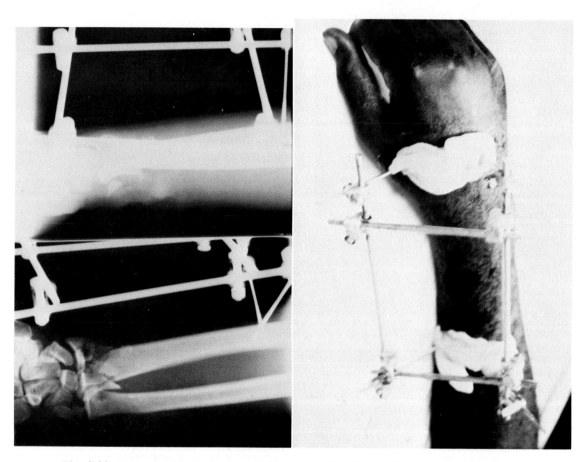

Fig. 7-77. Comminuted, intra-articular fracture of radius in biplane external skeletal fixation.

HAND FRACTURES

Fractures in the hand may occasionally require external fixation. Either the Hoffmann Mini-Fixator, the small Roger Anderson device usually applied in oral surgery (Fig. 7-78), or frames fashioned from dental acrylic or polymethylmethacrylate can be used to form external anchoring frames for percutaneously placed pins.

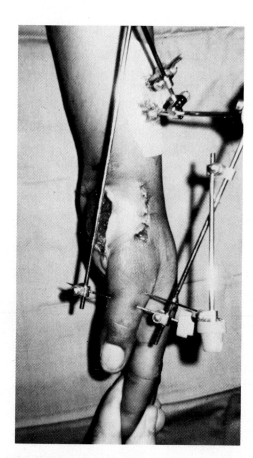

Fig. 7-78. Segmental defect of thumb metacarpal managed with biplane external skeletal fixation.

REFERENCES TO PART F—UPPER EXTREMITY

1. Burny, F., et al.: Traitement des fractures d'humérus par fixateur externe, Acta Orthop. Belg. **45:**47-56, 1979.
2. Cooney, Q.P., Linscheid, R.L., and Dobyns, J.H.: External pin fixation for unstable Colles' fractures, J. Bone Joint Surg. **61A:**840-846, 1979.
3. Grana, W.A., and Kopta, J.A.: Roger Anderson device in the treatment of fractures of the distal end of the radius, J. Bone Joint Surg. **61A:**1234-1238, 1979.
4. Green, D.P.: Pins and plaster treatment of comminuted fractures of the distal end of the radius, J. Bone Joint Surg. **57A:**304-310, 1975.

SUGGESTED READINGS TO PART F—UPPER EXTREMITY

Anderson, R.: Fractures of the radius and ulna, J. Bone Joint Surg. **16:**379, 1934.

Anderson, R., and O'Neil, G.: Comminuted fractures of the distal end of the radius, Surg. Gynecol. Obstet. **78:**434-440, 1944.

Jones, K.G.: A modification of the use of extraskeletal immobilization for comminuted fractures of the distal radius, Clin. Orthop. **123:**83-86, 1977.

Junkin, H.D.: The topography of pins: precision pinning of fractures, Industrial Med. **13:**387-395, 1944.

Part G

Treatment of infected nonunions and failed septic joints

DANA C. MEARS, M.D.
Pittsburgh, Pennsylvania

In recent years it has become evident that three complex fracture problems may be managed by remarkably similar principles. These three include complex open grade III fractures (Figs. 7-79 and 7-80) with extensive soft-tissue disruption, an infected nonunion, and a failed septic joint prosthesis. In all of these the general principles include early débridement and rigid stabilization. Subsequently, some technique is needed to encourage the invasion of granulation tissue over denuded bone, tendon, or ligament. Supplemen-

tary bone grafting frequently is required. Soft-tissue and cutaneous coverage likewise may be indicated. These and other stages are discussed in turn.

DÉBRIDEMENT

An adequate débridement of all necrotic and infected tissue is absolutely essential. Previously surgeons were reluctant to excise an adequate amount of bone in many of these cases in view of the anticipated problems that were provided by such a lengthy segmental osseous defect. With the advent of widely available external fixation, primary débridement of sufficient magnitude is possible and greatly hastens the course of treatment. Until such a step is adequately performed, multiple subsequent débridements with associated delay in the initiation of the reconstructive stages is inevitable. Generally such a wound is maintained in an open fashion for at least a few days after

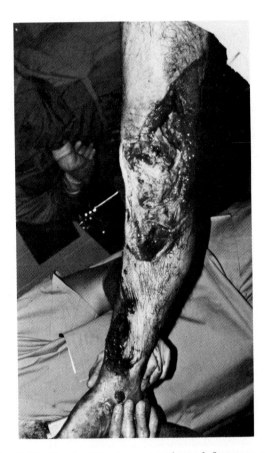

Fig. 7-79. Grade III open comminuted fracture of a femur and ipsilateral tibia. Extensive soft-tissue disruption with loss of skin and bone is evident.

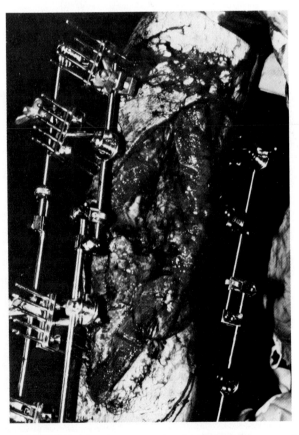

Fig. 7-80. Same extremity is shown after rigid external fixation with a complex external frame.

primary débridement. In most instances débridement is accompanied by the use of appropriate parenteral antibiotics in large doses. The duration of antibiotic therapy remains in debate. It certainly is maintained from the early preoperative period throughout the operation and for a few days after that surgery. Subsequently it may be maintained for variable periods depending on the severity of the infection, the severity of the septicemia, the presence of remote sites of infection, or other factors.

STABILIZATION

The application of external fixation for such an infected process frequently is complicated by the presence of segmental bone loss and of considerable osteoporosis of the residual osseous fragments (Fig. 7-80). For these reasons the external frame frequently requires modification to provide a much more rigid assembly. The number of pins may be increased substantially to provide adequate fixation. Also, a surgeon should consider the use of fixation pins of larger diameter usually in the range of 5 to 6 mm. In the presence of segmental bone loss a complex modular frame that provides good stabilization in the mediolateral and anteroposterior planes should be provided. At the completion of assembly, passive motion of the fracture site should be attempted by manipulation of the extremity. If motion is clinically evident, the frame should be altered or augmented until the presence of a rigid osseous framework is confirmed.

PROVISION FOR SOFT-TISSUE COVERAGE OF DENUDED BONE

In the presence of denuded bone, tendon, or ligament, some technique must be employed to encourage the ingrowth of granulation tissue. The principal ingredient is a continuous moist environment of physiologic saline solution possibly supplemented by some antibiotic. Many different regimens have been developed. I prefer to employ cotton mesh dressings that are moistened at 2-hour intervals by the use of physiologic saline with bacitracin, 50,000 units per liter. The antibiotic prevents bacterial overgrowth and the solution provides an adequate medium for the ingrowth of granulation tissue. Despite the use of this regimen, certain necrotic sites of bone may become evident and require supplementary débridement. In the presence of a continuously moistened environment and with adequate dé-

bridement, a continuous granulation layer should appear within 5 to 10 days. If the defect is a large one, other techniques to obtain soft-tissue coverage should be employed. These are described subsequently.

SUPPLEMENTARY AUTOGENOUS CANCELLOUS BONE GRAFT

In the presence of an osseous segmental defect, the application of autogenous cancellous bone graft should be employed. Only this type of bone graft can be used in these situations. If cortical bone or homologous cancellous bone graft is employed, the reactivation of the infection in the bone graft is extremely likely to occur. The autogenous cancellous bone graft is rapidly revascularized so that a substantial degree of resistance to further infection is provided. At the site of an exposed cavity of bone, the bone graft may be applied directly onto the host bone, provided that a continuous granulation layer has been restored. This technique has been popularized by Papineau though many other workers have used it. At the time of application of the bone graft to the granulation tissue bed, we apply a moistened cotton gauze dressing to the superficial surface of bone graft. The dressing is maintained in place for 3 to 5 days. During this time it is moistened with a similar antibiotic solution at 2-hour intervals. At the end of this time when the dressing is removed, dressing changes are begun every 8 hours while the bone graft is maintained in the moistened condition. Granulation tissue grows over the surface of the bone graft within a period of 1 to 2 weeks. Supplementary bone graftings may be undertaken as soon as another continuous granulation layer is evident. Also, split-thickness skin grafts may be applied to the cancellous bone graft once the granulation layer has been restored. This technique is particularly useful for application to an infected nonunion in the tibia or in the forearm. Usually it is unnecessary in the femur and the humerus in view of the superior soft-tissue envelope. Its principal liability is the prolonged period required to correct a lengthy segmental defect of greater than 2 inches. Also, it has a high likelihood for development of a chronic osteomyelitis or recurrent drainage with spontaneous elimination of small fragments of presumably necrotic bone graft. Although this may not be a functional problem, it is frequently a considerable cosmetic liability of the technique.

Supplementary autogenous bone graft also may

be applied at sites where there is good soft-tissue coverage. In the case of an infected nonunion of the tibia, this constitutes a posterior bone grafting or the application of a bone graft between the tibia and the fibula to provide a structural synostosis.

SERIAL BONE GRAFTING

About 6 weeks after the primary bone grafting, supplementary roentgenograms are taken of the fracture site. If a residual segmental defect in the bone of a partial or complete nature is confirmed, another bone grafting should be undertaken at that time. If such a bone grafting is deferred, the structural weakness will remain indefinitely. Ultimately, another bone grafting will be required though a great deal of time will be lost unnecessarily. Such time provides a greater likelihood for loosening of the pins with pin-track infection or other type of failure. For these stages, autogenous cancellous bone grafting or, in the presence of a closed fracture site with adequate soft-tissue coverage, corticocancellous strips may be employed. The surgical approach to such an extremity should be undertaken through a site of good skin coverage.

SOFT-TISSUE AND CUTANEOUS COVERAGE

Within a few days after the primary débridement and stabilization of the infected nonunion some methods for restoration of soft tissues and skin may be considered. In the case of an infected nonunion of the tibia, myoplasty by use of the medial head of gastrocnemius or the soleus muscle may be indicated (see Part D). I prefer to undertake the myoplasty about 1 week after débridement and stabilization. In these instances, generally the application of split-thickness skin graft and simultaneously of autogenous cancellous bone graft is undertaken about 1 week after myoplasty. Bone graft may be carefully inserted deep to the myoplasty, or it may be applied through a separate incision.

When the Papineau technique is employed, split-thickness skin graft may be used to cover the autogenous bone graft. The skin graft should not be applied until a continuous granulation layer is evident superficial to the bone graft. Comparable techniques for restoration of skin coverage and soft tissues such as muscle may be undertaken in the upper extremity or in the femur though they are less frequently indicated. Rarely for larger defects the use of free vascularized grafts such as the latissimus dorsi or an osseous and cutaneous free graft such as the anterior iliac crest may be employed. These complex procedures should not be undertaken until all evidence of active infection has vanished.

ALTERATION OF RIGIDITY OF THE FRAME

For the treatment of an infected nonunion an extremely rigid frame is necessary until the infection has been eradicated and until the soft tissues have been restored over denuded bone. Once the bone graft has been applied and the soft-tissue envelope around the fracture has been restored, a progressive diminution in the rigidity of the external frame may be initiated. A complex frame with the provision for anteroposterior stability as well as mediolateral stability may be modified back to a conventional mediolateral frame. At a somewhat later date, usually 3 to 4 months after the initial débridement of the nonunion site roentgenograms may show evidence of early consolidation of the fracture site. At this time a mediolateral frame may be converted to a unilateral frame. Alternatively, it may be replaced by a suitable cast or cast brace. The optimal timing for this change is still somewhat unclear. If it is undertaken prematurely before the fracture shows evidence of early consolidation, an active infection may be reactivated at the site of the previous nonunion. If an excessively rigid frame is maintained for a prolonged period, a very slow rate of osseous healing may be anticipated. Clinical judgment is the only widely available method to assess the timing for these changes in the rigidity of the frame.

In the management of many infected nonunions where adjacent soft tissues possess a precarious blood supply, the rate of healing of the fracture may be extremely slow. It can be anticipated that some type of cast or cast brace will be needed for a prolonged period of many months or occasionally a few years. Extensive remodeling of the bone at the fracture site is needed or a pathologic fracture is likely to transpire. In certain instances where the fracture healing is observed to be extremely slow, the surgeon may consider augmentation of the structural integrity of the bone by the application of an onlay plate. Such a procedure may be undertaken only if there is a suitable region of the bone under intact soft tissue that is amenable to exposure without the likelihood for severely denuding it. Such a method is most frequently undertaken in the femur where in many instances an infected nonunion of the diaphysis may be stabilized by the use of double-onlay plates. For an infected nonunion of the tibia the soft tissues are less well suited for this technique.

SUGGESTED READINGS TO PART G

Burri, C., Willenegger, H., et al.: Post-traumatic osteomyelitis Bern, 1975, Hans Huber Medical Publisher

Mears, D.C.: Percutaneous pin fixation. In Materials and orthopaedic surgery, Baltimore, 1979, The Williams & Wilkins Co.

Mears, D.C.: The management of complex pelvic fractures. In External skeletal fixation, Baltimore, 1979, The Williams & Wilkins Co.

Mears, D.C., and Fu, F.H.: Modern concepts of external skeletal fixation of the pelvis, Clin. Orthop. (151):65, Sept. 1980.

Mears, D.C., and Stone, J.P.: The management of open fractures, Orthop. Survey 3:247, 1980.

Meyer, S., Weiland, A.J., and Willenegger, H.: The treatment of infected nonunions in long bones, J. Bone Joint Surg. 57A:836, 1975.

Perren, S.M., and Rahn, B.A.: Biomechanics of fracture healing, Orthop. Survey 2:108, 1978.

Roy-Camille, R., Reignier, B., Soullant, G., and Berteaux, D.: Results of the Papineau operation with regard to 46 cases, Rev. Chir. Orthop. 62:347, 1976.

Slatis, P., and Karaharja, E.O.: External fixation of pelvic fractures, Injury 7:53, 1974.

Weber, B.G., and Cěch, O.: Pseudarthrosis: pathophysiology, biomechanics, therapy, results, New York, 1976, Grune & Stratton, Inc.

Part H

Complications of external skeletal fixation

FRED BEHRENS, M.D., F.R.C.S.(C)
St. Paul, Minnesota

Osteomyelitis secondary to pin-tract infections and the breakage of fixator components has prevented the widespread use of external fixation until the late 1960s. Purer metals, the development of stronger parts, and the increasing knowledge about the relative rigidity of various frame compositions have largely eliminated these serious complications.[1,5] Most of the remaining problems diminish as the surgeon becomes more familiar

□ Supported by Grant 8263 from the Medical Education and Research Foundation, St. Paul–Ramsey Hospital, St. Paul, Minnesota.

with a particular device and as he learns to take the extent of the injury and the patient's personality into account.

SYSTEMIC COMPLICATIONS

Since external fixators are often crucial for the early mobilization of a severely or multiply injured patient, they have become an important instrument in the prevention of such generalized posttraumatic complications as fat embolism, hypostatic pneumonia, and disuse osteoporosis.

Thromboembolism of the lower extremity is believed to be less frequent with fixators than after cast immobilization because free ankle and knee motion reduces venous stasis.[4]

LOCAL COMPLICATIONS

As external fixators are often applied to severely mangled extremities in only partially conscious patients, it is often difficult to separate deficits attributable to the traumatic event from those related to the application of the fixator. With a sound knowledge of the regional anatomy and some caution, most local complications are preventable.

Neurovascular complications

Threaded pins and transfixion are the biggest threat to vital structures. The tibia, femur, ulna, and ilium all have at least one border where the space between skin and bone is unencumbered by nerves and vessels, and the insertion of half pins therefore is safe. When necessary, the bony surfaces should be exposed operatively and the pins placed under direct vision.

Special caution is necessary in an extremity where one main artery has been severed by the initial trauma. Pin injury to the remaining vessel may precipitate an amputation.[10]

Compartment syndromes. Although only reported in the case of the anterior compartment of the tibia[8], a compartment syndrome is equally possible after pin insertion in the forearm and hand.

Arteries. Pin injury to the anterior tibial artery has been reported by two authors.[4,8]

Bony complications

Heat necrosis. In our view all pin sites should be predrilled using power and a sharp drill bit. If the drill bit is too small in relation to the pin, even manual insertion generates enough heat to form a cylinder of necrotic bone surrounding the hole.

This enhances the development of a pin-tract osteomyelitis (Fig. 7-81).

Refracture. This refers to a fracture of the same bone some time after the original break has healed. The incidence varies from none to 8%[4,6,7] in different series. Refractures are seen more often after single bar fixation and after primary bone healing. Apart from a break that goes through the area of the original lesion, which is most common, refractures can occur at other sites or through a pinhole. A break that goes through an infected pin tract constitutes an infected fracture and has to be treated accordingly.

Delayed and nonunions. There is a general impression that immobilization with an external fixator retards fracture healing. Although nonunions after severe open fractures are not unusual, reliable comparisons between different treatment methods are almost impossible. It appears, however, that for a closed tibial fracture, treat-

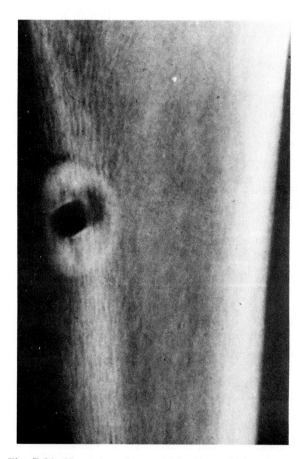

Fig. 7-81. Heat necrosis caused by manual insertion of a 5 mm pin into a predrilled hole of 3.6 mm diameter. No infection ensued. (Copyright Dr. F. Behrens.)

ment in a PTB (patellar tendon bearing) cast allows for unsupported weight-bearing about 4 weeks earlier than is possible after the use of an external fixator.[4,9]

Loss of reduction. The reasons for a loss of reduction are as follows:
1. *General causes*
   a. Lack of patient compliance (such as early weight-bearing)
   b. Falls, second accidents
2. *Local causes*
   a. Failure to control bony fragments (pins too close, not enough pins, pins too small, small fragments, pins too far from the fracture)
   b. Pin loosening
   c. Osteoporosis
   d. Osteomyelitis
3. *Fixator related*
   a. Component breakage
   b. Loosening of articulations

The loss of reduction can occur in up to 7% of fixator applications.[2] It is seen more often after single bar fixation and is frequently related to poor patient compliance. Breakage of components has become rare.

Most of the local and fixator related complications can be corrected by replacement of the defective parts, removal of the pins, and improved frame configurations. In other situations, a different treatment mode may be preferable.

Joint stiffness. This complication is preventable if pins are not impaling joint capsules or musculotendinous units. In the bedridden patient, careful splinting and daily active and passive range-of-motion exercises are paramount. The ankle joint is most frequently affected. Loss of dorsiflexion and, on rare occasions, residual equinus or equinovarus deformity have been noted in 18% of patients in one series.[3]

Pin-tract problems. With improved pin care and the development of more rigid frames, pin-tract problems have become rare. Irritation of pin-entry sites and "sterile" drainage, however, will occur in 10% to 20% of patients. Its frequency is directly dependent on how long the fixator remains in place.

Pin-tract infections. The following are causes of pin-tract infections:
1. *General*
   a. Poor host defense
   b. Poor hygiene

c. Irregular pin care
d. Increased activity
2. *Local*
   a. Increased pin-skin motion
   b. Insufficient fixation or frame rigidity
   c. Pins
      (1) Thin
      (2) Long
      (3) Loose
   d. Increased soft-tissue mobility
   e. Increased bone-skin distance
   f. Increased bone-clamp distance
   g. Near joints

Of all pin tracts, 5% to 10% eventually become infected and about one out of every 30 fixator frames has to be altered or removed for this reason[2] (Fig. 7-82).

General causes. Poor host defense is most often seen in older and debilitated patients. It is characterized by pin-tract inflammation early in the treatment course and often progresses to a generalized cellulitis of the whole area (Fig. 7-83). Although most of these episodes can be controlled with a short course of systemic antibiotics, the choice of a different treatment method for the fracture should be considered. Patients with poor hygienic habits and a frivolous neglect of daily pin care should be followed frequently in the clinic or regularly seen by a public health nurse. Increased pin drainage is often noted after a change in activity status and generally means that the rigid-

ity of the fixator frame or the degree of fracture consolidation has been misjudged. A temporary reduction in activity level invariably solves the problem.

Local causes. Increased motion between pins and surrounding soft tissues lies at the base of most locally caused pin-tract problems. This can be attributed to a frame configuration of insufficient rigidity or pins that are loose or not stiff enough. Other causes are increased soft-tissue mobility as seen around joints and the pelvis. A large bone-skin or bone-clamp distance has the same effect. It is important to become aware of local difficulties before soft-tissue or bony infection ensue. Appropriate management must be directly related to

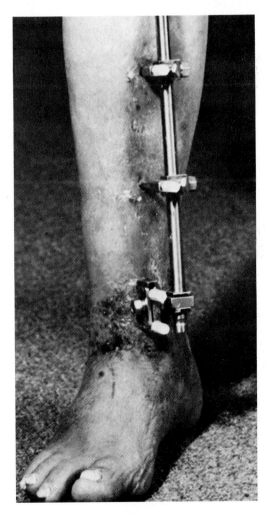

Fig. 7-83. Cellulitis involving whole lower leg. Responded to parenteral antibiotics for 72 hours. (Copyright Dr. F. Behrens.)

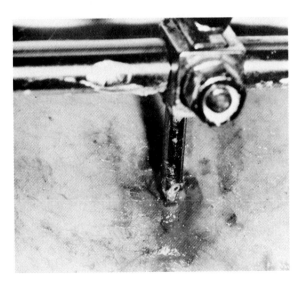

Fig. 7-82. Pin-tract infection. Resolved after more attentive pin care.

the underlying cause and may mean a decrease in patient activity, the use of a more rigid frame configuration or thicker pins, and more attentive pin care. If pins are loose or pin tracts infected, the offending pins should be removed. Draining subsides within a few days and curettage of the tract for osteomyelitis is rarely necessary. Pins can be replaced to provide for a sturdier frame configuration or a different method of immobilization can be chosen.

REFERENCES TO PART H

1. Adrey, J.: Le fixateur externe d'Hoffmann couplé en cadre, Paris, 1970, Editions Gead.
2. Burny, F.: Complications liées à l'utilisation de l'ostéotaxis, Acta Orthop. Belg. **41:**103-109, 1975.
3. Burny, F.: Elastic external fixation of tibial fractures: study of 1421 cases. In Brooker, A.F., and Edwards, C.: External fixation: the current state of the art, Baltimore, 1979, The Williams & Wilkins Co.
4. Burny, F.: Traitement par ostéotaxis des fractures diaphysaires du tibia: étude de 115 cas, Acta Orthop. Belg. **38:**280-300, 1972.
5. Chao, E.Y.S., Briggs, B.T., and McCoy, M.T.: Theoretical and experimental analyses of Hoffmann-Vidal external fixation system. In Brooker, A.F., and Edwards, C.: External fixation: the current state of the art, Baltimore, 1979, The Williams & Wilkins Co.
6. Karlström, G., and Olerud, S.: Percutaneous pin fixation of open tibial fractures: double frame anchorage using the Vidal-Adrey method, J. Bone Joint Surg. **57A:**915-924, 1975.
7. Lawyer, R.: Treatment of complex tibial fractures. In Brooker, A.F., and Edwards, C.: External fixation: the current state of the art, Baltimore, 1979, The Williams & Wilkins Co.
8. Raimbeau, G., Chevalier, J.M., and Raguin, J.: Les risques vasculaires du fixateur en cadre à la jambe, Rev. Chir. Orthop. **65**(suppl. II):77-82, 1979.
9. Sarmiento, A.: A functional below-the-knee cast for tibial fractures, J. Bone Joint Surg. **49A:**855, 1967.
10. Vidal, J., Buscayret, C.H., Connes, H., et al.: Traitement des fractures ouvertes de jambe par le fixateur externe en double cadre, Rev. Chir. Orthop. **62:**433-448, 1976.

FRACTURES ABOUT THE ELBOW

Chapter 8

Factors influencing elbow instability

HUGH. S. TULLOS, M.D.

GREGORY SCHWAB, M.D.

JAMES B. BENNETT, M.D.

G. WILLIAM WOODS, M.D.
Houston, Texas

Analysis of factors influencing stability of the elbow correlates questions as to the elbow's basic function in activities of daily living. The events in which elbow function is important include lifting (requiring flexion and extension) and the overhead activities, such as throwing or hammering. Sports (football, baseball, and tennis) and industrial occupations such as carpentry require elbow function to position the hand. They are not strictly flexion-extension activities. A review of stresses at the elbow in these activities suggest that valgus is the dominant force (Fig. 8-1). This basic predominance of valgus stress is reflected in the ligamentous anatomy of the elbow.

ANATOMY

A review of elbow anatomy indicates no lateral collateral ligament of the elbow per se. By definition a collateral ligament runs from one bone across the joint to its opposite partner bone. In the case of the elbow this is not true. The lateral collateral ligament arises from the epicondyle but inserts on the annular ligament (Fig. 8-2). Thus the only structure on the lateral aspect of the elbow that corresponds to a lateral collateral ligament is the anconeus muscle (Fig. 8-2). The primary function of this muscle may well be as a lateral stabilizer, taking the place of the absent underlying true lateral collateral ligament. In contrast, on the medial side there is a well-developed collateral ligament. This ligament is composed of

three basic components: an anterior oblique, a posterior oblique, and a small transverse nonfunctional ligament.

The anterior oblique ligament is band shaped and thick and runs from the undersurface of the medial epicondyle to a point on the medial aspect of the ulna just below the coronoid process. The posterior oblique ligament also arises from the undersurface of the medial epicondyle but inserts in a fan-shaped fashion across virtually the entire length of the olecranon process (Fig. 8-3).

The basic characteristics of the posterior oblique ligament are significant. First it is taut only in flexion, lax in extension, and absent in many primates (Fig. 8-4). This suggests that the posterior oblique is not the essential stabilizer of the medial aspect of the elbow. Indeed if the posterior oblique ligament in cadaveric specimens is sectioned and the anterior oblique ligament left intact, the elbow does not become unstable to valgus stress (Fig. 8-5). Thus the posterior oblique seems not to play a primary role in elbow stability.

The characteristics of the anterior oblique ligament are entirely different. It is taut both in flexion and extension, and throughout the entire arc of motion of the elbow because of the anatomic characteristics of both its origin and insertion. In extension the anterior fibers become tight and in flexion the posterior fibers become tight (Fig. 8-6). Thus the anterior oblique ligament functions throughout the range of motion. Likewise in ca-

185

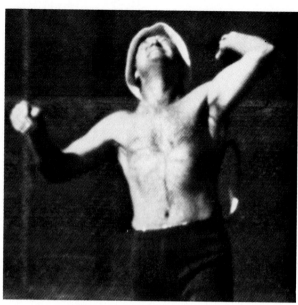

Fig. 8-1. High-speed photograph showing tennis player serving, demonstration valgus elbow stress.

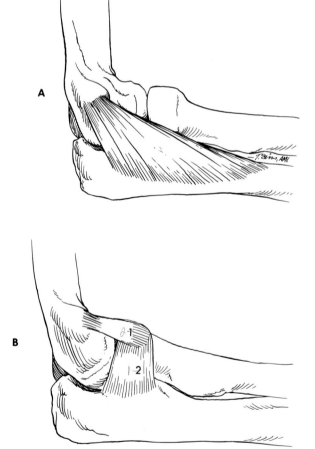

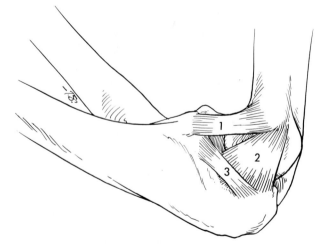

Fig. 8-2. A, Anconeus muscle. **B,** Lateral ligaments. *1,* Annular ligament; *2,* lateral collateral ligament.

Fig. 8-3. Medial elbow ligaments. *1,* Anterior oblique; *2,* posterior oblique; *3,* transverse oblique.

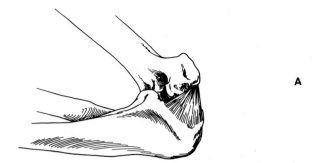

Fig. 8-4. A, Posterior oblique taut in flexion. **B,** Posterior oblique lax in extension.

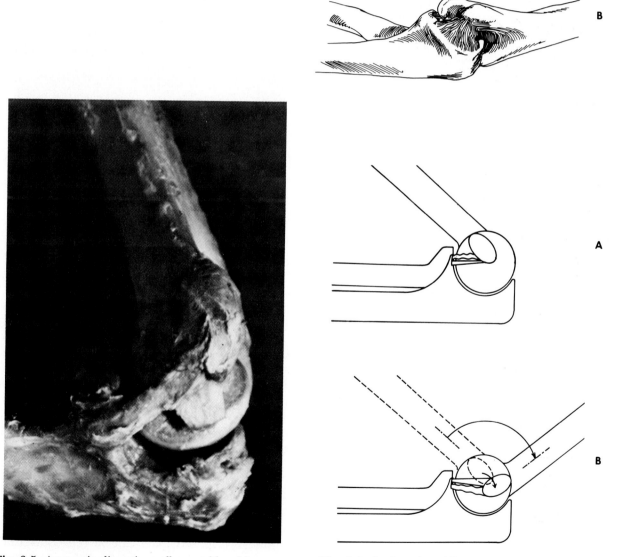

Fig. 8-5. Anatomic dissection: elbow stable with posterior oblique sectioned, anterior oblique intact.

Fig. 8-6. A, Anterior oblique taut throughout flexion. **B,** Anterior oblique taut throughout extension.

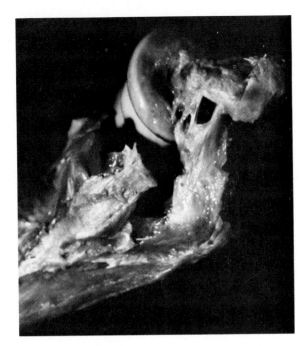

Fig. 8-7. Anatomic dissection: elbow unstable with anterior oblique sectioned; posterior oblique ligament is intact.

daveric specimens where the posterior oblique ligament is retained and the anterior oblique ligament is sectioned, the elbow becomes unstable (Fig. 8-7). It is therefore clear that the anterior oblique ligament is essential to the stability of the elbow throughout the entire range of motion.

ACUTE VALGUS INSTABILITY

Acute instability of the elbow to valgus stress is extremely uncommon. Rare cases of acute rupture of the anterior oblique ligament have been reported. This occurs primarily in javelin throwers. Other throwing athletes such as baseball pitchers can and do develop symptoms of acute anterior oblique ligament sprains though rarely of grade III.

The diagnosis of acute medial elbow instability is not difficult. Elbow arthrography will demonstrate extravasation of dye medially if ligament rupture is complete (Fig. 8-8). The characteristic physical findings of pain with valgus stress, and tenderness along the course of the anterior oblique ligament are generally sufficient to make a diagnosis.

Stress x-ray exam of elbows subjected to acute or chronic stress is essential. The elbow is inher-

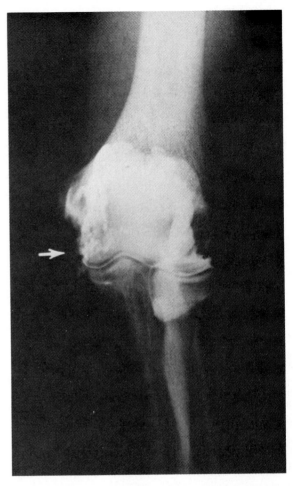

Fig. 8-8. Elbow arthrogram: extravasation of dye at medial joint line, *arrow,* indicative of complete rupture of medial collateral ligament.

ently stable in extension even in the absence of the anterior oblique ligament. The olecranon process locks into the olecranon fossa in extension making it technically difficult to produce a medial joint opening with valgus stress. If, however, the elbow is flexed 30 to 40 degrees to clear the olecranon process from its fossa, the elbow with insufficiency of its medial supporting structures can be both palpably and radiographically demonstrated to be unstable (Fig. 8-9).

Other tests useful in differentiating pain originating from the anterior oblique ligament as opposed to that from the flexor forearm mass are available. In the case of flexor forearm muscle ruptures or sprains, pain can be reproduced by resistive flexion of either the fingers or the wrist with the elbow held in neutral position (Fig. 8-10).

On the other hand with the forearm relaxed,

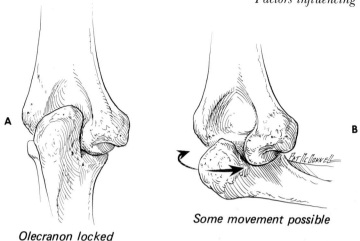

Fig. 8-9. A, Elbow in extension with olecranon locked in its fossa. **B,** Olecranon unlocked with elbow flexed 30 to 40 degrees. (**A** and **B,** Copyright Baylor College of Medicine, 1980.)

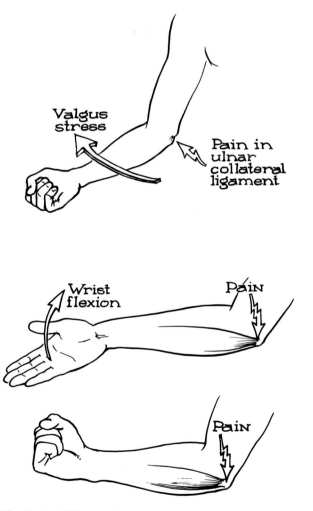

Fig. 8-10. Differentiation between medial collateral ligament strain and tear of the flexor of the forearm muscle by physical examination.

valgus stress on the elbow reproducing the pain along the course of the anterior oblique ligament is diagnostic (Fig. 8-10).

MEDIAL EPICONDYLE FRACTURES IN CHILDREN

Perhaps the most common example of acute valgus elbow instability occurs as medial epicondyle fractures in children. All are accustomed to treating these nondisplaced fractures conservatively. Not all these fractures, however, are undisplaced nor are they all stable. Several authors have suggested that when displacement occurs, surgery may be necessary. This has been based on millimeters of displacement.

We propose an alternate approach. It is not millimeters of displacement but rather degree of instability that is the determining factor as to whether the medial epicondyle should be surgically replaced.

It is significant that the medial epicondyle fragment usually contains the origin of the anterior oblique ligament, particularly if the fragment is large (Fig. 8-11). Therefore medial epicondyle fractures in children can represent a simple partial avulsion of the epiphysis or a complete fracture through the medial epicondyle with displacement or even entrapment of the fragment within the joint (Fig. 8-12). The anterior oblique ligament is the determining factor in these injuries. Failure to maintain the integrity of this ligament and its attached bone fragment can and does result in chronic instability, which persists throughout life.

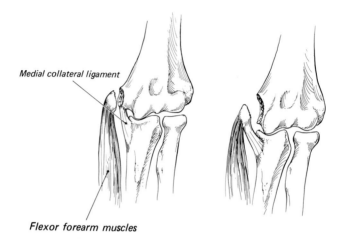

Medial collateral ligament

Flexor forearm muscles

Fig. 8-11. The larger the medial epicondyle fracture, the more likely the origin of the medial collateral ligament will be included with the fragment. (Copyright Baylor College of Medicine, 1980.)

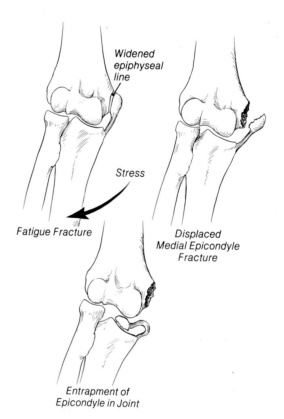

Widened epiphyseal line

Stress

Fatigue Fracture

Displaced Medial Epicondyle Fracture

Entrapment of Epicondyle in Joint

Fig. 8-12. Valgus stress in children. (Copyright Baylor College of Medicine, 1978.)

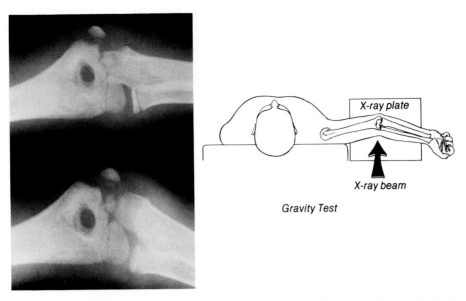

Fig. 8-13. Gravity stress roentgenogram of medial collateral ligament. (Copyright Baylor College of Medicine, 1980.)

A simple gravity stress test has been helpful (Fig. 8-13). The arm is brought into abduction and external rotation and lies unsupported off the edge of the x-ray table. This degree of gravity stress is not unduly painful. This x-ray view, obtained in the office without anesthesia, gives valuable information. If the elbow is unstable to valgus stress, that is, if the fragment moves significantly (Fig. 8-13), stability is best restored by surgical intervention. If the elbow is stable, surgery is unnecessary.

CHRONIC VALGUS INSTABILITY IN ADULTS

The most common example of chronic valgus instability is seen in the professional throwing athlete typified by the baseball pitcher. Chronic repetition of the throwing acts over many years results in attenuation of the medial supporting structures.

As the medial supporting structures become lax, the forearm drifts into valgus (Fig. 8-14). Valgus elbow deformity occurs in more than 30% of professional baseball pitchers.

With increased elbow valgus the mechanics of the joint are altered. The medial tip of the olecranon process may impinge on the wall of the olecranon fossa (Fig. 8-14). Loose body exfoliation occurs into the olecranon fossa. Loose bodies

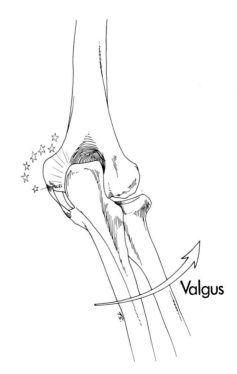

Fig. 8-14. Impingement of tip of olecranon in olecranon fossa with laxity of medial collateral ligament.

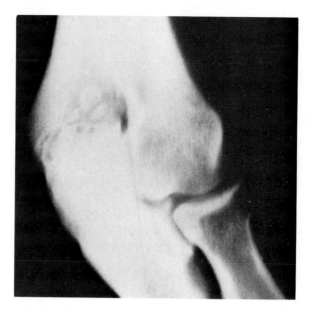

Fig. 8-15. Anteroposterior tomogram of elbow demonstrating loose bodies in olecranon fossa.

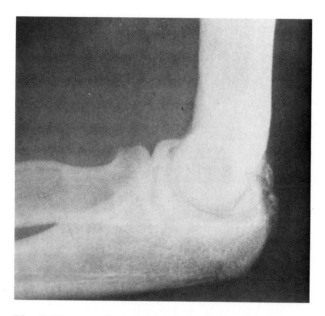

Fig. 8-16. Lateral roentgenogram of elbow in demonstrating loose-body exfoliation from tip of olecranon.

from this apparent site of origin are common and constitute the reason for approximately half of elbow surgery done in professional throwing athletes.

Tomograms of throwing athletes at varying stages in their career reflect corroborating evidence to this basic concept. Loose bodies are initially seen at the tip of the olecranon process (Fig. 8-15). With time they exfoliate filling the fossa with free fragments of bone and cartilage.

Routine lateral x-ray films of throwing athletes reveal fluffy calcification at the tip of the olecranon process (Fig. 8-16). This represents not triceps tendonitis but rather loose body exfoliation, since the tip of the olecranon process is intraarticular.

ROLE OF RADIOCAPITELLAR JOINT IN VALGUS STRESS

Basic to the understanding of elbow stability is the role of the radiocapitellar joint. Whereas the medial structures, particularly the anterior oblique, are the first line of defense in valgus stress, the second line of defense is the radiocapitellar joint. As the medial collateral ligament becomes attenuated or as force exceeds the capacity of the medial collateral ligament, the radiocapitellar joint is subjected to compressive forces (Fig. 8-17). These compressive forces induce loose bodies of either the radial head or capitellum of professional throwing athletes. Where stress exceeds the integrity of the medial ligament, as in dislocations, fractures of the radial head are common. Thus, in terms of valgus stress, radiocapitellar joint support is a secondary defense mechanism. The primary defense relies on the integrity of the anterior oblique ligament.

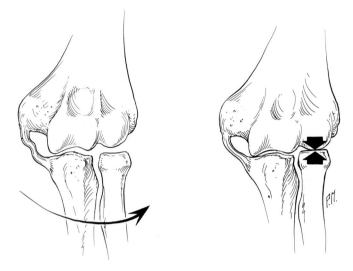

Fig. 8-17. Compression of radiocapitellar joint as a result of laxity of the medial collateral ligament. (Copyright Baylor College of Medicine, 1980.)

ANTEROPOSTERIOR INSTABILITY

The elbow joint is unique within the joints of the upper extremity. It begins in varus with full flexion and ends in valgus in full extension. This is caused by the lateral tilt of the joint surfaces of both the trochlea and the capitellum. It is also significant that as the elbow comes into complete extension the olecranon process locks into its fossa. There is no basic ligamentous support posteriorly. The stability of the elbow in terms of anteroposterior stress is dependent on the integrity of its collateral ligaments and on the coronoid process.

Much as been written of olecranon process fractures in regard to elbow stability after excision.

Anatomic studies indicate that where the olecranon process has been removed but the anterior oblique ligament remains intact, the elbow remains stable. Irrespective of whether the olecranon process is intact or not, if the anterior oblique is severed, the elbow becomes unstable (Fig. 8-18). The concept therefore is that it is the anterior oblique ligament and not the olecranon process that is essential for stability. With surgical excision of the olecranon process, as the anterior oblique ligament insertion is removed, the elbow will become unstable. And if the anterior oblique is absent, the elbow will be unstable even if the olecranon process is retained.

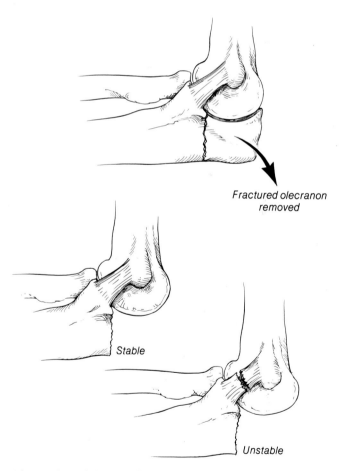

Fractured olecranon removed

Stable

Unstable

Fig. 8-18. Stability of elbow after olecranon excision if dependent on integrity of medial collateral ligament. (Copyright Baylor College of Medicine, 1978.)

ELBOW DISLOCATIONS

All orthopedic surgeons have experience with dislocations of the elbow. It is well known that the majority of these dislocations, once reduced, are stable and well managed with plaster immobilization followed by early motion. Although the preceding statement is generally accurate, it is not always so. Certain elbows, when reduced, are not stable and tend to redislocate within the first 7 to 10 days.

Insight into these unstable dislocations may be gained by an understanding of the mechanism of the dislocation.

The most reasonable, probably correct, theory of elbow dislocations is that it is an event of hyperextension (Fig. 8-19). As the elbow is hyperextended, the olecranon process is wedged into the fossa and then used as a fulcrum to bring the coronoid process under the trochlea. For this to occur, the anterior oblique portion of the medial collateral ligament must either be torn, stretched, or avulsed with a periosteal sleeve from the medial epicondyle.

At the point of reduction, if the ligament is fundamentally intact or avulsed with a periosteal sleeve, reduction may well produce a ligament that is functionally intact. If the ligament, however, has been torn either through its midsubstance or avulsed from bone so that continuity is not reestablished at reduction, the elbow has potential for, but not necessarily is, unstable.

Rupture of the medial collateral ligament alone in the course of elbow dislocation is probably common. In the face of an intact radiocapitellar joint, that is, with the secondary defense mechanisms intact, this type of elbow dislocation will do well after reduction with apparent healing of the medial ligament.

However, should both mechanisms be involved, that is, should the anterior oblique be ruptured and the radial head destroyed, then there is no basic stability either medically or laterally (Fig. 8-20). These elbows will be unstable and will redislocate. Surgical repair of one or both sides is justified.

Commonly restoration of joint integrity by replacement of the fractured radial head with a radial head prosthesis or spacer is sufficient. Recognition is the key to the injury (Fig. 8-20).

The use of intraoperative stress x-ray examina-

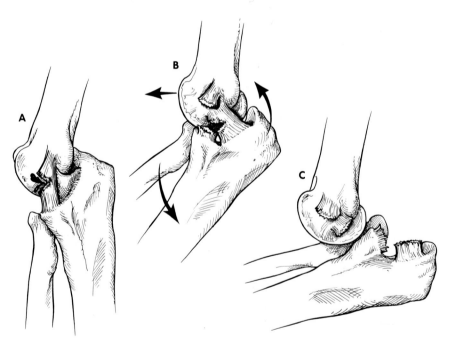

Fig. 8-19. Mechanism of elbow dislocation. **A,** Initial hyperextension ruptures or avulses medial collateral ligament. **B,** Levering of coronoid under trochlea by olecranon. **C,** Dislocated with torn medial collateral ligament. (**A** to **C,** Copyright Baylor College of Medicine, 1978.)

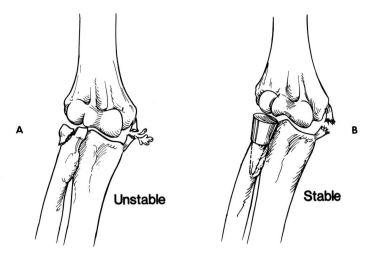

Fig. 8-20. A, Elbow is unstable with fracture of radial head and rupture of medial collateral ligament. **B,** Elbow may be stabilized by repair of medial collateral ligament, replacement of radial head, or both.

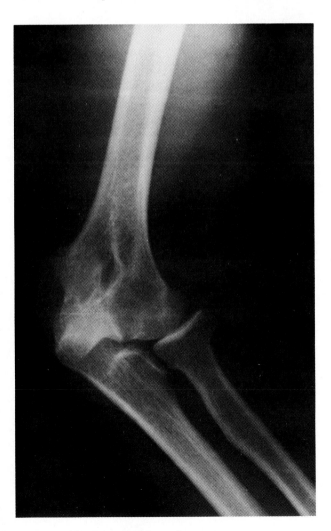

Fig. 8-21. Positive valgus stress test.

tions after elbow relocations, particularly those associated with fractures of the capitellum or radial head, is mandatory (Fig. 8-21). Should the elbow be unstable and the radial head fractured, the use of a radial head spacer is appropriate and will provide sufficient stability. However, should the lateral joint lesion be unrepairable (such as a comminuted fracture of the capitellum), attention must be directed to the anterior oblique ligament.

The approach to the medial collateral ligament is through an incision that traverses midway between the medial epicondyle and the tip of the olecranon process (Fig. 8-22). This is the same incision commonly used for transfer of the ulnar nerve. The ulnar nerve is identified and transferred anteriorly. The flexor forearm mass is identified, and beneath this the posterior oblique and anterior oblique components of the medial collateral ligament are identified.

The most common lesion in the anterior oblique ligament is avulsion from the medial epicondyle. This is repaired with a Bunnell suture passed through two drill holes in the medial epicondyle. An alternate approach where the ligament is torn from its midportion would be a simple end-to-end anastomosis (Fig. 8-23).

After repair of either the medial or lateral side of an elbow dislocation the postoperative plan is to manage the elbow in a cast brace with early motion but restricting varus-valgus stress forces. A posterior stop, limiting extension, is dependent on the position at which the elbow redislocates.

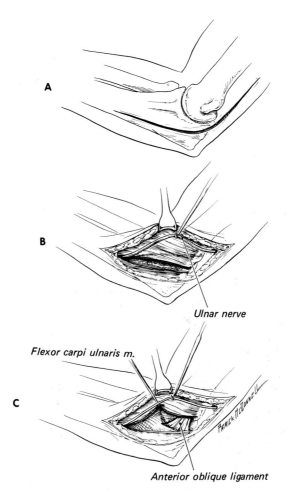

Flexor carpi ulnaris m.

Ulnar nerve

Anterior oblique ligament

Fig. 8-22. Surgical approach to medial collateral ligament. **A,** Skin incision halfway between medial epicondyle and tip of olecranon. **B,** Ulnar nerve released and transposed anteriorly. **C,** Flexor capri ulnaris retracted volarward to expose anterior oblique portion of medial collateral ligament. (Copyright Baylor College of Medicine, 1980.)

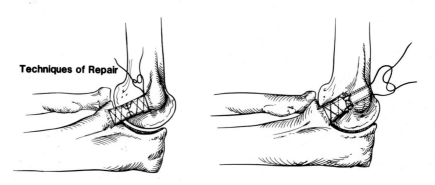

Techniques of Repair

Fig. 8-23. Techniques of repair and reattachment of medial collateral ligament.

CHRONIC ANTEROPOSTERIOR INSTABILITY IN RECURRENT ELBOW DISLOCATIONS

In those instances where anterior oblique ligament insufficiency is retained throughout life (particularly where the coronoid process is either congenitally shallow or the anterior third fractured with the initial dislocation) recurrence of the elbow dislocations can and does occur. It is, however, rare.

Our experience with the biceps tendon transfer (Fig. 8-24) is that although it is technically a feasible operative procedure, it is not directed at the basic pathologic process. It is not necessarily effective in preventing recurrence.

The bone-block procedures (Fig. 8-24) that build up the anterior third of the coronoid process are indicated where the coronoid process is deficient. It is, however, technically very difficult to get the bone block in exactly the right position, and I have had at least one instance where dislocation has occurred over the top of the bone block despite what appeared to be a stable and adequately fused graft.

Since the basic pathologic condition does not lie anteriorly in most instances (with the exception of coronoid fractures) but rather at the anterior oblique ligament, failure to repair this lesion results in an elbow that will remain susceptible to recurrent dislocations.

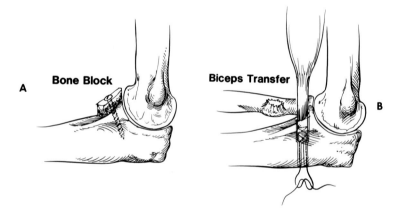

Fig. 8-24. A, Coracoid bone block transfer. **B,** Biceps tendon transfer.

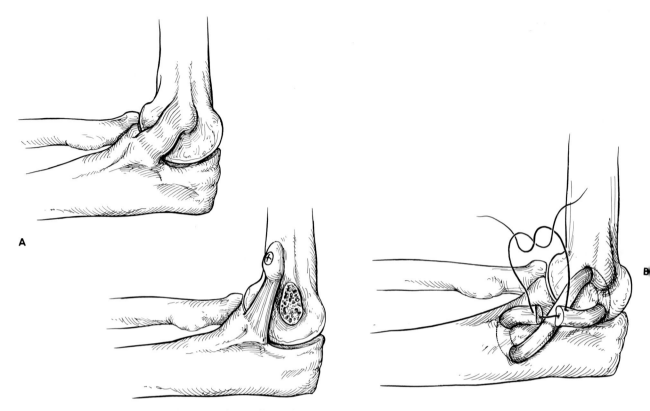

Fig. 8-25. A, Advancement of lax medial collateral ligament. **B,** Reconstruction of medial collateral ligament using palmaris longus tendon graft after Jobe. (**B,** Copyright Baylor College of Medicine, 1978.)

When the anterior oblique ligament is only attenuated, one can tighten it by removing the medial epicondyle and transferring it superiorly and anteriorly. This procedure performed on two or three occasions has resulted in no problems with rehabilitation and to date no documented evidence of recurrence of the dislocations.

Where the anterior oblique ligament is surgically absent because of remote trauma, reconstruction of the anterior oblique ligament becomes a technical problem. Our experience with prosthetic ligaments in this application has not been good. Recent communications with Jobe show that reconstruction of the ligament by use of a palmaris longus graft appears promising, making this now the procedure of choice. We have had no personal experience with this procedure (Fig. 8-25).

SUMMARY

Stability or instability of the elbow is contingent upon three distinct but interrelated conditions:

radiocapitellar articular continuity, coronoid process integrity and medial collateral ligament competency through an intact anterior oblique ligament. The latter, the anterior oblique ligament of the medial collateral ligament both in anatomic experimentation and clinical cases appears to be the most critical factor in elbow stability. The reconstruction of the unstable elbow must focus on this medial supporting ligament for a predictable result.

SUGGESTED READINGS

Adams, J.E.: Injury to the throwing arm: a study of traumatic changes in the elbow joints of baseball throwers, Calif. Med. **102:**127, 1965.

Adler, S., Fay, G.F., and MacAusland, W.R.: Treatment of olecranon fractures, indications for excision of the olecranon fracture, repair of the triceps tendon, J. Trauma **2:**597, 1962.

Allende, G., and Freytes, M.: Old dislocation of the elbow, J. Bone Joint Surg. **26:**691, 1944.

Anderson, L.: Fractures. In Crenshaw, A.H., editor: Campbell's operative orthopedics, ed. 5, St. Louis, 1971, The C.V. Mosby Co.

Barnes, D.A., and Tullos, H.S.: An analysis of 100 symptomatic baseball players, Am. J. Sports Med. **6:**62, 1978.

Brogdon, B.G., and Cros, N.F.: Little leaguer's elbow, Am. J. Roentgenol. **8:**671, 1960.

Colton, C.L.: Fractures of the olecranon in adults: classification and management, Injury **5:**121, 1976.

Conn, J., and Wade, P.: Injuries of the elbow: a ten year review, J. Trauma **1:**248, 1961.

DeHaven, K.E., and Evarts, C.M.: Throwing injuries of the elbow in athletes, Orthop. Clin. North Am. **1:**801, 1973.

DeHaven, K.E., Ferguson, A.G., Hale, C.J., Larson, R.L., and Tullos, H.S.: Symposium: throwing injuries to the adolescent elbow, Contemp. Surg. **9:**65, 1976.

Dunn, N.: Operation for fracture of the olecranon, Br. Med. J. **1:**214, 1939.

Eppright, R.H., and Wilkins, K.E.: In Rockwood, C.A., and Green, D.P., editors: Philadelphia, 1975, J.B. Lippincott Co.

Eriksson, E., Sahlin, O., and Sandah, U.: Late results of conservative and surgical treatment of fracture of the olecranon, Acta Chir. Scand. **113:**153, 1957.

Exarchou, E.J.: Lateral dislocation of the elbow, Acta Orthop. Scand. **48:**161, 1977.

Gosman, J.A.: Recurrent dislocation of the ulna at the elbow, J. Bone Joint Surg. **125:**448, 1943.

Gugenheim, J.J., Stanley, R.F., Woods, G.W., and Tullos, H.S.: Little league survey: the Houston study, Am. J. Sports Med. **4:**189, 1976.

Jacobs, R.L.: Recurrent dislocation of the elbow joint, Clin. Orthop. **74:**151, 1971.

James, S.: Discussion of pitching act. AAOS Post-Graduate Course, Committee on Sports Medicine, San Francisco, 1971.

Kapel, O.: Operation for habitual dislocation of the elbow, J. Bone Joint Surg. **33A:**707, 1951.

Kilfoyle, R.M.: Fractures of the medial condyle and epicondyle of the elbow in children, Clin. Orthop. **41:**43, 1965.

King, J.W., Brelsford, H.J., and Tullos, H.S.: Analysis of the pitching arm of the professional baseball pitcher, Clin. Orthop. **67:**116, 1961.

King, T.: Recurrent dislocation of the elbow, J. Bone Joint Surg. **35B:**50, 1953.

Knoflach, J.G.: Zur operation der habituellen Ellbogenluxation, Zentralbl. Chir. **62:**2897, 1935.

Linscheid, R.L., and Wheeler, D.K.: Elbow dislocations, J.A.M.A. **194:**1171, 1965.

Lou, I.: Olecranon fractures treated in orthopedic hospitals, Copenhagen 1936-1947: a follow-up examination, Acta Scand. **19:**166, 1949.

McKeever, F.M., and Buck, R.M.: Fracture of the olecranon process of the ulna: treatment by excision of fragment and repair of triceps tendon, J.A.M.A. **135:**1, 1947.

Milch, H.: Bilateral recurrent dislocation of the ulna at the elbow, J. Bone Joint Surg. **18:**777, 1936.

Osborne, G., and Cotterill, P.: Recurrent dislocation of the elbow, J. Bone Joint Surg. **48B:**340, 1966.

Reichenheim, P.P.: Transplantation of the biceps tendon as a treatment for recurrent dislocation of the elbow, Br. J. Surg. **35:**201, 1947.

Roberts, A.W.: Displacement of the internal epicondyle into the elbow joint, Lancet **2:**78, 1934.

Roberts, P.H.: Dislocation of the elbow, Br. J. Surg. **56:**806, 1969.

Slocum, D.B.: Classification of elbow injuries from baseball pitching, Texas Med. **64:**48, 1968.

Smith, F.M.: Surgery of the elbow, Springfield, Ill., 1954, Charles C Thomas, Publisher.

Sorrell, E.: Luxation récidivante du coude: opération, guérison, Bull. Mem. Soc. Chir. **61:**790, 1935.

Speed, J.S., and Boyd, H.B.: Fractures about the elbow, Am. J. Surg. **38:**727, 1937.

Spring, W.E.: Report of a case of recurrent dislocation of the elbow, J. Bone Joint Surg. **35B:**55, 1953.

Tachdjian, M.O.: Pediatric orthopedics, Philadelphia, 1972, W.B. Saunders Co.

Tullos, H.S., Erwin, W., Woods, G.W., et al.: Unusual lesions of the pitching arm, Clin. Orthop. **88:**169, 1972.

Tullos, H.S., and King, J.W.: Lesions of the pitching arm in adolescents, J.A.M.A. **220:**264, 1972.

Tullos, H.S., and King, J.W.: Throwing mechanism in sports, Orthop. Clin. North Am. **4:**709, 1973.

Wainwright, D.: Recurrent dislocation of the elbow joint, Proc. Soc. Med. **40:**885, 1947.

Waris, W.: Elbow injuries in javelin throwers, Acta Chir. Scand. **93:**563, 1946.

Warsick, R., and Williams, P.L., editors: Gray's anatomy, ed. 35, Philadelphia, 1973, W.B. Saunders Co.

Wheeler, D.K., and Linscheid, R.L.: Fracture dislocations of the elbow, Clin. Orthop. **50:**95, 1967.

Wilson, J.N.: The treatment of fractures of the medial epicondyle of the humerus, J. Bone Joint Surg. **42B:**778, 1960.

Wilson, P.D.: Fractures and dislocations in the region of the elbow, Surg. Gynecol. Obstet. **56:**335, 1933.

Winslow, R.: A case of complete anterior dislocation of both bones of the forearm at the elbow, Surg. Gynecol. Obstet. **15:**570, 1913.

Woods, G.W., and Tullos, H.S.: Elbow instability and medial epicondyle fractures, Am. J. Sports Med. **5:**23, 1977.

Woods, G.W., Tullos, H.S., and King, J.W.: The throwing arm: elbow injuries, J. Sports Med. **1**(Sports safety suppl.):4, 1973.

Chapter 9

Fractures about the elbow in adults

RICHARD S. BRYAN, M.D.
Rochester, Minnesota

The injured elbow joint presents more difficulty than almost any other because it really is three joints that move synchronously. Any alteration in the anatomic structure may cause impingement. The transverse axis of the humeroulnar articulation should be in line with the anterior surface of the humerus. So any change in angulation of the distal humerus affects flexion-extension if it is in the anteroposterior plane and affects the carrying angle if in the mediolateral plane. The carrying angle is normally established by the differential slope of the trochlea posteromedially, which forces the forearm into valgus in extension. Thus any change in either shape or alignment of the trochlea affects the carrying angle.

Because the capitellum has no articulation posteriorly and faces anteriorly and distally, it may be fractured by a longitudinal force in extension. With a loading of more than 4.5 kg (10 pounds), more than 50% of the force passes through the radiohumeral joint. Since the radius and ulna are fixed to each other by the annular ligament, any alteration in position or shape of the capitellum, radial head, or olecranon affects the range of motion by causing impingement.

Lastly, a point often not recognized is that the elbow must have a fossa both anteriorly and posteriorly to function properly. It is amazing that such a small, closely machined joint can accept the stress of three times body weight, which is its usual burden. Nonetheless, fractures about the elbow represent only 6% of all fractures treated, according to Eppright and Wilkins.[7]

SUPRACONDYLAR FRACTURES

Supracondylar fractures most commonly occur in children but again become common in the elderly as the bones become weaker than the ligaments. If the distal fragment is posterior, the fracture is of the extension type. The fracture is often caused by a fall on the outstretched hand. In this fracture, the posterior triangle formed by the medial and lateral epicondyles and the olecranon is intact.

Treatment may encompass any of several methods. Closed reduction and casting or splinting in flexion serves well for the extension type, and the consensus is in favor of pronation of the forearm, though debate still exists. The flexion type requires casting with a posteriorly directed force applied to the forearm, if conservative treatment is utilized. Percutaneous pinning may be used and is especially applicable to the unstable transcondylar fracture. Threaded Kirschner wires or Steinmann pins rather than smooth pins are usually better for this. Open reduction is indicated when there is vascular injury or the reduction is not acceptable. Internal fixation may be of several types, varying from the use of Y plates and screws, screws alone, and Kirschner wires, to the use of external fixators. The transcondylar fracture is particularly likely to cause problems because the fracture line passes through the fossae; the distal fragment is small, with only small extra-articular areas to control rotation; and the radiohumeral and ulnohumeral joints may dislocate during rotation. The humeral shaft may then block reduction by closed means. Furthermore, the amount of bone in contact for union, even in a perfect reduction, is small, and imperfect reduction may lead to large amounts of callus obliterating the fossae.

Radial nerve injury, which occurs in 10% to 15% of humeral shaft fractures (most commonly in the middle third), also occurs in supracondylar fractures. Packer and associates[16] and Sim and associates[18] have shown that the results of early exploration—within 2 weeks—are superior to observation with late exploration if recovery did not occur. The report of Fischer and House[8] also supports the concept of early exploration in complete

radial nerve palsy associated with fractures of the humerus.

Case 1

A 72-year-old woman fell on the ice, incurring a transcondylar fracture of her right elbow. A closed reduction was done, and the elbow was casted in extension for 10 days. The cast was then changed to 40 degrees, with some loss of position. The cast was removed 19 days after injury, and active range-of-motion exercises were begun. At 11 months, her elbow had 30 to 150 degrees of flexion-extension range, with full rota-

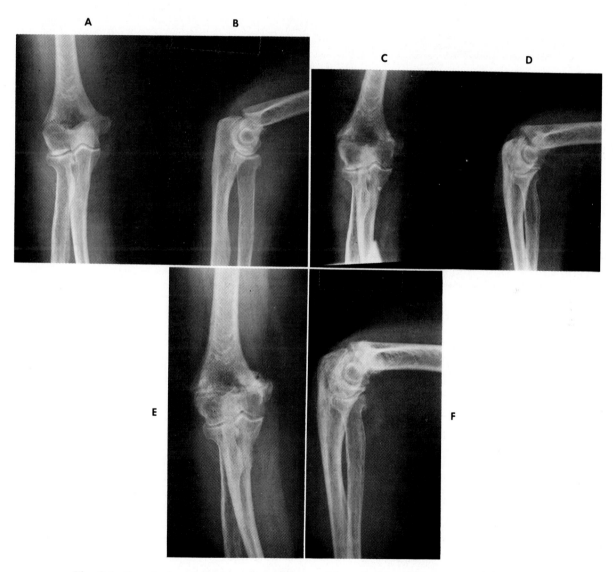

Fig. 9-1. *Case 1.* **A** and **B,** Anteroposterior and lateral views show transcondylar fracture of humerus. Mild displacement of distal fragment anteriorly. **C** and **D,** Six weeks later, fracture has slipped a little more but is healing. **E** and **F,** Four months later, fracture has healed.

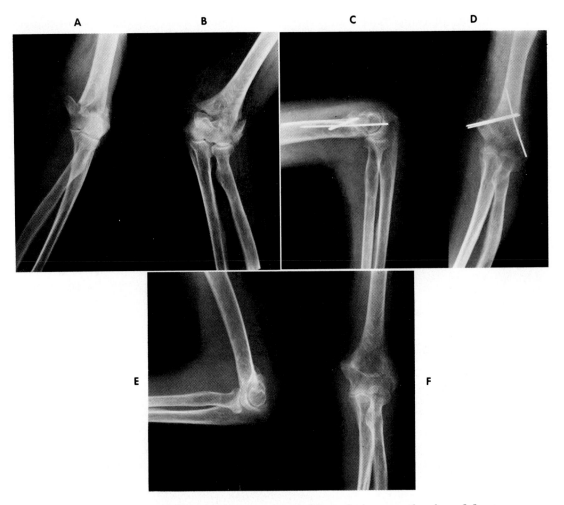

Fig. 9-2. *Case 2.* **A** and **B,** Anteroposterior and lateral views on the day of fracture show transcondylar fracture with some displacement and rotation. **C** and **D,** Anteroposterior and lateral views show fracture pinned with three Kirschner wires, but transverse axis of trochlea is posterior to anterior humeral cortex. Normal forward tilt of distal humerus has not been reconstituted. **E** and **F,** Fracture is well healed but with residual change in forward tilt.

tion and no pain. Roentgenograms are shown at the time of fracture, at 6 weeks, and at 4 months (Fig. 9-1).

Case 2

A 65-year-old woman fell on her left arm, fracturing the humerus transcondylarly. A splint was applied, but the reduction was lost at 14 days, and for that reason closed reduction and percutaneous pinning with three Kirschner wires were done. The wires were removed at 8 weeks, and at 4 months a range of extension-flexion of 35 to 145 degrees with full rotation was present. Roentgenograms at the time of fracture, at 5 weeks, and at 10 weeks are shown (Fig. 9-2).

INTERCONDYLAR T OR Y FRACTURES

Most of these fractures are caused by force transmitted directly through the olecranon to the trochlea by a fall. The position of the elbow at the moment of injury influences the extent and direction of the fracture line, and the muscular forces acting on the condyles produce the rotation that is so frequently seen. The prognosis in this rare fracture must be guarded. Radin and Riseborough[17] classified these fractures into type I, undisplaced (Fig. 9-3, *A*), which respond well to splinting; type II (Fig. 9-3, *B*), with mild displacement

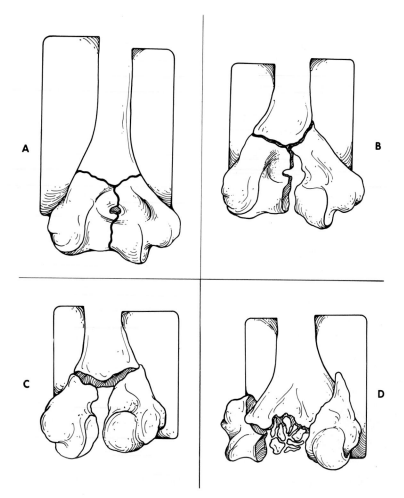

Fig. 9-3. A, Type I, undisplaced T condylar fracture of elbow. **B,** Type II, displaced but not rotated T condylar fracture. **C,** Type III, displaced and rotated T condylar fracture. **D,** Type IV, displaced, rotated, and comminuted T condylar fracture. (**A** to **D,** Copyright Mayo Clinic, 1980, Rochester, Minn.)

but no rotation; type III (Fig. 9-3, *C*), with rotation; and type IV (Fig. 9-3, *D*), with comminution. They favored conservative treatment for most patients with these fractures. However, Bickel and Perry,[3] Bryan and Bickel,[4] and Cassebaum[5,6] favored open reduction and internal fixation for most patients. These fractures are extremely difficult to treat, and poor surgical treatment can produce as much or more scarring and loss of function than the closed methods. Nonoperative methods are particularly applicable to the elderly, osteoporotic patient, who is often the one with a

type IV fracture. Fixation in these patients is poor at best, and the hazards of anesthesia may be excessive.

Closed methods of treatment

Casting with careful molding of the condyles and the elbow at 90 degrees is not a very effective method because it does nothing to reduce the fragments and it encourages the development of fibrosis.

Traction with early motion may increase rotation of the fragments though the use of a collar and cuff in acute flexion, with gradually increasing extension, uses the weight of the arm for traction and promotes the retention of motion in the needed range. This is an effective method for use in the elderly patient with a type IV fracture.

Operative methods

Closed pinning, followed by casting or splinting, though producing some fixation, usually does not permit accurate reduction, prevents early motion, and is usually only applicable to fractures of types I and II.

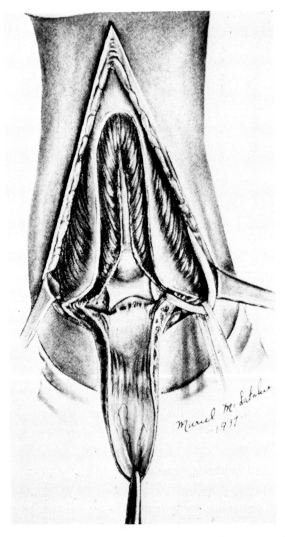

Fig. 9-4. Van Gorder or Campbell posterior approach to elbow. Triceps tendon is freed from muscle and turned down to olecranon. Muscle is then split and reflected medially and laterally for exposure.

Open reduction and screw fixation of the articular surface, with the treatment of the supracondylar fracture line by traction or casting, still is frequently used and may be all that can be done.

Rigid internal or external fixation, using screws, plates, Kirschner wires, or external fixators, has been used more frequently in recent years, as better instruments and exposures have become available.

There are three surgical approaches to this difficult fracture currently in use, all posterior. The Van Gorder, originally described by Campbell, utilizes a triceps-splitting approach, turning the lower triceps tendon, as a wide V based distally, down to the olecranon (Fig. 9-4). This approach gives good exposure of the supracondylar portion of the fracture and the medial and lateral condyles but only fair visibility of the trochlea and capitellum.

The Cassebaum or transolecranon approach divides the olecranon with an osteotome, after two holes are drilled from the tip through the cortex on each side (Fig. 9-5). The division is in the nonarticular portion. This approach permits excellent exposure of the trochlea and capitellum and of the anterior portion of the joint but removes a template against which the fractured parts can be reconstituted. Furthermore, it adds another fracture adjacent to the previous injury, which may cause increased adhesions. Nonunion also may result, and any malunion might be disastrous.

The Mayo approach was developed during the evolution of total elbow arthroplasty. We encountered five patients with triceps weakness after the Van Gorder approach or after a simple transection of the triceps during the exposure. Our approach was modified to a posterior incision, just medial to the olecranon, extending 10 cm above and 5 cm below the tip of the olecranon. The ulnar nerve is easily identified along the medial border of the triceps and is freed from the triceps down to the groove, where it is unroofed gently. The ulnar nerve is usually not disturbed but remains visible for protection (Fig. 9-6, *A*). The periosteum along the crest of the ulna, 2.5 to 5 cm below the tip of the olecranon, is incised and freed from medial to lateral, with the triceps retracted laterally and the ulnar periosteum also retracted laterally (Fig. 9-6, *B*). The insertion of the triceps and the capsule underlying it is released from the tip and sides of the olecranon (Fig. 9-6, *C*). Gradually this muscle with the tendon and periosteal flap and with the fat and capsule attached is mobilized laterally until the lateral condyle, trochlea, and capitellum are clearly seen (Fig. 9-6, *D*). In the presence of gross comminution, this mobilization may require freeing the lateral border of the olecranon and the anconeus origin and even detachment of the annular ligament from the ulna posteriorly. This extensive baring of the olecranon has resulted in no instances of necrosis in more than 50 patients.[15] After fixation of the fracture by the means selected, a transverse drill hole is placed in the olecranon, and two nonabsorbable sutures are placed as a horizontal mattress out through the distal triceps tendon and back to be tied at the bone hole. This puckers the tendon end against the olecranon tip and results in no loss of triceps strength. A lateral-to-medial approach also has been used, but this has the dis-

advantages of cutting across the triceps fibers that end laterally and not exposing the ulnar nerve as well for protection.

Methods of fixation of T condylar fractures vary with the experience of the surgeon, the degree of comminution, the osteoporosis present, and the extent of soft-tissue distortion. I prefer to use at least one screw to fix the trochlea and capitellum, with one additional wire or screw to prevent rotation. Occasionally the capitellum is a free fragment and must be fixed with Kirschner wires. If so, I prefer to use threaded wires and drill them to below the surface for removal posteriorly. Great care must be taken to remove any bone or pin that impinges on the fossae. Fixation of the distal fragments to the proximal humerus may be possible by screws or the use of a Y plate. Kirschner wires are less often satisfactory. External fix-

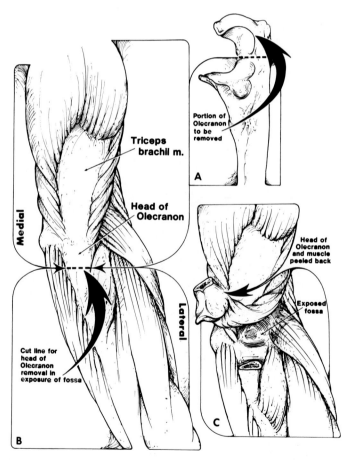

Fig. 9-5. Cassebaum[5,6] transolecranon approach. **A** and **B,** Osteotomy is through nonarticular area, and bone is drilled before division. **C,** Tip of olecranon and triceps are then reflected superiorly. (**A** to **C,** Copyright Mayo Clinic, 1980, Rochester, Minn.)

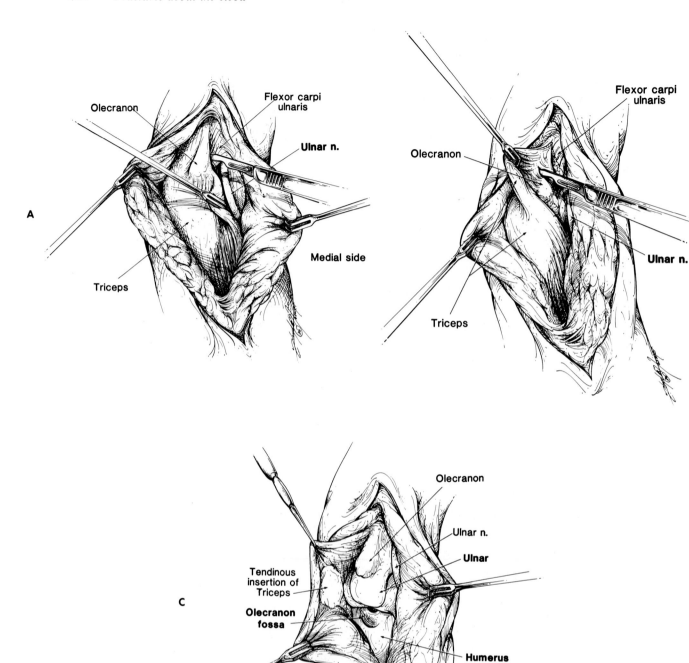

Fig. 9-6. A, Exposure is along medial border, protecting the ulnar nerve. **B,** Periosteum of ulna is reflected laterally, as is the triceps. **C,** Triceps insertion is severed, leaving the triceps in continuity with ulnar periosteum. Capsule and fat pad have been mobilized laterally to expose the fossa. (**A** to **C,** Copyright Mayo Clinic, 1980, Rochester, Minn.)

ators such as the Hoffmann apparatus may be very useful in these fractures, with two pins being placed across the distal fragment and three placed proximally. These have the disadvantage of communication from the exterior into an extensively damaged environment, but there have been no infections in our small series.[14]

The method of fixation should allow early motion at least by the third week after fracture if motion is to be regained. This fracture is most difficult to treat, and I have seen many patients with a severe loss of function from inadequate treatment. More of these patients can be salvaged, even after many months. Usually the patient retains good rotation and loses flexion-extension. Osteonecrosis is rare, as is neurovascular injury primarily. Nerve injury as a result of prolonged tourniquet time or manipulation during reduction is relatively more common. Eppright and Wilkins[7] enumerated a number of excellent principles for this fracture, and I repeat some of them.

1. The articular surface must be assembled and stabilized first.

2. Loss of articular surface can be accepted; incongruity cannot.

3. Any large separate fragments from the epithrochlear ridges should be fixed to the proximal shaft before an attempt is made to stabilize the articular condyles to the shaft because they act as buttresses.

4. Proximally directed screws must engage the opposite cortex in order to achieve fixation. The cancellous bone of the distal humeral shaft will not hold.

5. Screws are preferable to Kirschner wires.

6. The fossae must be clear of apparatuses, bone, and debris. The entire bone of the fossae may be excised, with impunity and even benefit. This emphasizes that stability depends on two stable columns of bone, the medial and lateral condyles.

7. The alignment of the axis of motion through the center of the capitellum and trochlea and in line with the anterior cortex of the humerus above the fossae is necessary to prevent loss of motion.

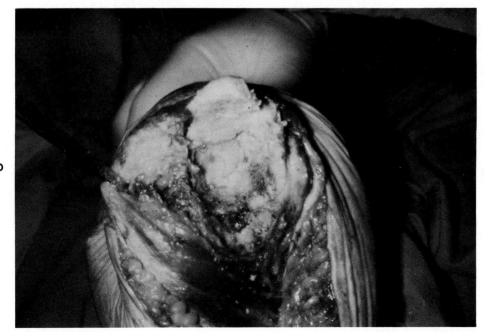

D

Fig. 9-6, cont'd. D, Surgical exposure in patient undergoing total elbow arthroplasty. Tip of olecranon has been excised for this reason, but exposure is the same.

Case 3

A 43-year-old woman fell from a chair and sustained a type III T condylar fracture of the left distal humerus (Fig. 9-7, *A* and *B*). An open reduction was performed the next day through a Van Gorder approach, using a Y plate and eight screws plus a transverse screw. The transverse screw was removed at 4 months. The roentgenogram at 3 months is shown in Fig. 9-7, *C* and *D*. Her range of extension-flexion was 35 to 95 degrees at 7 months, with full rotation. Two years later, she fell and incurred an undisplaced fracture of the olecranon (Fig. 9-7, *E* and *F*), which was treated with splinting for 3 weeks. Her range of motion increased to between 45 and 120 degrees. At 5 years, she fell again and fractured the olecranon. This was splinted for 3 weeks, and her range of motion increased to between 20 and 120 degrees, with full rotation (Fig. 9-7, *G* and *H*).

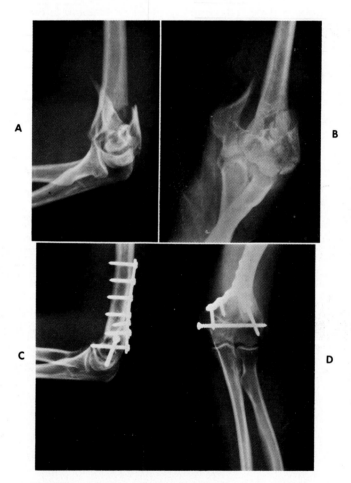

Fig. 9-7. *Case 3.* **A** and **B,** Type III fracture with displacement and rotation of condyles. **C** and **D,** Three months after open reduction. Joint is well aligned, but inferior lateral screw invades radial fossa.

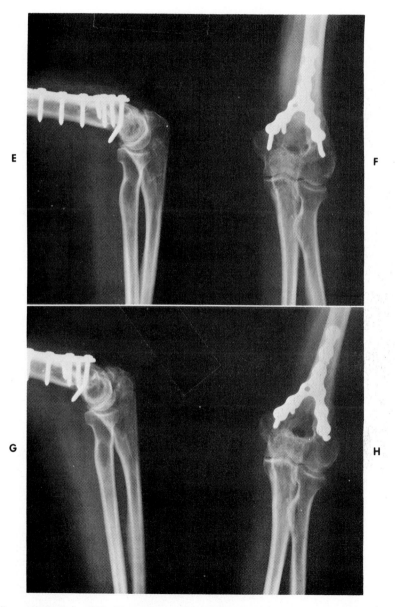

Fig. 9-7, cont'd. E and **F,** Two years after original fracture. Note healed olecranon fracture and bent screw. Transverse screw has been removed. **G** and **H,** At 5 years, note healing fracture of the olecranon and the bent screw.

Case 4

A 35-year-old woman was riding a snowmobile when it overturned; she sustained a type IV T condylar fracture of the left elbow (Fig. 9-8, *A* and *B*). An open reduction through a triceps-splitting approach was used, and four Kirschner wires were inserted, but non stabilized the articular surface (Fig. 9-8, *C* and *D*). The wires were removed at 3 months. Her range of motion at 4 months was only 50 to 95 degrees, and there was obvious malunion of the trochlea. At that time, the trochlea was replaced in its anatomic position and fixed with two Smille nails, one of which was too long (Fig. 9-8, *E* and *F*). The patient regained a range of motion of between 22 and 110 degrees, with full rotation, and the nail gradually wore a small groove in the ulna (Fig. 9-8, *G* and *H*). She remains pain free at 10 years.

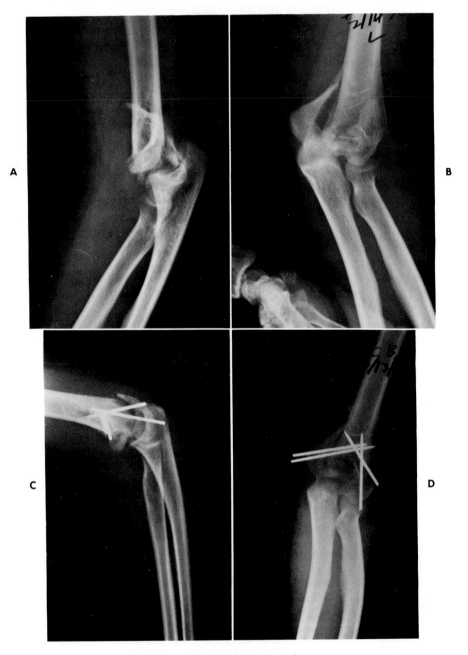

Fig. 9-8. For legend see opposite page.

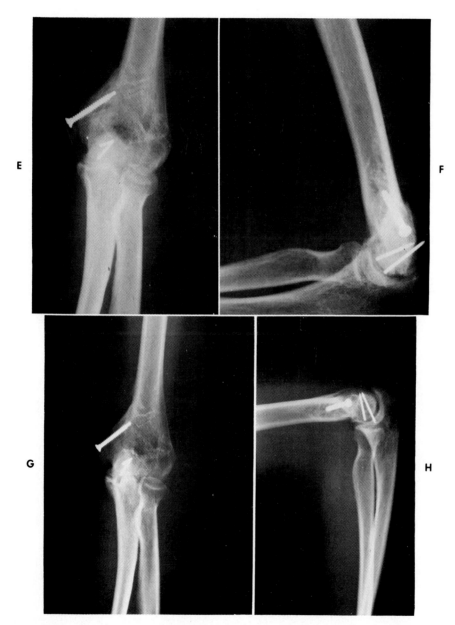

Fig. 9-8. *Case 4.* **A** and **B,** Type IV T condylar fracture. Note olecranon has sheared off medial condyle and rotation is caused by muscle pull. **C** and **D,** Wires fix supracondylar ridges well, but trochlea remains displaced and rotated. **E** and **F,** Trochlea has been repositioned, but one Smillie nail is too long. **G** and **H,** At 7 years, protruding nail has worn its own path in ulna.

Case 5

A 54-year-old man fell from a ladder, striking his right elbow and sustaining an open type IV T condylar fracture (Fig. 9-9, *A*). An open reduction was performed through a triceps-splitting approach, and the supracondylar fracture was fixed with a Y plate and seven screws. Roentgenograms postoperatively demonstrated displacement of the trochlea (Fig. 9-9, *B*), and a second procedure was performed 3 days later. The exposure extended the previous exposure by allowing re-

flection of the triceps insertion with the ulnar periosteum to either side (Fig. 9-9, *C*). The trochlea was secured to the lateral condyle with a screw and two threaded Kirschner wires, and the two mediodistal screws in the plate were repositioned to close the fracture line more accurately (Fig. 9-9, *D* to *F*). The arm was not casted, and it regained a range of flexion-extension of 40 to 120 degrees, with full rotation when the Kirschner wires were removed.

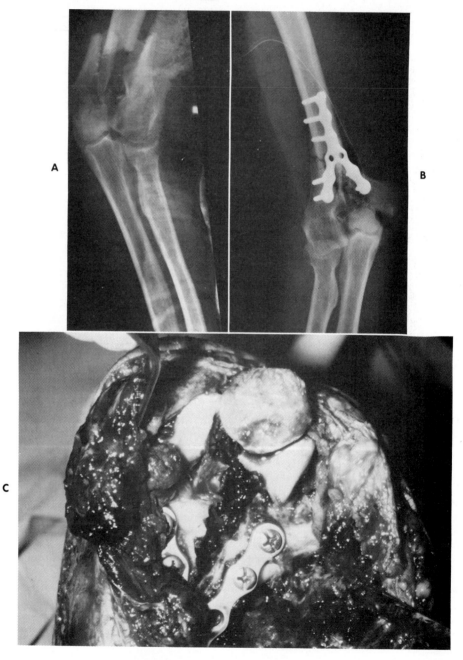

Fig. 9-9. For legend see opposite page.

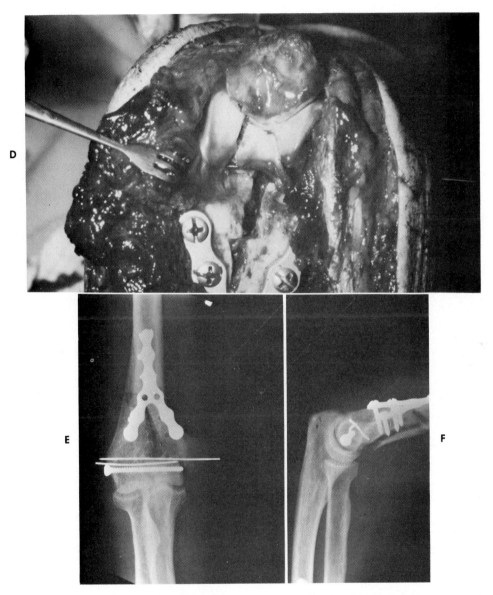

Fig. 9-9. *Case 5.* **A,** Type IV T condylar fracture. Trochlea is separate fragment with comminution. **B,** Anteroposterior view showing fixation of supracondylar portion of fracture, but note proximal displacement of trochlea and lack of attachment to either lateral or medial condyles. **C,** Humerus at bottom, olecranon at top, and fracture trochlea in middle. Plate is seen at bottom. This illustrates the exposure by the Mayo approach. **D,** Trochlea has been assembled and fitted to olecranon as a template. Ulnar nerve is at right, unroofed but not translocated. **E** and **F,** Anteroposterior and lateral views 1 week after second procedure. Articular surface has now been reassembled.

FRACTURES OF HUMERAL CONDYLES

The counterpart of the lateral condyle fractures seen in children occurs in the adult. This often is in combination with other injuries, such as a fracture of both bones of the forearm, which must be considered in the treatment. Milch[13] divided both medial and lateral condyle fractures into types I and II, with type II including the lateral trochlear ridge. Occasionally, percutaneous pinning or casting of an undisplaced fracture is possible, but usually the muscle pull has caused rotation, and open reduction with internal fixation is necessary. This permits accurate realignment and early motion.

Case 6

A 64-year-old woman was involved in an automobile accident in which she sustained a fracture of the lateral condyle of her left elbow (Fig. 9-10). An open reduction and insertion of one screw permitted motion to begin 8 days after her fracture, with return of a full range of motion quickly.

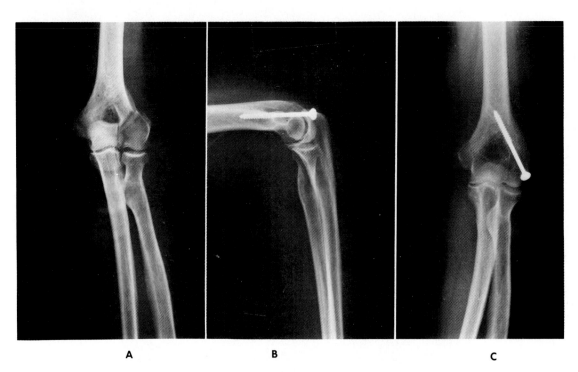

A   B   C

Fig. 9-10. *Case 6.* **A,** Anteroposterior view of elbow with fracture line from lateral trochlear ridge across lateral epicondylar column. **B** and **C,** Anteroposterior and lateral views showing screw in place, stabilizing the fracture.

FRACTURES OF CAPITELLUM

Fractures of the capitellum are divided into type I, which includes a large part of the capitellum, and type II, which includes articular cartilage with little bone. Impaction fractures also have been described. Type I fractures may result from a force passing from the radius to the humerus in extension, shearing off the capitellum anteriorly or from a direct lateral blow in flexion. Type II fractures are the result of shearing forces across the joint in varying degrees of flexion.

Damage to the capitellum is often related to the radial head. Milch[13] pointed out that fragments of radial head rarely displace proximally, which helps to identify capitellar injuries, but both surfaces must be scrutinized. The use of closed reduction in this fracture is very limited because the smallest displacement will limit function. A small incision posterolaterally, with removal of loose fragments, is easily achieved at small risk, and if the damage is severe, excision of the capitellum is preferable to malplacement.

The method for fixing a fragment as small as the entire articular surface presents a technical problem. I prefer small, threaded Kirschner wires, which are buried beneath the articular surface and which can be removed from the posterior aspect of the arm without the joint being reentered. Early motion by 3 weeks is again essential to a good result, and the radial fossa must be free of debris.

Alvarez and Shaftan,[2] in a report of 14 such fractures, found that the results in the 10 patients with excision were superior to the results in the three patients with closed treatment and the one patient with internal fixation. They summarized the results from cases reported in the literature as 78% good or excellent with excision, 51% good with internal fixation, and 63% good with closed treatment.

FRACTURES OF TROCHLEA

These fractures are very rare as an isolated fracture because the trochlea is supported by the ulna, which either fractures or transmits the force as a wedge, splitting the distal humerus. Because the trochlea does not have strong capsular attachments, avulsions are unlikely but shearing fractures may occur with dislocations.

Fractures of the epicondyles are rare in adults but occasionally occur as an avulsion or shear type of fracture.

FRACTURES OF CORONOID

These fractures are usually seen with posterior dislocation of the elbow. If the fragment is separated, it may occupy the fossa and block flexion. The brachialis does not insert on the tip of the coronoid but inserts at about 6 to 10 mm distal to the tip, along the anterior border of the ulna. The brachialis may be stripped from the ulna during dislocation or fracture in that area. The key structure in stability is the anterior portion of the medial collateral ligament, which attaches to the medial side of the coronoid and is often injured when the coronoid fractures.

Case 7

A 37-year-old woman fell off a haystack and sustained a chip fracture of her radial head and coronoid (Fig. 9-11, *A* and *B*). Motion was begun 5 days after injury, but a painful snap resulted, and roentgenograms revealed a posterior dislocation of the elbow (Fig. 9-11, *C* and *D*). A closed reduction and casting for 4 weeks permitted healing of the ligament, with stability; the bone chip remained ununited (Fig. 9-11, *E* and *F*). A range of extension-flexion of between 10 and 145 degrees, with full rotation, was achieved without pain.

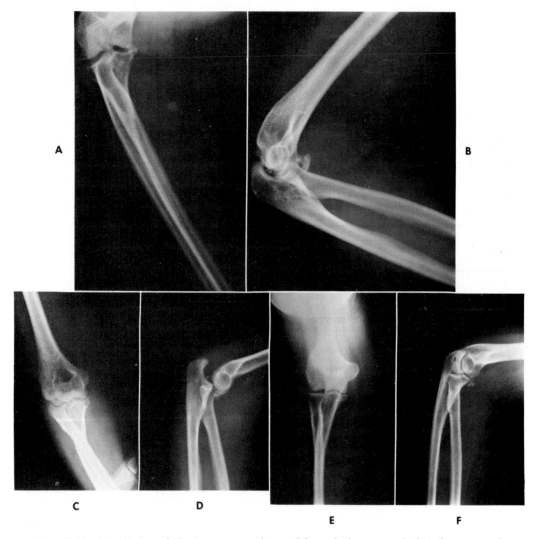

Fig. 9-11. *Case 7.* **A** and **B,** Anteroposterior and lateral views reveal chip fractures of radial head and coronoid. **C** and **D,** Anteroposterior and lateral views reveal posterior dislocation of olecranon. Anterior portion of the medial collateral ligament has been injured. **E** and **F,** Anteroposterior and lateral views demonstrate that fragment remains ununited, though joint relationships are now normal.

MONTEGGIA FRACTURES IN THE ADULT

These are essentially proximal ulnar fractures, with varying combinations of radial head dislocation or fracture. Almost all have a fracture of the radial head with the dislocation. The same varieties may be seen in adults as in children.

Case 8

A 23-year-old man involved in an automobile accident incurred fractures of the right tibia and fibula, maxilla, mandible, left humerus, and left ulna (segmented) and a dislocation of the left radial head anteriorly (Fig. 9-12, *A*). Three days later, along with treatment of his other fractures, a Rush rod was placed in the ulna and the annular ligament was repaired after dislocation of the radial head had been reduced (Fig. 9-12, *B*). A cross union developed (Fig. 9-12, *C*). The rod was removed at 6 months, and at 11 months the synostosis was excised and a Silastic radial head replacement was done. The replacement was removed 19 months later. The final motion was between 30 and 125 degrees, with 30 degrees of rotation.

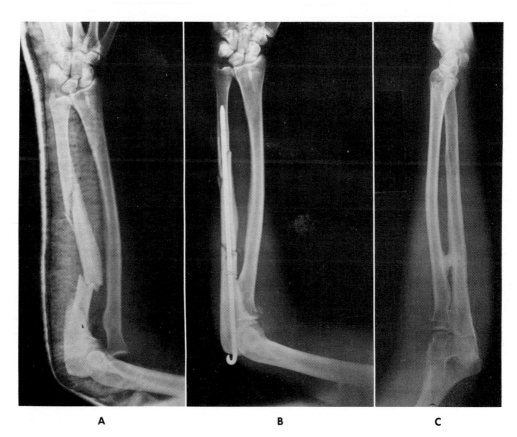

A	B	C

Fig. 9-12. *Case 8.* **A,** Lateral view shows segmental fracture of ulna, with anterior dislocation of the radial head. **B,** Similar view shows that Rush rod is maintaining reduction of fracture. Radial head is reduced. **C,** Rod has been removed, but patient has developed a synostosis at site of proximal ulnar fracture.

FRACTURES OF OLECRANON

Eppright and Wilkins[7] classify these fractures into two types: type I, or undisplaced, fractures and type II, or displaced, fractures (avulsion, oblique and transverse, comminuted, and fracture dislocations).

Undisplaced fractures may be treated conservatively, with splinting and early motion.

Avulsion fractures usually display a small proximal fragment and are most frequently seen in the elderly. The most effective treatment usually is excision of the fragment and reattachment of the triceps because the bone is often fragmented and osteoporotic and may block extension even if the fracture heals.

Oblique or transverse fractures have been treated by many methods of internal fixation, a that is, by cortical screws, wood screws, lag screws, wires, plates, tension wires, and pins. All these methods have their own problems. The Leinbach screws follow the medullary cavity, which angles toward the radius and then straightens, but they often break. The wood screws cannot follow the curves, and the Rush rods sometimes get jammed where the medullary cavity narrows, wires break, Kirschner wires back out, and so forth.

Currently the best two accepted methods seem to be tension wiring by use of either a screw or pins with a figure-of-eight wire posteriorly to convert the forces of the triceps into a compressive force and the use of a lag screw. Gartsman and his colleagues[9] at the Hospital for Special Surgery in New York have found that excision of even large fragments of the olecranon with repair of the triceps caused 20% fewer operative complications than did the screw-wire technique. Excision is the method of choice in the comminuted fractures, unless there is instability anteriorly. Kiviluoto and Santavirta[10] in a recent report of 35 patients found that 20 had lost some extension.

The most frequent complications of olecranon fractures are nonunion and loss of motion, usually in extension. Fracture dislocations involve fracture of the proximal ulna, specifically the olecranon, with dislocation of the humeroulnar joint. These fractures are often associated with fracture of the radial head or neck and dislocation of the radiohumeral joint. The counterpart of the Monteggia fracture in the child may be seen in the comminuted fracture of the proximal ulna, except that the radial head or neck is almost always fractured as well as dislocated. Nonunion may or may not be a problem. If the pseudarthrosis does not increase in size and does not limit motion by impingement in the fossa, the fracture often is not a problem and may heal slowly during a period of many months.

Case 9

A 78-year-old man fell on his left elbow. The fracture is seen in Fig. 9-13, *A* and *B,* which shows a stable elbow with fracture of the proximal third of the olecranon. The fractured portion was excised, with repair of the triceps insertion (Fig. 9-13, *C* and *D*). A full range of motion was regained.

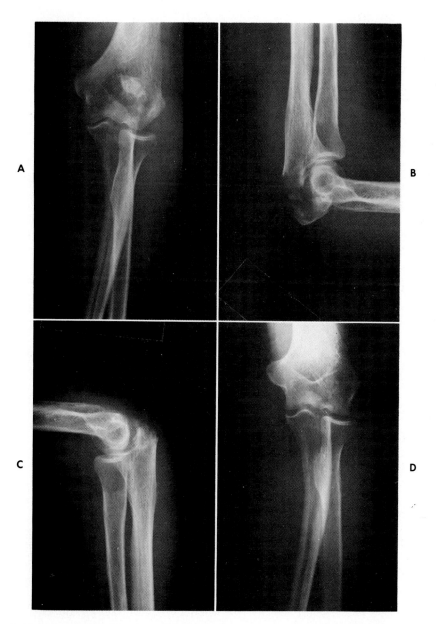

Fig. 9-13. *Case 9.* **A** and **B,** Anteroposterior and lateral views showing fracture of olecranon. **C** and **D,** Result after excision.

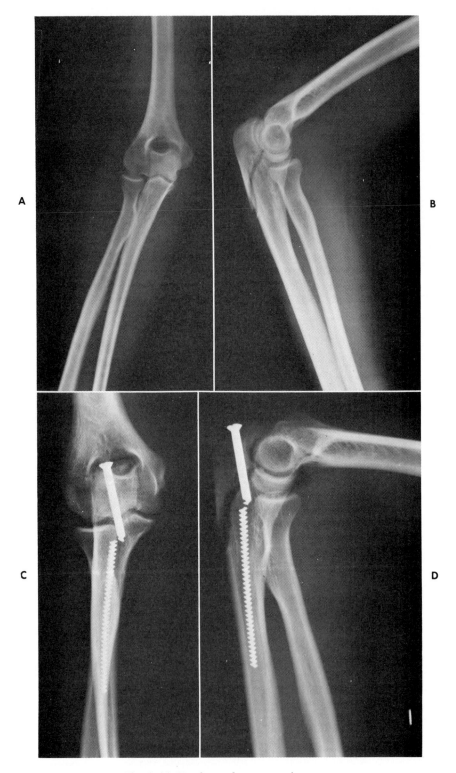

Fig. 9-14. For legend see opposite page.

Case 10

A 24-year-old woman was involved in an automobile accident and sustained an essentially undisplaced fracture of the olecranon (Fig. 9-14, *A* and *B*). She was also quadriparetic, with a severe cervical injury that required anterior removal of the fractured body and disk of C6, as well as fusion with halo stabilization. Ten days after the accident and after stabilization, an open re-

duction was performed. A Leinbach screw broke during insertion and distracted the fracture (Fig. 9-14, *C* and *D*). The screw was removed, and four Kirschner wires were used to stabilize the fracture (Fig. 9-14, *E* and *F*). The patient recovered a full range of motion (Fig. 9-14, *G* and *H*) and full neurologic function in this extremity but continued to have partial neurologic loss in the opposite arm and leg.

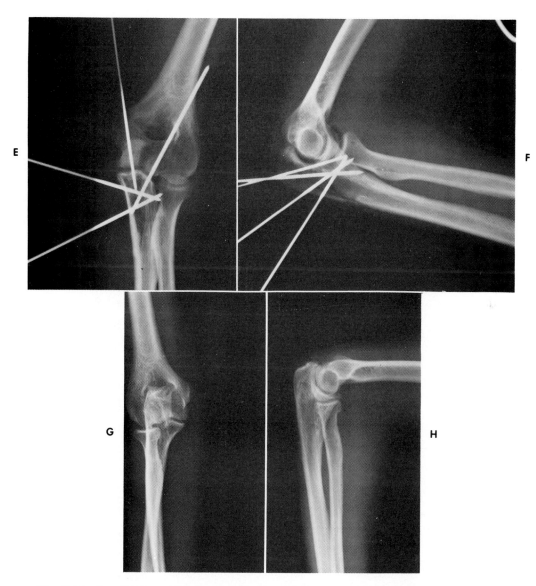

Fig. 9-14. *Case 10.* **A** and **B,** Anteroposterior and lateral views showing oblique olecranon fracture undisplaced. **C** and **D,** Fracture line had widened, and screw had broken at junction of thread shaft. **E** and **F,** Screw had been removed, and four Kirschner wires were inserted. **G** and **H,** Two years after fracture.

Case 11

A 31-year-old man jumped off a balcony and landed on his left elbow. This resulted in a comminuted fracture of the radial head and olecranon. The radial head was excised, and the olecranon was stabilized by two pins, tension wiring, and one screw (Fig. 9-15, *A* and *B*). Motion was begun at 2 weeks, and a full range of motion was achieved (Fig. 9-15, *C* and *D*).

RADIAL HEAD FRACTURES

These fractures usually result from direct force applied across the radiohumeral joint. Mason[11] classified three types: type I, undisplaced; type II, marginal with displacement; and type III, comminuted involving the entire head. Eppright and Wilkins[7] added a fourth type, fracture of the radial head in association with a dislocation of the elbow.

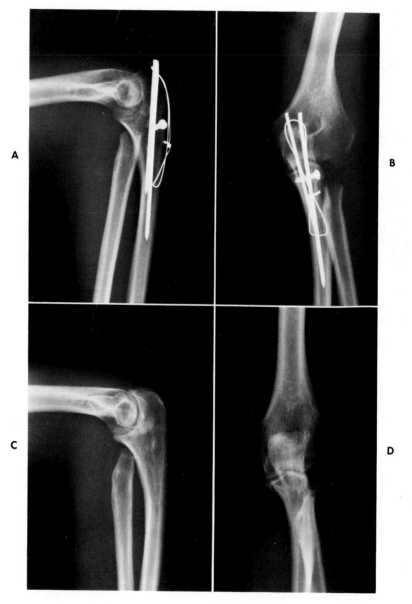

Fig. 9-15. *Case 11.* **A** and **B,** Lateral and anteroposterior views show radial head excised and olecranon fracture stabilized by pins and tension wiring with one screw. **C** and **D,** Lateral and anteroposterior views show result 2 years after fracture.

The fractures are sometimes difficult to see on standard roentgenograms, and their presence should be suspected when tenderness and effusion are centered laterally over the radial head, especially if rotation is more painful than flexion-extension. The posterior fat-pad sign is usually present, and often the anterior fat pad also is more evident in fractures of the radial head.

Type I, undisplaced fractures should be treated by rest and early gentle range of motion. These rarely need to be immobilized longer than 3 or 4 days, but they should be kept in a sling to discourage the forceful inadvertent use of the arm. Aspiration may be necessary in some patients but is used rarely.

Type II fractures are more difficult to evaluate. Mason[11] is quoted by Eppright and Wilkins[7] as advocating excision if more than one fourth of the head is involved; Radin and Riseborough[17] used two thirds. McLaughlin[12] believed that angulation greater than 30 degrees and depression of greater than 3 mm indicated that excision should be done. Adler and Shaftan[1] have favored a trial of early motion with excision, if motion is blocked at 8 weeks.

Type III, comminuted fractures are usually considered most effectively treated by early excision, yet some fractures present with minimal symptoms and limitation of rotation may be treated with early motion safely. The excision must extend to the neck, with coverage of the neck by a layer of synovium if possible.

Type IV fractures, with a posterior dislocation of the elbow in asssociation with a radial head fracture, must be promptly reduced, and the radial head then evaluated and treated as necessary.

CONCLUSIONS

Many different fracture patterns and methods of treatment involve the adult elbow. The principles to be followed in treatment may be summarized as follows: (1) adequate roentgenograms and examination for evaluation; (2) anatomic reduction if possible, implying closed treatment of stable fractures and adequate exposure and rigid fixation of unstable fractures if the patient's condition permits; (2) range-of-motion exercises to begin not later than 3 weeks after fracture; (4) extreme gentleness in the handling of the tissues; (5) excision of fragments not necessary for stability and not capable of being anatomically replaced; and (6) reconstitution of ligamentous stability of the joint.

REFERENCES

1. Adler, J.B., and Shaftan, G.W.: Radial head fractures, is excision necessary? J. Trauma **4**:115, 1964.
2. Alvarez, E., Patel, M.R., Nimberg, G., and Pearlman, H.S.: Fracture of the capitulum humeri, J. Bone Joint Surg. **57**:1093, 1975.
3. Bickel, W.E., and Perry, R.E.: Comminuted fractures of the distal humerus, J.A.M.A. **184**:553, 1963.
4. Bryan, R.S., and Bickel, W.H.: "T" condylar fractures of distal humerus, J. Trauma **11**:830, 1971.
5. Cassebaum, W.H.: Operative treatment of T and Y fractures of the lower end of the humerus, Am. J. Surg. **83**:265, 1952.
6. Cassebaum, W.H.: Open reduction of T and Y fractures of the lower end of the humerus, J. Trauma **9**:915, 1969.
7. Eppright, R.H., and Wilkins, K.E.: Fractures and dislocations of the elbow. In Rockwood, C.A., Jr., and Green, D.P., editors: Fractures, Philadelphia, 1975, J.B. Lippincott Co.
8. Fischer, D.A., and House, J.H.: Radial nerve paralysis associated with fractures of the humerus (abstract), J. Bone Joint Surg. **55**:1307, 1973.
9. Gartsman, G.M., Sculco, T.P., and Otis, J.: Operative treatment of olecranon fractures: excision or open reduction and fixation. Presented at the meeting of the American Academy of Orthopaedic Surgeons, Atlanta, Georgia, February 7 to 12, 1980.
10. Kiviluoto, O., and Santavirta, S.: Fractures of the olecranon: analysis of 37 consecutive cases, Acta Orthop. Scand. **49**:28, 1978.
11. Mason, M.L.: Some observations on fractures of the head of the radius with a review of one hundred cases, Br. J. Surg. **42**:123, 1954.
12. McLaughlin, H.L.: Trauma, Philadelphia, 1959, W.B. Saunders Co.
13. Milch, H.: Unusual fractures of the capitulum humeri and the capitulum radii, J. Bone Joint Surg. **13**:882, 1931.
14. Mitsunaga, M.M., Bryan, R.S., and Linscheid, R.L.: Treatment of nonunion in the vicinity of the elbow joint. Presented at the meeting of the American Orthopaedic Association, Honolulu, Hawaii, June 16 through 19, 1980.
15. Morrey, B.F., Bryan, R.S., Dobyns, J.H., and Linscheid, R.L.: Total elbow arthroplasty: a five-year Mayo Clinic experience 1973-1977. (Submitted for publication.)
16. Packer, J.W., Foster, R.R., Garcia, A., and Grantham, S.A.: The humeral fracture with radial nerve palsy: is exploration warranted? Clin. Orthop. **88**:34, 1972.
17. Radin, E.L., and Riseborough, E.J.: Fractures of the radial head: a review of eighty-eight cases and analysis of the indications for excision of the radial head and non-operative treatment, J. Bone Joint Surg. **48**:1055, 1966.
18. Sim, F.H., Kelly, P.J., and Henderson, E.D.: Radial-nerve palsy complicating fractures of the humeral shaft (abstract), J. Bone Joint Surg. **53**:1023, 1971.

Chapter 10

Transverse fractures of distal humerus in children

THOMAS B. DAMERON, Jr., M.D.
Raleigh, North Carolina

Transverse fractures of the distal humerus in children occur either through the epiphyseal plate or proximal to the epiphyseal plate in the supracondylar area. The supracondylar site is much more common.

Part A

Supracondylar humeral fractures

ANATOMY

Supracondylar humeral fractures occur immediately proximal to the condyles and proximal to the distal humeral epiphyseal plate. The distal end of the humerus is spade shaped, being broad in width and thin. The posterior surface is flat. The anterior surface is convex. The sagittal section of the elbow (Fig. 10-1) demonstrates the thinness of the bone in the supracondylar region. Supracondylar fractures occur at the thinnest area where the coronoid fossa is present anteriorly and the olecranon fossa posteriorly. The thin bone between the coronoid and olecranon fossae is congenitally absent in over 5% of the people. When the defect is present, it is covered by a membrane. It is of significance that in a study by Trotter the defect was more common on the left and more common in females.[12]

Serial sections through the distal humerus at 3 to 5 mm intervals demonstrate the significant change in contour of the distal humerus at different levels. The bone lateral to the fossae forms a

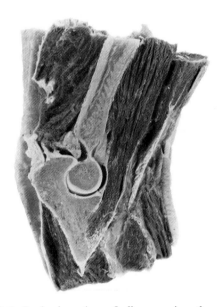

Fig. 10-1. Sagittal section of elbow region through the midportion of the distal humerus. Note the fat pads that are consistently present in the olecranon fossa and coronoid fossa.

column that is usually larger and stronger than the medial column (Fig. 10-2, *A* to *D*).

The neurovascular structures are shielded from the bone by a thin layer of muscle, the brachialis anteriorly and the triceps posteriorly.

DISSECTIONS

Eight arms from four postmature stillborn infants were dissected (Figs. 10-3 to 10-5). It was extremely difficult to produce supracondylar frac-

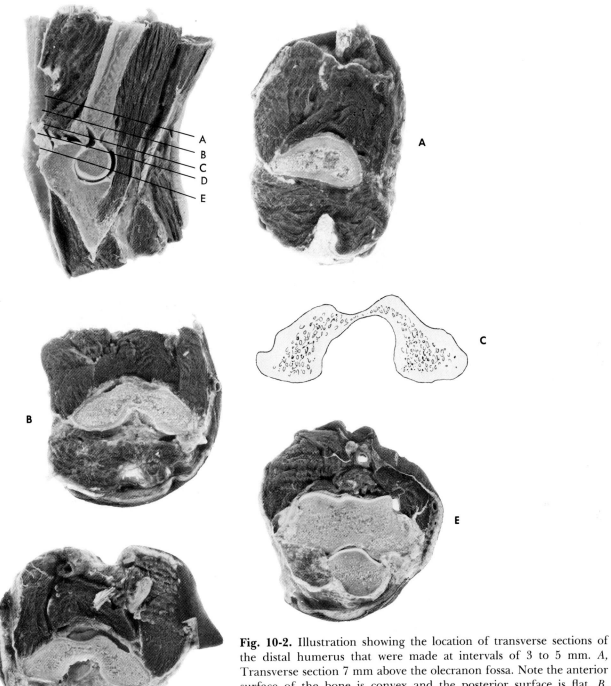

Fig. 10-2. Illustration showing the location of transverse sections of the distal humerus that were made at intervals of 3 to 5 mm. *A*, Transverse section 7 mm above the olecranon fossa. Note the anterior surface of the bone is convex and the posterior surface is flat. *B*, Transverse section through the proximalmost portion of the olecranon fossa. The anteroposterior dimension is greater in the lateral humeral condyle, and the medial humeral condyle is wider in the transverse dimension. *C*, Diagram of transverse section through the thinnest portion of the olecranon fossa. The actual cut through the bone comminuted the bone of the olecranon fossa because it was so thin. In the central portion of the fossa the bone is usually less than 1 mm thick. *D*, Transverse section of distal humerus 5 mm below the thinnest portion of the olecranon fossa. *E*, Eight millimeters below olecranon fossa through condyles. Note how the condyles are much thicker at this level. The section includes the olecranon.

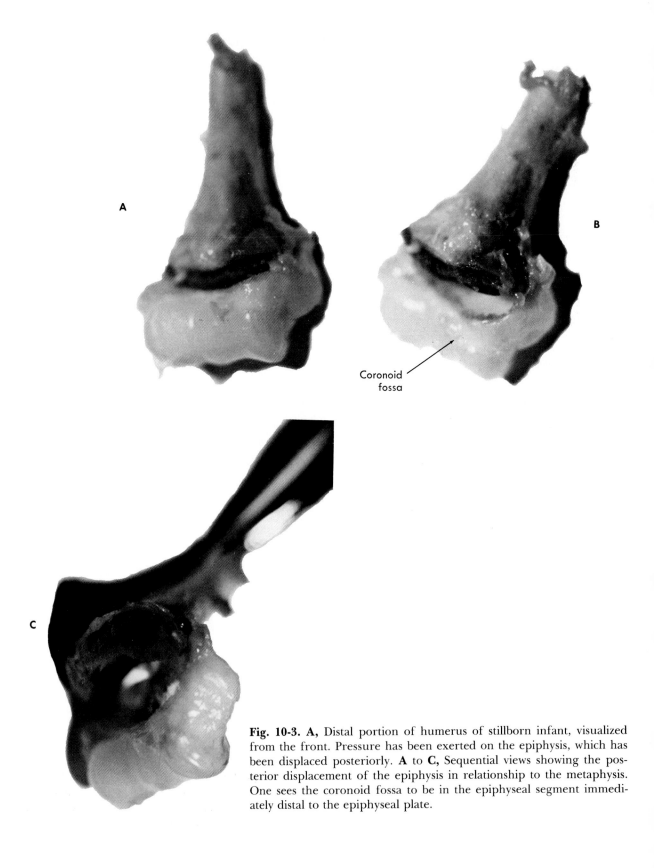

Coronoid
fossa

Fig. 10-3. A, Distal portion of humerus of stillborn infant, visualized from the front. Pressure has been exerted on the epiphysis, which has been displaced posteriorly. **A** to **C,** Sequential views showing the posterior displacement of the epiphysis in relationship to the metaphysis. One sees the coronoid fossa to be in the epiphyseal segment immediately distal to the epiphyseal plate.

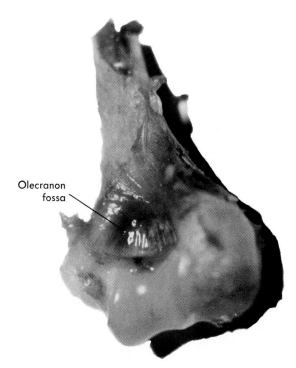

Olecranon fossa

Fig. 10-4. Posterior view of same specimen as that in Fig. 10-3. The epiphyseal fragment has been displaced slightly posteriorly. The olecranon fossa is immediately proximal to the epiphyseal plate in the metaphysis.

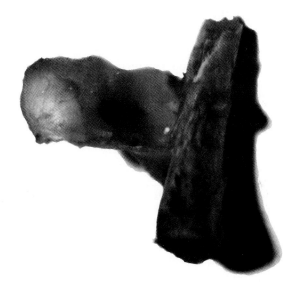

Fig. 10-5. Same specimen from the lateral view with further displacement posteriorly showing that the strong posterior periosteum causes the epiphysis to be turned back over the metaphysis.

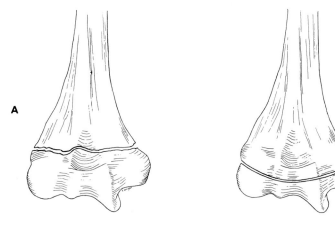

A   B

Fig. 10-6 A, Illustration showing the level of a typical supracondylar fracture on the left. **B,** The level of separation of the distal humeral transverse epiphyseal plate separation is shown on the right.

tures in these specimens. The distal transverse epiphyseal plate is much weaker than the distal humerus. When enough force was applied, the disruption consistently occurred at the interface between the epiphysis and the metaphysis. The dorsal periosteum was much stronger than the anterior. It was therefore much easier to displace the epiphysis posteriorly than to displace it anteriorly (Fig. 10-6).

THE INJURY

In addition to rotation, there are four directions in which a supracondylar fracture can be displaced. The distal fragment may be displaced posteriorly, anteriorly, medially, or laterally. It is essential that the treating physician recognize which direction the fracture is displaced before beginning treatment. One must evaluate the patient and the patient's roentgenograms to determine accurately what the deformity is and what mechanism should be instituted to correct the deformity before beginning manipulative treatment. There is no one formula to reduce and treat all supracondylar fractures. The posteromedial displacement is most common.[2] Anterior displacement of the distal humeral fragment is rare but the mechanism of treatment of those cases is very different from the more common posteriorly displaced fractures.

Rotational displacement is an important consideration. This often cannot be accurately ascertained until the arm is anesthetized and examined by palpation. Rotational displacement of supracondylar fractures leads to deformity because of the asymmetry of the medial and lateral columns of bone.[6]

MANAGEMENT

Supracondylar fractures through the distal humerus in children should be treated as emergencies. The neurovascular condition of the arm must be observed carefully.

Supracondylar fractures of the humerus have much information published about their treatment that is conflicting. Positive statements have been made about the treatment of supracondylar fractures that pertain to displacement in one direction only, without consideration of the fact that displacement is three dimensional. There are methods of treatment recommended that are at complete variance. Among the popular methods

of treatment that have been proved effective in certain authors' hands and have been accepted are the following:

1. Side arm skin traction described by John Dunlop.[8]
2. Overhead traction using an olecranon pin as popularized by Lyman Smith in 1960.[2,4,7] He emphasized the importance of recognizing the bone landmarks of the olecranon, medial epicondyle, and lateral epicondyle and monitoring the position of the fracture by alignment of these three bony landmarks the same as the uninjured elbow. He described this as the "visual method" of treatment. He emphasized the point that since supracondylar fractures are usually oblique, settling of the fracture causes rotation and angulatory deformity. Multiple modifications of this overhead traction technique have been published.[19]
3. Various forms of spica casts, either with the arm by the side or elevated from the side to varying degrees, have been recommended.[1]
4. Closed reduction with percutaneous unthreaded Kirschner wires has been recommended by several authors, some recommending one wire through each condyle and some recommending insertion of both through the lateral condyle to avoid irritation to the ulnar nerve.[10,11,14,19,21] When this technique is used, it is most helpful to have a pistol-grip power drill for Kirschner wire insertion. It is difficult to insert the pin through the paper-thin central area above the condyles.
5. Longitudinal transolecranon Steinmann pin as has been recommended by Childress.[5]
6. Open reduction with Kirschner wire fixation continues to be recommended.[13,27]
7. Closed reduction has been recommended[9] with immobilization of the arm in a cast and keeping the elbow extended and forearm supinated.
8. Closed reduction and postmanipulation immobilization in a collar and cuff with the elbow acutely flexed is recommended by many.[26]
9. Most authors recommending closed reduction prefer immobilization with the forearm at a right angle to the humerus or with more flexion. A majority recommend keeping the

forearm pronated in the cast though some state that keeping the arm supinated is necessary.

To reduce a fracture, one must recognize the anatomic displacement that has occurred and then decide which forces and which direction must be used to reduce the displacement. Treatment should not be begun until the displacement is clearly understood. Roentgenograms, unfortunately, picture only two planes. After studying the rotengenograms, the treating physician must stop and think a bit to understand accurately the position of the fragments.

The treatment that I most often prefer for acute supracondylar fractures is similar to that described by Sir John Charnley in his book *The Closed Treatment of Common Fractures*. Adequate anesthesia is important. Because the time of reduction is also important, axillary block or even hematoma block anesthesia may be used if there is a contraindication for general anesthesia.

The surgeon should plan what he is to do before he begins and then proceed with confidence. The upper arm must be held near the axilla by an assistant for countertraction. After adequate anesthesia, the elbow is gently extended and strong traction is exerted when one grips the patient's wrist and pulls it in line with the humeral shaft. By this means, the fragments are disengaged and any important structures incarcerated between them are released. In this maneuver, it is hoped that the distal end of the humerus will retrace its path and fall back into the periosteal sleeve from whence it emerged anteriorly. In this position of full extension under traction, the distal fragment should be moved in line with the shaft of the humerus so that the lateral or medial displacement is anatomically corrected by the tension of the surrounding soft parts. It is important, however, to pause at this stage to assess whether the lateral or medial displacement has indeed been completely overcome before any attempt is made to go on to the next step of the reduction. If necessary, gentle lateral and medial pressure, while the elbow is still extended, usually completes the reduction of the lateral or medial displacement. In the extended position, the carrying angle of the elbow can be obliterated. Rotation is the next consideration. Most commonly, the medial condyle is displaced more posteriorly than the lateral; therefore, while traction is being maintained with the elbow ex-

tended, the forearm is firmly supinated to correct the internal rotation deformity of the distal fragment. Then the thumb of the fixing hand is applied over the olecranon, and with the active hand still applying longitudinal traction to the forearm, the active hand now flexes the elbow. Before the elbow reaches the right angle, the fingers of the passive hand pull the shaft of the humerus backward while the ctive hand is directly pulling the forearm and the distal fragment forward. After the elbow reaches a right angle, the forearm is pronated to rock the condylar fracture fragment out of varus. The fracture reduction is then held in position by having the elbow kept at a greater than right-angle position.

One cannot improve the position of the fracture by flexing the elbow beyond 90 degrees. Further flexion merely locks the fragments into position by drawing the triceps tendon and periosteum tightly around the posterior surface of the fracture. If the fracture has not been reduced at the right-angle position, further flexion will be resisted and may do damage if forced. If lateral displacement has not previously been corrected or if there is rotary deformity, further flexion will impact the fracture in the displaced position.

There will never be as good an opportunity to reduce the fracture as with the first manipulation. I prefer to use a posterior plaster splint with cotton in the antecubital space to protect the skin. Tape is looped from the upper arm to the lower forearm to act as a check rein to prevent extension.

If there is concern about the stability of the fracture or about the swelling, percutaneous wires are used. The mechanism of reduction of the fracture is the same whether or not the wires are used. The pistol-grip power drill is necessary to best direct the wires.

When adequate reduction cannot be maintained or when, for other reasons, early ambulatory treatment is not used, I recommend the overhead traction-pin method of treatment described by Smith.[23]

BONE DEFORMITY COMPLICATIONS

One can find statements in the literature stating that one should always pronate the forearm, always supinate the forearm, always leave it in neutral, or vary these, depending on the fracture, displacement, and the periosteum remaining intact.[7,13,23] Use of variation must be the correct answer. Abnormal rotation does not prevent solid bony union but does cause angulatory deformities. Fracture texts[3,4,25] describe osteotomy treatment for cubitus varus, which is reported to occur as frequently as in 57%[17,25] of displaced supracondylar fractures. There is no mention of the proper technique to correct cubitus valgus because it is so rare.

The reports concerning the amount of deformity after supracondylar fractures appear to depend more on how carefully the follow-up study is done than on the method of treatment employed. As the normal elbow may have as much as 15-degree valgus, a 10- to 15-degree varus angulation of such an elbow is not clinically apparent or troublesome to such a patient. Although there may have been a 25-degree change in alignment of the arm, unless comparable roentgenograms are made of the patient's two elbows in complete extension and supination, such a deformity may not be apparent. The reported incidence of residual varus after supracondylar fractures varies from 10% to 57%. Residual valgus deformity after supracondylar fracture is very rare.

A mild varus deformity can be obscured by elbow flexion contracture, and hence true varus deformity may not be noted until many months after the injury when full elbow extension is obtained. Epiphyseal growth alterations cannot be incriminated if the deformities are not progressive. A mild varus deformity does not give any significant functional impairment. Salter[22] stated that the primary impairment of a varus elbow deformity is the inability to get one's hand to one's mouth without abducting the elbow. Little other functional impairment would result.

Cubitus varus resulting from rotary displacement cannot be anatomically corrected with closed-wedge lateral osteotomy. Connolly[6] illustrates this well in his paper emphasizing the importance of all three dimensions when one is dealing with three-dimensional structures such as bone.

OTHER COMPLICATIONS

Approximately 10% of displaced supracondylar fractures have nerve injury when first examined by a physician. Sixty percent of the nerve deficits involve the radial nerve, 30% the median nerve, and 10% the ulnar nerve.[15,16] The reported incidence of nerve involvement varies with the type of displacement and is skewed somewhat, since a majority of the reports are from tertiary care centers, which have a disproportionately high number of complicated cases in their series.

The long-term results of conservative management of nerve injuries are excellent if the fracture can be aligned properly or reduced. Case reports of persistent neurologic deficit after careful manipulation are minuscule. The development of neurologic deficits after careful manipulation is an indication for immediate surgical treatment.

Vascular complications are a concern. Usually the best treatment for circulatory compromise is early reduction of the fracture. Direct arterial injury in supracondylar fractures is, fortunately, rare.

Arterial spasm and venous stasis are the vascular problems most frequently encountered. Reduction and immobilization of the fracture are usually sufficient treatment when carried out early. Flexion of an already swollen elbow must be avoided.[26]

Flexor compartment fasciotomy is indicated when the pressure of the anterior compartment cannot be relieved by reduction of the bone fragments. The extensor and intrinsic muscle compartments may be involved and should be monitored as well as the anterior compartment.[18]

Postreduction order to record the involved radial pulse hourly is a good way to make certain that the patient is being monitored carefully. It is not the presence or absence of the radial pulse, however, but it is the amount of swelling within the muscle compartments that is most significant. Volkmann's contracture can occur with a full and bounding radial pulse if the anterior compartment is unduly compressed, but, on the other hand, the absence of a radial pulse does not necessarily mean that there is enough increased tissue pressure to cause irreparable muscle damage. It is therefore of paramount importance to evaluate the patient's muscle function carefully during the first 24 hours after supracondylar fracture treatment.

SIGNIFICANCE OF PRONATION AND SUPINATION

Rotary deformity of supracondylar fractures leads to varus-valgus deformity just as rotary deformity of fractured phalanges results in "crossing over of the fingers." One may have a rotary deformity of the distal humerus that is not evident with the elbow in extension but is evident when the elbow flexes and, to a lesser extent, vice versa. Because supracondylar fractures in children are slightly oblique fractures, there is the additional angular tendency if one column settles more than the other. Children's supracondylar humeral fractures have the tendency of the distal medial column of the humerus to settle more posteriorly than the lateral.

Let us assume that the elbow can move on the humerus in only one plane, flexion and extension, at the elbow joint. If then a supracondylar fracture occurs, varus-valgus and rotary forces on the ulna will then be transmitted to the supracondylar fragment. When the elbow is flexed to 90 degrees, a pronation force will rotate the supracondylar fracture into a valgus position (Fig. 10-7 A). Supination will force the supracondylar fracture into a varus position (Fig. 10-7 B). When the elbow is extended, however, these forces are exerted through a plane that is different by 90 degrees. The forces of pronation will rotate the lateral condyle forward (Fig. 10-8, A), and the forces of supination will rotate the medial condyle forward (Fig. 8-10, B).

The bone in the supracondylar area is quite thin. It is difficult to balance the fractured surfaces one edge against the other. Wainwright compared the end-on reduction of the supracondylar fracture to the balancing of two knife-blade edges one on top of the other.

The lateral column of bone is thicker than the medial column, and hence it is easier to balance the bone ends together on the lateral side. A medial condyle that is left in the posterior position will predispose the elbow to a varus deformity. (If length is maintained, this varus deformity will not

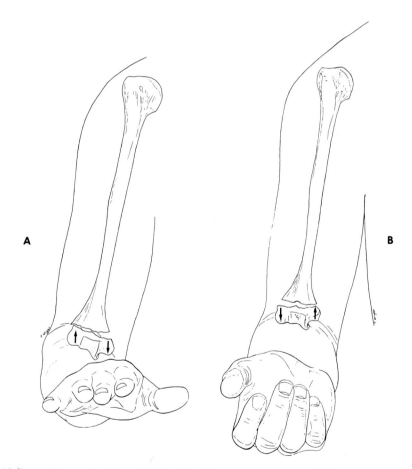

Fig. 10-7. A, Demonstration of deforming force on a supracondylar fracture with pronation when the elbow is flexed 90 degrees. **B,** Demonstration of deforming forces on a supracondylar fracture with supination when the elbow is flexed 90 degrees.

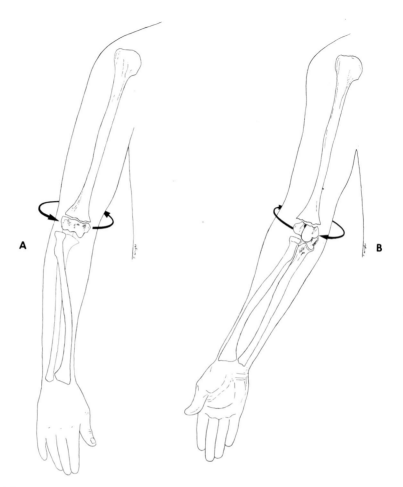

Fig. 10-8. A, Demonstration of the rotary force on the supracondylar fracture when the elbow is extended and the forearm is pronated. **B,** Demonstration of the rotary force on the supracondylar fracture when the elbow is extended and the forearm is supinated.

be evident in extension, but will be in flexion.) Symmetric displacement of both condyles posteriorly or anteriorly will not give rotary deformity and will be more acceptable than having only the lateral condyle reduced.

DISSECTIONS IN LABORATORY

Postmature stillborn infants' arms were used to study the effect of pronation and supination on the position of supracondylar fragments. Specimens were evaluated with the forearm flexor and extensor muscles left intact against those in which the forearm flexor and extensor muscles were removed. There was no apparent difference.

When the elbow was flexed to 90 degrees and the forearm pronated, the condylar fracture tilted into valgus (Fig. 10-7, *A*). Such did not rotate the fracture fragments. When the elbow was ex-

tended, however, forearm pronation displaced the medial condyle posteriorly (Fig. 10-8, *A*). This rotation did not change the angle of the arm so long as the elbow remained extended, but when the elbow was flexed, there was overriding of the medial fracture, and when the fragments were fixed in this displaced position, the varus deformity was apparent in both flexion and extension. From information based on this study, we now have modified our technique for closed reduction of supracondylar fractures of the elbow. When the patient is anesthetized and while traction is being exerted on the extended elbow, the forearm is supinated to help to bring the medial column of the supracondylar fragment anteriorly. Once the fracture is reduced and the elbow flexed to 90 degrees, the forearm is placed in pronation to help alleviate the varus strain on the medial column.

Technique of closed reduction

AFTERCARE

Supracondylar fractures heal quickly. Guarded motion can be begun with a collar-and-cuff sling after 3 to 5 weeks. The children can usually be allowed unrestricted activity 6 weeks after injury.

Passive exercises are contraindicated. Supervised physical therapy is not necessary. If the fracture has been adequately reduced and the soft tissue not traumatized enough to cause ectopic calcification, the child is most likely to have return of as much motion as the shape of the bone will allow. It may take 12 or more months to gain maximum motion. There is significant individual variation among patients in this regard.

ANTERIORLY DISPLACED SUPRACONDYLAR FRACTURES

The reported 1% to 4% of supracondylar fractures that are displaced anteriorly are the result of a hyperflexion injury in contrast to the posteriorly displaced hyperextension injuries.[24] The technique for reduction of these injuries is opposite to that for reducing posteriorly displaced fractures. General anesthesia is almost always required. Traction is exerted with the elbow flexed rather than extended, disengaging the fragments with the forearm supinated. Then gentle pressure is exerted on the posterior aspect of the distal humerus and forearm, and the supracondylar fragment is allowed to drift posteriorly. The arm is then immobilized in a posterior one-half cast with the elbow in slightly less than 90-degree flexion.

SUMMARY

Transverse fractures through the distal humerus in children should be treated as emergencies. Adequate roentgenographic evaluation is helpful. When taking roentgenograms, it is important to move the x-ray tube and cassette, and not the patient's arm, when getting different views. When the forearm and distal fragment are rotated between the times that the AP and the lateral roentgenograms are made, the fracture will have moved and the results will then be confusing. The hyperextension injury, with the distal condylar fragment being displaced posteromedially, is most common. It can usually be reduced by manipulation with the patient completely relaxed. First, traction is exerted on the extended elbow, the condyles manipulated, and the forearm supinated. With traction being maintained, the elbow is flexed and the distal fragment manipulated

manually anteriorly. Care is taken to make sure the medial condyle is reduced anteriorly. After the elbow is flexed slightly more than 90 degrees, the forearm is pronated to better control varus. Postreduction immobilization can be carried out, either with percutaneous pins or with posterior plaster-of-paris splint to maintain flexion at greater than 90 degrees. Open reduction is rarely indicated except for incarceration of the neurovascular structures. Careful surveillance of the intracompartmental pressures is imperative.

When reduction cannot be achieved or maintained by this method, overhead olecranon pin traction is indicated.

REFERENCES TO PART A

1. Altchek, M.: Treating displaced supracondylar fractures of humerus in children, Orthop. Rev. **8**(12):31-37, Dec. 1979.
2. Arnold J.A., Nasca, R.J., and Nelson, C.L.: Supracondylar fractures of the humerus, J. Bone Joint Surg. **59A**:589-595, July 1977.
3. Blount, W.P.: Fractures in children, Baltimore, 1954, The Williams & Wilkins Co.
4. Charnley, J.: The closed treatment of common fractures, Baltimore, 1961, The Williams & Wilkins Co.
5. Childress, H.M.: Transarticular pin fixation in supracondylar fractures at the elbow in children, J. Bone Joint Surg. **54A**:1548-1552, Oct. 1972.
6. Connolly, J.F.: Torsional fractures and the third dimension of fracture management, South. Med. J. **73**:884-891, 1980.
7. D'Ambrosia, R.D.: Supracondylar fractures of humerus: prevention of cubitus varus, J. Bone Joint Surg. **54A**:60-66, Jan. 1972.
8. Dunlop, J.: Transcondylar condylar fractures of the humerus in childhood, J. Bone Joint Surg. **21**:59-73, 1939.
9. El-Sharkawi, A.H., and Fattah, H.A.: Treatment of displaced supracondylar fractures of the humerus in children in full extension and supination, J. Bone Joint Surg. **47B**:273-279, May 1965.
10. Flynn, J.C., Matthews, J.G., and Benoit, R.L.: Blind pinning of displaced supracondylar fractures of the humerus in children, J. Bone Joint Surg. **56A**:263-272, March 1974.
11. Fowles, J.V., and Kassab, M.T.: Displaced supracondylar fractures of the elbow in children, J. Bone Joint Surg. **56B**:490-500, Aug. 1974.
12. Grant, J.C.B.: An atlas of anatomy, ed. 4, Baltimore, 1956, The Williams & Wilkins Co.
13. Gruber, M.A., and Hudson, O.C.: Supracondylar fractures of the humerus in childhood, J. Bone Joint Surg. **46A**:1245-1252, Sept. 1964.
14. Haddad, R.J., Jr., Saer, J.K., and Riordan, D.C: Percutaneous pinning of displaced supracondylar fractures of the elbow in children, Clin. Orthop. **71**:112, 1970.
15. Holmes, J.C., Skolnick, M.D., and Hall, J.E.: Untreated median-nerve entrapment in bone after fracture of the distal end of the humerus, J. Bone Joint Surg. **61A**:309-310, March 1979.

16. Lipscomb, P.R., and Burleson, R.J.: Vascular and neural complications in supracondylar fractures of the humerus in children, J. Bone Joint Surg. **37A:**487-492, June 1955.
17. Mann, T.S.: Prognosis in supracondylar fractures J. Bone Joint Surg. **45B:**516-522, Aug. 1963.
18. Mubarak, S.J., Carroll, N.D.: Volkmann's contracture in children: etiology and prevention, J. Bone Joint Surg. **61B:**285-293, Aug. 1979.
19. Palmer, E., Niemann, K.M.W., Vesely, D., and Armstrong, J.H.: Supracondylar fractures of the humerus in children, J. Bone Joint Surg. **60A:**653-656, July 1978.
20. Prietto, C.A.: Supracondylar fractures of the humerus, J. Bone Joint Surg. **61A:**425-428, April 1979.
21. Rockwood, C.A., and Green, D.P.: Fractures, Philadelphia, 1975, J.P. Lippincott Co.
22. Salter, R.B.: Problem fractures in children. A.A.O.S. Instructional course lecture. Read at the annual meeting, Dallas, Texas, Jan. 1974.
23. Smith, L.: Deformity following supracondylar fractures of the humerus, J. Bone Joint Surg. **42A:**235-242, March 1960.
24. Soltanpur, A.: Anterior supracondylar fracture of the humerus (flexion type), J. Bone Joint Surg. **60B:**383-385, Aug. 1978.
25. Tachdjian, M.O.: Pediatric orthopaedics, Philadelphia, 1972, W.B. Saunders Co.
26. Watson-Jones, R.: Fractures and joint injuries, ed. 4, Baltimore, 1962, The Williams & Wilkins Co.
27. Weiland, A.J., Meyer, S., Tolo, V.T., Berg, H.L., and Mueller, J.: Surgical treatment of displaced supracondylar fractures of the humerus in children, J. Bone Joint Surg. **60A:**657-661, July 1978.

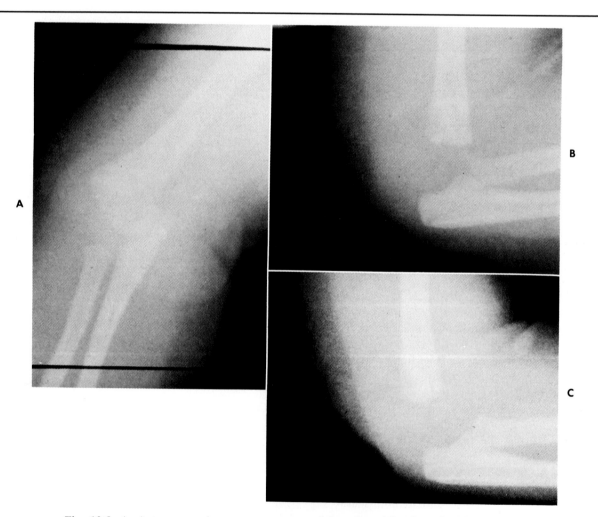

Fig. 10-9. A, Anteroposterior roentgenogram of the elbow of a 6-week-old child with suspected child abuse appearing as swollen, painful elbow. **B,** Lateral roentgenogram of the affected elbow with force exerted through the forearm posteriorly. **C,** Lateral roentgenogram of the child's elbow with force being exerted anteriorly on the forearm.

Part B

Transverse distal humeral epiphyseal fractures

The distal transverse epiphyseal plate is the weakest area of the distal humerus in the very young. This is particularly true in children less than 2 years of age. A dorsally directed force on the distal humerus can cause a fracture through the transverse epiphyseal plate. In older children, this same force usually causes a fracture through the supracondylar area.[2,4] The dorsal periosteum has been found, in anatomic specimens, to be a great deal stronger than the anterior. Fractures displacing the distal epiphysis anteriorly must be extremely rare. This injury is, at times, misdiagnosed (Figs. 10-9). When there is no ossification in the trochlear epiphysis, orientation can be difficult. Although most frequent in children less than 2 years of age, the injury has been reported in persons as old as 8 years. It can occur at the time of delivery. Child abuse as a cause of this type of injury is not uncommon.

In examining full-term stillborns' arms, I was unable to produce a supracondylar fracture in any of the 8 arms tested. In each case, the break would occur at the distal humeral epiphysis (Figs. 10-3 to 10-5). In children older than 2 years of age with this fracture, there will usually be a metaphyseal fragment of the Salter-Harris type II injury.[2,4]

If ossification of the capitellum is present, dislocation of the elbow and displaced fractures of the lateral condyle can be diagnosed more easily.[4]

When the shaft of the radius does not point toward the transverse axis of the capitellar ossification center, there has been a dislocation. If the capitellar ossification center has been rotated in relationship to the humerus, there has been a fracture of the lateral condyle.

Clinically a fracture-separation of the distal humerus that is manipulated produces a so-called muffled crepitus, which was described by Poland as being diagnostic of the injury.[2] The fracture can be difficult to diagnose without a high index of suspicion. These fractures should be treated as are supracondylar fractures. The stability of the reduced fracture is dependent on the amount of periosteal stripping that has taken place. If there has not been a great deal of displacement and periosteal stripping, the distal humeral epiphysis can be brought back into its anatomic position and locked there by the tethering force of the intact posterior periosteum when the elbow is flexed 90 degrees. These injuries are more stable than are supracondylar fractures because the bone is thicker and the injury more transverse in this area.[1]

REFERENCES TO PART B

1. DeLee, J.C., Wilkins, K.E., Rogers, L.F., and Rockwood, C.A.: Fracture-separation of the distal humeral epiphysis, J. Bone Joint Surg. **62A**:46-51.
2. Holda, M.E., Manoli, A., and LaMont, R.L.: Epiphyseal separation of the distal end of the humerus with medial displacement J. Bone Joint Surg. **62A**:52-57, Jan. 1980.
3. Mizuno, K., Hirohata, K., and Kashiwagi, D.: Fracture-separation of the distal humeral epiphysis in young children, J. Bone Joint Surg. **61A**:570-573, June 1979.
4. Silberstein, M.J., Brodeur, A.E., and Graviss, E.R.: Some vagaries of the capitellum, J. Bone Joint Surg. **61A**:244-247, March 1979.

SHOULDER

Chapter 11

Lesions of musculotendinous cuff of shoulder: diagnosis and management

Part A

Tears of rotator cuff

ROBERT J. NEVIASER, M.D.
THOMAS J. NEVIASER, M.D.
Washington, D.C.

Although it is accepted that tears of the rotator cuff of the shoulder occur, most orthopaedic surgeons remain uncomfortable when faced with a patient complaining of pain or loss of motion in the shoulder. The most common diagnoses applied in these instances are "adhesive capsulitis" or "bursitis." Even if a tear is suspected, however, the patient often is managed with skillful neglect, an approach arising from the considerable confusion surrounding treatment of this entity. Unfortunately, this course leads to many poor results and an unjustifiably bad reputation for the surgical repair of these tears.

The rotator cuff tear usually occurs in patients in their forties and older. It is seen in younger patients—even those in their late teens and early twenties—but not often. The increased incidence in the older patient is attributable to degeneration of the cuff tendons with associated loss of elasticity in the hypovascular area just proximal to the tendons' insertion into the tuberosities of the humerus.

Tears of the rotator cuff may be partial or complete. Partial or incomplete tears are generally of two types: the intratendinous tear or the deep surface tear. Either type may heal with nonoperative treatment. It is obvious therefore that the most important step before one embarks on a treatment program is to differentiate between an incomplete and a complete tear of the rotator cuff.

Complete tears are those that involve the full thickness of the cuff tendons, exposing the humeral head. The most commonly involved tendon is the supraspinatus, though the infraspinatus and teres minor also are frequently torn. The subscapularis is seldom ruptured.

There are five ways in which a tear of the rotator cuff can occur:

1. After injury to the shoulder without a fracture or dislocation
2. After anterior dislocation of the glenohumeral joint
3. After anterior dislocation of the glenohumeral joint with an associated fracture of the greater tuberosity
4. Chronically, with or without history of injury
5. After a seemingly innocuous avulsion fracture of the greater tuberosity

ROTATOR CUFF TEAR AFTER INJURY WITHOUT FRACTURE OR DISLOCATION

In the acute phase after this injury, the patient's ability to initiate, as well as maintain, abduction of the arm must be established. If he is unable to perform these functions, one cannot assume that the "drop-arm" test is positive; this inability may result from pain rather than from a musculotendinous deficit. Therefore the pain reflex should be eliminated. This can be accomplished by injection of the subdeltoid space with 8 to 10 ml of 1% plain lidocaine. After the pain has been alleviated by the local anesthetic, if the patient still is unable to perform the aforementioned maneuvers, the drop-arm test can be considered positive and the diagnosis of a complete rotator cuff tear enter-

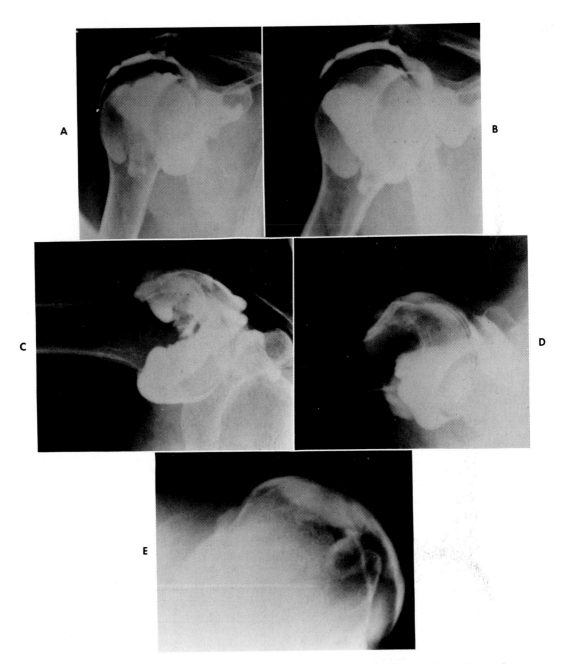

Fig. 11-1. The five standard views obtained during arthrography. A diagnosis can be made from any one. **A,** Anteroposterior in external rotation—dye seen in subdeltoid bursa. **B,** Anteroposterior in internal rotation—dye in the subdeltoid bursa consistent with a rotator cuff tear. **C,** Anteroposterior in abduction—obliteration of the axillary fold forcing dye into the bursa through any tear in the cuff. **D,** Axillary view—dye covering the entire head of the humerus because of the communication with the bursa. **E,** Bicipital groove view—dye in the bursa obscures the groove and biceps tendon.

tained. If, however, under the effect of the local anesthetic the patient can initiate abduction and maintain it against some resistance, the diagnosis of an incomplete tear should be considered. The treatment for the latter is rest in a sling for 2 to 3 weeks followed by progressive return to function. In either case, rest in a sling and repeated examinations over the ensuing 10 to 14 days are indicated. At the end of this period, if the patient still has a positive drop-arm test, arthrography should be done. On the arthrogram,[5,10] if the dye appears in the subdeltoid bursa on any of the five standard views (Fig 11-1), the diagnosis is established and operative repair should be undertaken. Repair of these massive complete tears should be done within the first 2 to 3 weeks. A longer wait can produce a significant defect in the tendons with fixed retracted edges—a very difficult reconstructive problem.

Repair of these acute complete or massive tears within the prescribed time period should provide good results. The surgical approach is the anterosuperior incision at the level of the acromioclavicular joint. At the same landmark, the deltoid is split in line with its fibers. It is then elevated subperiosteally from the superior surface of the lateral portion of the clavicle, the acromioclavicular joint, and the acromion. This is done posteriorly as far as the posterior margin of the acromioclavicular joint. If necessary, the deltoid and periosteum can be elevated sharply from the acromion both laterally and posteriorly to provide increased exposure.[8] An acromioclavicular arthroplasty[2] is performed by resection of the intra-articular meniscus and the lateral 0.5 to 1 cm of the clavicle. This provides increased exposure to the rotator cuff. An anteroinferior acromioplasty is also done. The coracoacromial ligament is resected in its entirety. The subdeltoid bursa can then be seen and is incised in line with the cuff tendons and retained, after being tagged. It is carefully dissected from the underlying cuff and overlying deltoid to which it may be adherent, thus exposing the tear of the rotator cuff (Fig. 11-2, *A*). In the acute phase, the edges of these tendons are healthy and fresh. Nonabsorbable traction sutures of 0 gauge are placed in the edges of the cuff tendons, and through these sutures traction is applied to the rotator cuff while it is being mobilized. The tendons are brought laterally and secured in a groove made with a gouge just medial to the tuberosities. The tendons are anchored to the bone with nonabsorbable sutures (Fig. 11-2, *B*). When the repair is complete, the cuff should be watertight. The bursa is repaired with plain catgut and the deltoid brought back to its normal resting position. The deltoid-splitting incision can be reinforced with inverted 0 nonabsorbable sutures as well. The skin is closed routinely. The arm is immobilized at the side and in internal rotation in a sling and swathe for 3 weeks postoperatively. The extremity is then placed in a sling and the patient begins pendulum exercises in the fourth week. After this he is started on a formal program of rotator cuff rehabilitation under the direction of the treating physician and a compe-

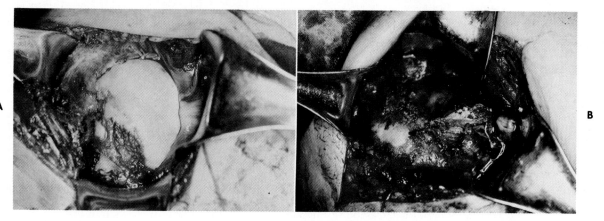

Fig. 11-2. A, A large recent tear of the subscapularis. **B,** Direct repair of the tear. (**A** and **B,** From Neviaser, R.J.: Orthop. Clin. North Am. **11**:295-306, 1980.)

tent physical therapist. The important aspect of retraining the rotator cuff is strengthening abduction, especially from the position of 90 degrees and beyond. The arm is not permitted to dangle freely at the side for 3 months postoperatively.

ROTATOR CUFF TEAR AFTER ANTERIOR DISLOCATION OF SHOULDER

Although this injury is more common in the older patient, it can occur in the younger one as well. It is frequently missed because of confusion with axillary nerve palsies. It has commonly been assumed that a frequent complication of anterior dislocation of the shoulder is an axillary nerve palsy; in our experience, a tear of the rotator cuff is a far more frequent associated injury. Nevertheless, many orthopaedists have mistaken the patient's inability to abduct the arm after anterior dislocation as a stretch palsy of the axillary nerve. There are two significant findings with rotator cuff tears after anterior glenohumeral dislocation. The first can be detected on physical examination. After the dislocation has been reduced and the acute effects of the injury have subsided for 10 to 14 days, the ability to initiate abduction should be assessed. If there is inability to abduct or maintain the arm in abduction, a rotator cuff tear should be suspected. When testing the patient's ability to abduct, one should be able to palpate the deltoid muscle as it contracts; if contraction can be felt, injury to the axillary nerve can be eliminated as a

potential diagnosis. At this stage an arthrogram should be done to confirm the rotator cuff tear. The second finding is roentgenographic. The humeral head may be superiorly displaced in relationship to the glenoid on the postreduction films (Fig. 11-3). This results from two structural mechanisms: the deltoid acting unopposed to pull the humeral head cephalad when there are no rotator cuff tendons interposed between the humerus and the acromion, and the loss of the depressing and stabilizing action of the supraspinatus on the humeral head against the glenoid. The same guidelines apply to tears associated with dislocation as to those without dislocation. Complete massive tears under either set of circumstances should be repaired within the first 3 weeks to avoid the problem of difficult late reconstruction.

ROTATOR CUFF TEAR AFTER ANTERIOR DISLOCATION WITH FRACTURE OF GREATER TUBEROSITY

If there is a fracture of the greater tuberosity associated with an anterior glenohumeral dislocation, one can assume that there is some type of rotator cuff tear. The key to appropriate treatment of these injuries lies with the roentgenographic evaluation of the tuberosity, which can assume one of three positions. It can remain opposite the glenoid in its normal anatomic position, it can follow the head of the humerus, or it can retract posterosuperiorly beneath the acromi-

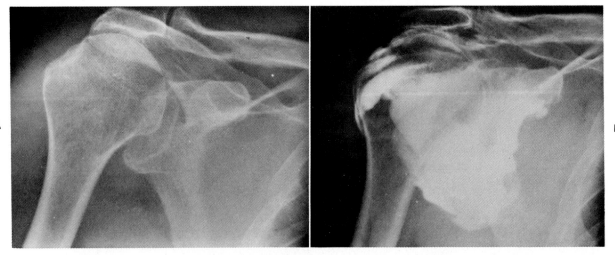

A

B

Fig. 11-3. A, Superior subluxation or migration of the humeral head in relation to the inferior margin of the glenoid. **B,** Arthrogram confirms the presence of a cuff tear. (**A** and **B,** From Neviaser, R.J.: Orthop. Clin. North Am. **11:**295-306, 1980.)

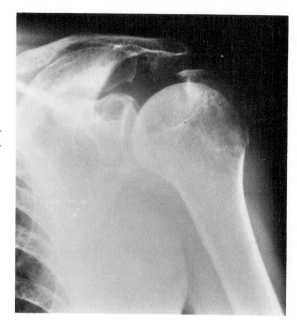

Fig. 11-4. Tuberosity fracture retracted posterosuperiorly under the acromion. (From Neviaser, R.J.: Orthop. Clin. North Am. **11:**295-306, 1980.)

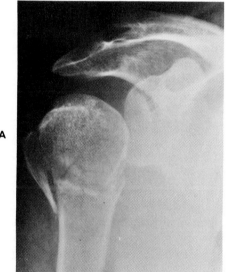

A

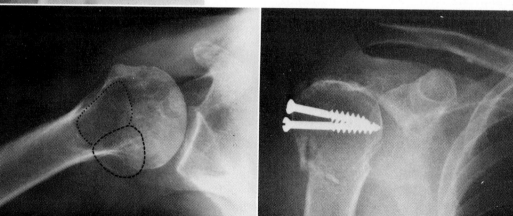

B

C

Fig. 11-5. A, Apparently satisfactory reduction of the tuberosity fragment. **B,** Axillary view reveals fragment, *dashes,* to be posteriorly displaced from normal position, *dots.* **C,** Screws fix the tuberosity fragment to the head. This was accompanied by a repair of the rotator cuff. (**A** to **C,** From Neviaser, R. J.: Orthop. Clin. North Am. **11:**295-306, 1980.)

on. In either of the first two positions, the fracture fragment may reduce satisfactorily after replacement of the humeral head in the glenoid. If the position is satisfactory, the longitudinal tear usually associated with this kind of fracture can heal, and treatment by immobilization is all that is required. If the tuberosity assumes a position posterosuperiorly beneath the acromion (Fig. 11-4), it will not heal, even with repositioning of the humeral head to its normal anatomic location. Assessment of the position of the tuberosity upon reduction of the dislocation must be based on roentgenograms taken in two planes: anteroposterior and axillary. Many of these fractures appear to be in a satisfactory position on the anteroposterior view (Fig. 11-5, *A*), but the axillary view reveals an unacceptable position with external rotation and posterior displacement (Fig. 11-5, *B*). Therefore the axillary view is the more important one for deciding about the need for surgery.

If the tuberosity is not in an acceptable position with the dislocation reduced, placing the arm in abduction will not accomplish a better reduction[5]—it will only displace the fragment further. The only satisfactory means for accomplishing anatomic reduction of the displaced tuberosity fragments is surgery, which must be done early to avoid having the fragment heal in an unacceptable position, thus blocking abduction and producing weak rotator cuff function. The surgical approach is the same as described previously. Certain facets of the operation differ, however, because of the bony involvement. The fragment usually is found externally rotated and displaced, and the cuff tear should be readily identified. The fragment is lined up in its anatomic position and fixed with one or two screws (Fig. 11-5, *C*). It is important to suture the cuff defect as well, in order to restore cuff function. In the rare instance where the tuberosity fragment is severely comminuted or extremely thin, it may be discarded and the cuff itself simply fixed to the cancellous defect in the bone. The postoperative course is similar to that previously described for cuff tears without bony involvement. It should be emphasized that abduction or airplane splints have no place in treatment of rotator cuff tears. Any repair immobilized in abduction runs a significant risk of pulling apart when the arm eventually is brought to the side. If a repair cannot be accomplished without undue tension with the arm at the side, then interposition grafting techniques (which are discussed later) should be utilized.

CHRONIC ROTATOR CUFF TEARS WITH OR WITHOUT HISTORY OF INJURY

These tears are the ones most commonly misunderstood, misdiagnosed, and poorly treated. The patient usually has been treated for adhesive capsulitis, bursitis, or tendinitis of the rotator cuff. His history often spans several months, if not years. He may have been examined by several physicians, taken anti-inflammatory medications (both local and systemic), and undergone a long course of physical therapy. These modalities usually provide minimal, if any, relief, often of only short duration. Most of these patients have good, if not virtually normal, ability to abduct, and it is this finding that is most confusing. Physicians often are taught that a patient must have loss of abduction as well as pain, if he has a tear of the rotator cuff. In the chronic condition, however, this does not hold true. Most patients with chronic tears of the rotator cuff complain of pain primarily, especially of pain waking them at night, but they retain the ability to abduct the arm to greater than 150 degrees and occasionally have complete abduction. Therefore any patient in middle age or older who has shoulder pain with significant night symptoms and who has satisfactory ability to abduct but has pain on palm-down abduction,[7] must be suspected of having a rupture of the rotator cuff. In these patients a simple, minimally invasive diagnostic procedure is arthrography of the shoulder. This will establish a diagnosis in a straightforward manner with minimal inconvenience and risk to the patient. As with arthrography in any shoulder condition, it is best done by the attending surgeon himself in order to obtain the greatest understanding of the pathophysiologic condition.[5,10]

The treatment of the patient with a chronic rupture of the rotator cuff can follow one of two courses. If the pain is tolerable and the patient can function in a satisfactory manner, he can be left untreated. This condition is not a life-threatening one, and the decision for surgical repair should be entered into jointly by the surgeon and the patient. The latter should understand all the ramifications of the nonoperative as well as the operative approach. It has been our experience that prolonged physical therapy and anti-inflammatory medications do not provide long-term satisfactory relief. In addition there is the risk of a superimposed second "injury" that would cause a massive acute extension of this tear.

The alternative therapeutic course is surgical

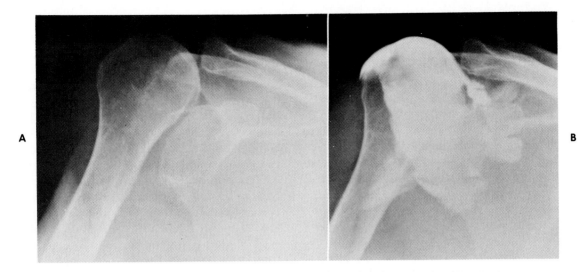

Fig. 11-6. A, A patient who had a complete acromionectomy and a failed cuff repair by someone else has a detachment of the deltoid. The head has herniated through the cuff and deltoid defects. **B,** Arthrogram confirms the cuff tear. (**A** and **B,** From Neviaser, R.J.: Orthop. Clin. North Am. **11:**295-306, 1980.)

repair. The type of operation performed depends on what is found when the cuff tear is exposed. These cases are approached through the anterosuperior incision at the level of the acromioclavicular joint, and the deltoid-splitting incision is used. After resecting the coracoacromial ligament and performing an anteroinferior oblique acromioplasty and an acromioclavicular arthroplasty, as well as incising and tagging the bursa, the surgeon should easily visualize the rupture of the rotator cuff. If the tear is large, one can obtain proved exposure by sharply dissecting the deltoid's subperiosteally from the superior aspect of the acromion as far laterally and posteriorly as necessary. The aponeurosis between the trapezius and the deltoid along with the superior acromioclavicular ligament can also be incised to permit reflection of the entire deltoid from the acromion. Additional posterior incisions are unnecessary. Since the deltoid is not incised from its origin, any concern about postoperative detachment of this muscle is eliminated. Complete acromionectomy is never done.[1,8] Removal of the entire acromion results in a short lever arm of the deltoid, reducing the patient's ability to abduct. It also frequently results in detachment of the deltoid in the postoperative period (Fig. 11-6) because the tissue remaining medial to the acromion to which the deltoid can be sutured is of such poor quality. As noted earlier, subperiosteal dissection of the deltoid from the superior surface of the clavicle and

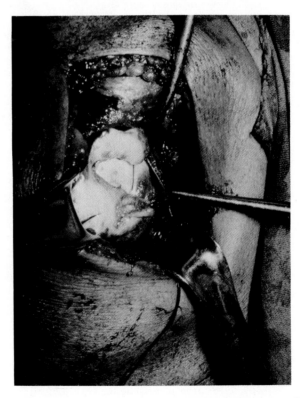

Fig. 11-7. Old cuff tear with whitish, avascular, scarred edges.

acromion eliminates the need for deltoid repair except for reinforcing of sutures in the deltoid-splitting incision.

With chronic tears, there is a noticeable difference in the tissue quality from that in acute tears. In the late stages the tendons are usually scarred, thickened, and avascular at their ends (Fig. 11-7). Often they are fixed and retracted, a condition making it difficult, if not impossible, to mobilize them so that they can be brought laterally to their anatomic insertion near the greater tuberosity. The objective of any operation on the rotator cuff is not only to close the defect but to reestablish anatomic continuity between the tendons and the tuberosities. Therefore, by using traction sutures and extensive mobilization with a periosteal elevator or the surgeon's finger, the tendons often can be freed enough from the neck of the glenoid

and scapula to bring them laterally. They should then be sutured to bone with 0 nonabsorbable sutures. This, however, must be done with the patient's arm at his side—the physiologic position. As indicated before, the use of abduction splints is not only unnecessay but increases the risk of pulling apart the repair when the arm is brought to the side. If it is impossible to close the cuff defect anatomically with the arm at the side and there is a residual gap in the tendons, there are several techniques that can be used. In the presence of a small or moderate-sized residual defect (Fig. 11-8, *A*), the best technique is to utilize the intra-articular portion of the long head of the biceps.[4,8] After fixing the biceps tendon in the intertubercular groove, the intra-articular portion is resected. This tendon is then split in a booklike fashion (Fig. 11-8, *B*) and used to bridge the re-

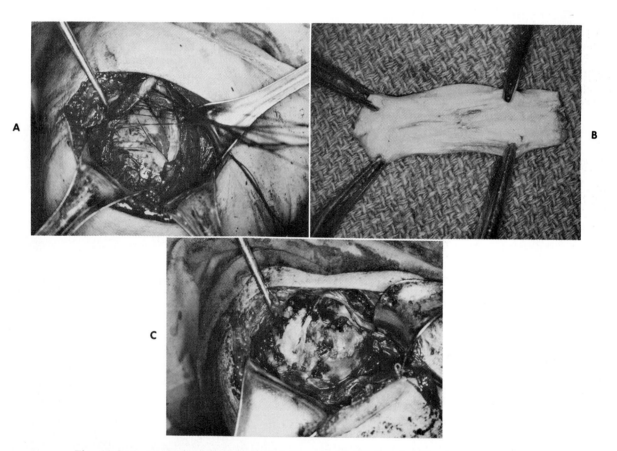

Fig. 11-8. A, Moderate-sized residual defect in a professional softball player who had an unrecognized cuff tear after an anterior dislocation. Traction applied through sutures does not close the defect. **B,** Biceps tendon is split to be used as a graft. **C,** The graft in place. The patient is playing professionally again. (**A** to **C,** From Neviaser, R.J.: Orthop. Clin. North Am. **11:**295-306, 1980.)

maining defect in the cuff (Fig. 11-8, *C*). The smooth or uncut surface is placed toward the humeral head, whereas the rough or cut portion is placed extra-articularly. This graft is sutured to the edges of the cuff first and then secured in the groove made in the anatomic neck of the humerus near the tuberosities. The closure of this capsular defect should be watertight. Postoperative management is the same as previously described except that the arm is kept in a sling-and-swathe for 6 weeks rather than 3.

With large residual defects for which the biceps graft is too small, the procedure of choice is the freeze-dried cadaver rotator cuff graft.[6,8] Since it is not possible to predict the need for a special reconstructive procedure preoperatively, one should be familiar with and have the ability to utilize any of these techniques. Although the arthrogram is extremely valuable in establishing the diagnosis, it will not indicate the size of the tear. The amount of dye that extravasates from the joint into the subdeltoid bursa merely indicates the size of the bursa. When large defects are found after exposure of the cuff in the manner already described, and if extensive mobilization and traction have failed to bridge the gap ade-

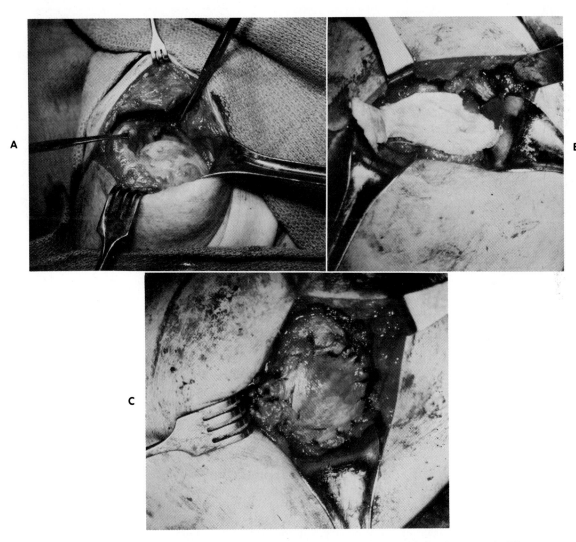

Fig. 11-9. A, Large residual tear, which had been misdiagnosed for 2 years. **B,** The reconstituted freeze-dried cadaver graft lying free in the wound. **C,** The graft secured to the cuff and tuberosities. (**A** to **C,** From Neviaser, R.J.: Orthop. Clin. North Am. **11**:295-306, 1980.)

quately, the type of reconstruction necessary can then be determined. One should reserve the use of freeze-dried cadaver grafts for defects that are too large for the biceps graft (Fig. 11-9, *A*). The freeze-dried tissue can be reconstituted in sterile saline solution over a period of 30 minutes (Fig. 11-9, *B*). Once reconstituted, it will be soft and pliable and can be sutured appropriately. It should first be anchored to the freshened ends of the torn cuff tendons. The graft should then be brought laterally and fixed in the groove made in the naturally occurring sulcus between the greater tuberosity and the articular surface of the hu-

merus. This graft is secured to bone through drill holes, and the knots should be tied external and inferior to the tip of the greater tuberosity (Fig. 11-9, *C*). Again, the capsular repair should be watertight. After routine closure, the postoperative course is the same as indicated before, but the arm is immobilized for a period of 6 weeks rather than the routine 3; this period ensures adequate incorporation of the freeze-dried graft. Currently the other options to using either the free biceps graft or the freeze-dried cadaver rotator cuff graft include use of fascia lata (which usually stretches out and gives a poor result) or inserting

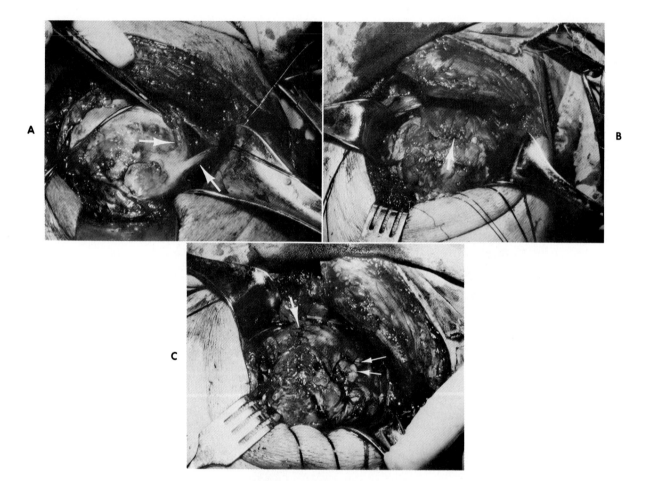

Fig. 11-10. A, Subscapularis, *right arrow,* has been separated from underlying capsule, *left arrow,* just prior to detachment of it from its insertion. **B,** Subscapularis and teres minor have been transferred superiorly and secured to tuberosities, *arrow.* **C,** Subscapularis and teres minor have been sutured together, *single arrow,* and new interval between lower border of subscapularis and the remaining anterior capsule has been closed, *two arrows.* The same closure is done posteriorly between the teres minor and the capsule. (**A** to **C,** From Neviaser, R.J., and Neviaser, T.J.: Transfer of the subscapularis and teres minor for repair of massive, chronic defects of the rotator cuff. In Bayley, J.I.L., and Kessel, L., editors: Shoulder surgery, Heidelberg, 1981, Springer-Verlag.)

the tendons into a groove made in the humeral head at whatever point the tendons happen to reach.[3] Although this can result in a capsular closure and relief of pain, it frequently leaves the patient with pronounced weakness in abduction. Simple acromioplasty and resection of the coracoacromial ligament without repairing the cuff rarely results in satisfactory relief of pain or improvement of function, and many patients treated in this way come to further reconstruction.

Although freeze-dried cadaver grafts give highly successful results, the graft material is becoming increasingly difficult to obtain because of the stringent criteria for its procurement; that is, it must come from a cadaver that is under the age of 45, with no history of infection or malignancy. An acceptable alternative has recently been developed by transferal of the subscapularis and teres minor to cover the defect.[9] The tendons of the subscapularis and teres minor are separated sharply and with care from the underlying capsule (Fig. 11-10, *A*) and detached at their insertions. The underlying capsule is left undisturbed, both anteriorly and posteriorly. After mobilization of these tendons proximalward, they are transferred to the superior aspect of the humeral head and tuberosities to cover the defect (Fig. 11-10, *B*). The new interval between these tendons is then sutured, and the tendons are secured to a groove made in the sulcus just medial to the tuberosities. The resulting spaces between the inferior margins of the subscapularis anteriorly, the teres minor posteriorly, and the remaining capsule from which they were previously separated, are sutured directly (Fig. 11-10, *C*). This results in a watertight closure. To date, 17 patients have undergone this operation and have been followed from 2 to 6 years. Seventy percent of them have achieved a good to excellent result, meaning that they can abduct more than 90 degrees and have less pain. As the technique has been refined, the incidence of good to excellent results has increased. Most of the failures have been in patients who had a deltoid detachment from previous unsuccessful surgery. As with other reconstructive procedures, the postoperative immobilization is 6 weeks rather than 3. Although some patients will achieve an excellent result of abduction greater than 120 degrees and relief of pain, the more typical outcome is a patient who can abduct up to 120 degrees and has less pain—a "good" rating. These results compare well with but do not equal those of the freeze-dried cadaver grafts.

ROTATOR CUFF TEARS AFTER AVULSION FRACTURE OF GREATER TUBEROSITY

Since avulsion fractures of the greater tuberosity often appear relatively uncomplicated, it is not commonly appreciated that a rupture of the rotator cuff may accompany this fracture, and the tendency is to treat the fracture as an isolated injury. The patient often may complain of persistent pain that exceeds the normal period of fracture discomfort. Again, a tear of the rotator cuff is not suspected because the patient can abduct the arm well. Physical therapy does not improve his symptoms. Arthrography should be considered when the patient's pain continues despite adequate treatment of an otherwise insignificant injury. This should apply also to those patients who have fractures of the acromion.

SUMMARY

The diagnosis of a torn rotator cuff can be readily established by arthrography. The key to making the correct diagnosis is a high degree of suspicion in any patient with shoulder pain, with or without a history of injury. In circumstances where spontaneous healing cannot be expected to occur, early surgical repair should provide consistently satisfactory results. Undue delay in repair leads to a more difficult reconstructive procedure, but the availability of the free biceps tendon graft and the freeze-dried rotator cuff graft has increased the good results even with late reconstructions. A promising new technique has been developed utilizing transference of the subscapularis end teres minor tendons as an alternative to the freeze-dried cadaver graft when the latter is unavailable.

REFERENCES TO PART A

1. Bakalim, G., and Pasila, M.: Surgical treatment of rupture of the rotator cuff tendon, Acta Orthop. Scand. **46:**751, 1975.
2. Bateman, J.E.: The shoulder and neck, ed. 2, Philadelphia, 1978, W.B. Saunders Co.
3. McLaughlin, H.L.: Reconstruction of the shoulder joint. Muscular and tendinous defects at the shoulder and their repair. In Thompson, J.E.M., editor: The American Academy of Orthopaedic Surgeons' lectures on reconstruction surgery, Ann Arbor, Mich., 1944, J.W. Edwards.
4. Neviaser, J.S.: Ruptures of the rotator cuff of the shoulder: new concepts in the diagnosis and operative treatment of chronic ruptures, Arch. Surg. **102:**483, 1971.
5. Neviaser, J.S.: Arthrography of the shoulder. The diagnosis and management of the lesions visualized, Springfield, Ill., 1975, Charles C Thomas, Publisher.

6. Neviaser, J.S., Neviaser, R.J., and Neviaser, T.J.: The repair of chronic massive ruptures of the rotator cuff of the shoulder by use of a freeze-dried rotator cuff, J. Bone Joint Surg. **60A:**681, 1978.

7. Neviaser, R.J.: Anatomic considerations and examination of the shoulder, Orthop. Clin. North Am. **11:**187, 1980.

8. Neviaser, R.J.: Tears of the rotator cuff, Orthop. Clin. North Am. **11:**295, 1980.

9. Neviaser, R.J., and Neviaser, T.J.: Transfer of the subscapularis and teres minor for repair of massive, chronic defects of the rotator cuff. In Bayley, J.I.L., and Kessel, L., editors: Shoulder surgery, Heidelberg, 1981, Springer-Verlag.

10. Neviaser, T.J.: Arthrography of the shoulder, Orthop. Clin. North Am. **11:**205, 1980.

Part B

Lesions of long head of biceps tendon

THOMAS J. NEVIASER, M.D.
ROBERT J. NEVIASER, M.D.
Washington, D.C.

The purpose of this section is to review the anatomy, pathomechanics, symptoms, and physical examinations of certain lesions of the biceps tendon. The discussion includes ruptures of the long head of the biceps tendon, dislocations, subluxations, and biceps tenosynovitis.

ANATOMY

The long head of the biceps brachii tendon and its synovial lining are an extension of the shoulder joint. The entire shoulder joint is superiorly covered by an arc of structures known as the acromial arch, including the coracoacromial ligament, the acromioclavicular joint, the acromion itself, and the coracoid process. The soft-tissue structures between the acromial arch and the bony portion of the shoulder joint include the rotator cuff, the subacromial bursa, and the long head of the biceps tendon. These soft-tissue structures fit snugly between the humeral head and the acromial arch. This relationship must be snug, since there is very little inherent stability in the glenohumeral joint. The biceps tendon originates at the superior lip of the glenoid labrum and exits the shoulder through a groove between the lesser and greater tuberosities. The lesser tuberosity normally is higher than the greater tuberosity and thereby, in effect, allows the biceps tendon to pass centrally in the groove so that there is a smooth gliding action of the biceps. As it exits from the shoulder joint, the biceps tendon passes under the rigid transverse humeral ligament, which prevents it from subluxating and dislocating and directs it distally onto the anterior surface of the humerus.

RUPTURES OF LONG HEAD OF BICEPS

Ruptures of the long head of the biceps can occur in the younger as well as in the older age group. The treatment, however, varies greatly in the two groups. The ruptured biceps in the healthy vigorous athlete should be repaired to establish as much power to the biceps as possible, since the athlete stresses the upper extremities well past the limit of daily activities. The older patient with an acute ruptured biceps tendon need not have any specific treatment other than watchful waiting and protection because of pain. No repair is indicated, since he will not be stressing the arm past his daily functional needs. The pain will subside within 10 days to 2 weeks. A ruptured biceps, however, can be associated with a rupture of the rotator cuff and repair of the cuff may well be necessary. It is not necessary to repair the biceps at the time of the rotator cuff surgery unless the distal end is easily found. The repair of the tendon does not consist of suturing the ends together since the quality of the tissues would preclude successful repair. The distal end is sutured into the bicipital groove with the elbow at 80 to 90 degrees of flexion. This repair is immobilized for approximately 3 to 4 weeks and then gradual flexion and extension exercises are started.

DISLOCATIONS OF BICEPS TENDON

Dislocation of the biceps tendon is the complete displacement of the tendon from the groove. The dislocation is always medial and usually presents as pain in the anterior aspect of the shoulder. The patient may often complain of a snapping sensation in abduction and external rotation causing a reflex dropping of the arm and subsequent relocation of the tendon. Many patients are often misdiagnosed as having a recurrent anterior subluxating shoulder since the history with that condition is somewhat similar to the dislocation of the biceps tendon. Surgery performed for a recurrent subluxating shoulder rather than a dislocating biceps tendon may make the dislocation more prominent.

There are three types of dislocations of the biceps tendon. The first is found with ruptures of the rotator cuff and the transverse humeral liga-

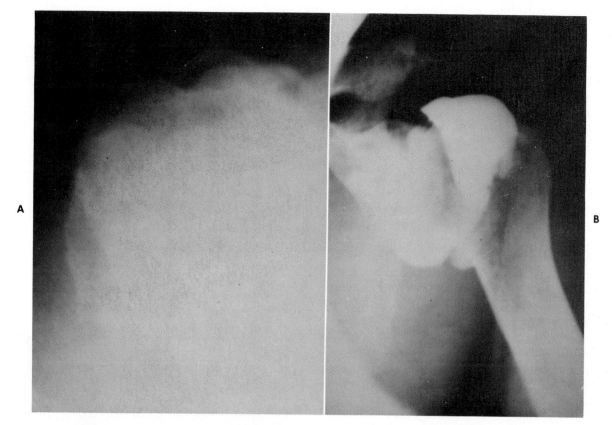

Fig. 11-11. A, Bicipital groove view showing medial dislocation of the biceps tendon. **B,** Anteroposterior view showing medial dislocation. Findings here are more difficult to visualize.

ment through attrition. The second is attrition of the transverse humeral ligament with only attenuation of the subscapularis at its insertion on the superior aspect of the lesser tuberosity. In these cases, no full-thickness cuff tear is present. The third type is the acute, traumatic rupture of the transverse humeral ligament. This is unusual. The diagnosis of a dislocating biceps tendon is not easy to establish. Arthrography is helpful in visualizing displacement of the biceps tendon medially[4,6] (Fig, 11-11). At arthrography, the bicipital groove view is the best one to demonstrate the dislocation, if present. It is more difficult to recognize a dislocated biceps tendon on the anteroposterior shoulder film with arthrography. If symptoms persist and arthrography is not helpful, an examination under anesthesia, followed by surgical visualization of the biceps tendon during an exploration of the shoulder joint may be needed. This occasionally is the only means to differentiate between the dislocating biceps tendon and a subluxating shoulder.

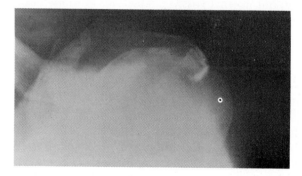

Fig. 11-12. Medial subluxation of the biceps tendon against the wall of the bicipital groove.

SUBLUXATION

Subluxation of the biceps tendon is incomplete displacement in the groove. Subluxation of the biceps tendon is easily seen on arthrography (Fig. 11-12). The biceps tendon is pressed against the medial wall of the bicipital groove. Plain roentgenograms may reveal a shallow groove. This physical displacement of the biceps tendon in an abnormal groove can be the causative factor of biceps tenosynovitis, which is discussed later. Classical signs of subluxation of the biceps tendon are usually tenderness over the bicipital groove, pain with forward flexion of the shoulder with elbow fully extended, and pain with abduction with the palm up. The patient also has pain with abduction with the palm down as in pushing down on the lock of a car door.

BICEPS TENOSYNOVITIS

The biceps tenosynovitis does not occur as an isolated entity. It is part of the acromial arch syndrome, which also includes a rotator cuff tendinitis and a subacromial bursitis, and presents as pain in the shoulder, often of long duration. Clinically, the pain of the acromial arch syndrome is insidious with aching and throbbing over the deltoid or its insertion radiating to the elbow and occasionally to the wrist. The pain is increased with overhead motion or forward flexion against resistance, and positional night discomfort may be present. Many patients complain that locking the car door on the opposite side of the car will reproduce the symptoms as well as when they reach behind themselves. Some will also complain of a catch or an acute pain either during abduction or coming down from the abducted position. Physical examination reveals decreased active abduction but normal passive abduction. Pure glenohumeral motion is normal, but external rotation by the side and external rotation in abduction, as well as internal rotation, are limited with pain usually centered at the anterior aspect of the shoulder. The biceps tendon is always tender, and, in fact, the most tender area is just below the transverse humeral ligament. The biceps resistance test is positive. This test is performed with the elbow in full extension and the forearm supinated while forward flexion of the shoulder is carried out against resistance. One percent lidocaine in the subacromial space reduces much of the pain and increases the motion because the accompanying rotator cuff tendinitis is anesthetized. The biceps tenosynovitis persists, however, since it is an extension of the intra-articular synovium rather than being extra-articular where the anesthetic agent has been injected. Roentgenograms may be normal, but some irregularities can be seen. Degenerative changes in the acromioclavicular joint, osteophytes on the inferior joint surface

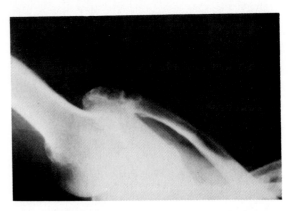

Fig. 11-13. Degenerative changes of the acromioclavicular joint with inferior traction osteophyte.

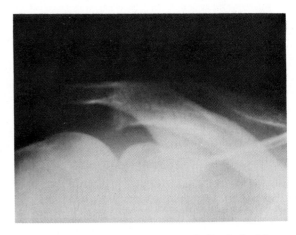

Fig. 11-14. Inferior subluxation of distal clavicle encroaching upon the subacromial space.

from traction on the ligaments secondary to chronic synovitis (Fig. 11-13), and inferior subluxation of the acromioclavicular joint combine to encroach upon the subacromial space (Fig. 11-14), irritating the rotator cuff and biceps tendon in abducted and external rotated motion. One may see a shallow bicipital groove, which readily produces tenosynovitis (Fig. 11-15). Medial and lateral bicipital groove osteophytes are traction spurs resulting from chronic synovitis producing traction on the transverse humeral ligament (Fig. 11-16). A flattened medial wall of the groove can lead to medial biceps subluxation. Acromial irregularities

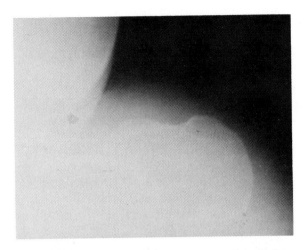

Fig. 11-15. A shallow bicipital groove and slanted medial wall.

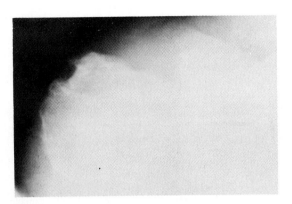

Fig. 11-16. Medial bicipital groove osteophyte caused by tenosynovitis and traction on the transverse humeral ligament.

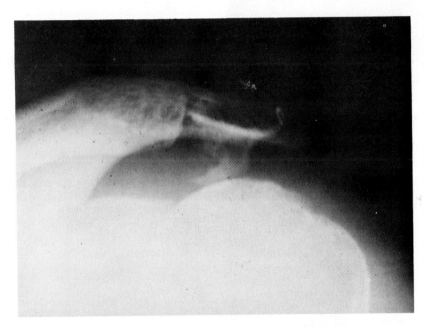

Fig. 11-17. Acromial osteophyte seen encroaching upon subacromial space.

such as osteophytes (Fig. 11-17) or old acromial fractures may be evident on roentgenograms. Arthrography is most important in the diagnosis of a biceps tenosynovitis.[4,6] It presents with many faces and must be evaluated on multiple arthrographic films to assure that this diagnosis is accurate. Arthrographic signs of a biceps tenosynovitis will include (1) a narrowed attenuated tendon, vacuolization of the biceps tendon, which represents filling defects of the tenosynovium caused by villous formation (Fig. 11-18), (2) elevation of the biceps from the groove as a result of a thickened tenosynovium (Fig. 11-19), (3) elevation of the biceps origin suggesting synovitis extending proxi-

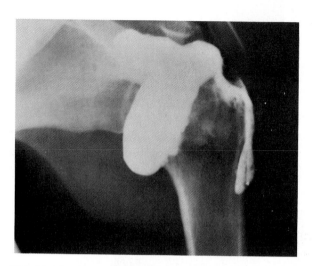

Fig. 11-18. Filling defects or vacuolization of the biceps tendon consistent with a biceps tenosynovitis.

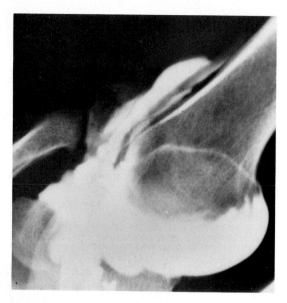

Fig. 11-19. Elevation of the thickened biceps sheath from the cortex of the humerus. (From Neviaser, R.J.: Orthop. Clin. North Am. **11**:343-348, 1980.)

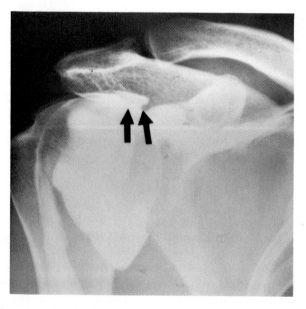

Fig. 11-20. Arthrogram showing elevation of the origin of the biceps, *arrows,* and post-stenotic dilatation of the tenosynovium.

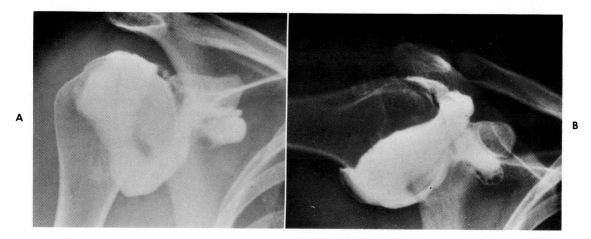

Fig. 11-21. A, Note that there is no dye expressed through the bicipital groove. **B,** Even on abduction, no dye is seen in the sheath. (From Neviaser, R.J.: Orthop. Clin. North Am. **11**:343-348, 1980.)

mally to the origin, elevating the biceps from the superior glenoid labrum and poststenotic dilatation of the tenosynovium seen distal to the transverse humeral ligament (Fig. 11-20), and (4) poor filling of the sheath especially under the transverse humeral ligament (Fig. 11-21). Occasionally one will see no dye expressed through the biceps groove because of complete obliteration of the groove by the tenosynovitis.

PATHOMECHANICS

Because the biceps tendon passes through the groove between the tuberosities, it undergoes the same motions as the tuberosities, rotator cuff, and subacromial bursa. Since the sheath of the biceps tendon is an extension of the shoulder-joint synovial lining and the synovium is intimately related to the rotator cuff, an inflammatory process involving any of these structures will affect the others as well. Factors contributing to the production of the acromial arch syndrome include degenerative changes in the acromioclavicular joint with capsular bulging inferiorly and osteophytes or inferior subluxation of the acromioclavicular joint, all of which encroach upon the subacromial space. By reducing the subacromial space, these factors increase rotator cuff and biceps tendon irritation leading to a tenosynovitis of the biceps tendon and a rotator cuff tendinitis. The inflammatory process that is caused in an acromial arch syndrome can develop from anywhere within the arch including the acromioclavicular joint, the ac-

romion, and the rotator cuff, as well as the biceps tendon. It is assumed that in order to treat the symptoms ·produced by this combination of factors successfully, one must correct all of the causes of the disease process.

TREATMENT

Initially, therapy includes anti-inflammatory medications, wet heat, restricted exercises, and avoidance of the abducted and external rotated position, especially in sports such as racquetball, baseball, football, and tennis. Injections of a local anesthetic with a small dose of refined steroid in the subacromial space or the bicipital tendon sheath, or both, may alleviate most of the pain and allow the patient to return to his activity. It is our feeling that the biceps tendon is the most prominent soft-tissue structure producing pain in the acromial arch syndrome. The rotator cuff tendinitis may respond readily to anti-inflammatory medications and injections. The biceps tenosynovitis, however, is usually more resistant. The reason for this is the rigid transverse humeral ligament that covers the bicipital groove between the tips of the lesser and greater tuberosities. The inflamed biceps tendon glides under this rigid structure, which does not allow expansion of the biceps tenosynovitis. The continuous compression of the tendon and its lining produces a chronic inflammatory state. Injections into the biceps sheath are difficult, since many patients have thick subcutaneous tissue as well as large deltoid muscle over this area hampering the ability of the surgeon to find the groove by palpation. Also, injections in this area must be precise, with the needle point placed not within the tendon but only within the tendon sheath. This is a technically difficult procedure. If symptoms persist and the normal lifestyle is disturbed, surgery is indicated. Surgery in the past has included stapling and K-wiring of biceps in the groove. This is an inadequate means of tenodesing the biceps, since the metal above the cortex level can cause an irritation of soft tissue with recurrence of symptoms. The surgical procedure of choice is the "four-in-one-arthroplasty for the acromial arch syndrome and biceps tenosynovitis." The four procedures performed are excision of the coracoacromial ligament, an acromioclavicular arthroplasty,[1,8] an anteroinferior oblique acromioplasty,[3] and tenodesis of the biceps tendon.[5] No claim is made for any originality of these procedures, but they have all been combined in this approach because of the pathomechanics already described.

SURGICAL PROCEDURE

The patient is positioned in a barber-chair position and the shoulder prepped and draped as usual. A superoanterior incision is made extending from the posterior aspect of the acromioclavicular joint forward and down over the proximal biceps tendon. Through a deltoid-splitting approach, the anterior aspect of the shoulder joint is exposed. The coracoacromial ligament is excised completely. The inferior capsule of the acromioclavicular joint is then incised up to but not including the superior periosteum and acromioclavicular ligament. These structures are dissected subperiosteally from the superior aspect of the distal clavicle and proximal acromium and retracted gently posteriorly to expose the entire acromioclavicular joint. The distal 1 cm of the clavicle is removed with a reciprocating saw and all the edges are rasped smooth. The retracted structures are then allowed to fall back into place. Attention is then turned to the anterior acromium where an oblique acromial osteotomy is carried out, including the inferior half of the articulating surface of the acromium. The undersurface of the acromium is then rasped smooth. The two osteotomy sites are then lavaged with saline solution. The humerus is then slightly externally rotated and forward flexed with the elbow at 90 degrees. The interval between the subscapularis and supraspinatus is incised longitudinally to expose the intra-articular portion of the biceps tendon. The incision is carried to but not including the transverse humeral ligament. With a blunt hook, the biceps tendon is pulled superiorly revealing the tenosynovitis of the biceps tendon un-

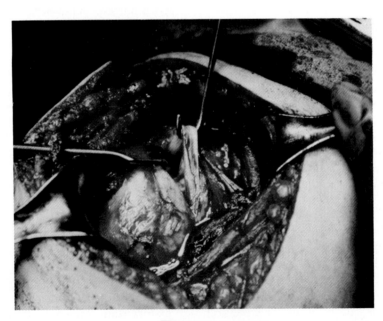

Fig. 11-22. Operative photograph of a biceps tenosynovitis being pulled up from under the transverse humeral ligament.

der and distal to the transverse humeral ligament (Fig. 11-22). The tendon is then allowed to retract to its original position in the groove and sutured in the groove to the surrounding soft tissues with 0 nonabsorbable sutures (four in number). This tenodesis is performed with the elbow at 80 to 90 degrees of flexion. The proximal intra-articular portion is then excised, and the rotator-cuff incision is closed with inverted 0 nonabsorbable sutures. The bursa is sutured over the repair with plain catgut, and the wound is closed in the usual manner. A stockinette sling and swathe is applied after the compression dressing.

The sutures are removed at 10 days, and the stockinette is changed weekly for 3 weeks. In the fourth week, pendulum exercises are started in a sling, and the patient is advised not to extend the elbow in order to give 4 full weeks for the tenodesis to heal. After 4 weeks, all immobilization is discontinued and gradually increased activities and exercises are started. Wall-walking and pendulum exercises are then followed by external and internal rotation exercises. Once progress is satisfactory, abduction and external rotation exercises are added. Pain medication is given, if needed, to reduce discomfort during periods of exercises. Passive exercises with pendulum and pulley are alternated with the shoulder wheel.

The rehabilitation time ranges from 3 to 9 months depending on the motivation and threshold of pain of the patient. Encouragement and close follow-up are crucial in the rehabilitation. Occasionally the patient will overdo the exercise program and need rest, wet heat, and an anti-inflammatory regimen to reduce his discomfort.

DISCUSSION

There has been some discussion as to whether all four procedures are needed in treating this syndrome. There is no question that the coracoacromial ligament and acromion have been proved to be offending agents.[2,3,7,9] Excision of the coracoacromial ligament and the oblique acromioplasty have been discussed many times. A tenodesis of the biceps tendon is necessary to eliminate biceps motion under the transverse ligament, and a release of the transverse humeral ligament

would increase the chances of subluxation and dislocation of the biceps tendon. An acromioclavicular arthroplasty is carried out because many of our cases had rotengenographic changes or disease at surgery in the acromioclavicular joint.[1] In those cases where rotengenograms show no abnormalities, early degenerative changes and inferior capsular swelling with abutment of the rotator cuff and biceps were noted at surgery. In the beginning, we did not perform the arthroplasty of the acromioclavicular joint on several cases and had to return later to perform the arthroplasty to eliminate residual symptoms. We have also had to perform the acromioclavicular arthroplasty on patients referred to us after having undergone various decompressive procedures that have failed.

Overall, the physician must be atuned to the patient's complaints about his shoulder on adequate physical examination with a basic understanding of the anatomy and pathomechanics of the shoulder. All conservative measures must be tried before arthrography and subsequent surgery are warranted. The four-in-one-arthroplasty of the shoulder has been most successful in over 80 cases and is believed to be the surgical procedure of choice for the acromial arch syndrome with rotator cuff tendinitis and biceps tenosynovitis.

REFERENCES TO PART B

1. Bateman, J.: The shoulder and neck, Philadelphia, 1972, W.B. Saunders Co.
2. Kessel, L., and Watson, M.: The painful arc syndrome, J. Bone Joint Surg. **59B:**166-172, 1977.
3. Neer, C.: Anterior acromioplasty for the chronic impingement syndrome in the shoulder, J. Bone Joint Surg. **54A:**41-50, 1972.
4. Neviaser, J.: Arthrography of the shoulder: the diagnosis and management of the lesions visualized, Springfield, Ill., 1975, Charles C Thomas, Publisher.
5. Neviaser, R.J.: Lesions of the biceps and tendinitis of the shoulder, Orthop. Clin. North Am. **11**(2):343, April 1980.
6. Neviaser, T.J.: Arthrography of the shoulder, Orthoped. Clin. North Am., vol. 11, no. 2, April 1980.
7. Pujadas, G.M.: Coraco-acromial ligament syndrome, J. Bone Joint Surg. **52A:**1261-1262, 1970.
8. Taylor, G.M., and Tooke, M.: Degeneration of the acromioclavicular joint as a cause of shoulder pain, J. Bone Joint Surg. **59:**507, 1977.
9. Watson, M.: The refractory painful arc syndrome, J. Bone Joint Surgery, **60B:**544-546, 1978.

Chapter 12

Tears of rotator cuff

ROBERT H. COFIELD, M.D.
Rochester, Minnesota

VARIATIONS IN PATHOLOGIC LESIONS

Any discussion of tears of the rotator cuff will become confusing and recommendations for treatment will seem vague unless the type and extent of pathologic change in the cuff are known. Much uncertainty in this area is caused by collective consideration of all pathologic lesions of the rotator cuff when, in reality, many different problems exist. This practice has generated statements in the literature that have seemed contradictory but may not have been confusing if the pathologic condition being considered had been well defined. For example, in 1934 Codman[9] recommended, "Not only is exploration indicated but . . . it should be strongly urged . . . ," and likewise Bateman[4] suggested, "If there is a definite defect completely through the cuff . . . operative repair is the method of choice." In contrast, Rowe[29] wrote, "The more experienced the surgeon, the more emphasis he will place on the conservative management . . . ," and McLaughlin,[22] in describing his experience, stated, "The author formerly favored early operation until experience demonstrated that the results of early and later repair were essentially the same . . . an imponderable number of these patients who had an early operation would have recovered spontaneously."

A full spectrum of pathologic conditions exists. Neer[24] described the concept of subacromial arch impingement with early edema and inflammation, progressing to fibrosis with fraying, and finally continuing to partial or full-thickness tearing of the tendons. An acute tear may occur with an injury in the presence of mild chronic tendon disease, or an acute disruption may occur when a severe long-term attrition of tendons has been present. Tears may be chronic by virtue of existing without an acute injury having occurred, or they may be present after a period of conservative management for a specific injury.

Almost all lesions affect the supraspinatus tendon near its attachment to the humeral tuberosity. This may be the only tendon affected, or extension may occur proximally with splitting of the tendon and muscle fibers, posteriorly with tearing of the infraspinatus, or anteriorly with rupture of the subscapularis. With scarring of the tissue, a fixed retraction of the ends of the tendon may occur, and further subacromial impingement may erode the torn edges of the tendon.

Other structures in the area may have coexistent disease. The biceps can be inflamed, frayed, torn, or dislocated. Nonetheless, severe disease of the long head of the biceps is not so frequent as the literature suggests. The acromioclavicular joint may be arthritic and painful, and the inferior acromioclavicular osteophytes may further compromise the subacromial space and add to tendon impingement. Finally, with long-standing severe cuff disease and glenohumeral instability, loss of cartilage may result in traumatic or secondary osteoarthritis of the shoulder.

The type and extent of the existing pathologic condition should be understood as fully as possible before a treatment program is outlined or initiated.

PHYSIOLOGY

The function of the rotator cuff is becoming better understood as a result of the accelerated interest in biomechanics. Simplistically, one can consider the cuff as a dynamic stabilizer of the shoulder joint and also as a motor for active movement of the arm. The rotator cuff mechanism centers the humeral head on the shallow gelnoid and prevents excessive motion in all directions: superiorly,[17] anteriorly or posteriorly,[13,18,19,28,30,34] and inferiorly.[3] During abduction of the arm, forces that attempt to subluxate the humerus are directed most superiorly between 60 and 90 degrees,[38] and inability to raise the arm past this position in the presence of anterosuperior instability of the humeral head is evident clinically in patients with large tears of the rotator cuff.

The rotator cuff contributes to the power of arm movement in all directions. Using cross-sectional area as an index to muscle strength, Walker[38] measured the rotator cuff as consisting of 31% of the total cross section of the shoulder musculature. The contribution of the rotator cuff to the power of abduction and external rotation is appreciable. Using selected nerve blocks and strength tests, Colachis and co-workers[10,11] found that the rotator cuff muscles contributed 45% of the available power to abduction and an incredible 90% or more to the power of external rotation. Using cross-sectional measurements of muscle and by defining moment arms, Chao,[8] with use of data from Fick,[14] calculated that the rotator cuff supplied 30.9% of the power of abduction and 79.2% of the available power of external rotation.

This basic information is relevant as an aid in the diagnosis of inadequate function of the rotator cuff. It also provides a focus for planning a reconstructive program to correct disease of the cuff mechanism.

DIAGNOSIS

Pain is the most frequent symptom of a tear of the rotator cuff. Often associated with pain are weakness and a corresponding loss of active motion.

Physical findings will vary with the size of the tear and its duration. In the presence of a moderate to large chronic tear, a full range of findings will be present, whereas a frayed supraspinatus with a full-thickness split in the line of its fibers will demonstrate only the findings usually associ-

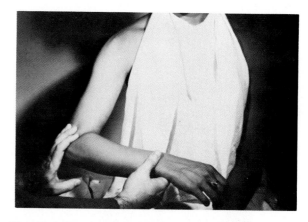

Fig. 12-1. Testing for weakness in direction of supraspinatus.

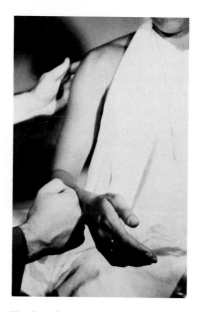

Fig. 12-2. Testing for weakness of external rotators of arm.

ated with subacromial impingement. Observing the shoulder, the physician may see diffuse muscle atrophy or selective atrophy of the supraspinatus or infraspinatus (or both). An old biceps tear may be present, and the humeral head may be slightly forward and superiorly subluxated.

Movement may be full, or flexion and abduction may be restricted. If passive movement exceeds active movement, loss of power in the direction of abduction is suggested. Loss of active external rotation is an unusual finding. Weakness in the direction of the supraspinatus is usually present (Fig. 12-1). If weakness of external rotation is also noted (Fig. 12-2), a large tear with ex-

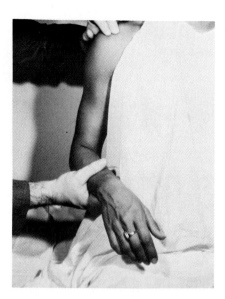

Fig. 12-3. Palpating for rotator cuff irregularity. Examiner should use index finger and long finger of one hand to palpate rotator cuff and other hand to manipulate patient's arm.

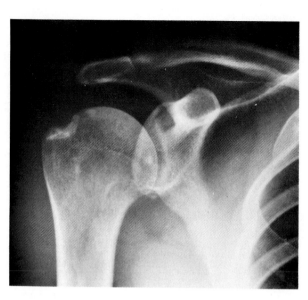

Fig. 12-4. Sclerosis of greater humeral tuberosity, with notch between tuberosity and articular surface of humeral head.

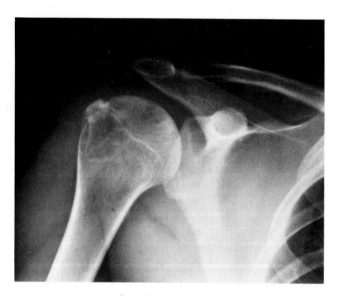

Fig. 12-5. Cyst formation and some sclerosis in region of greater humeral tuberosity.

tension into the infraspinatus is probably present. Palpation usually confirms the presence of cuff irregularity; crepitation and often a negative defect can be detected (Fig. 12-3). Tenderness of the acromioclavicular joint suggests the presence of synovitis or arthritis.

Although standard roentgenograms may be normal, more often nonspecific changes associated with disorders of the tendons of the rotator cuff and occasionally diagnostic changes are seen. The greater tuberosity may be sclerotic, with a notch present between the humeral articular surface and the tuberosity (Fig. 12-4). Alternatively, the greater tuberosity may have a cystic appearance (Fig. 12-5). The acromion may show sclerosis with spur formation or may lose its normal inferior convexity and appear concave (Fig. 12-6). The interval between the acromion and the hu-

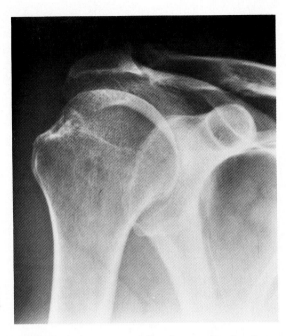

Fig. 12-6. Inferior convexity of undersurface of acromion has become concave. Slight upward subluxation of humeral head, sclerosis of greater tuberosity, and acromioclavicular arthritis are also seen.

meral head may be decreased by upward humeral subluxation. An acromion-humeral interval of less than 9 mm suggests the presence of rotator cuff disease, and an interval of less than 6 mm implies that a tear in the rotator cuff is probably present.[40] Upward subluxation is almost always more pronounced on external rotation than on internal rotation views (Fig. 12-7). The axillary view may confirm the presence of forward subluxation (Fig. 12-8)—again indicative of cuff and capsular insufficiency. Acromioclavicular arthritis may be present.

For absolute confirmation of the diagnosis, arthrography of the shoulder can be done. Double-contrast studies yield more information about the synovial lining and the thickness of the glenohumeral cartilage; occasionally, these studies (especially combined with tomography) may outline the size of a cuff tear. To demonstrate the presence or absence of a tear of the rotator cuff, however, a single-contrast study will suffice and probably is associated with fewer false-negative results.

Consistently good arthrograms can be obtained with the use of fluoroscopy. Our technique is to position the patient supine on a fluoroscopy table in the x-ray department; surgically scrub, prepare, and drape the anterior aspect of the shoul-der; inject 1% lidocaine a fingerbreadth infero-lateral to the coracoid process; and then direct a 20-gauge spinal needle to the anterior shoulder-joint line through this point. The position of the needle is confirmed by fluoroscopy and adjusted if necessary. A 30-ml syringe is filled with 25 ml of a contrast medium and 5 ml of a local anesthetic agent. The syringe is then connected to intravenous extension tubing, which is connected to the spinal needle, and the solution is injected while it is visualized by means of fluoroscopy. The contrast medium should be visualized almost immediately along the joint line; if it pools around the needle, the position of the needle must be altered. If dye is seen to flow into the subacromial bursa from the glenohumeral joint, a tear of the rotator cuff is confirmed, and the following permanent roentgenograms should be obtained: anteroposterior views with internal and external rotation, a lateral scapular view, and an axillary view. If the findings seem normal at fluoroscopy, the shoulder is exercised before the final films are taken. Fig. 12-9 shows a normal shoulder arthrogram with the subscapularis recess, the axillary pouch, the biceps sheath, and the sharp cutoff of dye at the superior and lateral edges of the humeral articular surface. Fig. 12-10 shows a small

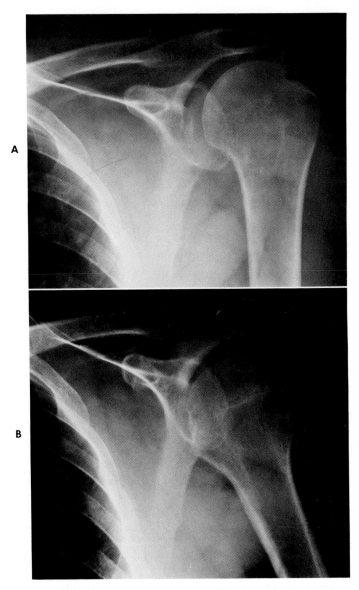

Fig. 12-7. Anteroposterior roentgenographic views of external, **A,** and internal, **B,** rotation of humerus. **A** shows upward humeral subluxation.

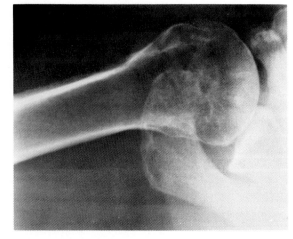

Fig. 12-8. Axillary roentgenographic view, demonstrating forward subluxation of humeral head in presence of rotator cuff disease.

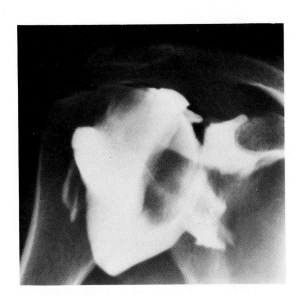

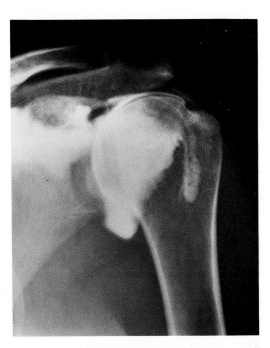

Fig. 12-9. Normal shoulder arthrogram, showing x-ray dye within glenohumeral joint with irregular extensions into axillary recess, subscapularis bursa, and biceps tendon sheath. Note abrupt cutoff of dye at superior edge of humeral articular surface.

Fig. 12-10. Shoulder arthrogram, showing streak of x-ray dye in rotator cuff substance; this finding suggests presence of a partial-thickness tear of rotator cuff.

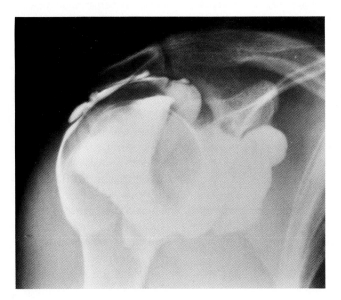

Fig. 12-11. Shoulder arthrogram, showing x-ray dye in both shoulder joint and sub-acromial bursa, an indication of a full-thickness tear of rotator cuff.

amount of dye above a notch that is present on the greater tuberosity, an indication of a partial-thickness tear of the rotator cuff. Visualization of dye in the joint and also in the bursa confirms a full-thickness disruption of the capsule and rotator cuff (Fig. 12-11).

ACUTE TEARS OF ROTATOR CUFF

McLaughlin[22] has convincingly argued that a trial of conservative treatment is indicated when a tear of the rotator cuff is associated with an acute injury. He offered the following reasons for his position:

1. A substantial incidence of ruptures is noted in cadavers, and palpable quiescent ruptures occur frequently in elderly persons.
2. In clinical practice, numerous ruptures heal spontaneously.
3. Ruptures occur through unhealthy tendons. The lesion is long standing when rupture occurs.
4. Early diagnoses may be uncertain.
5. Experience has demonstrated that early repair and later repair have produced similar results.

Other reports of a high frequency of spontaneous recovery from tears of the rotator cuff (Table 12-1) seem to support McLaughlin's views.[22] A secure diagnosis of a full-thickness cuff tear, however, was not forthcoming for any of these described patient groups whose frequency of recovery was better than 50%. Also, the amount of recovery of muscle power was seldom carefully described.

On the other hand, several authors, including Heikel,[16] have suggested the desirability of early repair on the basis of the following factors: acute tears have a worse prognosis than do chronic

tears; with time, tendon edges retract and become frayed; surgical repair yields good or excellent results; and early repair produces better results than late repair.

We studied our patients with an acute injury and a full-thickness tear of the rotator cuff who had operative treatment within 3 months after injury. This group included 43 patients with 43 injured shoulders. Thirty-seven patients were available for follow-up examination; the duration of follow-up averaged 7 years and ranged from $1\frac{1}{4}$ to 21 years. Twelve patients had surgical intervention from 0 to 3 weeks after injury, 6 from 3 to 6 weeks after injury, and 19 from 6 to 12 weeks after injury. The ages of the patients, amount of preoperative active abduction, size of tear of the rotator cuff, methods of operative repair, use of postoperative external support, and type and duration of physiotherapy were comparable for the three groups. Pain relief was satisfactory for all three groups, but patient satisfaction was better for those who underwent repair within 3 weeks after injury ($P = 0.05$). This difference in satisfaction was related to the striking postoperative difference in muscle strength and active abduction. When the repair was done less than 3 weeks after injury, active abduction postoperatively averaged 168 degrees; however, when surgical correction was done from 3 to 6 weeks or from 6 to 12 weeks after injury, active abduction postoperatively averaged only 126 and 129 degrees, respectively. The difference in postoperative active abduction between the first group (who underwent earliest repair) and the other two groups was statistically significant ($P = 0.03$). This study was not designed to determine whether conservative treatment is better than operative repair; however, it does point out that if surgical treatment is necessary, the best result is obtained if the operation is done within 3 weeks after the injury.

These results and other information lead us to make the following recommendations: Very active patients should have early confirmation of the diagnosis of an acute tear of the rotator cuff and should undergo surgical repair as soon as possible. Moderately active patients should be given conservative treatment for 10 to 14 days; if there is no dramatic improvement, arthrography should be done and surgical repair should be considered. If the patient is inactive, an extensive trial of conservative treatment is warranted; operative treatment should be reserved for relief of pain.

Table 12-1. Spontaneous recovery from tears of the rotator cuff

Study	Recovered (%)
Bakalim and Pasila,[2] 1975	88
Brown,[6] 1949	
Mild injury	87
Moderate injury	59
Severe injury	53
Samilson and Binder,[32] 1975	59
Takagishi,[36] 1978	44
Heikel,[16] 1968	23

CHRONIC TEARS OF ROTATOR CUFF

When a tear of the rotator cuff is diagnosed in a patient who has presented with shoulder pain or weakness but does not recall an acute injury and may or may not have had a prolonged history of minor shoulder symptoms, the treatment options depend on the patient's individual requirements for use of his arm and, to a lesser degree, on the extent of the pathologic damage. Many patients can be treated conservatively with analgesics, heat, massage, gentle range-of-motion exercises, muscle strengthening, and occasional subacromial injections of a corticosteroid. These patients are typically elderly and have nuisance pain and variable degrees of weakness. There are prudent arguments for nonoperative treatment. A natural progressive degeneration of all elements of the rotator cuff occurs with aging.[5] Additionally, tears of the rotator cuff have been found at autopsy; presumably, these patients were mildly symptomatic or asymptomatic during life (Table 12-2).

Nevertheless, a few patients with tears of the rotator cuff have severe pain and nocturnal symptoms that prevent sleep. Weakness and loss of active motion may vary from mild to extreme. After a trial of conservative, nonoperative measures, these patients deserve a surgical treatment option. The reported results of surgical repair of chronic tears of the rotator cuff[12,15,16,21,23-25,32,39] justify operative intervention. General results are excellent to good in 70% to 95%. Pain is relieved in 75% to 95%. Abduction motion and strength may be improved, and external rotation strength is usually augmented after surgical treatment.

One notable exception to the above discussion exists. Some elderly patients with minimal or no pain have extreme weakness and active abduction often less than 60 degrees. If diagnostic measures disclose a massive tear in the rotator cuff, operative treatment for the sole purpose of improvement of function is in serious question, as this may not be accomplished by the surgical intervention.

SURGICAL TECHNIQUE

Four potential operative approaches for repair of a torn rotator cuff are (1) anteromedial, with release of the anterior deltoid; (2) anterior, with a T incision of the deltoid and with or without excision of the distal clavicle or anterior acromioplasty; (3) superior, with partial or total acromionectomy; and (4) posterosuperior, with osteotomy of the acromion in the frontal plane. For extensive tears, the anteromedial approach may be best, but this magnitude of injury is unusual. The posterosuperior approach, popularized in Europe, may be used in the treatment of lesions of the greater tuberosity or isolated lesions of the external aspect of the rotator cuff, but the exposure is limited and the more anterior area of chronic impingement and attrition of tendons is not optimally visualized. Lateral acromionectomy or acromioplasty is obviously unnecessary and undesirable. This approach has many inherent actual or potential problems: deltoid detachment and retraction, ectopic bone, abduction weakness, severe instability of the humeral head, and unacceptable cosmesis.

The anterior approach with release of the deltoid from the anterior acromion and distal 2 to 3 cm of the clavicle is adequate for repair of almost all tears of the rotator cuff (Fig. 12-12, *A*). The deltoid is split distally from the acromioclavicular joint for 4 cm, and the fascia lateral to the conjoined tendons of the coracobrachialis and short head of the biceps and inferior to the coracoacromial ligament is incised (Fig. 12-12, *B*). The coracoacromial ligament is excised from its acromial attachment and reflected medially (to be excised later, if necessary); an anterior acromioplasty can be performed and the distal part of the clavicle can be excised, if necessary (Fig. 12-12, *C*), to treat acromioclavicular arthritis or to enlarge the exposure to the supraspinous fossa.

With an acute injury, the tear occasionally may be only a linear split but usually is a transverse avulsion involving the supraspinatus tendon with possible extension anteriorly or posteriorly (Fig. 12-13, *A*). If the avulsion is combined with a longitudinal split, an L-shaped tear is produced (Fig. 12-13, *B*). In contrast to these linear or angular

Table 12-2. Tears of the rotator cuff found at autopsy or during anatomic dissection

Study	Shoulders (number)	Cuff tear (%)
Smith,[33] 1835	40	18
Akerson,[1] 1931	200	32
Keyes,[20] 1933	73	19
Wilson,[41] 1943	—	20
Yamada,[42] 1969	154 (>40 years)	32
	42 (<40 years)	0

Fig. 12-12. A, Exposure through deltoid for repair of tear of rotator cuff. Origin of deltoid is incised along anterior acromion and distal 2 to 3 cm of clavicle, and deltoid is split distally from acromioclavicular joint for 4 cm. **B,** Exposure of subacromial space. Incision is made in fascia lateral to conjoined tendons and inferior to acromioclavicular ligament. Subacromial space is mobilized with a blunt elevator. Acromioclavicular ligament is excised from anterior acromion. **C,** Anterior acromioplasty and excision of distal part of clavicle, *dotted line,* may be done, if necessary. (**A** to **C,** Copyright Mayo Clinic, 1979, Rochester, Minn.)

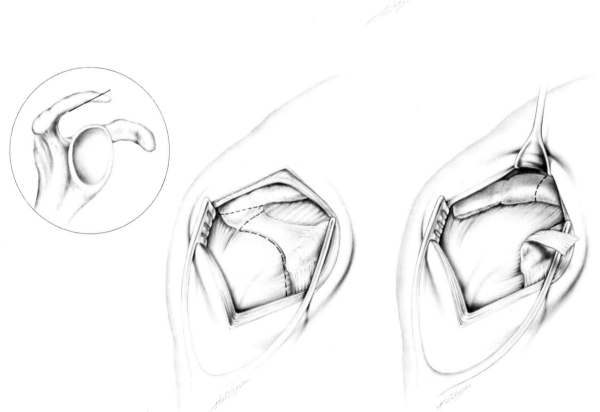

B

C

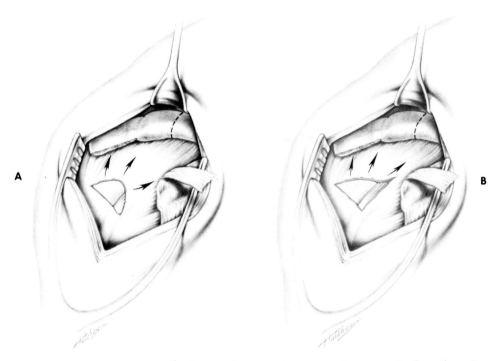

Fig. 12-13. A, Transverse avulsion of supraspinatus tendon near its insertion. **B,** Transverse avulsion of supraspinatus combined with linear split of tendon just posterior to biceps tendon. (**A** and **B,** Copyright Mayo Clinic, 1979, Rochester, Minn.)

Fig. 12-14. *Crosshatch,* Usual site of tendon deficit in chronic tear of supraspinatus. *Vertical markings,* Site of chronic tear of rotator cuff with posterior extension involving infraspinatus. *Horizontal markings,* Site of chronic tear of rotator cuff with anterior extension involving subscapularis. (Copyright Mayo Clinic, 1980, Rochester, Minn.)

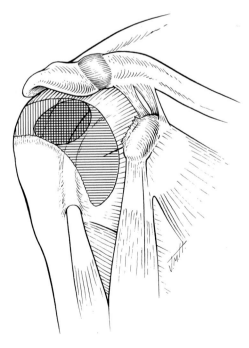

acute tears, chronic tears appear more rounded or oval. The usual area of apparent tendon loss is in the supraspinatus (Fig. 12-14), but it may extend posteriorly into the infraspinatus or anteriorly into the subscapularis. In the last situation, the proximal constraints to the long head of the biceps may be torn and the tendon dislocated anteriorly or medially.

For any tear, the surgical sequence after exposure is as follows: excision of the overlying bursa and degenerated or frayed tendon, careful definition of the tendon defect and trimming of the edges if necessary, assessment of tissue mobility, mobilization of the tendons by manipulation of the shoulder and freeing of the upper and lower surfaces of the tendons from scar tissue and the contracted capsule, and, last, planning for and executing closure of the defect.

Closure of the cuff may be achieved by direct suture of the tendon, suture of tendon to bone, or a combination of these two methods. Often, though, anatomic reconstitution is impossible because of contracted tissue and absolute loss of tendon substance. In this situation, the standard techniques of plastic surgery for dealing with loss of skin form a basis for development of a plan for tendon repair. The alternatives are listed in Table 12-3. If a primary closure is not feasible, the simplest method of repair is *pedicle advancement,* which could be used for a supraspinatus avulsion through an area of degenerated tendon (Fig. 12-15).

More complex tendon ruptures necessitate *triangulation* of the oval defect (Fig. 12-16), with partial side-to-side suture and suture of the unapposed tendon edges to cancellous bone, or side-to-side suture until tension is achieved and then rotation and transposition of tendon tissue (such as the subscapularis) into the defect. Fig. 12-17 illustrates an oval defect in the supraspinatus tendon, which in the acute phase was a transverse avulsion of the tendon attachment with a linear split in the tendon substance proximally just posterior to the long head of the biceps. Partial side-to-side closure was done, and the unapposed tendon edges were sutured to prepared cancellous bone on the humeral head. A patch of coracoacromial ligament was used to reinforce the repaired area and to smooth the repaired surface.

Use of *direct, local flaps* has been minimally beneficial in the repair of a torn rotator cuff. Neviaser[26] and Bush[7] have recommended the ad-

Table 12-3. Surgical alternatives for mobilizing and repairing tears of the rotator cuff

Direct suture of tendon
Suture of tendon to cancellous bone
Pedicle advancement
Rotation flap
Transposition flap
Direct flap
   Biceps tendon
   Trapezius
   Levator scapulae
   Pectoralis minor
   Deltoid
Free graft
   Coracoacromial ligament
   Fascia lata
   Freeze-dried rotator cuff
Neurovascular "island flap"
Free muscle and tendon transplant with microvascular
   anastomoses

junctive use of the biceps. Certainly the tendon can be an efficient constraint to upward migration and instability of the humeral head. Although use of flaps can complement tendon repair and may be incorporated in the closure of the tendon, it is no substitute for mobilization of the rotator cuff and the more standard methods of repair outlined above. Use of the trapezius, the levator scapulae, the pectoralis minor,[31] or the deltoid[35] has been suggested, but anatomic dissection leads one to believe that their use would seldom be practical.

Use of *free grafts* has been attempted. The coracoacromial ligament is an easily obtainable, local free graft and can be used as a patch for a defect as large as 1 by 1.5 cm; however, it will not cover an area larger than this, and it is relatively thin.[16] Fascia lata has been used in multilayered patch grafts or in strips as a mesh or suture for reconstruction of the rotator cuff.[4] In patients with rheumatoid arthritis who have limited demands on the upper extremities, the fascia can be used to strengthen an area that has been severely affected by rheumatoid synovitis with resultant local tissue friability. With careful postoperative protection, upper humeral stability can generally be achieved. Fascial strips can be obtained more easily than fascial patches by use of a stripper and with only a small incision on the lateral side of the thigh just above the knee. These strips can also be used as reinforcement in areas of tendon degen-

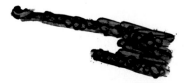

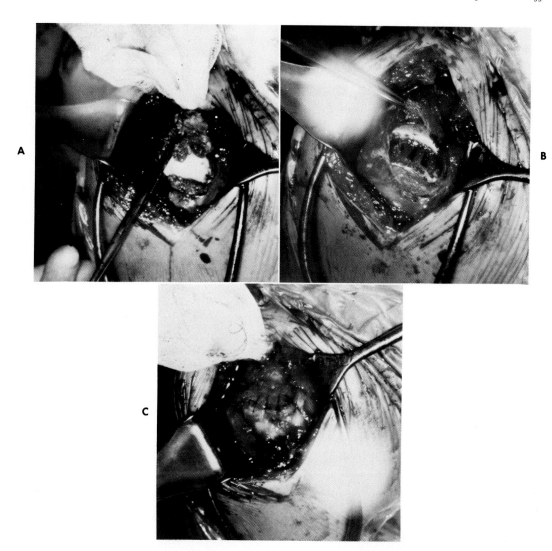

Fig. 12-15. Avulsion of supraspinatus of right shoulder in a 56-year-old man. Three months elapsed before surgical repair. **A,** Appearance of frayed end of avulsed supraspinatus. **B,** Tendon end has been trimmed, anteroposterior edges of tendon have been incised proximally, cancellous bony trough has been made to accept new tendon end, and suture holes have been made in the bone. **C,** Tendon has been advanced laterally and attached to bone with horizontal mattress sutures. A few simple superficial stitches have been placed to make upper surface of repair smooth.

eration. The Neviaser group[27] have suggested the use of freeze-dried rotator cuff for difficult repairs, and their results have been generally satisfactory.

Debeyre and co-workers[12] described an advancement of the supraspinatus based on its neural and vascular supply. This graft is essentially a *neurovascular "island flap,"* which is familiar to hand surgeons. Although they have been successful in repairing almost all rotator cuff defects with this method, improvement in function has not been greater than for more conventional methods. Experimental studies of this type of procedure in animals have shown a substantial loss of muscle power after such a surgical maneuver.[37]

Lastly, the possibility exists for use of *free muscle and tendon transplants with microvascular anastomoses* to replace lost rotator cuff tissue, but to date this alternative has not been considered to be practical.

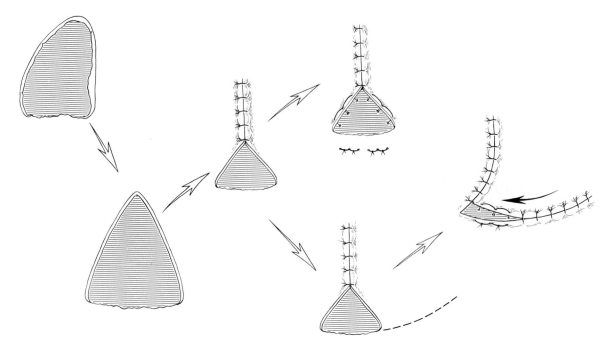

Fig. 12-16. Diagram of oval defect of rotator cuff. Tendon ends are trimmed and made triangular. Defect is partially closed, to point of tension, with side-to-side tendon suture. Unclosed tendon edges are then sutured to cancellous bone of humeral head, or additional tendon tissue is rotated into defect to effect a closure. (Copyright Mayo Clinic, 1980, Rochester, Minn.)

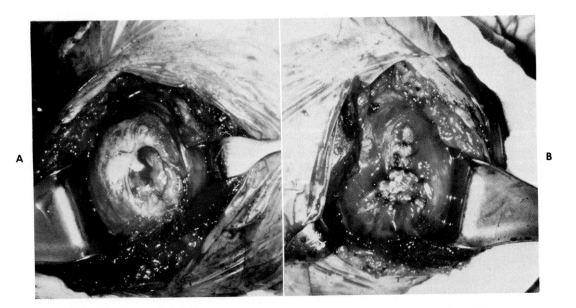

Fig. 12-17. Chronic tear of rotator cuff in area of supraspinatus tendon in a 60-year-old woman. **A,** Initial appearance of tendon tear. Edges were trimmed and partially triangulated, and upper and lower surfaces of rotator cuff in area of tear were freed from scar and contracted capsule. **B,** Tendon defect was closed by partial tendon-to-tendon suture. Remaining unclosed portion of defect was sutured to cancellous bone of humeral head. Irregularity of repair was covered with a coracoacromial ligament patch, both to reinforce and to smooth the cuff repair.

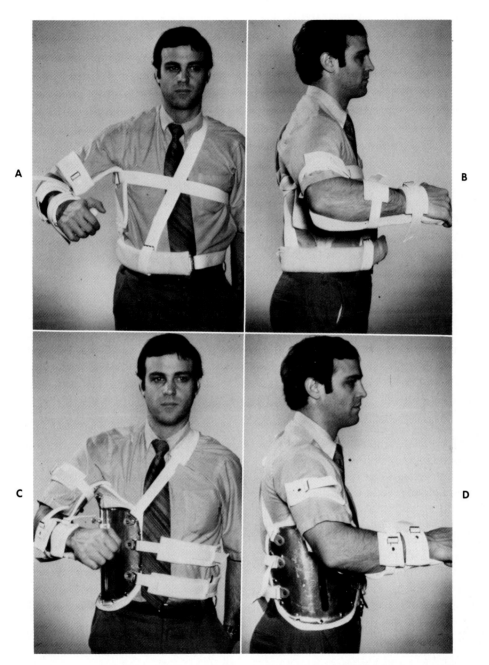

Fig. 12-18. A and **B,** Simple, relatively inexpensive, but nonadjustable humeral abduction splint (Bremer Brease Brace Co., Macon, Ga.). **C** and **D,** More complex humeral abduction splint that will allow varying degrees of abduction and either flexion or extension of arm (Rochester Orthopedic Appliances, Inc., Rochester, Minn.).

POSTOPERATIVE MANAGEMENT

Integrated postoperative management, including variations in the type of external support and the rate of progression of physiotherapy, is not only necessary but crucial to success with rotator cuff repairs. The tendon repair should generally be done with the arm positioned near the side and with the tendons under only slight tension when they are sutured. In some instances, however, the most secure tendon repair can be achieved with the arm slightly abducted and flexed. If the sutured tissues (tendon to tendon or tendon to bone) do not have normal strength because of disease or disuse, more than a sling and swathe or shoulder immobilizer should be used to protect the surgical repair. A humeral abduction splint can provide relaxation to the repaired tissues; it may be a simple abduction splint that protects the abductors and external rotators (Fig. 12-18, *A* and *B*) or a more substantial adjustable splint that will also protect the anterosuperior aspect of the rotator cuff by swiveling the arm attachment into more flexion (Fig. 12-18, *C* and *D*). The splint should be worn for 2 to 8 weeks (an average of 4 weeks), depending on the type and security of the repair.

Occasionally, an extremely difficult repair necessitates even more support. For these patients, a plaster pelvic band and an arm cylinder, with the elbow flexed 90 degrees, can be applied in the operating room. The arm should be positioned to provide maximal relaxation of the repaired tendons; the two plaster units are connected with wooden struts, which are secured with plaster. This type of cast offers the advantages of easy application in the operating room with the patient supine and observation of the operative site. After 7 to 10 days, this somewhat cumbersome support can be exchanged for a lightweight, plastic, single-shoulder, spica cast.

The physical therapy program will also vary according to the extent and security of the surgical repair. When the repair is secure and the extent of the repair of the external rotators is minimal, a shoulder immobilizer is used initially. On postoperative day 1, hand motion exercises are begun, and on days 2, 3, and 4, wrist, forearm, and elbow motion exercises are added. By the fourth or fifth postoperative day, the extremity distal to the shoulder should be supple and free of swelling and the operative discomfort should have diminished so that passive motion exercises within the

limits of the repair could be started for the shoulder. During the second postoperative week, isometric strengthening for the nonsurgically violated muscles is added to the program. Passive and assisted range-of-motion exercises and limited strengthening exercises are continued for 4 to 6 weeks. At that time, active motion with stretching is added, as are strengthening exercises for all muscle groups.

For patients with humeral abduction splints, the program is similar but the arm is not allowed to hang down or to be positioned below the level of the arm support. Patients with casts are limited to hand exercises until the cast is removed.

SUMMARY

Tears of the rotator cuff can be very challenging for the surgeon. He should be aware of the variations in the pathologic lesions that can be encountered and should understand the functions of the cuff-capsule mechanisms so that deficiencies can be appropriately defined and treated. A definite diagnosis, based on the history, physical examination, roentgenography, and arthrography, should be made. In some patients with acute tears of the rotator cuff, early operative treatment is warranted. Chronic cuff disease is often treated conservatively. When operative invervention is justified, the anterior or anterosuperior surgical approach is most useful, and the classic plastic surgery flap techniques provide a model for planning and executing the repair. Postoperative external support and the physical therapy program should be tailored to the complexity and the security of the cuff repair.

REFERENCES

1. Akerson, I.B.: Cited by Codman, E.A.: See reference 9.
2. Bakalim, G., and Pasila, M.: Surgical treatment of rupture of the rotator cuff tendon, Acta Orthop. Scand. **46**:751, 1975.
3. Basmajian, J.V., and Bazant, F.J.: Factors preventing downward dislocation of the adducted shoulder joint: an electromyographic and morphological study, J. Bone Joint Surg. **41**:1182, 1959.
4. Bateman, J.E.: The shoulder and neck, ed. 2, Philadelphia, 1978, W.B. Saunders Co., pp. 280 and 286.
5. Brewer, B.J.: Aging of the rotator cuff, Am. J Sports Med. **7**:102, 1979.
6. Brown, J.T.: Early assessment of supraspinatus tears: procaine infiltration as a guide to treatment, J. Bone Joint Surg. **31**:423, 1949.
7. Bush, L.F.: The torn shoulder capsule, J. Bone Joint Surg. **57**:256, 1975.

8. Chao, E.Y.S.: Personal communication, 1979, Rochester, Minnesota.
9. Codman, E.A.: The shoulder: rupture of the supraspinatus tendon and other lesions in or about the subacromial bursa, Boston, 1934, T. Todd, pp. 65 and 134.
10. Colachis, S.C., Jr., and Strohm, B.R.: Effect of suprascapular and axillary nerve blocks and muscle force in upper extremity, Arch. Phys. Med. Rehabil. **52:**22, 1971.
11. Colachis, S.C., Jr., Strohm, B.R., and Brechner, V.L.: Effects of axillary nerve block on muscle force in the upper extremity, Arch. Phys. Med. Rehabil. **50:**647, 1969.
12. Debeyre, J., Patte, D., and Elmelik, E.: Repair of ruptures of the rotator cuff of the shoulder: with a note on advancement of the supraspinatus muscle, J. Bone Joint Surg. **47:**36, 1965.
13. DePalma, A.F., Cooke, A.J., and Prabhakar, M.: The role of the subscapularis in recurrent anterior dislocations of the shoulder, Clin. Orthop. **54:**35, 1967.
14. Fick, R.: Handbuch der Anatomie und Mechanik der Gelenke unter Berücksichtigung der bewegenden Muskeln. In von Bardeleben, K., editor: Handbuch der Anatomie des Menschen, Jena, 1911, Gustav Fischer, vol. 2, p. 280.
15. Godsil, R.D., Jr., and Linscheid, R.L.: Intratendinous defects of the rotator cuff, Clin. Orthop. **69:**181, 1970.
16. Heikel, H.V.A.: Rupture of the rotator cuff of the shoulder: experiences of surgical treatment, Acta Orthop. Scand. **39:**477, 1968.
17. Inman, V.T., Saunders, J.B.deC.M., and Abbott, L.C.: Observations on the function of the shoulder joint, J. Bone Joint Surg. **26:**1, 1944.
18. Jens, J.: The role of the subscapularis muscle in recurring dislocation of the shoulder (abstract), J. Bone Joint Surg. **46:**780, 1964.
19. Joessel, D.: Ueber die Recidive der Humerusluxationen, Dtsch. Z. Chir. **13:**167, 1880.
20. Keyes, E.L.: Observations on rupture of the supraspinatus tendon: based upon a study of seventy-three cadavers, Ann. Surg. **97:**849, 1933.
21. McLaughlin, H.L.: Lesions of the musculotendinous cuff of the shoulder. I. The exposure and treatment of tears with retraction, J. Bone Joint Surg. **26:**31, 1944.
22. McLaughlin, H.L.: Repair of major cuff ruptures, Surg. Clin. North Am. **43**(6):1535, 1963.
23. Moseley, H.F.: Ruptures of the rotator cuff, Br. J. Surg. **38:**340, 1951.
24. Neer, C.S., II: Anterior acromioplasty for the chronic impingement syndrome in the shoulder: a preliminary report, J. Bone Joint Surg. **54:**41, 1972.
25. Neviaser, J.S.: Ruptures of the rotator cuff, Clin. Orthop. **3:**92, 1954.
26. Neviaser, J.S.: Ruptures of the rotator cuff of the shoulder: new concepts in the diagnosis and operative treatment of chronic ruptures, Arch. Surg. **102:**483, 1971.
27. Neviaser, J.S., Neviaser, R.J., and Neviaser, T.J.: The repair of chronic massive ruptures of the rotator cuff of the shoulder by use of a freeze-dried rotator cuff, J. Bone Joint Surg. **60:**681, 1978.
28. Reeves, B.: Experiments on the tensile strength of the anterior capsular structures of the shoulder in man, J. Bone Joint Surg. **50:**858, 1968.
29. Rowe, C.R.: Ruptures of the rotator cuff: selection of cases for conservative treatment, Surg. Clin. North Am. **43**(6):1531, 1963.
30. Saha, A.K.: Dynamic stability of the glenohumeral joint, Acta Orthop. Scand. **42:**491, 1971.
31. Saha, A.K.: Mechanics of elevation of glenohumeral joint: its application in rehabilitation of flail shoulder in upper brachial plexus injuries and poliomyelitis and in replacement of the upper humerus by prosthesis, Acta Orthop. Scand. **44:**668, 1973.
32. Samilson, R.L., and Binder, W.F.: Symptomatic full thickness tears of the rotator cuff: an analysis of 292 shoulders in 276 patients, Orthop. Clin North Am. **6**(2):449, 1975.
33. Smith, J.G.: Pathological appearances of seven cases of injury of the shoulder-joints, with remarks, Am. J. Med. Sci. (old series) **16:**219, 1835.
34. Symeonides, P.P.: The significance of the subscapularis muscle in the pathogenesis of recurrent anterior dislocation of the shoulder, J. Bone Joint Surg. **54:**476, 1972.
35. Takagishi, N.: The new operation for the massive rotator cuff rupture, J. Jpn. Orthop. Assoc. **52:**775, 1978.
36. Takagishi, N.: Conservative treatment of the ruptures of the rotator cuff, J. Jpn. Orthop. Assoc. **52:**781, 1978.
37. Terzis, J.K., Sweet, R.C., Dykes, R.W., and Williams, H.B.: Recovery of function in free muscle transplants using microneurovascular anastomoses, J. Hand Surg. **3:**37, 1978.
38. Walker, P.S.: Human joints and their artificial replacements, Springfield, Ill., 1977, Charles C Thomas, Publisher, p. 87.
39. Weiner, D.S., and Macnab, I.: Ruptures of the rotator cuff: follow-up evaluation of operative repairs, Can. J. Surg. **13:**219, 1970.
40. Weiner, D.S., and Macnab, I.: Superior migration of the humeral head: a radiological aid in the diagnosis of tears of the rotator cuff, J. Bone Joint Surg. **52:**524, 1970.
41. Wilson, C.L.: Lesions of the supraspinatus tendon: degeneration, rupture and calcification, Arch. Surg. **46:**307, 1943.
42. Yamada, M.: Cited by Takagishi, N.: See reference 36.

KNEE

Chapter 13

Reconstruction of the difficult arthritic knee

Part A

An articulated knee prosthesis for treatment of severe mechanical knee joint disease

LARRY S. MATTHEWS, M.D.
HERBERT KAUFER, M.D.
Ann Arbor, Michigan

The recent popularization of total joint replacement has encouraged a large group of patients with varying degrees of knee joint arthritis to seek orthopaedic consultation. The majority of these patients believe that the surgeon should perform an operation to relieve their discomfort and to return them to a previous pain-free activity level. The fact that this is rarely possible is generally not immediately recognized by the usual patient. This initially disappointing first encounter with the patient is an opportunity to present a description of the range of disease and treatment, to outline a prognosis, and to recommend a program or approach to maximize lower extremity function for the patient. The patient should come to understand that total knee arthroplasty almost never provides normal painless knee function, and that the service duration of a replacement joint is limited. Although we do not know the service limits for an average result, we do know that there are many failures and revisions before 10 years. Often the thought of failure within this time frame is sobering to the patient who cannot, forewarned, accept the possibility of a sometimes irreversible failure. This patient then becomes more amenable to accepting alternate treatment programs and is more willing to take a reasonable position in the concurrent development of his or her knee disorder and better methods of treatment.

NONOPERATIVE MANAGEMENT

An active, working patient, most frequently with single-compartment arthritis, symptomatic only after a hard day or unusual sports activities, must be treated nonoperatively. Often a program of salicylates, warm water soaks, and moderate activity limitations will eliminate much of the discomfort. We specifically recommend two aspirin tablets every 4 hours around the clock, two warm soaks, and a limitation of activity level. The patient should be warned that although there may be tinnitus and gastric irritation at this dosage level, 12 aspirin per day, there are, however, few complications. The clearest indication of an appropriate activity level is as follows. If an activity causes increased levels of pain during its performance, but if the following day the level of discomfort is back to the usual tolerable levels, then this activity is believed to have been appropriate. If, however, the following day, the pain is still present and more severe than usual for the patient, then the exercise level of the previous day was excessive and should not be repeated. The joint stress relief afforded by the use of a cane has been stressed for the hip. The benefit for the knee is probably as great. At times the patient will not take the cane to public places but will nonetheless benefit from its use on weekends and evenings.

PROXIMAL TIBIAL OSTEOTOMY

For the relatively young patient, usually under 60 years of age and usually with unicompartmental disease, proximal tibial osteotomy has proved beneficial. The patient selection should follow the

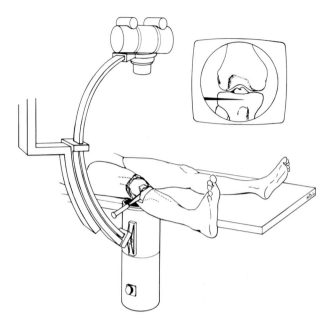

Fig. 13-1. The electronic-memory image intensifier allows direct monitoring of the direction, depth, and angular magnitude of a high tibial osteotomy during the operation.

guidelines of Coventry.[2] Osteoarthritic knees should be selected. Varus deformities of 12 degrees or less treated with laterally based wedge osteotomies are associated with the best results. Preoperative standing anteroposterior roentgenograms demonstrate the maximum angular deformity to be corrected and will sometimes eliminate tibial osteotomy as a treatment of choice for a specific patient. Because of a series of mechanical operative complications[10] often involving fracture into the medial tibial plateau or into the tibial spine region, and because of osteotomy saw cuts entering the joint itself, we now utilize the electronic-memory image intensifier (Fig. 13-1) to guide the production of the osteotomy and its closure. The intensifier is positioned with the receiver tube located at the level of the operating table just lateral to the patient's knee. Repeatedly, the surgeon can check on progress by moving the limb with an osteotome in the osteotomy site to demonstrate the progress, direction, and completeness of the production of the wedge defect. A medial incision is sometimes beneficial for easy completion of the cuts under direct vision. The portable image intensifier is then used to demonstrate complete closure of the osteotomy site and appropriate final angular correction of the deformed limb.

While tibial osteotomy has served some patients very well, the complication rate and the incomplete and unreliable pain relief in some cases has encouraged us to be very cautious in patient selection. Each patient is advised that a total knee arthroplasty may be required in the indefinite future and that this should be considered a delaying procedure.

UNICOMPARTMENTAL ARTHROPLASTY

Results with unicompartmental arthroplasty have been relatively inconsistent, and the operation subjects the patient to nearly the same serious complications as standard resurfacing total knee arthroplasty. Unicompartmental arthroplasties are rarely performed by us at present.

TOTAL KNEE ARTHROPLASTY

Patients, generally over 60 years of age, with multiple-compartment arthritis and whose symptoms cannot be adequately controlled by a conscientiously applied conservative treatment program are candidates for resurfacing total knee arthroplasty. The specific disease cause, whether rheumatoid arthritis or osteoarthritis, is not a limiting factor, with nearly equal results to be expected from resurfacing arthroplasty in both cases. Varus or valgus deformities of up to 20 degrees can usually be managed with the nonlinked resurfacing prostheses. Likewise, fixed flexion contractures of up to 30 degrees can be corrected dependably with resurfacing procedures. Medial and lateral collateral ligament function is essential.

Patients who are potential candidates for total knee arthroplasty should recognize the magnitude of their decision and should be impressed with the honest uncertainty regarding the duration of function that can be expected. It is better not to make arrangements for the surgery after only one consultation. The patient and the family should have the time to freely discuss the merits of the proposed surgery and to formulate questions that could not have been asked at the first meeting. The person who will be responsible for the patient if serious complications occur should optimally take part in the final decision process. Although quantitative descriptive physical and roentgenographic criteria are useful for selection of patients for resurfacing arthroplasty, it is also helpful to consider the patient's perception of his or her functional status. A person who cannot effectively shop for food at a supermarket is severely handicapped in our society. Likewise, difficulty with independent passage to and from home bathroom facilities is a serious incapacity of sufficient degree to warrant consideration of total knee arthroplasty. Pain quantitation and characterization is difficult for the physician and patient alike. It is unique to the patient and often dependent on time and place. Still, when the patient and the family feel that the patient's pain is impairing his or her ability to relate effectively with family members and is interpreted as causing a change in personality, there is a relative indication for definitive treatment.

No patient should undergo total knee arthroplasty who has not been warned of the potential dangers and complications specifically related to the procedure. Wear is inevitable and progressive. Although wear seems primarily related to particulate methyl methacrylate trapped in the polyethylene of the tibial component, often secondary to poor cement technique even with optimal cement technique, the millions of steps per year will lead to wear. Obviously wear will be a more important factor for the relatively young individual. Loosening is also a complication of such frequency and importance that it should be explained to the potential arthroplasty patient and family. During this generally second consultation loosening of the

prosthesis can be likened to the recognized vagaries of prosthetic dentistry. A crown will sometimes remain secure for years but at any time may become loose and displaced. The patient usually appears to understand this comparison and its implications. Finally, although infrequent, infection remains the most dreaded complication of total joint replacement. Despite efforts of air quality control, prophylactic antibiotics, and reduction in operating room traffic and conversation, the incidence of infection remains about 1%. Each preoperative patient must recognize the risk and the magnitude of the discomfort, inconvenience, and danger should a deep infection occur. An infection would certainly mean a long period of serious illness, perhaps septicemia, almost always the removal of the prosthetic components, an indefinite period of wound care, and most frequently the necessity for surgical fusion or permanent usage of a long leg brace.

If the patient's discomfort and disability are of sufficient magnitude, if the patient understands the implications of the surgery, if the general factors are appropriate (age, weight, activity level), if the radiographic films document a sufficient extent of joint destruction, and if the physical examination demonstrates satisfactory collateral ligaments and a competent posterior cruciate-posterior capsule, then resurfacing total keen arthroplasty is recommended.

For the past 5 years we have used the Geopatellar-Geotibial Retainer resurfacing combination for this patient population. This prosthesis (Fig. 13-2) is comparable to the Townley, Total Condylar, and ICLH. It has a patellofemoral flange that can optionally be mated to a patellar polyethylene prosthesis. Unique to this prosthesis is the metal endoskeleton, which provides a metal-cement-bone rather than a polyethylene-cement-bone fixation interface for the tibial component. This same tibial endoskeleton supports the polyethylene perpendicular to the major stresses transferred from the femur and thus minimizes the chances of plastic cold-flow deformation. Finally a ramp element designed for the tibial component bearing surface itself allows for 20 degrees of internal and external rotation of the tibia on the femur while maintaining a congruent bearing surface. This greatly decreases torsional loading on the prosthesis and secondarily on the all-important prosthesis-cement-bone interfaces. These

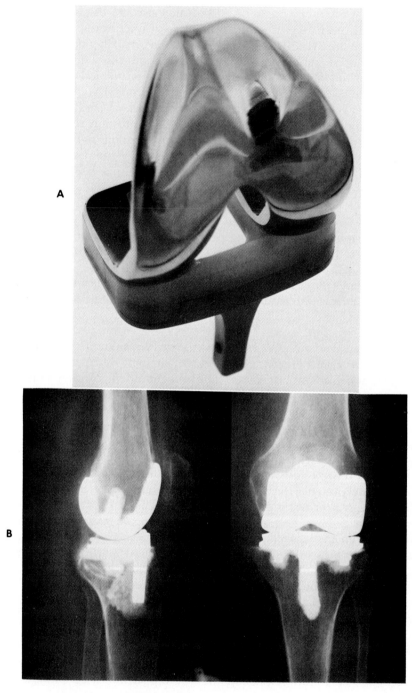

Fig. 13-2. A, The Geopatellar-Geotibial Retainer resurfacing prosthesis with the tibial component metal endoskeleton. **B,** Roentgenograph of implanted Geopatellar-Geotibial Retainer prosthesis.

special design characteristics of the Geotibial Retainer should limit the incidence of tibial-component loosening. Our early experiences with this prosthetic combination have been very satisfactory and will be reported at a later date.

SOFT-TISSUE RELEASE

In cases where the deformity of the knee is considerable, where there is more than 20 degrees of varus or valgus deformity or where there is a flexion contracture in excess of 20 degrees, it becomes increasingly difficult to achieve a normal limb alignment and range of motion by use of resurfacing total knee prostheses. A variety of soft-tissue releases[9] have been described. In expert hands they can extend the usage of resurfacing prostheses beyond these limits. The greater the extent of soft-tissue disruption and the manipulation required, the less certain the outcome is, and in some cases (Fig. 13-3) a satisfactory postoperative result is impossible with a resurfacing procedure.

SURGICAL ARTHRODESIS

If the arthritic destruction is widespread and severe, if conservative care provides inadequate relief of discomfort, and if because of youth, activity level, or work status the patient is not a candidate for resurfacing arthroplasty, surgical arthrodesis can be a wise treatment recommendation. Although functionally limiting, a solid arthrodesis is usually pain free. Unlimited walking and weight-bearing stresses can be tolerated. The outcome is highly predictable and very durable. For the patient with high functional demands this is an excellent choice.

SPHEROCENTRIC ARTHROPLASTY

Severe cases of instability with no or often only one collateral ligament functionally present cannot dependably be treated by resurfacing prosthetic arthroplasty. Some of these cases may have resulted from an inadvertent transection of a collateral ligament at previous surgery, or alternatively, early trauma may have been so severe that ligament reconstruction was not possible. In other situations there has been such bone loss as to grossly disturb the normal kinematics of the knee. In these cases the ligaments, though intact, are so deformed, scarred, or malpositioned that they cannot be developed into normal functional units. If previous prosthetic arthroplasty has failed for any of a variety of reasons primarily involving mechanical failure or loosening, there may be considerable loss of trabecular or cortical bone. In such cases it is extremely difficult to create a suitable foundation for resurfacing arthroplasty.

For the specific indications of extreme deformity, gross instability or failure of a previous prosthesis, Spherocentric (Fig. 13-4) arthroplasty has

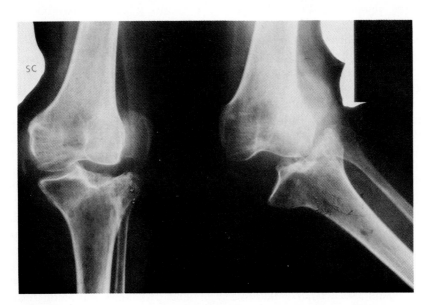

Fig. 13-3. Roentgenograph of a patient with posttraumatic arthritis and complete medial instability.

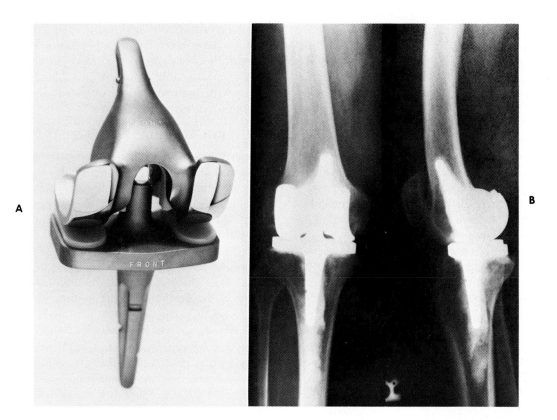

Fig. 13-4. A, The Spherocentric prosthesis. **B,** Roentgenograph of implanted Spherocentric prosthesis.

become a satisfactory alternative to fusion and has proved superior to hinge arthroplasty, the previous approach to this demanding clinical situation.

In 1971 it had become evident that the concepts that Charnley had successfully developed for total hip arthroplasty—low-friction bearings, metal-on-polyethylene bearing surfaces, and methyl methacrylate fixation of components—could be advantageously applied to the knee. Although a variety of resurfacing total knee prostheses proved generally satisfactory in the treatment of moderate degrees of knee joint arthritis, there was no intrinsically stable knee prosthesis that utilized these important principles. Our group at the University of Michigan recognized this need and began the development of a stable knee prosthetic system for the treatment of these patients with severe degrees of knee-joint destruction. The result of this effort, the Spherocentric knee, is based on a contained or trapped ball-in-socket articulation, which provides security against dislocations or subluxations while at the same time allowing triax-

ial rotation. Flexion, extension, internal and external rotation of the tibia on the femur, and varus-valgus flexibility are allowed by the ball and socket and modulated by the tracks and runners to nearly mimic the motions of a normal knee. Hinge prostheses loosened with high frequency[3] partly because their metal extension stops impacted against each other at full knee extension therefore impact loading the supporting bone, and because there was no provision for the tibial rotation. A condylar cam mechanism allows the Spherocentric knee to progressively decelerate at end extension, minimizing the maximum loadings encountered at the prosthesis-cement-bone interfaces. Metal-on-plastic bearing surfaces, an inverted socket to allow for gravity elimination of wear particles, all-plastic components supported by metal, and metal-cement-bone interfaces with the patient seemed beneficial design characteristics for an intrinsically stable total knee prosthesis.

The prosthesis has been tested in the biomechanics laboratory to evaluate its motion, strength, fixation stability and fatigue characteristics. These studies have demonstrated that fresh human specimens incorporating the Spherocentric prosthesis are equal or superior to the normal knee in strength, or in energy absorption to failure, when tested in extension, varus, valgus, or compression. Fatigue evaluations led to design changes that minimzed the chances of fatigue failure under normal usage.

Clinical material. Since 1973 we have performed 134 Spherocentric arthroplasties for 113 patients on the clinical services of the University of Michigan. The patients' average age at operation was 66 years, with a range of 36 to 84 years. Thirty-six were men and 98 were women. Rheumatoid arthritis was the cause in 72, whereas the remaining 62 patients had degenerative arthritis. The specific known causes of degenerative arthritis were trauma, gout, pseudogout, hemochromatosis, and neuropathic arthropathy. Forty-four knees had had previous operations to include 21 prior arthroplasties and three arthrodeses. These patients were elderly, systemically ill, and multiply operated on and had severely damaged knees.

The average follow-up for the entire group is 34 months (with a range of 12 to 66 months). We have been unable to contact four patients. This report thus presents information from 130 arthroplasties in 109 patients. Our indications for surgery remained uncorrectable flexion contracture of 30 degrees or more, varus-valgus instability of greater than 20 degrees, or failure of a previous prosthesis with considerable metaphyseal bone loss. Operations were performed in a standard operating room using standard Simplex cement technique according to the procedure as described previously.[14] Vacuum wound drainage was used for 24 to 48 hours. A soft knee splint was used until the patient was confident of being able to stand and walk with supports. Flexion of the knee was allowed when the wound was securely closed and there was little chance of separation of the wound edges. This usually was at the tenth to the fourteenth day. Patients were examined and roentgenograms obtained at 6-month intervals. Eight of the patients died during the follow-up period.

Results. Fifty-eight patients had a preoperative varus deformity of an average of 25.3 with a standard deviation of ±10 degrees (range 3 to 50 degrees of varus). The average postoperative follow-up position for these patients is 5 degrees of valgus (range 5 to 11 degrees of valgus) representing an average of 23 degrees of correction. Valgus deformity was an indication for Spherocentric arthroplasty in 48 knees with an average preoperative position of 25.5 ±10.3 degrees of valgus (range 12 to 55 degrees of valgus). These knees were corrected an average of 20 degrees for a final postoperative position of 6 degrees of valgus (range 5 to 11 degrees of valgus). Fifty knees with an average 35.6 ±15.1 degrees of flexion contracture (range 20 to 90 degrees of flexion contracture) were corrected to an average 3 ±4.9 degrees of flexion contacture (range 0 to 20 degrees). Instability was the indication for arthroplasty for 61 knees with an average varus-valgus arc of 27.0 ±7.7 degrees (range 20 to 45 degrees). All knees were stabilized by the procedure. At final follow-up six knees demonstrated a detectable varus-valgus arc. All six had definite loosening of the femoral, tibial, or both components. Before surgery the average patient had rest pain with severe pain on extended periods of walking. At follow-up the average patient had no rest pain and little pain after a day's activities. The average preoperative patient could not leave the house alone and could not shop independently. The average postoperative patient uses a cane for outside independent activities. Of the 103 patients reported, 91 used no supports or a cane when walking at the last examination.

Complications A radiolucent line was noted for 37% of the femoral components and 40% of the tibial components. Definite aseptic loosening, a shift in component position with time or stress demonstrated on roentgenograms, was present in 10 knees (7.7%). Two of these patients had definite trauma with fracture of the metaphyseal bone that precipitated the loosening. Five patients with loosening had successful revisional long-stem Spherocentric arthroplasty and had final results equal to the group as a whole. Two had no disabling symptoms. One had been revised to another type of prosthesis and was considered a failure. Two patients were symptomatic but do not presently want revision. Twelve knees with loosening, including two cases of septic loosening, provided a total loosening rate of 9.2%. A reoperation rate for the entire group of 130 arthroplasties was 7.7%. There were three deep knee joint infections (2.2%). Two required removal of the prosthesis, and one was finally treated with amputation. All are considered failures.

One hundred and twenty-six knees with a functional Spherocentric prosthesis in living patients at the last follow-up were symptomatically and functionally better than before surgery (96.9%).

Discussion and summary. A 97% success rate, a 7.7% loosening rate, a 7.7% reoperation rate, and a 2.2% infection rate after a 34 month follow-up on more than 100 cases demonstrates that Spherocentric arthroplasty is superior to other stable knee prosthetic arthroplasties when used for the treatment of patients with severe deformity, gross instability, or failure of previous prostheses.[3,5,8,12-14] Our patients after Spherocentric arthroplasty are comparable both subjectively and objectively to initially less seriously affected patients treated with resurfacing arthroplasty.[1,4,6,7,11]

While the standard Spherocentric prosthesis is appropriate for use in patients described here, there are some patients with yet greater deformity or bone loss, some with severe metaphyseal destruction after removal of the previous prosthesis, and some with tumors or nonunions of metaphyseal fractures, for which long-stem Spherocentric components have been designed and used. In 20 cases performed by the authors these custom components utilizing the basic design characteristics of the Spherocentric prosthesis have provided a functional limb for a yet more severely damaged group of patients.

REFERENCES TO PART A

1. Bargren, J.H., Freeman, M.A.R., Swanson, S.A.V., and Todd, R.C.: ICLH (Freeman & Swanson) arthroplasty in the treatment of arthritic knee. A 2-4 year review, Clin. Orthop. **120:**65-75, 1976.
2. Coventry, M.B.: Osteotomy about the knee for degenerative and rheumatoid arthritis, J. Bone Joint Surg. **55A:**23-47, Jan. 1973.
3. Deburge, A., and GUEPAR: GUEPAR hinge prosthesis. Complications and results with two years of follow-up, Clin. Orthop. **120:**47-53, 1976.
4. Evanski, P.M., Waugh, T.R., Orofino, C.F., and Anzel, S.H.: UCI knee replacement, Clin. Orthop. **120:**33-38, 1976.
5. Freeman, P.A.: Walldius arthroplasty. A review of 80 cases Clin. Orthop. **94:**85-91, 1973.
6. Ilstrup, D.M., Combs, J.J., Jr., Bryan, R.S., Peterson, L.F.A., and Skolnick, M.P.: A statistical evaluation of Polycentric total knee arthroplasties, Clin. Orthop. **120:**18-26, 1976.
7. Ilstrup, D.M., Coventry, M.B., Skolnick, M.P., and Matthew, D.: A statistical evaluation of Geometric total knee arthroplasties, Clin. Orthop. **120:**27-32, 1976.
8. Insall, J.N., Ranawat, C.S., Aglietti, P., and Shine, J.: A comparison of four different total knee replacements. In Proceedings of the American Orthopaedic Association, J. Bone Joint Surg. **56A:**1541, Oct. 1974.
9. Insall, J., Scott, N.W., and Ranawat, C.S.: The Total Condylar knee prosthesis. A report of 220 cases, J. Bone Joint Surg. **61A:**173-180, March 1979.
10. Kaufer, H.: Peaked plateaus. A complication of proximal tibial osteotomy. Presented at the 1975 AAOS meeting in San Francisco, California.
11. Lacey, J.A.: A statistical review of 100 consecutive UCI low friction knee arthroplasties with analysis of results, Clin. Orthop. **132:**163-166, 1978.
12. Murray, D.G., Wilde, A.H., Werner, F., and Foster, D.: Herbert total knee prosthesis. Combined laboratory and clinical assessment, J. Bone Joint Surg. **59A:**1026-1032, Dec. 1977.
13. Phillips, H., and Taylor, J.G.: The Walldius hinge arthroplasty, J. Bone Joint Surg. **57B:**59-62, Feb. 1975.
14. Sonstegard, D.A., Kaufer, H., and Matthews, L.S.: The Spherocentric knee: biomechanical testing and clinical trial, J. Bone Joint Surg. **59A:**602-616, July 1977.

Part B

Treatment of the difficult arthritic knee

DONALD B. KETTELKAMP, M.D., M.S.
Indianapolis, Indiana

As a prelude to a discussion of the treatment for the difficult arthritic knee, a brief presentation of the indications and patient selection for treatment alternatives provides necessary perspective. Different surgeons will have considerable variation in their indications and treament selection. Such variation is to be expected until a sufficiently long follow-up of the varying procedures defines the objective reasons for the selection of each. Until that time, each surgeon must to a degree approach the problem based on his own philosophy.

PRINCIPLES

In the next few paragraphs I will briefly give my indications for selecting the various reconstructive procedures used in degenerative and rheumatoid arthritis of the knee. The selection of these procedures is based upon two principles. The first is to save functional structures whenever possible, particularly ligaments and bone. To date, no replacement will perform the functions of either bone or ligaments as well as the original structures. Therefore I do not believe they should be sacrificed if correction can be obtained without that sacrifice.

The second principle is to select the best procedure based on the status of the knee, the disease process, the occupational needs of the patient, the patient's age, and, to a lesser degree, the patient's size.

This selection process implies that the surgeon must be prepared to perform a variety of reconstructive procedures dependent on these variable factors.

PROCEDURES
Proximal tibial osteotomy

Proximal tibial osteotomy, though not resulting in as high a percentage of initially good results as implant replacement, has the advantage of permitting the patient to return to any activity or occupation that the knee tolerates.[7] An osteotomy is easily revised by either arthrodesis or implant replacement.

For these reasons I believe that proximal tibial osteotomy is the procedure of choice for unicompartmental degenerative arthritis of the knee. It is most useful for varus deformity and for valgus deformity that will not result in more than 10 to 15 degrees of obliquity of the tibial surface.[4] Flexion contracture should be less than 15 degrees with an additional flexion range of 70 degrees or more. The cruciate and collateral ligaments must be intact. Osteotomy is not size dependent, though gross obesity should be corrected before operation if possible. Successful proximal tibial osteotomy will permit the patient to return to moderate and heavy activity. Osteotomy is increasingly applicable the younger the patient is. In patients greater than 65 to 70 years of age, joint replacement may be a workable alternative.

The goals in proximal tibial osteotomy are to correct a varus deformity to 2 to 4 degrees of valgus mechanical angle and a valgus deformity to 0 to 2 degrees of varus mechanical angle.[10] With a successful result, the patient should be able to do the same activity with less discomfort or perform greater activity before pain recurs. One can expect 80% satisfactory results with 3 to 5 years of follow-up and, based on current information, in excess of 60% satisfactory results between 5 and 10 years.[4,6,9]

Unsuccessful osteotomy may occasionally be saved by joint débridement, when the cause of additional symptoms is secondary to intra-articular derangement, or by arthrodesis or implant surgery depending upon the patient's age, needs, and status of other joints.

Arthrodesis

Arthrodesis must be considered as an alternative method of treatment in a relatively young individual with single joint involvement, who must continue with moderately heavy to heavy work. The usual indications are joint destruction with secondary pararthrosis, severe ligamentous instability, infection, failed implants, and neurotrophic joints.[3]

The goal is to obtain a stable painless limb. Arthrodesis is best accomplished with compression techniques using multiple pins. Supplemental bone graft is desirable when not precluded by active infection.

The fusion is 90% or better except for the failed implants and Charcot joints. Multiple operative procedures including bone grafts may be necessary in the latter circumstances.[2]

Knee implants

In the next few paragraphs I will give general indications for the use of nonconstrained, semiconstrained, and constrained implants. Each of these areas are covered in more detail elsewhere in this text. In line with the philosophy expressed in the beginning of this section, I choose a nonconstrained implant, currently either the Anametric or Duopatellar, when there is multiple joint disease involving both knees or knees and hips, usually less than 20 degrees of flexion contracture, and intact collateral and posterior cruciate ligaments. In degenerative arthritis, tibial osteotomy would preferentially be performed for single compartment disease unless bone loss from the tibial plateau contraindicates osteotomy because of the potential for a teeter effect.[9] I prefer to have the patient's weight less than 170 pounds. Preferentially I use the metal-stemmed tibial tray available with the Anametric prosthesis because the laboratory studies indicate that this configuration is less likely to become loose.[14]

My goals for all knee implants are fundamentally the same. I prefer that the patients restrict themselves to light activities and would anticipate minimal symptoms with 80% to 90% good results over a 3- to 5-year period.

Semiconstrained implants

My preferential choice for a semiconstrained implant has been the Variable Axis design.[12,13] Occasionally for some problem cases I will use the Total Condylar implant.[5] My indications for this group of implants are multiple joint disease, either rheumatoid or degenerative; greater than 20- to 30-degree knee flexion contracture; cruciate ligament loss; a deformity so severe that the cruciates must be sacrificed to gain alignment; or severe bone loss, usually of sufficient degree to necessitate sacrifice of the cruciate ligaments. Frequently severe bone loss occurs with a failed nonconstrained or semiconstrained implant.[1] Collateral ligaments must be intact. A more detailed discussion of this group of implants is presented subsequently. In general the goals and results are similar to those for nonconstrained patients.

Constrained implants

To date, my choice of constrained implants has been the Spherocentric knee. This implant is discussed in detail elsewhere by Matthews. My primary reservation with this particular design has been the large volume of bone that must be removed from the distal femur, which would cause increased difficulty with fusion or other salvage should the need arise. As a result, I have had only very limited use of this implant over a rather long period of time. I think the primary indication for constrained implants is severe ligamentous instability with or without concomitant flexion deformity and severe bone loss. The short-term results over 3 to 5 years and the goals are similar to those of other implants.

Treatment of difficult arthritic knee with a Variable Axis prosthesis

During the past 5 years the Variable Axis knee prosthesis, developed by Murray and Shaw, has been very useful for salvage of the difficult arthritic knee.[1,8,12] The designed features of this implant are unconstrained rotation, large-stemmed metal tibial component, which provides good fixation, particularly in cases where bone loss has been present, and constraint against fore-and-aft and side-to-side subluxation.[12] This implant does require intact collateral ligaments.

The primary advantages of this implant are the technical ease of implantation and no loosening to date despite the use in patients with bone loss and of large size. There are however some disadvantages. Patellar subluxation has been a problem for us.[8]

Subluxation of the tibia can occur with more than 90 degrees of flexion unless the prosthesis is inserted with optimum tension on the collateral ligaments in flexion.[8]

Because of the long stems, cement removal for infection is a problem and may require windowing distally and proximally to obtain complete cement removal.[8] This implant does require resection of the posterior cruciate. Our indications for use of this prosthesis have been weight in excess of 170 pounds, instability or deformity that would necessitate sacrifice of the cruciates or in knees where the cruciates are already nonfunctioning, and bone loss, whether primary, secondary to deformity, or scondary to failed previous implants.

From a technical standpoint the use of this implant in patients weighing in excess of 170 pounds presents no problem, nor would it for other types of implants.

Cruciate ligament loss may be secondary to disease with instability, secondary to deformity, particularly flexion deformities of severe degree where the cruciates must be sacrificed to regain extension, and in salvage situations where a previous implant has failed. There are no technical problems associated with the use of this implant when it is used for instability caused by cruciate loss secondary to disease.

Bone loss, with or without cruciate ligament loss secondary to severe varus, valgus, or flexion deformities, or secondary to a failed implant, does present a difficult problem. It is for this indication, bone loss with or without cruciate ligament loss secondary to deformity or for salvage of a failed implant, that we are primarily concerned at this time.

Reconstruction of severe arthritic deformity or failed implant

There are two principles that must be observed in reconstruction of the severe arthritic deformity or failed implant. The first principle is to release all tight structures so that, if possible, alignment can be obtained before bone resection.[5,12] The second principle is to resect minimal bone. The next few paragraphs will illustrate and elucidate these two principles.

Release of tight structures. In a varus deformity during the approach, the superficial portion of the medial collateral ligament can be stripped from the proximal tibia extending deep to the pes anserinus if necessary (Fig. 13-5). The deep oportion of the medial collateral ligament is released from its tiabial insertion. When necessary the re-

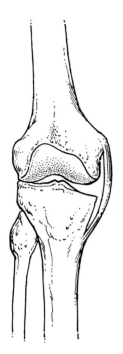

Fig. 13-5. Soft-tissue release for a varus deformity consists of subperiosteal elevation of the superficial portion of the medial collateral ligament and release of the deep medial collateral ligament and capsule. Release may be extended around the posterior medial corner if necessary.

lease can be carried around the posterior medial corner. Usually approximation of the anterior periosteum to the periosteum in the area of the tibial tubercle and the distal patellar tendon is all the repair that is necessary. If more fixation is required, the superficial portion of the medial collateral ligament can be stapled to the tibia. I have found the correction of a varus deformity considerably less difficult than the correction of a valgus deformity.

In a valgus deformity, the first of the tight structures that requires release is the iliotibial band (Fig. 13-6). There are two primary methods of doing this. Insall and co-workers[5] have described a section of the iliotibial band at or just proximal to the lateral femoral condyle from the anterior incision. This approach is also used for release of the lateral retinaculum if the patella is laterally subluxated. This leaves a rather large subcutaneous flap on the lateral side, which may communicate with the knee joint. On occasion hematoma under this flap has created difficulties. Therefore, I have preferred a Yount fasciotomy through a separate incision, thus avoiding wide

lateral dissection. The tibial insertion of the iliotibial band should be preserved because it contributes to lateral stability.

When more relaxation is needed, the lateral collateral ligament and popliteus tendon can be separated from the lateral femur with a piece of underlying bone and permitted to retract. Care must be taken to avoid injury to the superior lateral genicular vessel.[5] Patellar subluxation must be corrected by release of the lateral retinaculum. This can be done from within the knee at the termination of the procedure.

In knees with deformity secondary to the tight type of rheumatoid arthritis, and previously operated knees, the suprapatellar pouch and surrounding synovium are usually scarred, with diminished joint space and motion. When this situation exists, the suprapatellar pouch should be recreated with release of the synovium and scar from the medial and lateral femoral condyles.

Resecting minimal bone. The second principle, that of resecting minimal bone, can usually be accomplished by adequate soft-tissue release to restore alignment of the knee before the initial bone cuts are made. Restoration of passive alignment cannot always be obtained in the particularly difficult knee. An example of the inability to obtain complete realignment with only soft-tissue release is shown in Fig. 13-7. This patient had a severe varus deformity with a large osteophyte on the medial femoral condyle and severe bone loss from the posterior medial portion of the medial plateau. Soft-tissue release alone will not permit correction of alignment with this type of deformity. Relsease of the medial collateral ligament from the proximal tibia was carried out as described earlier. The large medial osteophyte was then resected. This effectively provided additional relaxation for the medial collateral structures. Because of the posterior bone loss on the medial side, the projection anterior rim of the tibia was resected. This permitted access to the femoral condyles when the knee was flexed. The posterior portion of the femoral condyles were then resected. In each case only sufficient bone was removed to permit realignment. Release of the medial collateral ligament, resection of the osteophyte from the medial femoral condyle, resection of the anterior lip of the residual bone from the tibia, and resection of the posterior portion of the medial and lateral femoral condyles permitted realignment of the extremity. At this point the use of the

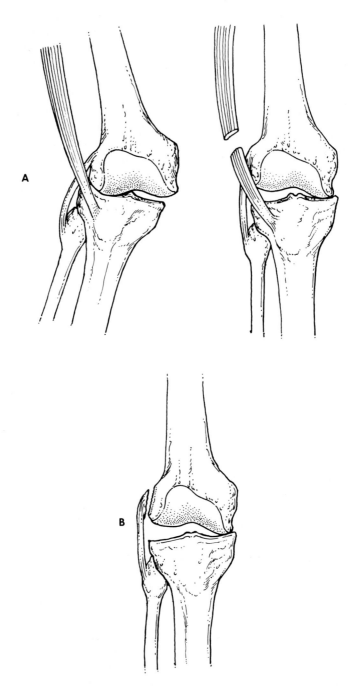

Fig. 13-6. Soft-tissue release to correct a valgus deformity starts with section of the iliotibial band proximal to the lateral femoral condyle. This release may be through the anterior incision as described by Insall and co-workers (1979) or through a separate lateral incision as described by Yount, **A.** The lateral collateral ligament and popliteus tendon may be released with the underlying bone if more correction is required, **B.**

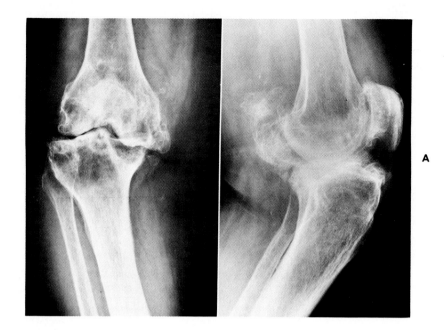

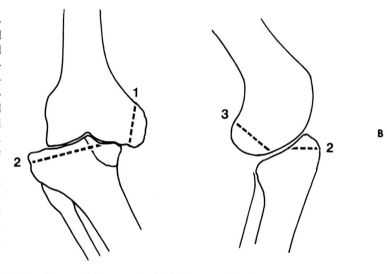

Fig. 13-7. This patient had a severe varus deformity with bone loss from the posteromedial tibial plateau and large osteophytes, **A.** Medial release alone would not allow passive correction. The initial bone cut was to resect the medial femoral osteophyte, which provided additional medial relaxation, **B,** *line 1.* Minimal bone was then removed from the proximal tibia lateral to the defect in the medial plateau, **B,** *line 2.* The knee was then flexed, and the posterior condyles were resected, **B,** *line 3.* Medial release and minimal bone resection permitted reduction of the tibia under the femur with correct alignment. Insertion of a Variable Axis prosthesis was accomplished in the usual manner without further difficulty, **C.**

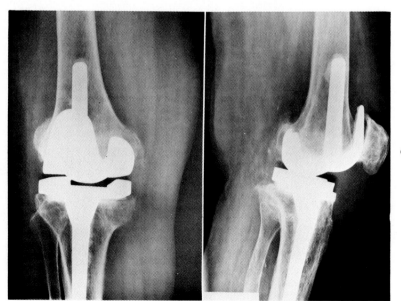

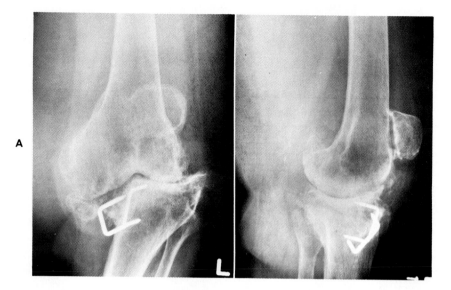

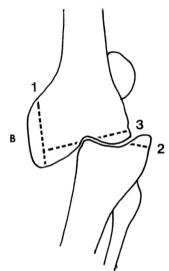

Fig. 13-8. This lady had a problem somewhat similar to that in Fig. 13-7. Aseptic necrosis with collapse and loss of the medial tibial plateau followed a closing wedge osteotomy for degenerative genu valgum, **A.** Varus deformity with lateral subluxation of the tibia resulted. After subperiosteal release of the medial collateral ligament, the large medial osteophyte was resected, **B,** *line 1.* The projecting lateral tibial rim was then removed, **B,** *line 2,* with care being taken to preserve the insertion of the iliotibial band. Resection of a portion of the medial femoral condyle, **B,** *line 3,* permitted placement of the tibia under the femur in satisfactory alignment. A small Variable Axis prosthesis was then inserted without difficulty, **C.** The tibial stem hole was made by the bit being turned back and forth rather than drilling to avoid penetration of the tibial cortex. Despite this the lateral tibial cortex was infracted, but it healed without difficulty.

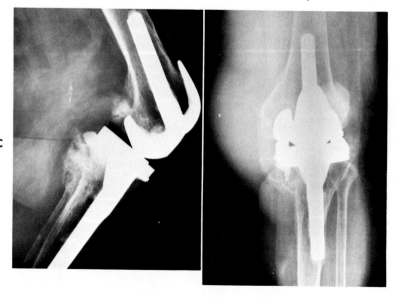

standard jigs and spacer was possible and a Variable Axis knee was implanted without difficulty.

A second patient (Fig. 13-8) had a somewhat similar compound problem. This patient developed degenerative genu valgum, which was treated with a proximal tibial osteotomy. Lateral subluxation of the tibia persisted, however, and the patient's medial tibial plateau underwent aseptic necrosis and collapse resulting in a severe varus deformity with loss of the entire medial tibial plateau. A stress view demonstrated improvement of the varus deformity but did not restore the an-

atomic angle to 0. This was at least partly caused by residual lateral tibia secondary to the initial valgus deformity. In this patient the initial approach was that of elevation of the medial collateral ligament from the tibia followed by resection of the large medial femoral osteophyte as a second releasing procedure. The second bony cut removed the projecting lateral cortical margin from the tibia to permit seating the tibia under the femur. To complete repositioning of the tibia under the femur, a third osseous cut was made along the distal femur. This combination of soft-tissue re-

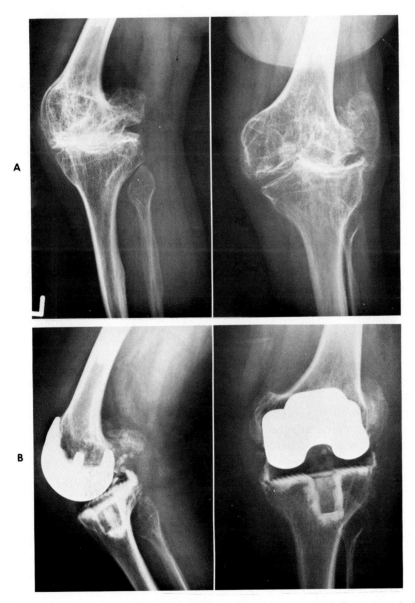

Fig. 13-9. The taper of the anterior tibial cortex in this dwarfed patient precluded the use of the Variable Axis prosthesis, **A.** A custom-made small Total Condylar implant satisfactorily met the needs of this knee, **B.**

lease and resection of minimal bone permitted placement of the tibia under the femur. From this position the necessary jigs and cuts could be made for implantation of a small-sized Variable Axis knee. The patient had a laterally subluxed patella secondary to her original valgus deformity, which required release of the lateral retinaculum.

It is important that the surgeon not be so wedded to a given implant that he attempts to use it when, because of the anatomic or structural deviation, it is not suitable for a given knee. The next case emphasizes this point. This patient was a dwarf, secondary to metaphyseal dysplasia of a recessive type. The small Variable Axis implant might have been suitable as far as knee size was concerned. However, the lateral roentgenogram (Fig. 13-9) shows that the anterior cortex of the tibia deviates posteriorly such that it would be impossible to implant a Variable Axis knee with the standard stem position. For this reason a very small custom-made Total Condylar implant was used. This implant met the requirements for this patient.

Bone loss and secondary scarring. So far I have dealt primarily with the problems of bone loss secondary to deformity. The second circumstance in which bone loss is a primary problem is the salvage of a previously failed prostesis. In this situation the surgeon is faced with bone loss, often of a significant degree, and scarring secondary to the initial surgery. In addition to other necessary soft-tissue releases, the development of a suprapatellar pouch and release of scarring from about the femoral condyles is mandatory as part of the exposure.

Fifteen to twenty years ago the Massachusetts General Hospital femoral prosthesis was in some vogue. When this prosthesis was used, one could resect sufficient bone to overcome severe flexion deformities by leaving the femoral attachment of the medial and lateral collateral ligaments with an osteoperiosteal flap attached to the proximal femur (Fig. 13-10). This is an important point to be remembered and is illustrated by the next patient.

This patient had rheumatoid arthritis with varus deformity that had been treated by a Geometric prosthesis about a year and a half earlier. His new implant performed very well for about a year and four months. At that time he noted increased pain, increasing instability, and increasing varus deformity. The appearance of the knee is shown in Fig. 13-11. The anteroposterior view shows not

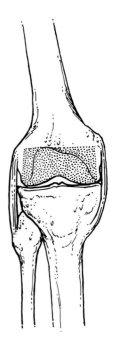

Fig. 13-10. Severe flexion deformity or salvage of a failed implant may require resection of femoral bone proximal to the attachments of the collateral ligaments. Collateral stability can be retained if the collateral ligaments are left attached to the femur by an osteoperiosteal flap.

only varus deformity, but collapse of the medial tibial plateau with fragmentation. What may not be so well appreciated is that the lateral view shows considerable posterior bone loss with settling of the tibial implant into the cancellous bone. This situation makes exposure of the implant for removal difficult. Resection of a minimal amount of the anterior lip from the central and lateral portion of the tibia provided adequate exposure for removal of the loose implant. Once this had been accomplished, insertion of the Variable Axis knee posed no particular difficulties. In salvaging failed implants there is frequently a problem in using the jigs provided. Most often the marking jigs for the holes for the intramedullary stems will not penetrate the hard residual bone. Resection to good cancellous bone is not possible without sacrificing collateral ligaments. For this reason it is important that the surgeon be well versed in knee anatomy, knee alignment, and the use of this implant so that these holes can be properly positioned based primarily on experience and gross visualization.

A second case further illustrates the problems of salvage of failed implants (Fig. 13-12). This pa-

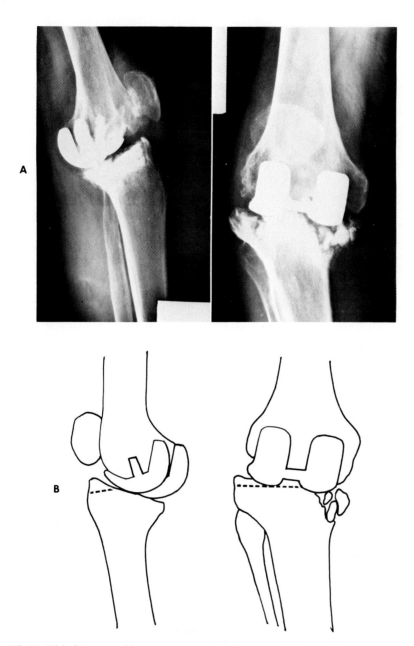

Fig. 13-11. This 71-year-old man presented with a painful bowed leg 2 years after Geometric arthroplasty for rheumatoid arthritis. The knee had functioned well for the first 1½ years before the bowing started. The roentgenograms showed fragmentation of the medial plateau, **A.** The lateral view showed depression of both the tibial and femoral components into the adjacent cancellous bone. Resection of the anterior lip of the tibia, **B,** provided sufficient exposure for removal of the old implant. Resection of the distal femur as shown in Fig. 13-6 was necessary to obtain space for the Variable Axis implant.

Continued.

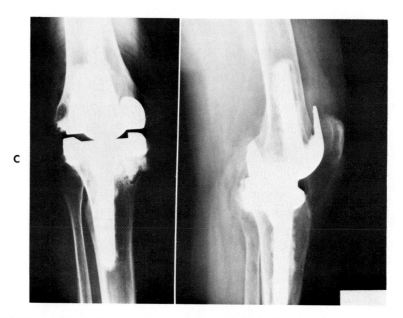

Fig. 13-11, cont'd. C, This implant functioned well until the patient's death 4½ years later.

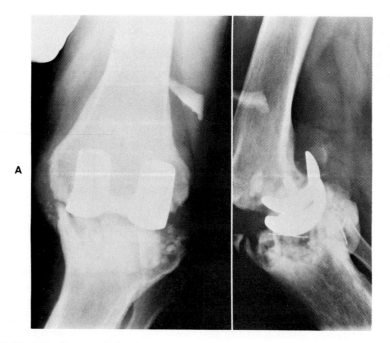

Fig. 13-12. This Geometric implant became loose after 1½ years of hard use by a 230-pound man, **A.** As in the previous case, resection of the anterior lip of the tibia was necessary for implant removal.

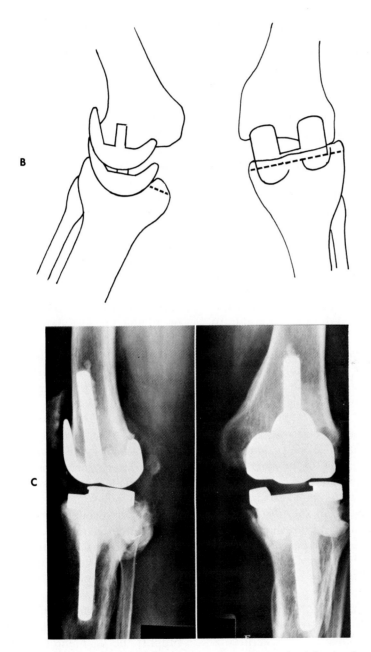

Fig. 13-12, cont'd. B, No additional bone resection was required for implantation of a Variable Axis prosthesis, **C.** The implant is stable 4 years later.

tient had a degenerative varus knee, weighed 230 pounds, and was treated elsewhere with a Geometric prosthesis. One and a half years after he returned to his trucking firm and with recreational activities, which included water-skiing, the implant broke loose. A severe varus deformity resulted with loosening of both the femoral and tibial components, and depression of the tibial component deep into the proximal tibia. The approach, once soft-tissue exposure had been obtained, required resection of the anterior lip of the tibia, with care being taken to avoid resection of no more than would be desirable for implant replacement, for removal of the loose components. Once this was accomplished, the Variable Axis implant could be used without undue difficulty except that all bony landmarks were absent, thus necessitating the use of experience rather than a jig for making the holes for the femoral and tibial stems.

Loosening has not been a problem despite cementing into the defects left by the removed prosthesis. I believe that this is primarily the result of unconstrained rotation and the long tibial stem with the associated firm metal base.

Complications. As might be expected in patients with severe deformity, there have been complications. There was one case of infection with enterococcus that did not respond to débridement and antibiotic treatment and required implant removal and arthrodesis. The primary technical difficulty was cement removal, which required windowing of both the femoral the tivial coritices. Fusion did finally occur but it took more than 1 year.

Posterior subluxation of the tibia with the knee in the flexed position occured in one patient. This patient regained 120 degrees of flexion, which was sufficient, since her collateral ligaments loosened secondary to her rheumatoid arthritis, to permit posterior subluxation of the tibia with irritation of the peroneal nerve. With the Variable Axis implant this problem can be treated relatively easily by removal of the standard-sized polyethylene insert and insertion of a thicker polyethylene tibial component.

Hyperextension subluxation occurred in one patient. This problem was the result of a poor choice of implants. This knee had severe preoperative valgus-hyperextension deformity. The valgus deformity was corrected at the time of surgery with soft-tissue releases, and the implant was inserted without difficulty. Three months postoperatively the patient complained of a loud popping in the knee with walking. She hyperextended when walking, and the popping was caused by posterior subluxation of the ball of the femoral component out of the polyethylene insert with hyperextension. Subsequently this patient was treated for 3 months in a plaster cylinder in a flexed position followed by a polyethylene night splint holding the knee in flexion and a long-leg double upright knee brace with fixed flexion of 10 degrees. The knee currently is asymptomatic but does require the external support.

Patellar subluxation has been a problem. This usually has occurred late and has not been prevented by extensor realignment at surgery. I believe the problem is most likely related to gradual stretching of the medial retinaculum secondary to tibial rotation. Use of a patellar button may decrease this problem.

Stress fractures have occurred in three patients after knee replacement. One lady (Figure 13-7) developed an ipsilateral subcapital femoral neck stress fracture, which was treated with a prosthesis. After total knee replacement of her opposite knee she developed a nondisplaced stress fracture in the subtrochanteric area on that side. A second patient developed stress fractures across the base of all the metatarsals in the contralateral leg a year after revision for a failed Geometric. Two and a half years later she developed a stress fracture of the contralateral distal tibia and fibula. She also has had a problem with subluxation of her patella on the Variable Axis side and eventually stress fractured her patella, which required patellectomy. A third patient who had a Variable Axis to replace a loose Geometric prosthesis fell 6 months after revision and sustained a high transcervical femoral neck fracture, which was treated with a prosthesis. A fourth patient had a comminuted intertrochanteric fracture of the ipsilateral hip 8 months after knee implant, which was treated with a nail plate. To date, all the stress fractures have healed, with the exception of the patellar stress fracture, which was treated by patellectomy.

Collateral ligament instability occurred in two patients. Both were initially treated with braces to support the ligamentous laxity, and both over a period of 2 years discontinued use of their braces as the ligamentous laxity tightened. This was an error in judgment as well as a technical error.

One patient was a very small lady of East Indian origin who had bowed femurs and tibias, probably secondary to rickets, and degenerative genu varum. Insufficient relaxation was obtained at the medial collateral ligament, and as a result, after implant replacement, the knee falls into varus with opening on the lateral side. A year after arthroplasty she had a stroke involving the contralateral side. She was given a brace after surgery. She has since discontinued the brace and is asymptomatic in that knee.

REFERENCES TO PART B

1. Brady, T.A., Ranawat, C., Kettelkamp, D.B., and Rapp, G.F.: Salvage of the failed total knee arthroplasty, Orthop. Trans. J. Bone Joint Surg. **1:**101-102, May 1977.
2. Brodersen, M.P., Fitzgerald, R.H., Jr., Pederson, L.F.A., Coventry, M.B., and Bryan, R.S.: Arthrodesis of the knee following failed total knee arthroplasty, J. Bone Joint Surg. **61A:**181-185, 1979.
3. Charnley, J.: Arthrodesis of the knee, Clin. Orthop. **18:**37-42, 1960.
4. Coventry, M.B.: Osteotomy about the knee for degenerative and rheumatoid arthritis, J. Bone Joint Surg. **55A:**23-48, 1973.
5. Insall, J., Scott, W.N., and Ranawat, C.S.: The Total Condylar knee prosthesis, J. Bone Joint Surg. **61A:**173-180, 1979.
6. Insall, J., Shaji, H., and Mayer, V.: High tibial osteotomy: a five year evaluation, J. Bone Joint Surg. **56A:**1397-1405, 1973.
7. Kettelkamp, D.B.: A review of proximal tibial osteotomy for degenerative arthritis, J. Cont. Ed. Orthop. **7:**11-19, April 1979.
8. Kettelkamp, D.B., Pryor, P., and Brady, T.A.: Selective use of the Variable Axis knee, Orthop. Trans. J. Bone Joint Surg. **3:**301-302, 1979.
9. Kettelkamp, D.B., Wenger, D.R., Chao, E.Y.S., and Thompson, C.: Results of proximal tibial osteotomy: the effects of tibiofemoral angle, stance-phase flexion-extension, and medial plateau force, J. Bone Joint Surg. **58A:**952-960, 1976.
10. Maquet, P.G.J.: Biomechanics of the knee, Heidelberg, 1976, Springer-Verlag.
11. Matthews, L.S., Kaufer, H., and Sonstegard, D.A.: The Spherocentric knee: current developments and experiences, AAOS Symposium on Reconstructive Surgery of the Knee, St. Louis, 1978, The C.V. Mosby Co.
12. Murray, D.G., and Shaw, J.A.: Variable Axis total knee prosthesis: design considerations, testing, and clinical experiences, AAOS Symposium on Reconstructive Surgery of the Knee, St. Louis, 1978, The C.V. Mosby Co.
13. Murray, D.G., and Webster, D.A.: Variable Axis total knee replacement–clinical experience with a 2 year follow-up, Orthop. Trans. J. Bone Joint Surg. **2:**193-194, Nov. 1978.
14. Walker, P.S., Greene, D., Ben-Dov, M., Thatcher, J., and Ewald, F.C.: Fixation of tibial components of knee prostheses, Trans. Orthop. Res. Soc. **4:**95, Feb. 20-22, 1979.

Part C

Place of nonconstrained total knee replacement unit in reconstruction of the difficult arthritic knee

LEE H. RILEY, Jr., M.D.
Baltimore, Maryland

RESULTS OF KNEE RECONSTRUCTION

Physician-related factors. There are several physician-related factors associated with the quality of results obtained after reconstruction of the difficult arthritic knee with a nonconstrained total knee unit (see below):

Physician-related factors associated with quality of results after total knee arthroplasty

1. Selection of proper operation for patient
2. Selection of proper prosthesis for patient
3. Technical skill of surgeon

These factors include the selection of the proper operation for the patient, selection of the proper prosthesis for the conditions imposed by the abnormalities of the arthritic knee, and the skill of the surgeon. Nonconstrained total knee replacement should only be considered when no other surgical procedure can be expected to achieve the goals of a painless, stable, and movable knee. In particular, total knee replacement should never be considered when indications for osteotomy are present. When total knee replacement is indicated, selection of a prosthesis compatible with the pathologic anatomy of the diseased knee is crucial; that is, a nonconstrained prosthesis is often contraindicated by the extent of bone destruction or ligamentous instability. One should never choose an unconstrained knee prosthesis when a more constrained unit or arthrodesis of the knee is indicated.

The quality of results that may be expected after unconstrained total knee arthroplasty, and in particular the longevity of the results to be anticipated, depend on proper insertion of the unconstrained unit. The technical skill of the surgeon in achieving correction of axial malalignment, in centering the extensor mechanism, and in achieving a stable and firm bone acrylic interface are crucial to the achievement of gratifying long-term results.

Patient-related factors. There are also patient-related factors associated with the results to be expected after unconstrained total knee replacement (see below):

Patient-related factors associated with quality of results after total knee arthroplasty
1. Bone loss, ligamentous instability, and fixed deformity of knee
2. Soft-tissue abnormalities around knee
3. Weight of patient
4. Disease necessitating total knee arthroplasty

As a general rule the results to be anticipated are inversely related to the extent to which the anatomic and physiologic conditions of the diseased knee vary from normal preceding the surgical procedure; that is, the more closely the anatomic and physiologic condition of the knee approximates normal before total knee arthroplasty, the better the result that can be anticipated. I have found that the best results after nonconstrained total knee arthroplasty are seen when the procedure is carried out for the patient with rheumatoid arthritis in whom the absence of articular cartilage is the only variation from the normal anatomic and physiologic condition of the knee.[2] The worst results are to be expected when unconstrained total knee arthroplasty is performed for treatment of a Charcot knee with pronounced bone loss and instability. Anticipated results for patients with degenerative arthritis and posttraumatic arthritis fall between those two extremes. As a general rule the patient with rheumatoid arthritis will have multiple joint involvement that will result in the reconstructed joint being used less than one in the patient in whom a reconstructed posttraumatic knee is the only abnormal joint.

It has been my experience that more satisfactory long-term results are achieved in those patients who weigh less than 175 pounds than in those patients who weigh more than 175 pounds. However, no objective data are available at this time to substantiate that subjective impression.

Bone loss and ligamentous instability are factors that may contraindicate the use of a nonconstrained total knee unit. As a general rule, fixed deformity will not contraindicate the use of a nonconstrained unit so long as there is sufficient bone of the femur and tibia upon which to seat the units. Fixed varus or valgus deformities of the knee are corrected by selective soft-tissue releases before the initial osteotomies are carried out and should pose no difficulty when one is performing

the procedure. Fixed varus deformities of the knee are corrected by selective release of the medial capsule and the medial collateral ligament from the tibia until passive correction to the desired axial alignment is possible whereas fixed valgus deformities are corrected by release of the femoral origin of the lateral collateral ligament, and lengthening of the iliotibial band proximal to the joint line until the knee can be corrected to the desired axial alignment before the initial osteotomies are made. I have found that bone loss contraindicates the use of the nonconstrained total knee unit of the Anametric type when there is not sufficient bone in the distal femur or proximal tibia upon which to seat the prosthetic units. Units should be seated on bone and fixed with acrylic bone cement, and acrylic bone cement should not be used to compensate for major bony deficiencies or improperly designed or constructed osteotomies. In particular, it is important to seat the tibial unit on the cortical rim of the proximal tibia if at all possible and to seat the femoral unit on bone of the distal femur, and if that is not possible, a more constrained unit should be chosen. The presence of the medial collateral ligament and the more posterior fibers of the posterior cruciate ligament are necessary for stability of an unconstrained unit of the Anametric type. The nonconstrained design depends on the posterior fibers of the posterior cruciate ligament to provide anteroposterior stability of the tibia under the femur while permitting the greater range of motion inherent in a nonconstrained unit. The femoral unit of the Anametric knee unit has been designed with decreasing radii of curvature of the posterior condyles to permit flexion beyond 90 degrees, with the posterior cruciate ligament guiding the tibia posteriorly as the knee is flexed beyond 90 degrees while providing stability in the anteroposterior plane. If the posterior fibers of the posterior cruciate ligament are absent or if the medial collateral ligament is absent, a more constrained total knee unit should be chosen. The design features of the Anametric total knee unit and the surgical technique for insertion have recently been described.[1]

RESULTS OF UNCONSTRAINED TOTAL KNEE REPLACEMENTS

Between November 1976 and December 1977 I performed unconstrained total knee replacement using the Anametric total knee unit in 20 knees of

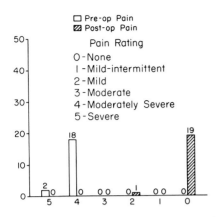

Fig. 13-13. Preoperative and postoperative pain rating of Anametric total knee unit.

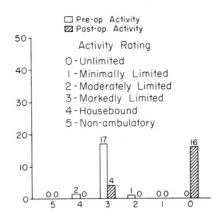

Fig. 13-14. Preoperative and postoperative activity levels of Anametric total knee unit.

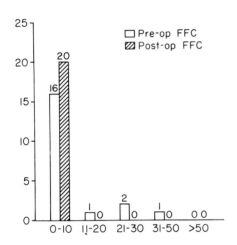

Fig. 13-15. Preoperative and postoperative fixed flexion contracture of Anametric total knee unit.

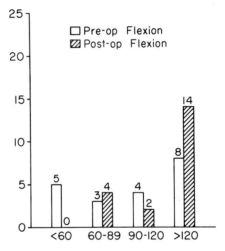

Fig. 13-16. Preoperative and postoperative arc of flexion of Anametric total knee unit.

16 patients. The underlying disease was degenerative joint disease in 2 and rheumatoid arthritis in 18. There were no immediate postoperative complications in this group and only one late complication, a secondary infectious synovitis after a gastrointestinal infection that occurred in a patient with rheumatoid arthritis receiving maintenance prednisone daily. The synovial infection with *Staphylococcus aureus* was diagnosed within 24 hours of onset, and the knee was surgically drained and immobilized until soft-tissue healing had aoccurred. Bactericidal antibiotic levels were maintained for 8 months. At the time of her death from unrelated causes approximately 7

months later there was no evidence of recurrent infection.

Nonconstrained total knee arthroplasty was effective in greatly reducing knee pain in all patients for whom it was done (Fig. 13-13). The activity level increased significantly in this patient group despite the fact that most of the patients had rheumatoid arthritis with multiple joint involvement (Fig. 13-14). Fixed-flexion contractures were corrected at the time of operation (Fig. 13-15), and postoperative flexion was greater than 90 degrees in 16 of the 20 knees (Fig. 13-16). These patients are included in a larger group of patients recently reported.[1]

SUMMARY

Nonconstrained total knee replacement of the Anametric type can be expected to result in a stable, painless, and movable knee for many patients with far advanced arthritic changes within the joint. Patient-related factors associated with good results after unconstrained total knee replacement include the disease necessitating total knee replacement (with the best results being achieved in those patients with rheumatoid arthritis), the patient's weight being less than 175 pounds., and only moderate deviation from the normal anatomic and physiologic condition of the diseased knee before surgical reconstruction. The presence of the medial collateral ligament and the posterior fibers of the posterior cruciate ligament are essential if a nonconstrained unit of the Anametric type is to be chosen.

Physician-related factors associated with an acceptable result after nonconstrained total knee arthroplasty of the Anametric type include selection of the proper operation for the patient: selection of the proper prosthesis for the degree of bone loss, deformity, and instability present: and the skill of the surgeon to insert the knee units properly so as to correct axial malalignment of the leg, center the extensor mechanism across the knee, and produce a stable acrylic resin–bone interface.

REFERENCES TO PART C

1. Finerman, G.A.M., Coventry, M.D., Riley, L.H., Turner, R.H., and Upshaw, J.E.: Anametric total knee arthroplasty, Clin. Orthop. **145:**85-90, 1979.
2. Riley, L.H., and Hungerford, D.S.: Geometric total knee replacement for treatment of the rheumatoid knee, J. Bone Joint Surg. **60A:**523, 1978.

Chapter 14

Total knee replacement

Part A

Stability characteristics of total knee designs

A. SETH GREENWALD, D.Phil.(Oxon)
JAMES D. BLACK, M.Sc.
MARY-BLAIR MATEJCZYK, M.D.
Cleveland, Ohio

Understanding the consequences of mechanical environment on the behavior of normal human joints is of first importance in the development and long-term clinical success of joint-replacement systems. The knee joint, the "middle link" of the lower extremity, holds a particular fascination because of the prevalence of degenerative arthritis in this joint, as such the knee has become a prime candidate for joint-replacement arthroplasty.

The increasing sophistication of total knee replacement design has led to a refined appreciation of the interactions among implant system, mechanical environment, and stabilizing soft-tissue elements.

MECHANICAL ENVIRONMENT

Kinematic features. Several features of knee-joint mechanics are importantly related to rational implant design. Motion of the normal knee is kinematically complex. Through the range of flexion extension, the articular surfaces experience gliding, rocking, and rotation with respect to one another.[7] The sagittal axis of knee motion is not constant, but changes throughout the range of motion because of the changing radius of curvature of the femoral condyles (Fig. 14-1).

Rotation about the longitudinal axis of the tibia, guided by the anatomy of the joint and controlled

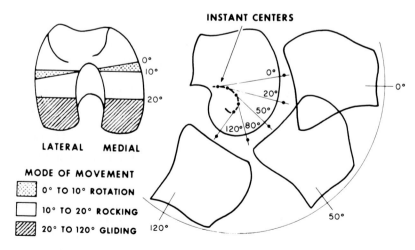

Fig. 14-1. Motion of the normal knee. (From Gunston, F.H.: J. Bone Joint Surg. **53B:**272, 1971.)

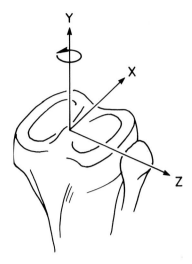

Fig. 14-2. Rotation about the long axis of the knee. (From Greenwald, A.S.: In Savastano, A.A., editor: Total knee replacement, New York, 1980, Appleton-Century-Crofts.)

Table 14-1. Forces across knee during activity.

Activity	Maximum joint force per body weight (average value)
Level walking	3.03
Ramp climbing	3.97
Ramp descending	3.95
Stair climbing	4.25
Stair descending	3.83

Modified from Morrison, J.B.: J. Biomechanics **3:**51, 1970.

by muscles and ligaments, is about 15 degrees during normal walking.[12,13] Appreciation of the influence of rotation has contributed greatly to design improvements of current knee systems (Fig. 14-2).

Knee-joint forces. The forces of functional activity to which knees and their replacements are subjected are of considerable magnitude. During such routine activities as stair climbing, Morrison's estimates of peak load exceed body weight by several times (Table 14-1).[15] Forces of the same order of magnitude are also generated in the patellofemoral joint.

A more recent analysis by Seireg and Arvikar[16] suggests even higher peak joint reaction forces for the knee, including anteroposterior and mediolateral shear components of force equal in magni-

tude to the body weight. It is plain that the mechanical environment of the knee joint is rather severe, a fact that challenges the success of knee-joint replacement arthroplasty (Fig. 14-3).

MECHANICAL FEATURES OF TOTAL KNEE DESIGNS

Mechanical features to be considered in total knee design include functional range of motion in either uniaxial or multiaxial planes, stability, fixation, dimensions, load transfer areas, and materials.

Historically, two extremes of design philosophy are evident. Uniaxial designs, typified by the early hinges, restrict motion to a single flexion-extension axis. In the light of present knowledge of knee kinematics, such designs are inadequate for long-term function because of their excessive constraint. Multiaxial hinged and nonhinged devices permit displacement in multiple directions. Virtually all currently used designs fall into this latter category.

The stability required of a knee replacement is a combination of extrinsic stability, provided by anatomic or bone and soft-tissue support, and intrinsic stability, provided by implant design.

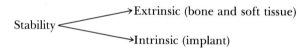

Intrinsic design stability is defined as the capacity of the knee implant system alone to resist displacement in the anteroposterior, mediolateral, and horizontal rotational directions. These displacements represent components of knee motion (Fig. 14-4).

Most current total knee systems rely on condylar bearing surfaces and require functional collateral ligaments. Some designs allow preservation of the cruciate ligaments as well. Stability of the reconstructed knee is achieved by interaction between implant and muscular, capsular, and ligamentous structures. Load sharing results in a balance between intrinsic and extrinsic stability.

Hinged total knee replacements. Hinge type of knee systems are designs in which the components are mechanically linked together, providing great intrinsic stability. The older hinged long-stem designs, such as the GUEPAR, gained a bad reputation because of problems such as the case shown in Fig. 14-5. Gross loosening of this cemented GUEPAR prosthesis is shown on push-pull films.

MECHANICAL FORCES

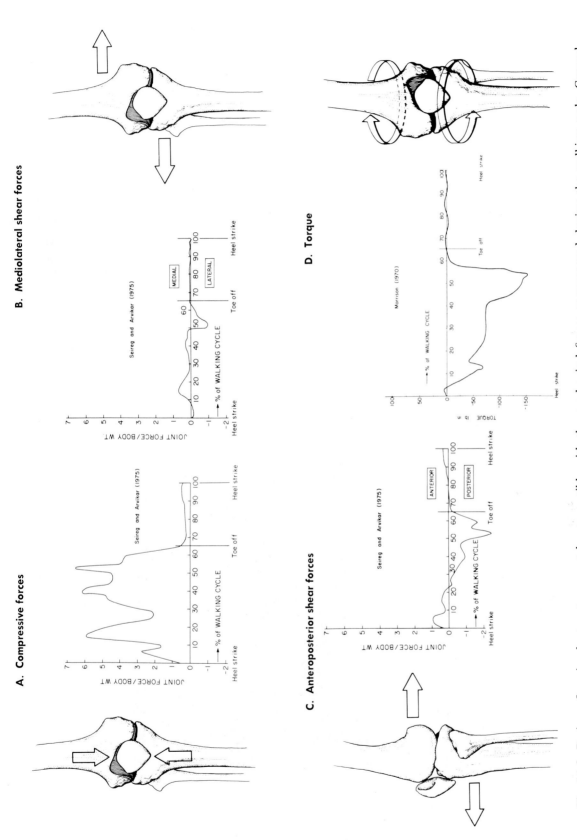

Fig. 14-3. Design of an implant system must be compatible with the mechanical forces encountered during the walking cycle. Ground reaction, gravitational, ligamentous, and muscular forces act to produce significant compressive (**A**), shear (**B** and **C**), and torsional loads (**D**) at the knee. (**A** to **C**, From Seireg, A., and Arvikar, R.J.: J. Biomechanics **8**[2]:89, 1975; **D**, from Morrison, J.B.: J. Biomechanics **3**:51,1970.)

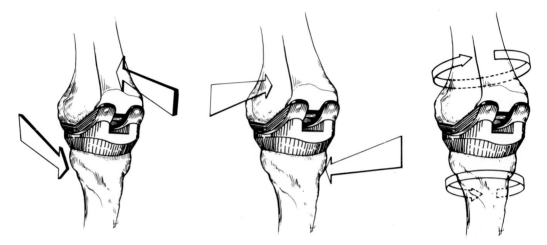

Fig. 14-4. Intrinsic design stability is reflected by the capacity of the implant to resist anteroposterior, mediolateral, and rotational displacements.

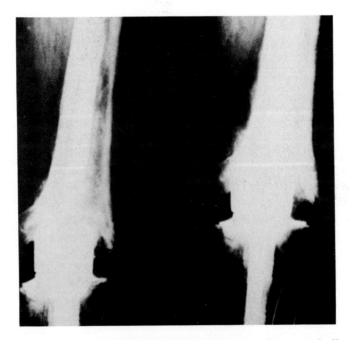

Fig. 14-5. Push-pull films of a cemented GUEPAR knee replacement indicating loosening. (Courtesy Dr. H. Kaufer, Ann Arbor, Mich.; from Greenwald, A.S.: In Savastano, A. A., editor: Total knee replacement, New York, 1980, Appleton-Century-Crofts.)

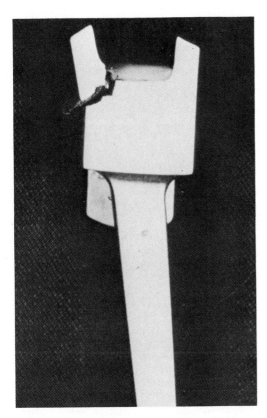

Fig. 14-6. Structural failure of a Herbert knee in an area of localized stress concentration.

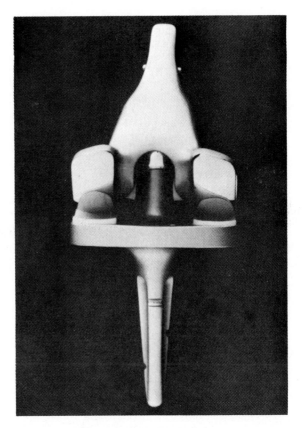

Fig. 14-7. Spherocentric knee.

Uniaxial hinge implants with long rigid intramedullary stems are prone to failure because, regardless of fixation, the degree of constraint generates interface stresses far in excess of the capabilities of interface strength.

The Herbert design allowed some rotation in flexion, but again loosening as well as structural failure occurred because of design constraint in a severe dynamic loading environment (Fig. 14-6).

Nonetheless, there is a clinical need for an implant that provides significant intrinsic stability in patients with severe deformity and uncorrectable laxity.

The Spherocentric (Fig. 14-7) and Attenborough designs represent constraint-relieving modified hinge systems with sufficient intrinsic stability for this clinical situation. Although in some patients the amount of bone resection must be a consideration in their selection when one anticipates salvage fusion. The ideal answer to the problem of gross instability awaits evolving design concepts.

Nonhinged total knee replacements. Nonhinged total knee replacements are resurfacing devices that approach simulation of normal knee motion with varying degrees of constraint. Compared to hinge devices, nonhinged systems are relatively unconstrained, but still exhibit a significant incidence of loosening, as long-term clinical experience is accumulated.

Table 14-2 summarizes early experience with various nonhinged designs. Even at only 2 years, it is apparent that the problem of loosening cannot be ignored. The magnitude of this problem will be even greater for the younger patient with monoarticular osteoarthritis.

Many factors in component loosening have been identified. Proper cement and surgical technique is of basic importance. Failure to correct deformity can place large and uneven stresses on implant-bone interfaces. Inadequate bone support and malalignment of components, as well as excessive patient demand, have similar effects. Obviously, prosthesis design plays a central role in determining successful long-term use of knee replacement arthroplasty.

Knee implant–design geometry is a prime fac-

Table 14-2. Reported incidence of loosening*

Prosthesis†	Series	Component loosening	Percent
Geometric[a]	Coventry et al.	8/33 OA	25
	(Mayo Clinic)	0/42 RA	0
Geometric[b]	Wilde et al.	6/41 OA	15
	(Cleveland Clinic)	2/47 RA	4
Freeman-Swanson[c]	Freeman et al.	8/116	3
	(The London Hospital)		
Modular[d]	Marmor	11/126	9
Polycentric[e]	Gunston	10/89	11
Polycentric[f]	Bryan et al.	12/143 OA	9
	(Mayo Clinic)	5/276 RA	2
UCI[g]	Waugh et al.	6/83	7

*Follow-up greater than 2 years.
†References are as follows: (a) Ilstrup, D.M., et al.: Clin. Orthop. **120**:27, 1976; (b) Greenwald, A.S., et al.: AAOS Slide Sound no. 715, 1978; (c) Bargren, J.H.: Clin. Orthop. **120**:65, 1976; (d) Marmor, L.: Clin. Orthop. **120**:86, 1976; (e) Gunston, F.H., and McKenzie, R.I.: Clin. Orthop. **120**:11, 1976; (f) Ilstrup, D.M.: Clin. Orthop. **120**:18, 1976; (g) Evanski, P.M., et al.: Clin. Orthop. **120**:33, 1976.

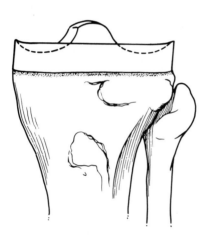

Fig. 14-8. Cup-shaped tibial plateau design.

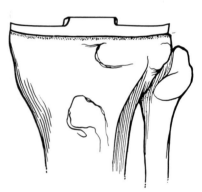

Fig. 14-9. Flat tibial plateau design.

tor in determining the stresses to which implant fixation interfaces are exposed. Designs in which the geometry of components limits rotation and anteroposterior and mediolateral displacement generally have cup-shaped depressions in the tibial plateaus. Higher interface stresses are necessarily experienced during activity because of inherent design constraint (Fig. 14-8).

On the other hand, implants that are not geometrically constrained, such as those in flat tibial plateau designs, offer only frictional constraint. Soft-tissue elements must then serve a greater load-sharing function to provide stability. The optimum design for a specific clinical situation depends on assessment of ligamentous stability and severity of deformity to be corrected (Fig. 14-9).

LABORATORY EVALUATION OF IMPLANT SYSTEMS

To understand the contribution of design geometry to the function of a total knee system, investigators have studied the intrinsic stability of 10 knee designs (Fig. 14-10).

Rotational tests. Implants articulated in 15-degree flexion were loaded in compression to simulate forces occuring during walking. The torque required to produce 5 degrees of rotation in the transverse plane was recorded, providing a measure of the ability of the system to constrain rotation (Fig. 14-11).

Constraint of rotation varies with implant geometry. The less-constrained (low-torque) systems require greater participation of soft tissue–stabilizing structures. The more inherently stable (high-torque) designs transfer greater stresses to fixation interfaces (Fig. 14-12).

Rotation test results for these systems are all lower than the maximum torque generated at the normal knee, as reported by Morrison.[15] Similar tests, previously reported,[3,4,6] showed values above 150 inch-pounds for the old geometric designs. It is interesting to correlate these results with the unacceptably high incidence of loosening reported for the geometric designs (Table 14-2).

It was noted in additional tests that slight intentional malalignment of components resulted in much higher torque values and rapid deformation of tibial components similar to tibial component deformation observed at revision operations for loosening.

Shear tests. Knee systems under compressive loads were tested for anteroposterior and mediolateral stability by application of shear forces in

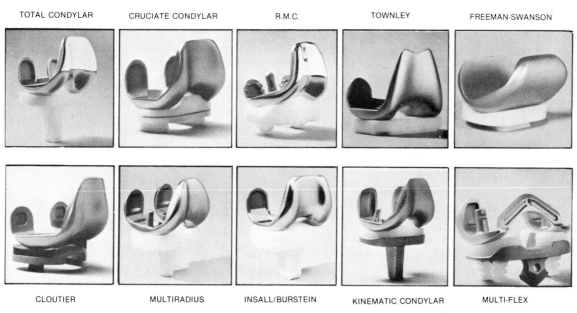

TOTAL CONDYLAR   CRUCIATE CONDYLAR   R.M.C.   TOWNLEY   FREEMAN-SWANSON

CLOUTIER   MULTIRADIUS   INSALL/BURSTEIN   KINEMATIC CONDYLAR   MULTI-FLEX

Fig. 14-10. Varying degrees of intrinsic stability are provided in the spectrum of available designs.

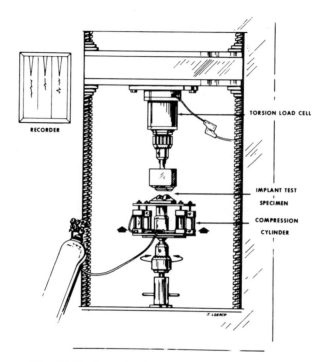

Fig. 14-11. Knee implant rotation test apparatus.

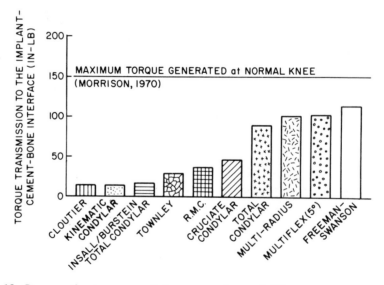

Fig. 14-12. Comparative torques at 5-degree rotation and 575-pound axial load. (From Greenwald, A.S.: In Savastano, A.A., editor: Total knee replacement, New York, 1980, Appleton-Century-Crofts.)

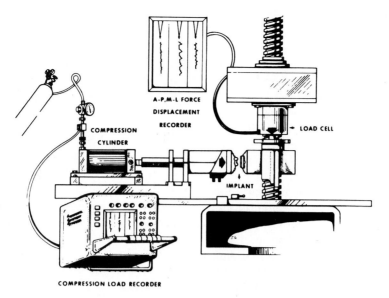

Fig. 14-13. Knee implant anteroposterior and mediolateral test apparatus.

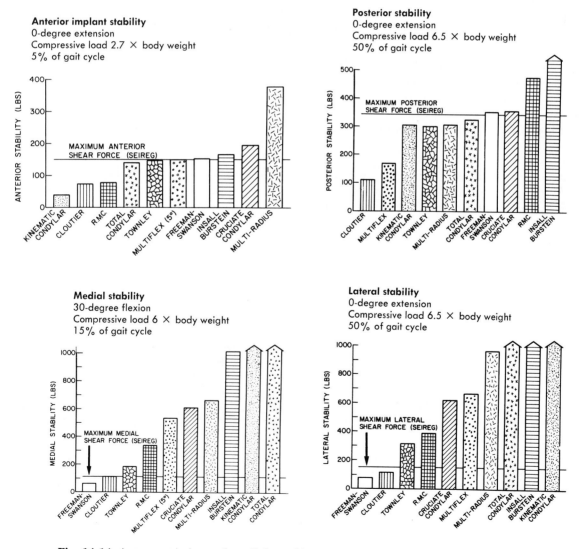

Fig. 14-14. Anteroposterior and mediolateral intrinsic stability of total knee systems for 150-pound person.

these directions. Compressive loads were chosen to represent those points in the gait cycle where maximum shear forces act (Fig. 14-13).

Relative stability of the systems tested varies according to implant geometry and with test direction. The maximum shear forces generated during gait in the normal knee are indicated for comparison (Fig. 14-14).

In general, geometrically stable implants may compensate to some degree for ligamentous insufficiency, but such relatively constrained designs may transfer higher stresses to fixation interfaces. On the other hand, the less-constrained designs require greater soft-tissue involvement in the load-sharing process. Ideally, a balance should be achieved by use of the least constrained design compatible with ligament integrity in a given patient.

ROLE OF CRUCIATE LIGAMENTS

From the description of the interplay between stability and constraint, a concept of ligamentous load-sharing has emerged (Table 14-3). Total knee implant systems, in combination with ligaments and muscles, absorb and control forces generated during function. Sound ligamentous structures matched with geometrically unconstrained implants allow ligament-implant load-sharing and reduce implant cement-bone interface stresses.

Should the cruciate ligaments, if present and competent, be preserved?[11] In normal knee function the anterior and posterior cruciate ligaments act to control backward and forward gliding, respectively, of the tibia and assist the medial collateral ligament in limiting rotation of the femur on

the tibia. The studies by Morrison[15] indicate significant load-sharing roles for both the posterior and anterior cruciate ligaments during daily activities.

CLINICAL CORRELATION

It is evident from the laboratory studies reported that varying degrees of intrinsic stability are offered by the spectrum of available designs. Analysis of clinical failures illustrates some of the considerations of knee implant design and correlates with the laboratory parameters described.

Fig. 14-15 shows a failed medial hemiarthroplasty that was revised to a Total Condylar knee replacement. The intrinsic stability of this system is compromised by incomplete correction of the varus deformity, causing progressive lateral instability.

Progressive radiolucency under the tibial component (Fig. 14-16) may have resulted from uneven stresses generated by the posterior cruciate ligament in the presence of this relatively constrained Cruciate Condylar design (Fig. 14-14). Components designed for cruciate preservation should be relatively unconstrained because forces generated in these ligaments will be transferred to the bone-cement interface if the prosthesis is excessively constrained.

Despite the use of the relatively constrained Total Condylar system designed for cruciate sacrifice (Fig. 14-17), this patient has painful and disabling posterior instability. A thicker tibial component to tighten posterior capsular structures, or a design with greater intrinsic posterior stability, possibly achieved by an anterior lip, might have avoided this situation.

Table 14-3. Cruciate ligaments and load-sharing

Activity	Ligament force (in approximate pounds)			
	Anterior cruciate	Posterior cruciate	Medial collateral	Lateral collateral
Level walking	40	80	20	50
Walking up ramp	15	140	15	160
Walking down ramp	100	60	20	60
Walking up stairs	6	275	10	160
Walking down stairs	20	100	20	80

Modified from Morrison, J.B.: J. Biomechanics **3:**51, 1970.

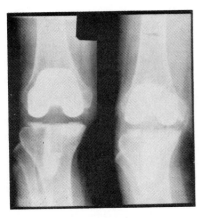

Fig. 14-15. Incomplete correction of varus deformity caused lateral instability in this Total Condylar revision.

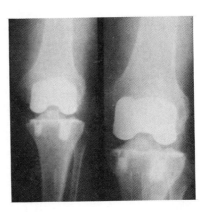

Fig. 14-16. Loosening of relatively constrained Cruciate Condylar implant may have resulted from the presence of a competent posterior cruciate ligament.

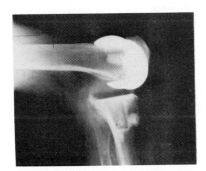

Fig. 14-17. Posterior subluxation of a total condylar system designed for cruciate sacrifice.

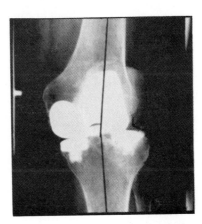

Fig. 14-18. This patient has posterolateral rotatory instability caused by avulsion of the posterior cruciate ligament.

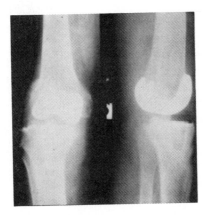

Fig. 14-19. This patient has developed anterolateral rotatory instability presumably because of progressive cruciate insufficiency.

A functional posterior cruciate ligament is essential to the stability of minimally constrained systems such as the Cloutier system shown in Fig. 14-18. After initially successful arthroplasty, this patient sustained a twisting injury resulting in posterolateral rotatory instability. At revision, avulsion of the posterior cruciate ligament from the femur was found.

The gradual development of anterolateral rotatory instability occured after modified total condylar type of arthroplasty with posterior cruciate cutout (Fig. 14-19). In this unusual case, the flat configuration of the tibial component, together with progressive cruciate insufficiency, necessitated revision to a stabilized hinge design.

These clinical problems illustrate the importance of proper interaction between implant design and soft-tissue stabilizing structures. The price of design stability in implant systems is increased interface stress with increased risk of component loosening. These concepts are summarized in the following diagram:

$$\uparrow \text{Stability} = \frac{\uparrow \text{Implant}}{\text{constraint}} = \frac{\uparrow \text{Interface}}{\text{stresses}}$$

$\quad(\downarrow \text{Dependence} \qquad\qquad (\uparrow \text{Risk of loosening})$
$\quad\;\; \text{on extrinsic}$
$\quad\;\; \text{support})$

whereas

$$\downarrow \text{Stability} = \frac{\downarrow \text{Implant}}{\text{constraint}} = \frac{\downarrow \text{Interface}}{\text{stresses}}$$

Obviously then functional cruciate ligaments contribute to the stability of a replacement system that provides for their retention. It may be, however, that the presence of cruciate ligaments places uneven stresses on implant components and may contribute to loosening in certain designs.

SUMMARY

We have considered some features of knee joint mechanics as related to evaluation of knee implant design. Clearly, many factors influence the outcome of knee replacement arthroplasty. These include patient selection, surgical technique, correction of deformity, sound fixation in good bone stock, and patient demand. Appreciation of knee implant design capabilities and critical evaluation of clinical successes and failures will contribute to the evolution of optimum systems.

ACKNOWLEDGMENT

Contributions of clinical material from Clement B. Sledge, M.D., Edward T. Habermann, M.D., and Jean-Marie Cloutier, M.D., are gratefully acknowledged.

REFERENCES TO PART A

1. Bargren, J.H., Freeman, M.A.R., Swanson, S.A.V., and Todd, R.C.: ICLH (Freeman-Swanson) arthroplasty in the treatment of arthritic knee, a 2-4 year review, Clin. Orthop. **120:**65, 1976.
2. Evanski, P.M., Waugh, T.R., Orofino, C.F., and Anzell, S.H.: UCI knee replacement, Clin. Orthop. **120:**33, 1976.
3. Greenwald, A.S., and Matejczyk, M.B.: Knee joint mechanics and implant evaluation. In Savastano, A.A., editor: New York, 1980, Appleton-Century-Crofts.
4. Greenwald, A.S., Matejczyk, M.B., and Black, J.D.: Selection of nonhinged total knee replacements, AAOS 45th Annual Meeting Scientific Exhibit, Dallas, Texas, 1978.
5. Greenwald, A.S., Matejczyk, M.B., and Wilde, A.H.: Properties of methyl methacrylate and high density polyethylene: analysis of failures in total knee replacement, AAOS Slide-Sound no. 715, Chicago, 1978.
6. Greenwald, A.S., Matejczyk, M.B., Black, J.D., and Wilde, A.H.: Rotational characteristics of non-hinged total knee replacements, Transactions of the 29th Annual Conference on Engineering in Medicine and Biology **29:**248, 1976.
7. Gunston, F.H.: Polycentric knee arthroplasty, J. Bone Joint Surg. **53B:**272-277, 1971.
8. Gunston, F.H., and McKenzie, R.I.: Complication of Polycentric knee arthroplasty, Clin. Orthop. **120:**11, 1976.
9. Ilstrup, D.M., Coventry, M.B., and Skolnick, D.: A statistical evaluation of Geometric total knee arthroplasties, Clin. Orthop. **120:**27, 1976.
10. Ilstrup, D.M., Combs, J.J., Jr., Bryan, R.S., Peterson, L.F.A., and Skolnick, M.D.: A statistical evaluation of Polycentric total knee arthroplasties, Clin. Orthop. **120:**18, 1976.
11. Kettelkamp, D.B., and Insall, J.N.: Excision of the cruciate ligaments in total knee replacement (Letters to the editor), Clin. Orthop. **131:**308, 1978.
12. Kettelkamp, D.B., Johnson, R.J., Smidt, G.L., Chao, E.Y.S., and Walker, M.: An electrogoniometric study of the knee motion in the normal gait, J. Bone Joint Surg. **52A:**775-790, 1970.
13. Levins, A.S., Blosser, J.A., and Inman, V.T.: Transverse rotation of the segments of the lower extremity in locomotion, J. Bone Joint Surg. **30A:**859, 1948.
14. Marmor, L.: The modular (Marmor) knee case report with a minimum follow-up of two years, Clin. Orthop. **120:**86, 1976.
15. Morrison, J.B.: The mechanics of the knee joint in relation to normal walking, J. Biomechanics **3:**51-61, 1970.
16. Seireg, A., and Arvikar, R.J.: The prediction of muscular load sharing and joint forces in the lower extremities during walking, J. Biomechanics **8:**89-102, 1975.

Part B

Evaluation of patients for knee arthroplasty

RICHARD S. BRYAN, M.D.
Rochester, Minnesota

The evaluation of a patient for knee surgery of any type is an art, not a science. In sports medicine, there has evolved a series of tests, all with names attached, that is purported to be associated with various instabilities that are suitable for capsular and ligamentous repair. However, considerable disagreement still exists concerning the meaning of these various tests and the efficacy of the various repairs.

In patients who are considered to be candidates for arthroplasty, the pathologic state has passed the point where mild dysfunction during athletic activities must be searched for, and most of the patients have severe pain and gross dysfunction while walking. These terms, however, are purely subjective and must be interpreted by the surgeon. Hippocrates taught us to do no man ill, and premature arthroplasty is surely one of the violations of this teaching.

No one can conceive of a patient with a total knee repair as a football star, a hockey star, a basketball star, or a tennis star—all activities functionally dependent on knee agility. Indeed, our knee replacements at present are barely adequate for walking—that most prosaic and first-learned technique of mobility. Such an achievement is not to be decried because relief of pain alone may immensely improve the quality of life, but one must be sure that the patient's expectations do not exceed the capabilities of the procedure. In this age of instantaneous satisfaction of desires and overselling of the image, this is a real problem. The public often interprets a cautious, rational discussion as inexperience and opts for the surgeon with the golden promises.

PRIMARY CONSIDERATIONS

Pain and loss of function. The problem patient is one who is in the third decade of life, who has always been active in sports activities, and who presents with "severe" pain, which has caused a change in life style. First, the patient really has no means by which to measure his pain because he has not had previous pain. Second, the patient

wants the situation corrected so that he may resume the activities that have caused the pain—and often the pathologic condition. Such a patient probably will not achieve a satisfactory result in his own view. Therefore the two primary indications for knee arthroplasty are pain and loss of function sufficient that the patient might benefit by arthrodesis. Most of the patients fulfill these requirements, and there is no problem in the decision; but in others, even with these qualifications, there may be contraindications. A patient with rheumatoid arthritis who has many joints involved and who is receiving a lot of love and attention in a wheelchair may not wish to give it up by undergoing knee arthroplasty and extensive rehabilitation in order to walk around the house with painful feet.

A low pain threshold may be a contraindication to surgery because rehabilitation of the knee is painful. Similarly, some patients who can tolerate pain cannot tolerate a cast and should not have tibial osteotomy. If in doubt, let them try a cast for 24 hours. After all, if they have never worn a cast, it is a very disconcerting experience, even though intellectually they accept it.

Radiographic and arthroscopic studies that do not sufficiently explain the severity of pain should alert the surgeon to the patient's low pain threshold. This is the single greatest contraindication to arthroplasty in the younger age groups. These patients are treated conservatively by physical medicine and rehabilitation if possible, and I do not hesitate to use steroid injections at intervals of 3 to 4 months and salicylates or other antiarthritic drugs to alleviate their symptoms if necessary. Arthroscopy has been extremely useful in defining the cause of pain in patients with evidence of only mild changes on routine roentgenograms, often revealing areas that are totally denuded of cartilage.

Débridement. In relatively young 40- to 60-year-old patients, there is a place for débridement of the joint and drilling of eburnated areas. Many patients have been without severe pain for 6 to 8 years after débridement, with modification of their activities. Usually, however, this procedure yields at best satisfactory results in 50%; so it is not a substitute for replacement if the proper conditions are present. However, time may be gained, just as synovectomy may sustain the rheumatoid patient, and débridement is far less damaging to the knee than is arthroplasty. Properly done, débridement removes all the osteophytes, drills the eburnated areas, removes any frayed bits of cartilage, and often includes a partial synovectomy. This probably denervates the joint to some extent and, whether by placebo or physiologic action, often improves symptoms for several years, but only 50% of patients achieve any lasting relief. Surprisingly, even in patients with moderately severe degenerative changes, the remnant of a torn meniscus may be responsible for the current symptoms.

CONTRAINDICATIONS

Neurologic disease. Many neurologic diseases produce neurotrophic changes in joints, especially in the lower extremity. Diabetes, amyotrophic lateral sclerosis, Charcot-Marie-Tooth syndrome, and syphilis are examples of these disorders and are contraindications to knee replacement arthroplasty, osteotomy, or débridement. However, undoubtedly many patients have undergone successful operation early before the diagnosis became clear. In these patients, some of the procedures subsequently have failed. I had such a patient who presented with the medial femoral condyle that was severely eroded but who had no hypertrophic bone. He had mild diabetes that was controlled by diet, and neurologically he was normal. A Polycentric knee arthroplasty was done but loosened at 4 months. The loose component was replaced, and the knee failed again; and at 18 months, the Polycentric arthroplasty was revised to a Geometric arthroplasty. This subsequently failed, and 2 years later, it was converted to a Total Condylar replacement, which, with bracing, remained satisfactory 18 months later. During this 6-year course of events, his diabetes remained mild but his ankle and subtalar joints developed the classic Charcot changes, despite his relatively normal neurologic status.

Unconstrained joint replacement with bracing, despite the inevitable deterioration with time, may be justified in the patient who has a stable, mild neurologic condition with joint pain. I have such a patient with amyotrophic lateral sclerosis who has been stable neurologically for 5 years and who had severe knee pain until replacement arthroplasty. Such a patient must be watched for effusion, must limit activities if effusion occurs, and may require bracing for protection.

Life expectancy. A short life expectancy is a contraindication for extensive surgery of any type and especially for surgery in which the primary purpose is improvement of mobility. However, chronologic age may not be an indication of the proximity of death. A careful medical evaluation is a part of every preoperative workup, and the risks and benefits of the procedure must be discussed with the patient and relatives.

Infection. Active infection in the joint is a contraindication to knee arthroplasty, and aspiration and culture in patients in which infection is suspected is helpful. Gallium scanning may be useful, especially in the revisions of knees previously operated on. A history of previous successfully treated infection in the joint is not a contraindication, but this must be differentiated from previous metaphyseal or epiphyseal osteomyelitis, which probably is a contraindication if bony areas affected by the disease will be invaded by the procedure. These patients should have a thorough débridement if arthroplasty is done, and careful selection of multiple cultures during the procedure is helpful in prophylaxis. There is no conclusive data on which to base a program of treatment in acute infection. Therefore, if one is in doubt, the procedure should be staged, with initial débridement followed by definitive care after the results of cultures have been reported. Arthrodesis usually is the procedure of choice in the presence of active infection, but even then, the procedure probably should be staged, with compression applied at a second stage 3 to 5 days after the initial débridement.

OTHER FACTORS

Age. A number of factors affect our ability and our willingness to do total knee replacement. There has been a reluctance to do total replacement in patients who are less than 60 years old and in those who are older than 80 years, but there are exceptions. For example, the juvenile rheumatoid patient may not be able to walk without arthroplasty. These patients are almost certainly going to need revision later, despite the reduced demands they make on their joints, but keeping them active and ambulatory benefits them in many ways and more than justifies the loss in muscle and bone stock incurred with the procedure.

Occupation. Occupation and avocation influence the choice of surgical procedure. Farmers, for example, are hard-working, industrious persons who get rehabilitated quickly after surgery but who are poor long-term risks for total knee arthroplasty because of the demands of their occupation. One could list many other activities that put patients with knee replacement at undue risk, but this knowledge must be tempered with an evaluation of the patient's needs. The patient's body habitus is also important in increasing the risk of failure. Obesity is probably more of a hazard than simply size, but stress is certainly increased in the person who is 198 cm tall and weighs 113 kg. There are no data available in relating weight and build to subsequent results of knee arthroplasty, though data are available for the hip, and these can be applied to the knee.

Bone stock. The term "bone stock" includes the quality and quantity of bone substance present. All of us have seen prostheses sink in the osteopenic tibia of the patient with rheumatoid arthritis and in the elderly. Technically, this affects the ligamentous stability that can be achieved at surgery, and ligaments may be avulsed on occasion when the joint is tightened by the insertion of a prosthesis, particularly if malpositioned. I can recall patients who have bone soft enough so that the tibial plateau can be dented by finger pressure. Surgery in such patients is not contraindicated, but the bone-cement junction must be protected with only partial weight-bearing until the bone is of better quality. No bone should be needlessly sacrificed.

Malunion. Malunion of a previous fracture, resulting in angulation affecting the knee, may be a problem. Correction should be made at the site of the angulation because any adjustment at the knee will result in unequal ligamentous stress or shear stress of the joint because of angulation from the horizontal plane. Similarly, arthrodesis of the hips produces a problem in total knee surgery because rotation must occur through the pelvis. This rotation imparts a rolling torque to the knee region, as well as increased varus-valgus stress.

Basic disease process. The basic disease process may afford either an indication or a contraindication to surgery. Rheumatoid arthritis responds well to total knee arthroplasty and very poorly to any other method of treatment when the articular cartilage is destroyed, though double osteotomy has enjoyed some popularity in Great Britain. Rheumatoid patients should not be operated on during an acute flare, however, because the disease-activity level may affect the rehabilita-

tion after total knee replacement. Steroids do not adversely affect the results of surgery, though healing may be prolonged.

OTHER CONSIDERATIONS

I have already mentioned neurologic disease, but Parkinson's disease and ataxic states and optic lesions such as cataracts, though not contraindications, require special evaluation, as do Paget's disease and hemophilia. Collagen diseases with a large vascular component may make arthroplasty inadvisable because of increased risk. A lack of capacity for immune response may make the risk of infection unacceptably high, as noted by MacLean and co-workers.[4] Dermatologic conditions also may preclude arthroplasty, and stasis problems encourage caution, though they are not absolute contraindications.

The vascular supply to the extremity is important in the consideration of knee arthroplasty. The surgery can be performed easily and without a tourniquet and is safer than osteotomy in the patient with absent pulses. Nonetheless, atherosclerosis is a progressive disease, and surgery should be avoided in many patients.

The most important factor in the final decision is the desire of the patient. It should always be a red flag of warning if a relative does the talking for the patient. The decision must be made by the patient and the surgeon, freely, after a full discussion of the risks and alternatives, and if the patient is not capable of such discussion, the surgeon must be very sure that such surgery is indicated for the patient's benefit and not the relatives'.

Upper tibial valgus osteotomy has a place in the treatment of posttraumatic and osteoarthritic knees. Bowman and Conventry[1,2] have shown that results last for 10 years in 62% of properly selected patients. The problem is to decide which patient will do best with osteotomy, unicompartmental replacement, and bicompartmental replacement. Varus osteotomy in the tibia and in the femur has proved to be not too successful, though we occasionally do varus osteotomy in the femur. I prefer valgus tibial osteotomy in the active, healthy patient with unicompartmental disease who is less than 76 years old and who has some medial cartilage left. The patient with a very loose knee does less well, however. I prefer unicompartmental replacement in patients with osteonecrosis of the femoral condyle, posttraumatic arthritis after plateau fracture, and valgus knees with no more than 15 degrees of deformity and in patients who are more than 76 years old with unicompartmental disease. I also prefer it in the varus knee that is loose if there is no medial cartilage left. The use of unicompartmental replacement has been justified by the results noted in a series of 56 patients with a 4-year follow-up reported by Marmor[5] and by Jones, Peterson, Ilstrup, and myself[3] in 209 patients followed up for 2 to 4 years. Based on my own experience, these patients exceed functionally anything I have achieved with any other type of total knee replacement.

I prefer bicompartmental replacement if the varus or valgus is more than 15° and if there is more than minimal involvement of the weight-bearing area of the good side of the joint.

ILLUSTRATIVE CASES

Here are illustrated with several patients the different choices.

Case 1 (Fig. 14-20)

A 67-year-old man with degenerative joint disease had had left knee pain for 2 years. He had 10 degrees of varus, and his range of motion was 0 to 120 degrees, with crepitus medially. There was mild medial laxity, and the knee shifted laterally during weight-bearing. His pulses were normal, and he used no aids. The knee was suitable for upper tibial valgus osteotomy, and this was done on March 15, 1976. He returned on November 2, 1978, to have his right knee operated on. The left knee still gave him mild discomfort if he walked a mile, and it had a range of motion of 4 to 118 degrees with 6 degrees of valgus. He was satisfied with his result since it permitted him to pursue hunting and the activities that he enjoyed. He continues to do well in 1981.

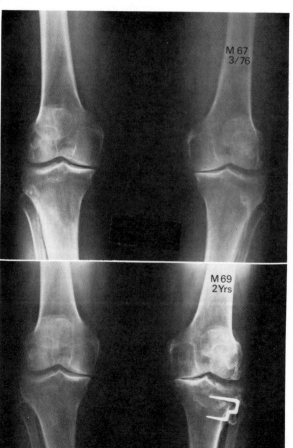

Fig. 14-20. *Case 1.* **A,** Medial narrowing bilaterally and slight lateral shift of tibia with lateral joint widening in left knee of 67-year-old man. **B,** At 2 years postoperatively, further narrowing medially but increased mineralization of lateral tibial trabeculas. The latter indicates that weight-bearing has been moved laterally. A fading of medial subchondral ossification occurs in many but is not seen in this patient.

Case 2 (Fig. 14-21)

A 73-year-old woman with degenerative joint disease had mild hypertension and a history of recurrent urinary tract infections. In 1974, a simple mastectomy was done for intraductal, papillary, grade 2 adenocarcinoma with negative nodes. She presented with painful grating medially in the left knee while walking. Her range of motion was 0 to 130 degrees, and the knee was only mildly loose medially. Her alignment was 0 degrees on a roentgenogram and was 5 degrees varus clinically, but she could walk 1 to 3 blocks without aids. Her pulses were good. She was 167.6 cm tall, and she weighed 77 kg. A valgus upper tibial osteotomy was performed on August 1, 1977. Her postoperative course was complicated by allergy to resin plaster, which necessitated early cast removal. In October 1978, she returned to have the same procedure done on the right knee. She had minimal discomfort in the left knee, despite roentgenographic evidence of a lack of cartilage space. She is well satisfied with the function of her knees at 3 years.

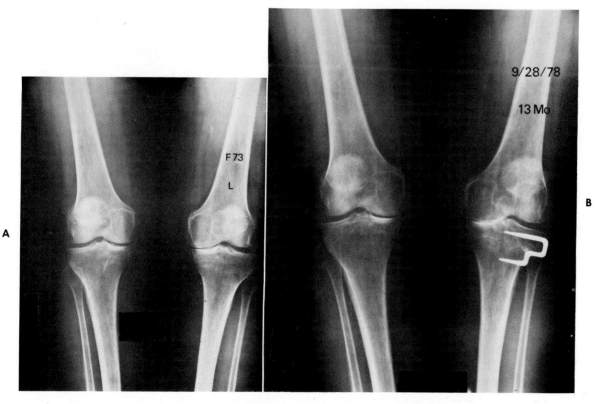

Fig. 14-21. *Case 2.* **A,** Medial narrowing worse on left than on right knee of 73-year-old woman. **B,** Thirteen months after valgus upper tibial osteotomy. Patient has minimal discomfort on left and is seen for pain of right knee.

Case 3 (Fig. 14-22)

A 54-year-old man gave a history of injury to his right knee 5 years before admission, with severe pain for the last year. He had had repeated injections of cortisone, including four during the preceding 3 months. Results of general examination were normal, except for his right knee, which had a moderate effusion. His range of motion was 15 to 95 degrees, and his alignment was a 5-degree varus. Arthroscopy on April 14, 1978, revealed severe chondromalacia of both femoral condyles, with the medial worse than the lateral. On June 30, 1978, arthrotomy with débridement and drilling of the entire weight-bearing area of the medial condyle and one small area of the lateral condyle was combined with valgus upper tibial osteotomy. His knee was placed in a cast brace, which was removed on August 16, 1978. His last visit on July 17, 1979, revealed a range of motion of 5 to 115 degrees, and he was walking with minimal discomfort without aids.

Case 4 (Fig. 14-23)

A 68-year-old woman with degenerative joint disease presented with a history of pain in both knees for 15 to 20 years. She weighed 79.5 kg and was 154 cm tall. Range of motion was 5 to 105 degrees in each knee, and she could walk 1 to 3 blocks using a cane. Her knees were rather loose medially, and this, plus the surgeon's opinion that because of her obesity she would not tolerate the cast and would need a long leg cast to keep it from sliding, resulted in bilateral unicompartmental arthroplasty. Her postoperative course confirmed her low pain threshold, but her result at 1 year revealed a range of motion of 0 to 105 degrees bilaterally without pain. She used no aids and walked an unlimited distance according to her desires.

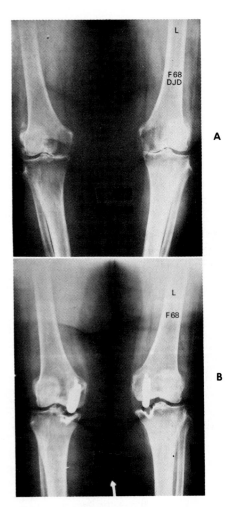

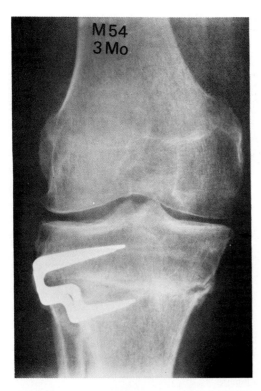

Fig. 14-22. *Case 3.* A 54-year-old man had débridement and osteotomy. *Arrow* points to osteophyte, but just above, on the femoral condyle, there are the patterned drill holes *à la* Pridie. Patient is pain-free at 1 year.

Fig. 14-23. *Case 4.* **A,** A 68-year-old woman with osteoarthritis has bilateral medial knee pain. She is obese and her knees are loose medially. *DJD,* Degenerative joint disease. **B,** Bilateral unicompartmental polycentric arthroplasty has been done, with good alignment of joints.

Case 5 (Fig. 14-24)

A 76-year-old woman with degenerative joint disease of both knees was originally seen in 1971 and was advised to have surgery on her knees. She had a diagnosis of temporal arteritis and polymyalgia rheumatica in 1976 and was treated with steroids, which were finally discontinued in April 1978. She had no signs of arteritis on examination in July 1978. She walked indoors using two canes and had a range of motion of 20 to 125 degrees on the right and 15 to 130 degrees on the left,

with a 5-degree varus bilaterally. Roentgenograms showed cystic changes and osteoporosis. She was 157.5 cm tall and weighed 72 kg. On August 2, 1978, bilateral Polycentric total knee arthroplasty was performed. Both femoral condyles were deficient in articular cartilage. On November 8, 1978, she had a range of motion of 20 to 90 degrees in the right knee and 15 to 105 degrees in the left knee, with 0-degree alignment, and she was walking with one cane and no weight-bearing pain. She continues to do well at 18 months.

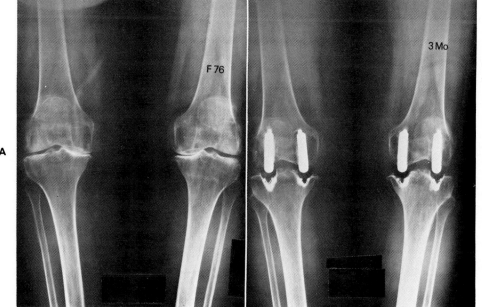

Fig. 14-24. *Case 5.* **A,** A 76-year-old woman with degenerative joint disease has no cartilage left medially in either knee; laterally, there are some changes. **B,** Replacements were done at one operation, and alignment is excellent at 3 months, with good joint separation.

Case 6 (Fig. 14-25)

A 66-year-old man with rheumatoid arthritis had had increasing pain in his left knee for 10 years and in the right knee for 1 year. He could walk only 1 block with a cane and was essentially confined to his house. His range of motion was 40 to 115 degrees on the left, with valgus of 5 degrees, and 25 to 130 degrees on the right, with valgus of 5 degrees. There was mild lateral insta-bility on the left and mild synovitis in both knees. The new Polycentric components were used in the right knee, and Cruciate Condylar components with a patel-lar button were placed in the left knee on July 18, 1979. At 3 months, he had a 0- to 120-degree range of mo-tion in both knees, with no pain in either. At that time, the left knee was a little less stable medially than the right. The knees functioned equally well when exam-ined at 18 months.

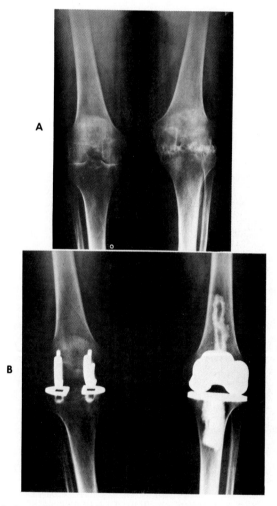

Fig. 14-25. *Case 6.* **A,** A 66-year-old man with severe rheumatoid arthritis. No cartilage remains and bone loss is more severe in the left knee. **B,** Left knee has been replaced with a Cruciate Condylar type and right with a revised type of Polycentric total knee arthroplasty.

Case 7 (Fig. 14-26)

A 52-year-old man with rheumatoid arthritis for 6 years presented in a wheelchair because of knee pain. He was 165 cm tall and weighed 83 kg. His range of motion was 10 to 105 degrees in the right knee and 10 to 110 degrees in the left knee, with a 6-degree valgus in each, but his instability in each knee was moderately severe. He walked indoors using two crutches. On August 4, 1978, bilateral Cruciate Condylar replacements were performed. On November 6, 1978, he had 0 to 105 degrees on the right and 0 to 110 degrees on the left, with 3 and 7 degrees of valgus, respectively. He was walking with no pain and no aids. He continues to do well at this time.

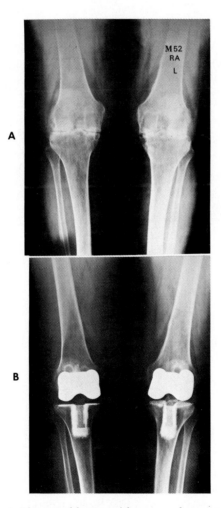

Fig. 14-26. *Case 7.* **A,** A 52-year-old man with severe rheumatoid arthritis. No articular cartilage remains and cystic changes are present. **B,** Cruciate Condylar replacement relieved his pain.

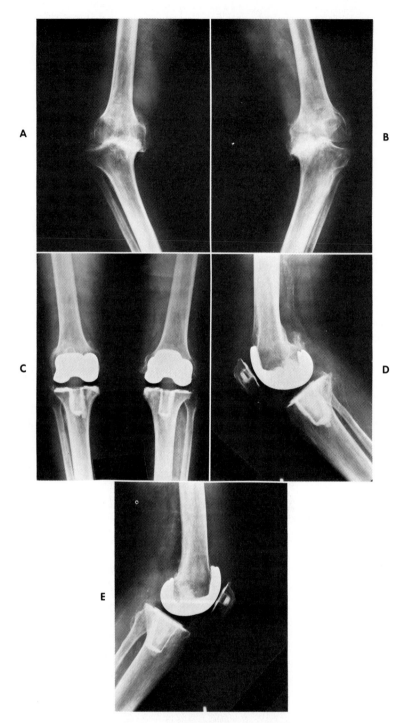

Fig. 14-27. *Case 8.* **A** and **B,** A 74-year-old man with degenerative arthritis and severe varus, with medial bone loss in both knees. These are standing views, which had to be taken on separate films. **C,** Cruciate Condylar replacements have been performed, with good alignment of extremities. **D** and **E,** Lateral views show correct placement of components.

Case 8 (Fig. 14-27)

A 74-year-old man with degenerative arthritis has had painful knees for 15 years and used crutches for 3 years. His range of motion was 7 to 95 degrees on the right and 10 to 100 degrees on the left, with roentgenographic evidence of a 28-degree varus on the right and 27 degrees on the left. There was moderate instability laterally in both and posteriorly on the right. Cruciate Condylar arthroplasties were used 5 weeks apart, without release of any ligaments and with an excellent early result in both.

Case 9 (Fig. 14-28)

A 29-year-old man was seen in October 1975, with a history that he had a twisting injury of his right knee resulting in a lateral meniscectomy in 1961. He did well but had occasional locking until 1964, when he reinjured the knee in baseball and required a right medial meniscectomy. He continued to have problems and was discharged from the U.S. Armed Forces because of pain and effusion in the right knee. His symptoms grew worse, and in May and August 1975 arthrotomy with shaving was performed.

On our initial examination, he complained of severe pain, ambulated with a cane or crutch, and had been out of work since 1975. His quadriceps was weak, and his gait was antalgic. His range of motion was 5 to 95 degrees with moderate effusion. A trial of casting was not helpful; so on February 6, 1976, the knee was explored. Medially, the cartilage surface was good but laterally no cartilage remained on the weight-bearing surface. A unicompartmental widetrack Polycentric arthroplasty was performed. Although he achieved a range of motion of 5 to 115 degrees, he continued to complain of pain. On March 18, 1977, the widetrack arthroplasty was revised to a standard Polycentric because the widetrack was subluxating. The patient now complained of popliteal pain, and on January 6, 1978, a bone spur was excised. When examined in October 1978, he still complained of pain, had a range of motion of 5 to 115 degrees, and had no effusion. He had not worked since 1975. This patient underwent arthrodesis and returned to work but continues to complain of knee "spasms."

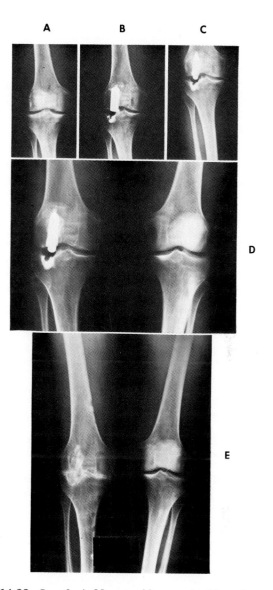

Fig. 14-28. *Case 9.* A 29-year-old man. **A,** After three operations. **B,** After fourth operation. **C,** After fifth operation. **D,** After sixth knee operation, at the age of 32 years, still with pain and scheduled for arthrodesis. **E,** Six months after arthrodesis.

I believe it is obvious that this patient should have been rejected for arthroplasty on the basis of his history. We are often led astray by our belief in our surgical ability to help people and must guard carefully against this enthusiasm. It is a rare patient with this many failed operations who can be helped by further surgery.

These cases illustrate the many factors other than the roentgenographic findings that enter into a decision in regard to the type of arthroplasty performed for the relief of a painful, malfunctioning knee joint.

SUMMARY

The indications for knee arthroplasty are pain and loss of function, but the art of the physician is in the consideration of all the other factors involved in leading the patient to the correct decision for or against surgery.

REFERENCES TO PART B

1. Bowman, P., and Coventry, M.B.: Upper tibial osteotomy: long-term results in the nonrheumatoid varus knee (abstract), J. Bone Joint Surg. **60**:437, 1978.
2. Coventry, M.B.: Upper tibial osteotomy for gonarthrosis: the evolution of the operation in the last eighteen years, and long term results, Orthop. Clin. North Am. **10**:191, 1979.
3. Jones, W.T., Bryan, R.S., Peterson, L.F.A., and Ilstrup, D.: Unicondylar knee arthroplasty, Orthop. Trans. **2**(2):202, 1978.
4. MacLean, L.D., Meakins, J.L., Taguchi, K., Dingman, J.P., Dillon, K.S., and Gordon, J.: Host resistance in sepsis and trauma, Ann. Surg. **182**:207, 1975.
5. Marmor, L.: Marmor modular knee in unicompartmental disease: mimimum four-year follow-up, J. Bone Joint Surg. **61**:347, 1979.

Part C

Technique of total knee replacement

JOHN NEVIL INSALL, M.D.
New York, New York

PRINCIPLES OF SURGICAL TECHNIQUE

Regardless of the type of prosthesis used, there are some common surgical principles that apply to the use of surface replacements of the knee. This type of replacement caps the end of the femur and tibia (though some models may possess intramedullary stems to aid fixation), and the components are not linked together, depending on the soft tissues for stability.

Surface replacement of knees without significant bone loss, deformity, or instability is relatively simple, involving sufficient resection of bone from both femur and tibia to provide room for the components. Earlier models (for example, the Duocondylar) complicated this procedure because the deep or bony surface of the femoral component was curved and required considerable "carpentry" skill to obtain precise placement. Also the tibial component was in two separate pieces (though the bony surface was flat) requiring the use of a jig to control positioning. Most current models do not have this type of configuration and possess a deep surface basically requiring right-angle bone cuts, which is, of course, considerably easier. The tibial component of most is usually of one piece so that a flat cut across the upper tibia can be made. In a knee that is straight and already correctly aligned, component placement is then not too difficult and can be done by eye, though the use of comprehensive instruments is recommended for the utmost precision and reproducibility. Although minor variations in component position may not have any apparent early effect upon the outcome of the arthroplasty, it is evident that malposition (for example, obliquity of the transverse joint axis) will produce uneven loading, which will shorten component life as a result of asymmetric wear. The recommended optimum position will produce a limb aligned in 5 to 10 degrees of valgus with the tibial cut exactly at a right angle to the long axis of the shaft of the bone (and thus parallel to the floor when the patient is standing), with the femoral component placed in 5 to 10 degrees of valgus relative to the long axis of the shaft of the femur when viewed from the anterior aspect, and with 0 to 20 degrees of flexion of the femoral component when viewed from the lateral aspect depending on the particular design of the prosthesis.

When instability, deformity, and contracture are encountered, it is necessary to understand the pathologic processes involved before one attempts correction.

PATHOLOGIC PROCESSES

Instability. In most arthritic knees, instability initially develops because of loss of cartilage and bone; this is more or less symmetric in rheumatoid arthritis and usually asymmetric in osteoarthritic knees. Instability by itself (that is, without any accompanying adaptive changes in the ligaments) can be managed by application of the standard surgical technique and principles. All that is needed to provide a stable arthroplasty is to remove relatively less bone when one is inserting the prosthesis so that the bulk of the prosthetic components themselves (the spacing effect) restores ligament length to normal. Instability that can be corrected by these means is known as "symmetric instability."

However, in advanced arthritis there are nearly always adaptive changes that take place in the ligaments. For example, in the usual varus deformity of osteoarthritis, the medial collateral ligament becomes shortened in part because of osteoarthritic overgrowth on the medial side of the knee and later because of actual contracture of the ligament. (Because its physiologic length is not maintained as a result of loss of medial bone, the process is akin to the contracture of the posterior capsule associated with a long-standing flexion deformity.) The effect of contracture of the medial ligament is a varus deformity that is fixed and cannot be passively corrected.

Additionally, in the same example, adaptive changes occur in the lateral ligament and capsule, which are stretched by the stresses of walking on a knee that is in a fixed varus position. Thus an "asymmetric instability" is now present, the elements of which are asymmetric loss of bone medially, contracture of the medial ligament, and stretching of the lateral ligament. It is obvious that this type of instability cannot be corrected simply by the spacing effect of the prosthesis because the collateral ligaments have become permanently altered, with one being shorter and the other longer than normal.

In valgus deformity there is the reverse occurrence with contracture of the lateral ligamentous capsule and iliotibial band and stretching of the medial collateral ligament. In fixed valgus deformity, particularly in rheumatoid arthritis, there may be, in addition, a fixed external rotation deformity of the tibia presumably caused by contracture of the iliotibial band (a situation analogous to the similar contracture seen in poliomyelitis).

Flexion contractures and instability. There may be in addition to angular deformities and contractures, flexion contracture, flexion instability, and restricted motion of the knee (this last may be thought of as an "extension contracture").

Flexion contracture is not usually very pronounced in osteoarthritis and seldom presents much of a technical problem. It is in rheumatoid arthritis that the more extreme degrees are seen. In patients who have been nonwalkers for years and who have spent most of their time sitting in a wheelchair, fixed flexion contracture of 90 degrees and sometimes more can occur. The contracture is attributable to shortening of the posterior capsule and therefore should be corrected by posterior capsulotomy. Although one can overcome lesser degrees by removing relatively more bone from the femur and tibia, there are disadvantages. The amount of bone that can be removed from the femur is limited by the attachment of the collateral ligaments. Excessive resection of the tibia produces a large gap between the bone ends in flexion, which is likely to produce flexion instability. Excessive bone removal, be it from femur or tibia, results in shortening of the leg and functional lengthening of the quadriceps and extensor mechanism (which may very well be already stretched), so that postoperatively there may be a permanent extension lag.

Flexion instability from primary disease is seen only in rheumatoid arthritis, but it may be caused secondarily during the course of surgery by ligament release or an inaccurate cut on the tibia that removes too much bone (see previously).

In rheumatoid arthritis sometimes more bone is lost from the posterior femoral condyles than from their distal aspect, so that when viewed laterally the lower femur looks like a drumstick or chicken leg. This condition therefore may be suspected from the roentgenographic appearance and may be confirmed at the time of surgery by distraction of the knee in flexion, at which point excessive separation of the joint surfaces will be seen. Paradoxically, flexion instability often coexists with flexion contracture, compounding the technical problem to be solved. Extra thick components are needed to fill the flexion gap and to make the knee stable in flexion, whereas thinner components than usual are required in extension to overcome the flexion contracture.

Flexion instability from excessive tibial resection is a technical mistake and, as such, of course, should not occur. Except in most unusual circumstances, the level of tibial resection is always immediately below the subchondral end plate, and if instruments indicate otherwise, it is usually attributable to improper positioning. The most frequent causes are that (1) the reference hole in the femur has been made in the wrong place (too far posteriorly) and (2) the knee is insufficiently flexed. The surgeon may also choose to make an excessively large tibial resection when there is considerable asymmetric bone loss from the tibia so as to obtain a flat tibial surface. This also is an error not only producing a wide flexion space but also placing the component on relatively weak cancellous bone (the density of cancellous bone decreases with distance from the end plate). Compensation for asymmetric loss of bone should be made with protruding screws, titanium mesh, or best of all an asymmetric tibial component (Fig. 14-41, *B*). The use of metal-enclosed plastic and an intramedullary prosthetic stem may also be helpful in obtaining adequate component anchorage.

The creation of an enlarged flexion space by ligament release for the purpose of correcting angular deformity may also require some amplification. As previously stated, the abnormal anatomy found in angular deformity is ligament asymmetry (one ligament contracted and the other stretched). The presence of a stretched ligament is normally readily perceived when the knee is examined in extension but may not be at all obvious once the knee is flexed because of the tethering effect of the contracted ligament. However, once the contracted ligament has been released, the joint is now free to open until the previously elongated opposite ligament becomes tight. Furthermore, in a severe deformity with loss of tibial bone, the contracted ligament may hold the femoral condyles into a tibial cavity when the knee is flexed. This in turn affects the location of the femoral reference point (the intramedullary location hole) with regard to the upper tibia, so that the instruments may indicate an excessively large tibial resection.

It is of critical importance that ligament asymmetry be assessed and corrected before any of the bone cuts are made. The extent of ligament contracture or stretching must be assessed also in two positions: as near to full extension as the knee will go and at 90 degrees of flexion. Once the knee is exposed, the joint must be levered apart until the ligaments become fully tight in both of these positions. which can be done most simply by insertion of a periosteal elevator into the sides of the joint alternately and by prying of the joint surfaces apart. Distraction instruments such as a rachet-handled laminar spreader are also extremely helpful but sometimes cannot be used for the initial assessment because when one side of the knee is extremely tight there may not be sufficient room to permit insertion. Thus a laminar spreader can be inserted to distract the loose side of a joint while the joint surfaces are pried apart by a manually held instrument on the tight side. By these means ligament asymmetry is identified and must now be overcome.

TECHNIQUE FOR SOFT-TISSUE RELEASE

A standard midline approach is used unless otherwise indicated (for example, a previous scar). The skin incision should be of adequate length so that retraction is not required during the procedure. The capsule incision into the extensor mechanism passes over the medial third of the patella and runs distally medial to the patellar ligament and tibial tubercle (Fig. 14-29). This incision is also virtually straight and permits a secure closure that will allow early motion without risk of disruption. By an overlapping closure, proximal

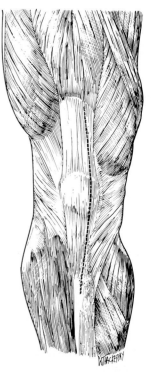

Fig. 14-29. The capsular incision is almost straight and crosses the medial edge of the patella. This type of incision allows a very secure closure and is unlikely to pull apart with early motion of the knee.

realignment can also be done to correct patellar tracking if this is required. The incision is extensile and can be continued both proximally and distally as needed for further exposure. In all cases the exposure must allow complete displacement of the tibia in front of the femur by freeing the collateral and capsular attachments to the tibia sufficiently to allow the tibia to be "button holed" forwards. Although the attachment of the patellar ligament to the tibial tubercle can be partially freed, avulsion must not be allowed, and the maintenance of continuity between the patellar ligament and distal periosteum is recommended.

Varus deformity (Figs. 14-30 to 14-32). Ligament balance is achieved by progressive release of the medial soft tissues until they reach the length of the lateral ligamentous structures. The extent of the release can be monitored by periodic insertion of the laminar spreaders and judgment of alignment with an aligning rod. The end point to be reached is a position in which the rod passes in a line from the center of the ankle over the tibial tubercle to the hip joint (Fig. 14-33) (a location

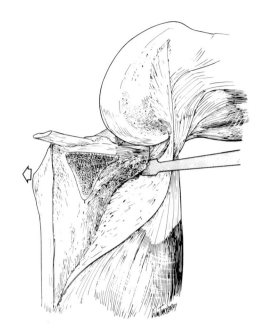

Fig. 14-31. The cruciates are removed and the tibia is externally rotated so that a dissection of the posterior capsule is allowed.

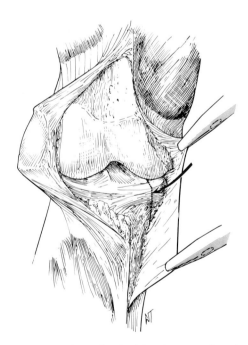

Fig. 14-30. The capsular incision is opened and a subperiosteal sleeve elevated from the medial tibia carrying with it the superficial medial collateral ligament. The medial osteophyte and medial protrusion of the upper tibia is removed. The amount of bone removed from this area depends on the correction desired and the width of the upper tibia that must remain to provide support for the tibial component.

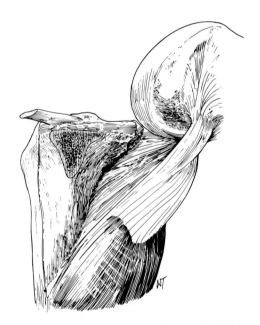

Fig. 14-32. The objective is to dislocate the tibia anteriorly so that the tibial component can be inserted directly upon the upper surface of the tibia. When ligament imbalance still remains despite this dissection, the *distal* insertion of the superficial medial collateral ligament is stripped from the tibia.

dependent on individual stature will be from one to three fingerbreadths medial to the anterosuperior iliac spine). The cruciate ligaments must be completely excised before the release is started because their presence will inhibit correction. The reason is that, after the lateral ligament has been stretched and is elongated, the end point of a medial release (when correct balance is obtained) is a lengthening of the medial structures beyond their original length. Cruciate ligaments being in the center of the knee usually retain approximately

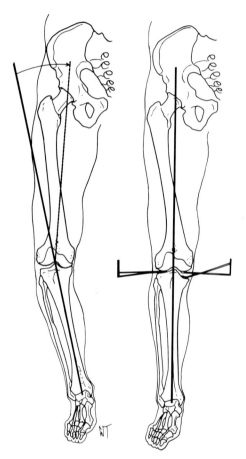

Fig. 14-33. Ligament balance is only considered satisfactory when, with both collateral ligaments placed on stretch, the alignment of the leg is correct. In the diagram laminar spreaders are inserted into the medial and lateral compartments of the knee to tense the collateral ligaments. The aligning rod passes from the center of the ankle joint over the tibial tubercle to the center of the hip joint. If the alignment rod still passes laterally to the hip joint, further medial dissection is required. The hip joint for practical purposes is considered to lie two fingerbreadths medial to the anterior superior iliac spine.

their original length regardless of alterations that occur in the collateral ligaments and thus, when intact, will not permit the stretching that is the objective of the release procedure.

The medial release is done by removal of the medial osteophytes from the femur and the tibia (including the protruding flare of the tibial plateau) and then by elevation of a sleeve of soft tissue from the upper medial tibia that is allowed to slide proximally. The sleeve consists of the periosteum, deep medial ligament, superficial medial ligament, and insertion of the pes anserinus tendons. More posteriorly at the joint surface the sleeve is continuous with the semimembranosus insertion and posterior capsule. Distally the release may include the deep fascia investing the soleus and the popliteus. The development of the sleeve is simply made by continuation of the standard approach distally on the anteromedial surface of the tibia for 8 to 10 cm and stripping of the periosteum medially from the tibia. The knee is flexed, and the leg is progressively externally rotated to gain posterior access. The distal attachment of the superficial medial ligament can be initially left intact, and in the less severe cases this will be the extent of the necessary release. Correct alignment after insertion of the spreaders will now be demonstrated (Fig. 14-33). When this is not the case, the release is continued posteriorly and distally by further subperiosteal stripping. Correction of deformity occurs gradually and is aided by the intermittent stretching action of the medial laminar spreader. With a progressive release, there is no discontinuity between the medial soft-tissue structures; the result is both balance and near normal stability, albeit with some overall lengthening of the limb (the amount of lengthening is dependent on the degree of preoperative stretching of the lateral structures).

The ideal postoperative alignment with regard to prosthetic placement and function is also not dependent on the original anatomy. This is to say that in a patient who has always been bowlegged and has later developed unilateral osteoarthritis, it is not sufficient to match the alignment of the replaced knee with that of the opposite "normal" (which in this case means varus). Whatever the original appearance may have been, the relationship of hip, knee, and ankle must be as described after prosthetic replacement (a femorotibial alignment between 5 and 10 degrees of valgus); otherwise the prosthetic components will be unequally loaded and will be subjected to excessive varus stress.

At the completion of varus release, the limb is already aligned in the proper position, no further correction is needed, and the bone cuts can be made in a standard manner to place the components in ideal position as previously defined. After insertion of components of the correct size, the knee is fully stable and does not require prolonged immobilization because of the ligament release. Motion can be strated at the usual time (when wound healing has progressed enough to allow it) and walking with full weight-bearing is allowed within a few days of surgery.

Valgus deformity (Figs. 14-34 to 14-37). The principles for the correction of fixed valgus are precisely the same as those for fixed varus; however, there are certain differences because the anatomic structure is not the same. The popliteal nerve passes on the lateral side of the knee and, along with other structures, is stretched often beyond its original resting length. (There is no cor-

responding structure to be concerned about on the medial side of the knee.) The ligamentous, capsular, and fascial attachments are also different, and for this reason the release must be done from the femur rather than the tibia.

The harmful effects of the inevitable stretching of the peroneal nerve can be partially mitigated by dissection of the nerve, especially the portion that passes around the fibular neck extending to and including the position where the deep portion of the nerve passes beneath a fibrous raphe into the anterior compartment of the leg. The rationale for this dissection is the belief that interference of nerve function is attributable not only to stretching but also to fascial compression, especially at the sites mentioned. The iliotibial band also has no counterpart on the medial side and, when contracted, not only maintains fixed valgus but also (because it remains tight even with flexion of the knee) a fixed external rotation of the tibia. The iliotibial band cannot be stripped and progressively lengthened as with the medial

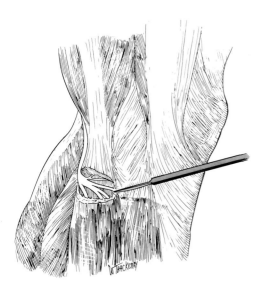

Fig. 14-34. Correction of fixed valgus deformity may result in peroneal nerve palsy attributable to a combination of stretching and compression of the nerve by overlying fascia. Although stretching of the nerve is unavoidable, one can eliminate the compressive effect of the fascia by a nerve dissection freeing the nerve around the neck of the fibula and tracing the nerve until the division into two main branches. The deep branch of the nerve passes through a fibrous tunnel to reach the anterior compartment, and the roof of the tunnel should be divided.

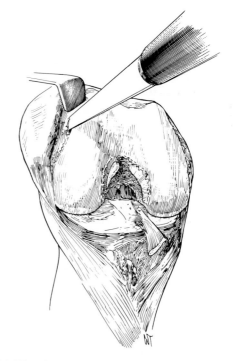

Fig. 14-35. After the nerve dissection is completed, the knee is opened through the standard medial capsular incision and the patella is dislocated laterally. The lateral capsule, lateral ligament, and popliteus tendon are stripped from the lateral femoral condyle.

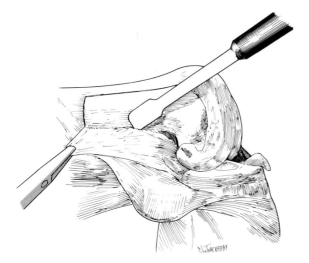

Fig. 14-36. Capsular dissection is continued by subperiosteal stripping 3 to 4 inches above the level of the knee joint, and the periosteum is incised transversely. The capsular and periosteal flap that is created is now completely separated from remaining attachments to the linea aspera of the femur by a posterior vertical cut that extends distally to the posterior tibia. Further correction when necessary is obtained when a transverse incision is made through the fascia lata. This cut is at the same level as the transverse periosteal cut (3 to 4 inches above the knee joint).

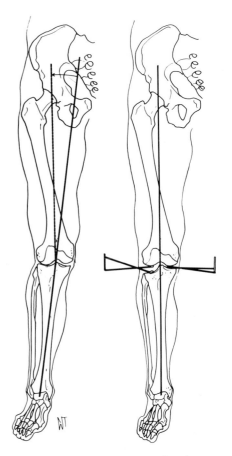

Fig. 14-37. The adequacy of correction is assessed just as after medial release by insertion of spreaders into each side of the knee, tension put on the ligaments, and use of the alignment rod for assessment of the position. The alignment rod should also in this instance pass from the center of the ankle joint over the tibial tubercle to the center of the hip joint.

sleeve, and often complete transection is required. Fixed valgus deformity may also be associated with lateral patellar subluxation. One can of course correct this by dividing the lateral patellar retinaculum at the patellar border, but if this is done, there is considerable interference with the blood supply. There is evidence that fatigue fracture of the patella may occur because of avascular necrosis. It is accordingly preferable to reposition the patella by a release that has the least effect upon patellar vascularity. By dissection in the interval between the iliotibial band and the biceps femoris, patella repositioning is possible, with preservation of all the vessels that arise from the lateral genicular artery, and at least some of those derived from the superior genicular artery.

These considerations dictate a modification to the surgical approach by allowing access to a more extensive area on the lateral aspect of the knee. Two alternatives exist: (1) a lateral parapatellar skin incision provides access to the peroneal nerve by subcutaneous dissection under the lateral flap, and by similar undermining of the other flap, one can make the usual medial arthrotomy incision

into the knee; (2) this method involves two incisions, the first placed anteriorly as before, and the second positioned posterolaterally over the peroneal nerve. Division of the iliotibial tract and forward release of the patellar retinaculum is then done blindly and subcutaneously by use of both incisions.

Whichever approach is chosen, the capsular incision is made in the usual manner and the patella dislocated laterally. The lateral capsule is removed from the femoral condyle, together with the lateral ligament and popliteus tendon. A periosteal sleeve in continuity is developed proximally on the femur 8 to 10 cm, at which point a transverse cut in the periosteum is made extending posteri-

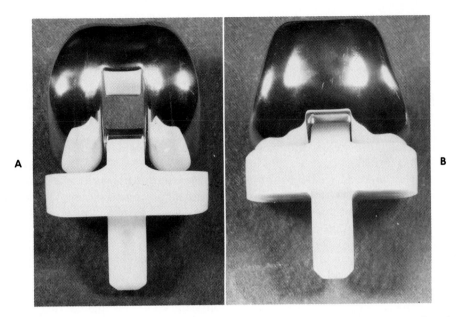

Fig. 14-38. The posterior stabilized condylar knee in which posterior cruciate function is assumed by a central cam on the tibial component, which articulates against a transverse bar on the femoral component. **A,** Prosthesis at 90 degrees and, **B,** in full extension. Note that in extension the tibial cam does not contact the femoral component anteriorly; thus an impact is avoided in terminal extension, which if occurring repetitively when the patient is walking might cause loosening.

orly to the linea aspera femoris. This attachment to the femur posteriorly must also be divided vertically until the sleeve is free from the femur. The most distal of the perforating arteries may be cut and should be ligated. At the level of the lateral femoral condyle, the posterior capsule (and sometimes the lateral head of the gastrocnemius) requires division. As is the case on the medial side, the amount of correction obtained at each stage is determined by insertion of laminar spreaders and an alignment check. Usually the amount of dissection so far described is sufficient to provide balance and correction. In severe cases, particularly those with associated external rotation deformity, the iliotibial band must also be divided in the manner previously described. When the release includes the iliotibial band, some permanent laxity may result. There is no functional significance in *extension* and does not cause instability when walking. However, there may be a functionally significant instability in *flexion* because, as was true for medial release, cruciate excision (particularly the posterior) is mandatory. Therefore, even when using the thickest components that will fit, there

is a tendency toward lateral rotatory subluxation in a posterior direction. Normally, in the process of healing, readherence of the lateral capsule and scar formation prevent this becoming a clinical problem, but some degree of unpredictability must be conceded. It is therefore safer in this situation to use components that assume posterior stability (total condylar II or posterior stabilized knee prosthesis) (Fig. 14-38).

Needless to say, the full lateral dissection as described will divide all the elements that contribute to associated external rotation contracture, with the exception of the biceps femoris. Very rarely partial or complete division of this muscle may also be required.

Flexion contracture. As previously discussed, unlike angular deformity, some degree of correction of flexion contracture is possible by bone resection. This must be done by resection of the femoral bone and is limited by the collateral ligament attachments. Beyond this point correction must be obtained by posterior capsulotomy. In a long-standing contracture, the normal posterior recess is obliterated, and the capsule is adherent to the femoral condyles. The recess must be recreated by stripping adherent capsule, though this alone seldom results in much correction. Cruciate ligament excision removes the central portion of the posterior capsule, leaving the medial and lateral segments lying anterior to the respective heads of the gastrocnemius. These segments must be separated from the contiguous *lateral* capsule by vertical incisions made at the medial and lateral posterior corners. (Because there are no important structures posterior to the capsule in these areas, the vertical incisions can be made blindly with confidence and safety.) The remaining medial and lateral segments of the posterior capsule can now be divided sharply and under direct vision. Often in rheumatoid arthritis the capsule is greatly thickened and intimately adherent to the gastrocnemius, which if this is the case, must also be divided. The objective is to cut all fibrous structures from one side of the knee to the other, with exposure of the popliteal layer of fat. Because the thickest capsule is in the medial or lateral recess, there is little likelihood of injury to a vital structure. However, needless to say, the division of the posterior capsule requires care and a light touch. The necessary exposure can be made easier by prior removal of bone from the upper tibia and posterior femoral condyles (unlike the correction of angular deformity when soft-tissue dissection must precede all the bone cuts). When flexion deformity is associated with fixed valgus, the approach is considerably simplified because the lateral release is done first, so that the posterior capsule can be approached from the side, allowing retraction of the popliteal vessels.

Correction of severe flexion contracture may also stretch and compress the peroneal nerve, and foot drop may occur. Decompression of the nerve through a separate posterolateral incision is recommended.

Correction of flexion contractures may be "springy," and to prevent recurrence during the postoperative period, one should splint the knee in extension for about 3 weeks.

Flexion instability. When the condition is primary, as in rheumatoid arthritis, it should be recognized by the initial ligamentous assessment. Then one must make an appropriate allowance in deciding the level of tibial resection. The condition is then self-correcting.

When caused by the effect of ligament release or by the error of excessive tibial resection, flex-

ion instability may not be recognized until the time comes to fit the trial components. There will be apparent excessive anteroposterior motion in flexion, which, if accepted, may lead to posterior subluxation of that tibia on the femur.

The remedies are (1) restoration of flexion stability by use of a thicker tibial component thereby filling the flexion gap and restoring collateral ligament tension. This means an appropriate adjustment to the extension gap, or the knee will not fully extend with the thicker component in place. Extra bone must be removed from the distal femur equal to the difference between the tibial component originally selected and the thickness now selected. (2) The alternative to respacing the knee is to use components that in themselves provide posterior stability. As was mentioned in regard to the correction of fixed valgus deformity, in some cases this may be the preferred solution.

Stiff knee and quadriceps contracture. Long-standing stiffness at or near full extension, even though caused primarily by intra-articular adhesions, inevitably leads to secondary quadriceps contracture.

The use of the standard midline approach may have disadvantages because excessive tightness in the rectus femoris can lead to an avulsion of the tibial tubercle during knee flexion. This is difficult to repair satisfactorily and is best avoided by early recognition that such a problem is likely. The inverted V incision (Coonse and Adams) is recommended in these circumstances and completely avoids the risk of distal avulsion. The quadriceps tendon and the patella are turned distally leaving a broad-based attachment to the tibia. Immediate and extensive exposure is obtained (Figs. 14-39 and 14-40).

The V incision may be closed as a Y, thus lengthening the rectus femoris or by selective reattachment of the vasti according to their degree of tightness. Usually very little V-Y lengthening is required, and sufficient quadriceps mobilization is obtained by reattachment of the vastus lateralis at a higher level. The result of the inverted V incision is that good motion is usually obtained at the expense of a mild extension lag (which usually diminishes with time).

Intra-articular adhesions. Posterior adhesions and contractures of the posterior cruciate ligament will cause the knee to "open like a book." Instead of the normal rolling and gliding motions, a posterior hinge is formed so that increased flex-

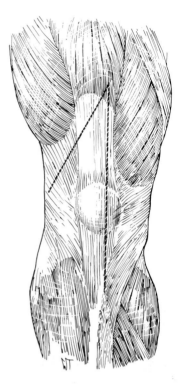

Fig. 14-39. When there is a quadriceps contracture associated with stiffness or ankylosis of the knee, the conventional exposure may be difficult and can cause avulsion of the patella ligament from the tibial tubercle. The solution is to make a second incision across the quadriceps tendon running distally at an angle of 45 degrees from the apex of the first incision.

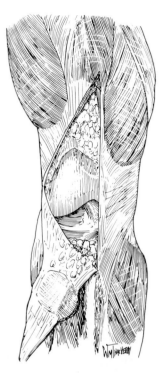

Fig. 14-40. The quadriceps tendon and the patella can then be turned laterally and distally so that an easy exposure is provided. On closing of this incision only the apex and medial limb of the incision need suturing. Postoperative immobilization for about 3 weeks is required to allow healing. Only seldom does an extension lag result.

ion is accompanied by a progressive anterior displacement of the tibia on the femur. For prevention of the same pattern of motion after replacement, the posterior cruciate must be excised and the normal posterior recess reestablished by capsular stripping. Vertical incisions medially and laterally are often needed to separate the posterior capsule from the collateral capsule.

Of all the techniques described, the release of "extension contracture" is perhaps the least satisfactory, and it is the uncommon case in which the result will be as good as that after other kins of release because of the failure to restore both normal motion and quadriceps strength.

SUMMARY

Soft-tissue release techniques are designed to restore normal alignment and motion with the preservation of sufficient ligamentous integrity to enable the use of a surface knee-joint replace-

ment. The techniques require cruciate ligament excision, so that anteroposterior stability after the arthroplasty is dependent in part on collateral ligament tension and in part on the surface geometry of the prosthesis, which must possess some degree of cupping. Additional anteroposterior stability can be obtained, when necessary, by use of prosthesis that possesses an intercondylar cam with a cruciate substituting function. The alternative to soft tissue release techniques is to obtain correction of deformity by additional bone resection. A constrained prosthesis that assumes ligament function is then required. However, constrained prostheses, in general, have been shown to possess higher rates of loosening, breakage, and infection, so that their use should be limited to as few cases as possible. With experience, soft-tissue release techniques make it possible to correct most deformities and to enable the use of a surface-replacement prosthesis (Fig. 14-41).

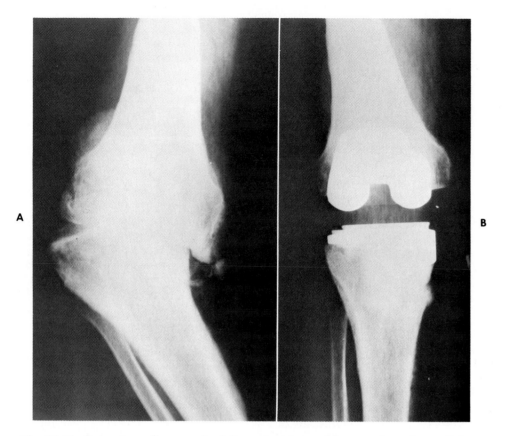

Fig. 14-41. Correction of a severely deformed and unstable varus knee by medial release. **A,** Standing roentgenogram with a measured angulation of 38 degrees; there is a severe erosion of the medial tibial plateau. **B,** Alignment in 10 degrees of valgus after medial stripping from the tibia and the insertion of the posterior stabilized condylar knee. In this case a metal tray with a medial buildup to compensate for the bone erosion was used.

Part D

Complications after knee replacement: prevention and management

ALAN H. WILDE, M.D.
Cleveland, Ohio

Inevitably after major surgery, even in the best of hands, complications will occasionally arise. Therefore, the mark of a good surgeon is not only his ability to avoid complications but, should they occur, to manage them effectively as well. The major complications after total knee replacement fall into several categories. There are diffi-culties with soft tissue, infection, the patella, limitation of motion, component loosening, thromboembolism and instability. The subjects of component loosening and instability are topics of substance to be discussed in other publications.

PROBLEMS OF SOFT TISSUE

Skin necrosis. The main difficulties with the soft tissues are necrosis of the skin, and sinus tract formation. Necrosis of the skin postoperatively can occur from several causes. Extensive under-mining of the flaps as in a straight anterior approach in order to reach both the medial and lateral sides of the joint must be performed with great caution. Such a practice may result in necrosis of one of the flaps, most often the lateral flap. It would be preferable to perform an approach

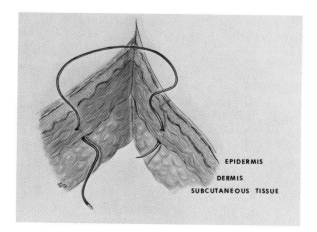

Fig. 14-42. In patients with poor subcutaneous tissue such as those with rheumatoid arthritis, one may need to place sutures at the junction of the dermis and subcutaneous layers to relieve tension on the skin margins.

either medially or laterally and not to dissect the flap on the opposite side if significant wound necrosis is to be avoided. Closure of the wound under tension increases the risk of wound necrosis. If there is inadequate suturing of the subcutaneous layer, all of the tension will fall on the skin itself. If the skin is sutured tightly, necrosis is likely to occur, particularly if hemorrhage occurs postoperatively. The more hemorrhage occurs, the greater the pressure on the wound closure. If the wound has not been sutured properly, the pressure will be transmitted to the wound margins. If the pressure becomes too great, the circulation of the skin becomes endangered and necrosis occurs. In an effort to control the amount of hemorrhage, it is our practice to meticulously coagulate or ligate all the major bleeding points or potential bleeding points in the knee throughout the procedure. Once the operation has been completed, the tourniquet is released and bleeding from the major sources is coagulated or ligated. We also use a suction catheter inserted into the knee joint in an effort to reduce the effect of pressure on the wound.

As mentioned, closure of the wound itself is important if necrosis is to be avoided. In the patient with rheumatoid arthritis, the subcutaneous tissues are often of poor quality. Under these circumstances sutures will not hold securely in the subcutaneous fat. A 3-0 suture placed in the dermis at the junction of the dermis and the subcutaneous layer will be secure and will also serve to relieve tension on the remainder of the skin (Fig.

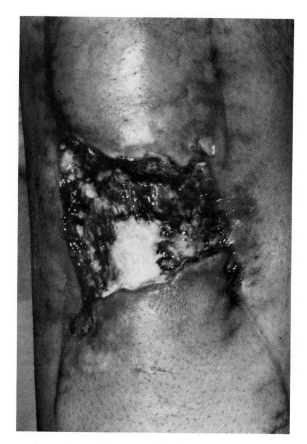

Fig. 14-43. Full-thickness loss of skin has occurred in the infrapatellar region when a median parapatellar incision was used after a recent lateral parapatellar incision. Reconstruction was performed by a split-thickness skin graft followed by a full-thickness flap.

14-42). The remainder of the skin can be repaired with 4-0 suture.

The matter of placement of the skin incision is important, particularly when there has been a previous operative scar on the knee. Generally, it is wisest to use a previous median parapatellar or lateral parapatellar approach if there is already a scar in that area. One should not use a median parapatellar approach where a lateral parapatellar approach has been used previously, or vice versa, because a large area of necrosis may occur in the infrapatellar area where the distal lines of the median and lateral parapatellar incisions converge[23] (Fig. 14-43). The surgeon should not make an incision that parallels a previous approach and leave a narrow strip of skin between the two incisions, which may undergo necrosis. When a transverse incision has been used previously and a greater exposure is needed to perform a knee replacement, it is preferable to use a longitudinal incision that crosses the transverse incision at 90 degrees. We have done this on several occasions and have utilized a median parapatellar incision after a transverse incision without any loss of skin. This is undoubtedly safer when the transverse incision has been made 1 year or longer before the new approach has been performed.

As far as operative approaches are concerned, we prefer the approach first described by Erkes in 1929.[9] This operative exposure allows the same degree of exposure as the median parapatellar approach but does not violate the tendon of the rectus femoris muscle or the aponeurotic insertion of the vastus medialis into the patella. It also allows the placement of the incision on the side of the knee where it is not so visible as a long straight anterior incision. It is well to keep the inferior limb of the incision away from the tibial tubercle so that patients can kneel on the knees postoperatively without discomfort. The incision begins at the midpoint between the medial intermuscular septum and the rectus femoris tendon and proceeds distally. It curves medially along the medial border of the patella and extends along the medial side of the tibial tubercle. The deep fasciae overlying the vastus medialis and medial articular capsule are incised. The fibers of the vastus medialis that attach into the medial intermuscular septum are released. This can usually be performed with a finger because the attachment is not firm. One has to be careful not to section the medial superior geniculate artery. If this occurs, it should be coagulated or ligated, otherwise significant hemorrhage can occur. The surgeon should also remember that the medial intermuscular septum forms the roof of Hunter's canal and the femoral artery and vein are immediately beneath the septum. The femoral artery can also be encountered proximally in the wound before it enters Hunter's canal. After the release of the fibers of the vastus medialis, the patella can be everted and the knee flexed. For a knee replacement to be performed it is usually necessary also to excise the infrapatellar fat pad. If further exposure is necessary, a few fibers of the attachment of the infrapatellar tendon can be released. No more than a third of these fibers should be released, however, because detachment of the infrapatellar tendon might occur. The full exposure provided by the Erkes approach is more than ample to perform a total knee replacement or other procedure

that requires a large exposure of the anterior aspect of the knee.

In some cases of rheumatoid arthritis where there is vasculitis, the skin may become very atrophic and discolored and is prone to breaking down with minor trauma. Although this type of skin is seen frequently over the distal tibia, at times it may extend over the anterior aspect of the knee itself. Major knee surgery carries an increased risk because the skin may undergo necrosis postoperatively or react poorly to minor trauma in later years. We do perform knee replacement with atrophic, vasculitic skin distal to the area of the proposed approach as long as the skin in the area of the approach is relatively normal. Atrophic skin will break down with minimal trauma; it must be handled with great care because lacerations can occur readily. If a laceration

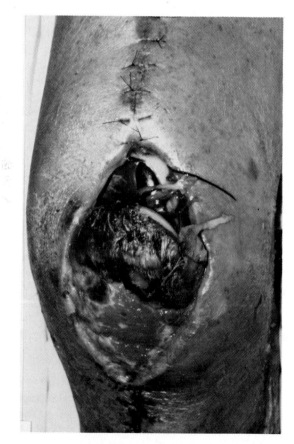

Fig. 14-44. A large area of skin necrosis has occurred exposing the patella and knee joint prosthesis. Infection has developed. Reconstruction required removal of the prosthesis, cement, and patella, and arthrodesis. Primary wound closure was accomplished.

occurs, it is difficult to suture because the skin is so friable that sutures pull out easily. In this situation the laceration can be repaired using Steri-Strips. These lacerations will eventually heal but will take longer than a usual laceration.

Once a skin necrosis has occurred, it should be treated promptly. Occasionally one sees a small area of necrosis of 1 to 2 cm, which can be excised and the wound closed. This should be accomplished before infection occurs. Marginal necrosis of the sides of the incision may be treated by excision of the necrotic tissue and split-thickness skin grafting if the residual defect cannot be closed primarily. If a larger area of necrosis occurs as in Fig. 14-43, a full-thickness flap may be necessary. This may be preceded by a split-thickness skin graft. We have encountered a few cases where the area of necrosis was large enough to expose the patella and the prosthesis (Fig. 14-44). In such a case where the prosthesis is exposed and there is deep infection present, it is necessary to remove the prosthesis, cement, and patella in order to perform an arthrodesis. It may be possible to close the wound after débridement and removal of the prosthesis and patella. If the wound is under tension, the tibial tubercle can be excised and the medial and lateral femoral epicondyles as well, to allow the wound to be sutured without tension.

Sinus tract formation. Sinus tract formation may occur in the early postoperative period. During the first 2 to 3 weeks after surgery the sinus tract can be recognized when the patient continues to discharge a large amount of bloody drainage through the wound, particularly after exercise. This usually indicates a separation of the deep suture line. The sinus tract may not spontaneously close even after the knee has been immobilized in a cast for a period of 3 to 4 weeks. The danger is that the knee joint can become infected secondarily it is recommended that if a sinus tract appears in the early postoperative period, the wound should be reopened and the defect in the capsular repair be resutured. A sinus tract that develops months or years after knee replacement when the wound has healed entirely, usually represents a deep infection, though a slight amount of drainage can be the result of suture granulomas in the subcutaneous space or in the capsule. Exploration is advised. If it is a suture granuloma, is should be excised and the wound can be closed. If there is a sinus tract that communicates with

the knee joint, one can assume that a deep infection is present and the infection will have to be treated accordingly. This is discussed in a later section.

PATELLAR PROBLEMS

Pain. The difficulties that are encountered with the patella are pain, subluxation, dislocation, and fracture. It should be recognized that there are a number of causes of anterior knee pain after knee replacement. Pain may result from quadriceps weakness, a neuroma of the infrapatellar branch of the saphenous nerve, a synovial hernia, infection, and component loosening, as well as patellar subluxation or dislocation. The scar itself, particularly if it is a straight anterior scar, may be painful. If the patellofemoral joint or the patella has not been replaced, there can be pain as a result of the resulting inflammation and patellar-prosthesis incongruity. The complaint of pain from the patellofemoral joint cannot be elicited from the patient unless he is asked if pain occurs on arising from a chair or climbing stairs, particularly on descending stairs. A review of my first 50 Geometric II knee replacements revealed that 32% of patients had pain on the patellar compression test that corresponded to the same kind of pain in the same location that they were experiencing during activities that required knee flexion.[24] The pain that occurs from residual patellofemoral arthritis is usually not disabling and does not often require revision of the knee replacement. In most instances, conservative treatment suffices. This type of pain can be managed by the use of a nonsteroid anti-inflammatory drug and the instruction in quadriceps extension exercises through a short arc of motion.

Subluxation. Patellar subluxation or dislocation is the result of failure to realign the quadriceps mechanism at the time of surgery. This is particularly unlikely to occur when the tibia has been externally rotated on the femur and also when there has been a valgus deformity. Before closure of the skin and after the suturing of the medial articular capsule, it is our practice to flex and extend the knee in order to observe the tracking of the patella on the femur or the femoral prosthesis. If there is a tendency toward patellar subluxation, a lateral retinacular release is performed. This can be performed from the inside by eversion of the patella. The lateral flap should not be dissected because doing so could lead to necrosis of the wound. The medial articular capsule is imbricated, and the knee is flexed and extended. If the subluxation continues, the vastus medialis insertion can be advanced onto the patella. If patellar subluxation still occurs (and I have had this experience in a patient with a severe external rotation deformity of the tibia and a valgus deformity of the knee), a Roux-Goldthwait or other type of patellar tendon realignment may be needed as well.

Fracture. There have been a few cases of fracture of the patella that have occurred after patellar resurfacing. Several factors may be responsible for this, aside from trauma. If the anchor hole for the stem of the patellar prosthesis penetrates the anterior cortex of the patella, a stress riser is created and it could lead to a fracture. If more than half of the substance of the patella has been removed or if the bone itself has been weakened by severe osteoporosis, a fracture can occur. Extensive release of the soft-tissue attachments of the patella may result in avascular necrosis. This may occur after the medial, superior, and lateral muscular insertions into the patella have been released as in the approach of Coonse and Adams.[4] If a fracture occurs and is undisplaced or minimally displaced, it can be treated simply by immobilization. If the fragments are widely separated, open reduction and internal fixation with a circumferential wire can be used. If adequate fixation cannot be obtained, patellectomy may be necessary. This should be avoided, if possible, because it not only may weaken the quadriceps muscle group by as much as one third, but it may also contribute to instability of the knee.

LIMITATION OF MOTION

Perhaps the most common reason for limitation of motion after knee replacement is lack of participation in an active rehabilitation program postoperatively. We start isometric quadriceps exercises on the day after surgery and begin isotonic exercises on the second postoperative day, once the postoperative dressing and the suction catheter are removed. We also employ a knee exerciser that is attached to an overhead traction frame. By using the knee exerciser, the patient can actively assist range-of-motion exercises. Occasionally we may discharge patients with 90 degrees of active motion and have them return 6 weeks later with only 60 degrees of motion. For this reason, if at all convenient, we schedule the patient to return to the outpatient physical therapy department on a once-weekly basis for a checkup on their progress. We will continue active range-of-motion exercises and progressive resistance exercises through a short arc of flexion, lifting no more than 25 pounds as long as there is improvement. We no longer employ manipulation in an effort to improve the range of motion. There are several undesirable complications from manipulation, including supracondylar fracture, patellar fracture, fracture of the proximal tibia, wound separation, capsular rupture, patellar tendon rupture, quadriceps mechanism rupture, hemarthrosis, and pulmonary embolism. Furthermore, it has recently been shown that manipulation has not been of value in increasing the range of motion postoperatively.

As a last resort, if the patient has not achieved a satisfactory range of motion after extensive physical therapy, we will consider an open release of adhesions in an effort to increase the range of motion. The possibility of another procedure is usually enough to motivate the patient to increase his efforts so that the operative procedure is unnecessary. In an open release of adhesions, scar is excised from the suprapatellar pouch, both collateral ligaments, and the cruciate ligaments.

THROMBOEMBOLISM

Thromboembolism is at least as common if not more common after knee surgery than after hip surgery. The incidence of deep vein thrombosis has been reported as 60% of patients after knee surgery and 50% of patients after hip surgery. Pulmonary emboli have been reported in 8% of patients after knee surgery and from 0.5% to 1.3% of these were fatal when no precautions were taken. The data are similar to that found after hip surgery, with an incidence of pulmonary emboli of 6% to 14%, of which from 1.8% to 3.4% were fatal.[3] Although there is definitely a group of patients who are subject to a high risk of thromboembolism, including those over 60 years of age, those with a previous history of thromboembolic disease, previous venous surgery, or known venous insufficiency, it seems prudent to protect all patients who undergo knee replacement. We are currently using aspirin 600 mg b.i.d. preoperatively and postoperatively in male patients who are not in the high-risk group.[11,14] Since aspirin is less effective in women and patients who are in the high-risk group, we use low molecular weight dextran in these situations. We start 500 ml of dextran intravenously before surgery and continue it during surgery and immediately postoperatively. It is continued at the rate of 25 ml/hour for 4 or 5 days until the patient ambulates.[8]

We also elevate the foot of the bed in the recovery room and place the patient in the semi-Fowler's position for the first day or two because this has been shown to decrease the incidence of thromboembolism.[12]

INFECTION

Incidence and etiology. The presence of infection after knee replacement is the most serious complication that the surgeon must face. The incidence of infection after the resurfacing type of knee replacement prothesis has been reported commonly as being 2%, whereas after the hinge type of prosthetic replacement the incidence may be as high as 8%.[13,17,18,20-22] Infections may result directly from surgery, or come from sources in the body outside the knee joint. Secondary infections may occur in the knee joint after pneumonia, urinary tract infections, dental infections, otitis media, pharyngitis, sinusitis or intestinal infections.[1,6,7,17] Obviously, all such secondary infections must be treated promptly. Since bacteremia may occur after dental extractions or genitourinary manipulations, we routinely advise patients to use prophylactic antibiotics for 5 to 7 days after such procedures.[23]

Prevention. The prevention of infection is a topic unto itself. The development of postoperative infection is multifactorial. We routinely search for possible sources of infection preoperatively. It is essential to elicit a careful history about symptoms of urinary tract infections or obstruction and obtain urine cultures if there is any suspicion of chronic or recurrent infection. In the case where there has been an operation on the knee previously, it is advisable to aspirate fluid from the knee joint preoperatively for culture and sensitivity.

The patient's skin is shaved only over the area of proposed incision in the operating room after the induction of anesthesia. We use a horizontal-flow laminar air flow room with side walls. Paper gowns, drapes, and hoods are used. An aspirator system removes the expired air from the nose and throat of the operating team. For a more detailed discussion of the operating room environment and the prevention of infection, refer to the excellent articles by J. P. Nelson.[17,18]

Treatment. The treatment of a patient with an infected total knee prosthesis is changing; therefore, it is difficult to be authoritative at this time. The following remarks will have to be regarded as the state of the art at the time of writing. Do understand that new information is becoming available and that treatment may change subsequently.

First of all, one must recognize that the mere presence of a deep infection in the knee joint of a patient does not require the automatic removal of the prosthesis and cement. There are a few patients who present with a chronic low-grade infection, which is in essence a chronic osteomyelitis. They may periodically undergo episodes when the infection may become active and drainage may occur. In the interim between acute attacks, the knee joint may be comfortable and functional. In such individuals it may be preferable to leave the prosthesis in place and treat the episodes of acute flare-up of infection. The patients that we have elected to treat in this way usually have had severe disabling polyarticular rheumatoid arthritis and may ambulate minimally with external aids or may be nonambulatory. This is particularly likely to be the case if a hinge replacement and arthrodesis would be difficult if not impossible to achieve. The conservative treatment given consists of rest, no weight-bearing on the involved extremity, immobilization of the leg in a long leg cast, and antibiotics. The antibiotics that are given are determined on the basis of cultures and sensitivities. If the patient becomes systemically ill, however, the prosthesis and cement must be removed.

In most cases the treatment of an infected total knee prosthesis is surgical. Because the management of orthopaedic infections is complicated, we prefer to manage these patients with specialists in infectious disease. We usually withhold antibiotics until cultures have been taken from the depths of the wound. It is preferable to culture the tissue at the bone-cement interface rather than to culture the pus alone. Both aerobic and anaerobic cultures should be obtained. It is our practice also to order cultures for fungi and acid-fast bacilli. *Staphylococcus aureus*, *S. albus*, and *S. epidermidis* have been the most common organisms. *Escherichia coli*, *Enterobacter*, *Streptococcus*, and *Pseudomonas* have also been found frequently.[2] The choice of antibiotics is decided once the sensitivities have been determined. The antibiotics should be given intravenously for a minimum of four weeks.

After the culture is obtained, the wound should be thoroughly debrided. The wound margins and subcutaneous tissue are debrided. The wound is lavaged with an irrigation system. For this purpose we use a solution of 0.005% neomycin. A more concentrated solution of neomycin may produce permanent damage to the vestibular apparatus or to the kidneys.[16] If an adequate débridement has been performed and the tissues that remain are healthy, there is probably little reason to use a suction irrigation system. If suction irrigation is for longer than 1 week, secondary infection may occur with organisms such as *Pseudomonas* or *Proteus,* which are difficult to treat.

The decision as to whether to remove the prosthesis and cement as part of the débridement may be difficult. If there is no sign of loosening at the time of surgery and there is no evidence of osteomyelitis roentgenographically and the infection is of recent onset (a matter of a few days or weeks), the prosthesis and cement may be allowed to remain in place.[5] Under these circumstances, when the infection appears in the early postoperative period or acutely many years later as a result of hematogenous seeding from a source outside the knee joint, there is evidence suggesting that the knee joint may be salvaged in one third of the cases.[19] In the presence of loosening at the bone-cement interface, the prosthesis, methyl methacrylate, and cement membrane must be completely removed. If there is radiographic evidence of osteomyelitis, it is probably wisest to attempt an arthrodesis of the knee. If there is no demonstrable evidence of bone infection clinically or radiographically, another attempt at replacement arthroplasty either immediate or delayed, might be considered.

Whether it is better to replace the knee joint with another prosthesis at the time of débridement or later as a second stage operation is not clear at this time. If there is a virulent organism present such as coagulase-positive staphylococcus or if the organism is unknown, it may be wiser to perform a two-stage procedure. One can immobilize the knee joint in a Hoffman apparatus while waiting to perform the second stage. If we are to follow the principles as outlined by Wilson, for reimplementation[25] after subacute sepsis after total hip replacement, the second-stage procedure can be done 2 to 6 weeks after the primary débridement, provided that cultures from the joint are negative.

If a knee prosthesis is to be reimplanted, it would appear prudent to mix antibiotics in powder form in the methyl methacrylate. Marks et al. found that oxacillin, cefazolin, and gentamicin are stable in cement and are released in a microbiologically active form. They found high bactericidal concentrations of oxacillin in the surrounding bone for 21 days after implantation. The antibiotic for admixture should be chosen on the basis of culture and sensitivity results.[15]

In addition to antibiotics in the cement and intravenous antibiotics postoperatively for at least 4 weeks, the patient should also take oral antibiotics for at least 3 months. There are some surgeons who feel that antibiotics should be given indefinitely in this situation.

There seems to be general agreement that the knee should be fused if recurrent infection has occurred after one attempt at salvage of an infected total knee replacement.[16] Obtaining a solid fusion may be difficult. Tullos et al. have reported successful fusion in 64% of patients after knee replacement.[10] The reasons for failure include lack of sufficient bone, inadequate fixation and deficiencies in operative technique. They reported that 80% fused with a double Charnley clamp and only 55% fused with a single Charnley clamp.[10] We are currently using the Hoffman apparatus for arthrodesis of the knee. The Hoffman apparatus also has the advantage that additional compression can be applied in the postoperative period. Immobilization may have to be prolonged to achieve fusion. The average time for fusion in one series is 5.3 months, but it is not unusual for it to take as long as 12 months.[10]

SUMMARY

The main complications after knee replacement are skin necrosis, sinus tract formation, patellar subluxation, dislocation or fracture, limitation of motion, thromboembolism, component loosening, instability, and infection. Many of these complications can be avoided by proper patient selection and attention to detail during and after surgery. When complications occur, the key to a successful outcome is prompt recognition and aggressive, well-outlined treatment.

REFERENCES TO PART D

1. Burton, D.S., and Schurman, D.J.: Hematogenous infection in bilateral total hip arthroplasty, J. Bone Joint Surg. **57A:**1004, 1975.
2. Burton, D.S., and Schurman, D.J.: Salvage of infected total joint replacements, Arch. Surg. **112:**574, 1977.

3. Cohen, S.H., Ehrlich, G.E., Kauffman, M.S., and Cope, C.: Thrombophlebitis following knee surgery, J. Bone Joint Surg. **55A:**106, 1973.
4. Coonse, K.D., and Adams, J.D.: A new operative approach to the knee joint, Surg. Gynecol. Obstet. **77:**344, 1943.
5. Coventry, M.B.: Treatment of infections occurring in total hip surgery, Orthop. Clin. North Am. **6:**991, 1975.
6. Cruess, R.L., Bechez, W.S., and Von Kessler, K.L.C.: Infections in total hip secondary to a primary source elsewhere, Clin. Orthop. **106:**99, 1975.
7. D'Ambrosia, R.D., Shoji, H., and Heater, R.: Secondarily infected total joint replacement by hematogenous spread, J. Bone Joint Surg. **58A:**450, 1976.
8. Evarts, C.M.: Thromboembolism. In Rockwood, C.A., Jr., and Green, D.P.: Fractures. Vol. 1: Complications, Philadelphia, 1974, J.B. Lippincott.
9. Erkes, F.: Weitere Erfahrungen mit physiologischer Schnittführung zur Eröffnung des Kniegelenks, Bruns Beitr. zur Klin. Chir. **147:**211, 1929.
10. Hagemann, W.F., Woods, G.W., and Tullos, H.S.: Arthrodesis in failed total knee replacement, J. Bone Joint Surg. **60A:**790, 1978.
11. Harris, W.H., Salzman, E.W., Athanasoulis, C., Waltman, A.C., Baum, S., and Desantis, R.W.: Comparison of warfarin, low-molecular weight dextran, aspirin and subcutaneous heparin in prevention of venous thromboembolism following total hip replacement, J. Bone Joint Surg. **56A:**1552, 1974.
12. Hartman, J.T., Altner, P.C., and Freeark, R.J.: The effect of limb elevation is preventing venous thrombosis, J. Bone Joint Surg. **52A:**1618-1622, 1970.
13. Insall, J.N., et al.: A comparison of four models of total knee replacement prostheses, J. Bone Joint Surg. **58A:**754-765, 1976.
14. Jennings, J.J., Harris, W.H., and Sarmiento, A.: A clinical evaluation of aspirin prophylaxis of thromboembolic disease after total hip arthroplasty, J. Bone Joint Surg. **58A:**926-928, 1976.
15. Marks, K.E., Nelson, C.L., and Lautenschlager, E.P.: Antibiotic impregnated acrylic bone cement, J. Bone Joint Surg. **58A:**358, 1976.
16. Petty, W., Bryan, R.S., Coventry, M.B., and Peterson, L.F.A.: Infection after total knee arthroplasty, Orthop. Clin. North Am. **6:**1005, 1975.
17. Nelson, J.P.: The operating room environment and its influence on deep wound infection. The Hip, St. Louis, 1977, The C.V. Mosby Co.
18. Nelson, J.P.: Operating room clean rooms and personnel isolator systems, AAOS: Instructional course lectures, **26:**52, St. Louis, 1977, The C.V. Mosby Co.
19. Petty, W., et al.: Infection after total knee arthroplasty, Orthop. Clin. North Am. **6:**1005-1014, 1975.
20. Riley, L.H., and Hungerford, D.S.: Geometric total knee replacement for treatment of the rheumatoid knee, J. Bone Joint Surg. **60A:**523-527, 1978.
21. Scott, W.N., Insall, J., and Ranawat, C.S.: Total Condylar prosthesis, Orthop. Trans. **1**(1):102, 1977.
22. Skolnick, M.D., et al.: Polycentric total knee arthroplasty, J. Bone Joint Surg. **58A:**743-748, 1976.
23. Wilde, A.H.: Management of complications after knee replacement. In Ahstrom, J.P., editor: Current practice in orthopaedic surgery, St. Louis, 1979, The C.V. Mosby Co.
24. Wilde, A.H.: Geometric II knee replacement prothesis. (Unpublished data.)
25. Wilson, P.D., Jr., Aglietti, P., and Salvati, E.A.: Subacute sepsis of the hip treated by antibiotics and cemented prosthesis, J. Bone Joint Surg. **56A:**879, 1974.

Chapter 15

Patella pain syndromes and chondromalacia patellae

JOHN NEVIL INSALL, M.D.
New York, New York

One of the difficulties in any discussion of chondromalacia patellae is that the term has several meanings. Correctly it describes pathologic changes in the patellar cartilage consisting of softening, fissuring, and fibrillation. Less accurately but still in a descriptive pathologic sense, chondromalacia is often used interchangeably with osteoarthritis in describing articular damage of a more severe degree. Articular erosions in which the underlying subchondral bone is exposed have sometimes been called a stage IV chondromalacia, and indeed the assumption has frequently been made that chondromalacia and osteoarthritis are only different stages of a degenerative process.

Chondromalacia has come to have other meanings. The familiar syndrome of patellar pain in adolescents is often called chondromalacia, though typical pathologic changes are not always found in these cases. Likewise, patellar pain after a direct injury (for example, contact with the dashboard in an automobile accident) is known as "traumatic chondromalacia." Patellar pain in certain athletes, notably runners, may be so described also. Clearly this lack of precision in the nomenclature causes confusion and makes communication misleading. Even the use of "chondromalacia" in the most strict and in the most correct sense as a pathologic description is not without problems. For example, many observers have noted that chondromalacic changes are frequently found in the knee joint and are seen when an arthrotomy is done for the purpose of performing a meniscectomy. The appearance of the articular degeneration often suggests that it has been long-standing, that is, long preceding the injury that caused the meniscal tear, thus existing at a time when the patient considered the knee to be "normal." Autopsy studies have shown that chondromalacia is a normal part of aging and is not uncommon over 30 years of age.[3] This can be confirmed by the examination of normal subjects: crepitus on motion of the knee is a frequent finding. It is therefore undeniable that even extensive chondromalacic change may exist in knee joints that are completely asymptomatic.

If this is so, how can it be explained that identical changes cause symptoms only in some people? Difficulty arises in attempting to explain the mechanism of pain in chondromalacic cartilage because nerve endings have never been found in either normal or abnormal cartilage. Moreover, attempts to explain pain through peripatellar routes (synovium or capsule) have never been convincing. It seems most likely that it is true bone pain and is identical in character to the pain of osteoarthritis in which the explanation of pain from denuded subchondral bone presents no difficulty.

We have then a situation in which chondromalacia is used to describe knee pain in certain people when it is known that similar pathologic changes exist in much of the normal population. The same term is also used to describe a frequently encountered clinical syndrome in young people in whom no pathologic changes at all may be found in arthrotomy.

342

HISTORICAL BACKGROUND

As far as it is known, the first description of chondromalacic cartilage was given by Budinger in 1906.[4] He described fissures that he believed were caused by trauma. The term "chondromalacia," however, was not used by Budinger himself and is attributed to Aleman (1928). Owre[26] (1936) studied the physiologic location of the changes in the patella. He reported that they were most frequently found straddling the patellar crest. Wiberg,[30] on the other hand, believed that chondromalacia was predominantly a disease of the medical facet. He attributed this fact to the convex shape of the medical facet and believed that there was a localized increase in stress in this region. He also believed that symptoms were dependent on the shape of the patella and were most common in those with small vertical and deeply convex facets. This finding is still unconfirmed. Karlson[17] (1939) studied cases that were followed in Aleman's clinic. These were patients in whom a clinical diagnosis had been made, but whose symptoms were insufficient to require surgery. He concluded that the majority continued to have moderately troublesome symptoms, though some improved and some worsened. MacNab,[21] in 1952, emphasized the frequent association of patellar chondromalacia with recurrent dislocation of the patella, an association that would seem to support a traumatic origin.

The following year Harrison, Schajowicz, and Trueta[12] suggested that far from being a manifestation of cartilage overload as Wiberg had supposed, chondromalacia might, in fact, be a disuse phenomenon. They based this observation on anatomic studies of the hip joint in which they observed that the earliest changes characteristic of chondromalacia were invariably found in noncontact zones. Because the nutrition of articular cartilage is derived from the synovial fluid, the penetration of which is aided by the pumping action of alternating pressure, they reasoned that the absence of joint contact might well lead to nutritional insufficiencies. Although the validity of their observations has not been questioned, the concept has not received wide support, even though the idea of disuse remains current at Oxford. Goodfellow and Bullough,[8] in 1967, also described chondromalacic changes in the elbow joint as existing in zones of habitual noncontact. In 1976, Goodfellow[9] described a form of chondromalacia characterized by an abnormal disk of

soft cartilage occurring at the junction of the medial and "odd" facets. The appearance of this disk he attributed to disuse because the odd facet makes contact with the medial femoral condyle only in extremes of flexion, and the full squat position is assumed only infrequently in Western man.

The Oxford group's theories, notwithstanding, most authors have agreed with Budinger that some form of trauma either direct or indirect is most likely responsible. Wiles, Andrews, and Bremner,[31] in an excellent review of the subject, concluded as early as 1956 that chondromalacia was but a precursor of osteoarthritis. They reported on the results of shaving of the patella and, in a further review[32] of the same patients published in 1960, concluded that shaving was a worthwhile procedure. In 1961, Outerbridge[25] described an abnormal ridge on the femur, which he felt made contact with the medial facet of the patella, and he recommended excision of the ridge. However, the constancy of the ridge has not always been confirmed. Ficat and Hungerford[7] believe that there are several forms of chondromalacia, and they describe an entity, the excessive lateral pressure syndrome (ELPS), that they believe is a cause of cartilage degeneration of the lateral facet. In 1976, Insall, Falvo, and Wise[13], noting the frequency of anatomic variants (increased quadriceps angle or high-riding patella) that were found in a group of patients treated for chondromalacia, believed that malalignment is an important cause of chondromalacia, which in fact may be a *forme fruste* of subluxation.

To summarize, the following etiologic factors have been described: trauma, both direct and indirect; habitual pressure, either too much or too little; a dysplasia, similar to that producing patellar dislocation; and premature aging.

DIAGNOSIS OF PATELLOFEMORAL PAIN

Typically, patients with patellar pain complain of an aching pain situated behind the patella, on the medial side of the joint, and sometimes posteriorly in the popliteal fossa. This pain is aggravated by activity, particularly stair climbing, and sometimes by sitting with the knees in a flexed position (the so-called movie sign). The onset of symptoms is usually gradual and unrelated to any significant traumatic episode, though one knee is usually worse than the other. There may also be nonspecific complaints of catching, giving-way, and even locking, but similar complaints can be produced by other "internal derangements." When the pain of chondromalacia is anteromedial and when it is associated with catching and locking, there may be confusion with a torn medial meniscus. Likewise, when there is instability with episodes of giving-way followed by painful swelling, the patellofemoral disorder may be confused with a chronic ligament injury (especially anterior cruciate ligament insufficiency). Diagnostic confusion may occur when an injury seems to have precipitated the onset of the symptoms. Therefore, the exact mechanism of the injury is important. The occurrence of a "pop" is highly suggestive of an anterior cruciate tear.

In obtaining a description of pain, the site is important, though anteromedial pain can occur both with patellar disorders and meniscal injuries. Bilaterality favors a patellar origin as does constant plan (instead of the more usual intermittent types of pain associated with a torn meniscus). It is also important to know whether the pain is provoked by activity or present all the time.

In the assessment of instability an exact description of what happens is important. Complaints of "sliding" or "coming apart" are more suggestive of anterior cruciate lesions. Patients who state "the knee dislocates" are most likely to have a patellar subluxation. Of course, some individuals will describe a kneecap dislocation with precision. Instability on pivoting or cutting movements are nonspecific and can occur from either aforementioned lesions.

Examination should begin with the patient standing with feet together. Any malalignment can then be observed, particularly the "squinting" associated with an increased quadriceps angle. The gait is then observed and the patient is asked to squat holding the halfway position briefly. Pain in this position is usually patellar in origin, whereas inability to perform a deep knee bend is characteristic of meniscal tears.

With the patient sitting on the examining table, active extension is observed from the flexed position. Patellar crepitus can be elicited at this time as well as painful catching. The tibial rotation test attributed to Steinmann is also performed in this position. Sharp external rotation of the flexed knee in a relaxed patient usually produces sharp pain if the meniscus is torn. This maneuver is probably the most reliable of the various rotation tests described for meniscal tears (McMurray, Apley).

With the patient lying down, range of motion is observed as one measures the heel-to-buttock distance in flexion. One can assess the degree of extension with the heel supported, or by positioning the patient prone and extending the feet over the edge of the examining table. The knee is examined for synovitis or effusion. Ligamentous stability is assessed. In this regard, I prefer to describe instability in the four basic quadrants of motion: anterior, posterior, medial, or lateral. Anteroposterior testing with the knee extended may be more informative than the same test done with the knee flexed. When positive, the pivot shift or jerk test is diagnostic of anteroposterior insufficiency.

Finally, specific tests for a patellar disorder are performed. (Abnormalities of patellar tracking and patellar crepitus will have been observed previously.) The knee is now flexed about 30 degrees (usually crossing one knee over the other is sufficient). With the patient as relaxed as possible, the patella is pressed *medially* with the thumbs. Pain thus produced is diagnostic of "chondromalacia." The same test is repeated with the patella being pressed laterally. This is the well-known "apprehension test" and, when positive, is diagnostic of patellar instability.

OTHER INVESTIGATIONS

Roentgenograms. Standard views are a standing anteroposterior (which is normal in patellar disorders), a lateral with the knee semiflexed, and the Merchant skyline view. The lateral view will reveal a high patella (Insall and Salvati ratio) (Figs. 15-1 and 15-2). It will also provide evidence of patellar arthritis, when present. From the Merchant view the sulcus angle and congruence angle are measured. The medial marginal fracture of the patella, diagnostic of patellar dislocation, will also be revealed.

Patellofemoral incongruence (Fig. 15-3). Merchant[24] (1974) described a method of obtaining a patellar "skyline" view. In this technique the patient lies supine with the lower leg over the end of the table with the knees flexed 45 degrees. The roentgenographic tube is placed proximally and angled 60 degrees from the vertical. The roentgenographic plate is positioned at the midtibial area. This technique produces a tangential view of the patellofemoral joint from which two measurements can be obtained: (1) the *sulcus angle* of the femur and (2) the *congruence angle,* which describes the fit of the patella in the femoral sulcus.

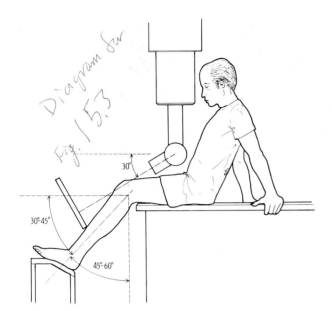

Fig. 15-1. Diagram of a lateral roentgenogram of the knee showing a normally positioned patella measured by the Insall-Salvati method.

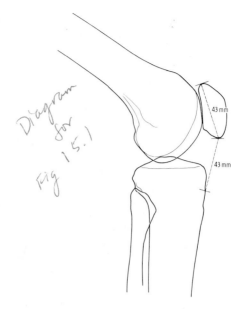

Fig. 15-2. In this diagram the patella is high-riding, and the length of the patella ligament is considerably greater than the diagonal length of the patella. To make the measurement of patella ligament length, one must clearly see the tibial tubercle in profile.

Because of the frequency of anatomic variants in patients with knee pain, Aglietti[1] has studied both normal and abnormal knees. The parameters he measured were (1) the quadriceps angle (Q angle), which is a clinical measurement of the angle formed by the pull of the quadriceps muscle and the inclination of the patellar ligament; (2) the patellar height, measured by the roentgenographic method suggested by Insall and Salvati (a method relating the diagonal length of the patella and the length of the patellar tendon measured to the tibial tubercle, with the measurements being made from the lateral roentgenogram taken in a semiflexed position; and (3) the sulcus angle measured by the Merchant technique; and (4) the congruence angle measured by the Merchant technique.

According to Aglietti, the normal quadriceps angle is 15 degrees, the Insall and Salvati ratio is 1, the sulcus angle 137 degrees (±6 degrees), and the congruence angle −8 degrees (±6 degrees).

Aglietti also measured 90 abnormal knees, 53 with chondromalacia and 37 with recurrent subluxation. He found that in the patients with chondromalacia, the patellar ratio and the sulcus angle were normal but the quadriceps angle was 20 degrees and the congruence angle −2 degrees. Both differences are statistically significant. In the patients with patellar subluxation, the quadriceps

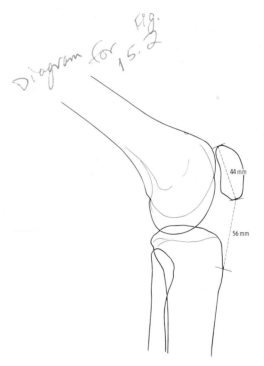

Fig. 15-3. Merchant's technique for obtaining a "skyline" view of the patella. When the patella tendon is of normal length, the angle of knee flexion should be 30 degrees. For high-riding patellas more flexion is required for a tangential view of the patella to be obtained.

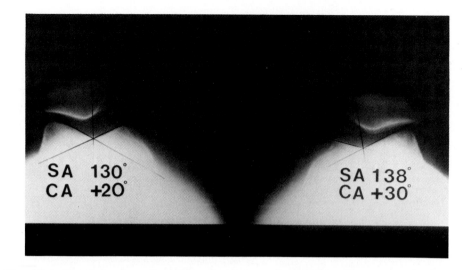

Fig. 15-4. Merchant view of patellas showing an abnormal congruence angle, *CA*, on both sides. The femoral sulcus is marked and a bisecting line drawn. The crest of the patella lies lateral to the bisection of the sulcus and is termed a "positive congruence angle." The normal congruence angle is −8 degrees (the crest of the patella lies medial to the bisection line of the sulcus). The roentgenogram shown is from a case of high-riding patella. Abnormal congruence associated with an increased quadriceps angle is less severe than this. *SA*, Sulcus angle.

angle was normal, the patellar ratio was 1.23, the sulcus angle was 147, and the congruence angle was +16 degrees. These differences are statistically significant. Both types of malalignment syndromes therefore result in significant alterations in the *patellar congruence angle* (Fig. 15-4).

Arthrography. Although direct evidence of chondromalacia by arthrography has been reported, it is not reliable. Arthrography is mainly of value in the diagnosis of meniscal tears where a very high degree of accuracy is possible. At The Hospital for Special Surgery (in New York), double-contrast arthrography is preferred. A poorly performed arthrogram is useless, and good-quality, tangential views of the meniscus are essential.

Arthroscopy. There is no doubt that in the hands of a skilled arthroscopist, a very high degree of diagnostic accuracy is possible. However, much experience is required to reach this level of competence, and the individual surgeon must be realistic about his own ability. When good-quality arthrography is available, arthroscopy is required less frequently. There is also a fundamental difficulty in using the arthroscope to diagnose patellar disorders because the extent of cartilage damage correlates poorly with symptoms. Although quite severe degeneration may be asymptomatic, severe

patellar pain and tenderness can occur in an apparently normal articular surface.

Stress radiography. Stress radiography is useful in documenting ligamentous instability.

Scintimetry. Scintimetry can be used to differentiate "chondromalacia" from osteoarthritis. The scintimetric pattern in the former is normal, whereas in the latter radioisotope uptake is usually greatly increased.

On the basis of a careful history, clinical examination, and the judicious use of ancillary testing, it should be possible to diagnose pain of patellar origin with a high degree of accuracy. It should also be possible to identify the cause of pain most frequently encountered: malalignment syndromes, osteoarthritis, direct trauma, or overuse associated with sports.

PAIN MECHANISMS

Patellar pain is the same in character whatever the cause and presumably arises from bone. When there is cartilage erosion exposing subchondral bone (osteoarthritis), the pain pathway is not difficult to explain. However, in other painful patellar syndromes, the cartilage is more or less intact and presumably the bone is then loaded above the pain threshold by (1) incongruence, (2) overuse, or (3) local cartilage abnormalities (such as fissures or discrete areas of softening). The evidence for the latter mechanisms is in each case theoretical, though tender areas in the patella have been demonstrated in patients under local anesthesia. A chemical or enzymatic pathway by the products of cartilage degeneration seems less likely than a mechanical explanation because (1) cartilage damage is not consistently present, (2) effusion and synovitis are usually absent, and (3) even in the presence of extreme cartilage degeneration (severe osteoarthritis), pain is mostly felt on weight-bearing.

TREATMENT

Because of the significant differences in the response and in the method of treatment selected, it is important to identify the cause of patellar pain.

Conservative treatment. It is standard practice to recommend certain nonsurgical measures in the initial management of patients with patellar pain. The patient's response to treatment will vary with the cause of the patellar pain. It is possible to divide the commonly used modalities into three categories:

Category 1—usually helpful

ACTIVITY. When the patellar pain is clearly related to specific activity (such as running), either the elimination or the altering of this activity can normally be expected to produce an improvement. The use of orthotics in runners has become popular and may be helpful to these patients. Activity change in the malalignment syndromes or when the pain is secondary to direct trauma, however, is much less helpful and the activity level can usually be left to the discretion of the patient, for there is no evidence that activity has any harmful long-term effects.

EXERCISES. An exercise program is recommended so long as care is taken to avoid exacerbation of patellar pain. This usually means performing muscle-strengthening exercises with the knee in extension and avoiding weight-lifting from the flexed position. Weight-lifting can be done from the flexed position provided that the knee is only moved through a painless arc, with extension being stopped as soon as pain is felt.[22] Pain secondary to patellofemoral osteoarthritis responds best. Straight-leg raises done several hundred times daily without weights will produce a dramatic improvement, which will continue for as long as the exercises program is maintained. There is often no discernible response, however, to exercises in the malalignment syndromes.

KNEE BRACES. In malalignment syndromes, a patellar cut-out brace with appropriate padding placed in a horseshoe fashion around the sides and upper pole of the patella is particularly helpful. It is not effective when the pain is secondary to direct trauma.

Category 2—doubtful. Aspirin, though often recommended on theoretical grounds because of a supposed healing effect on articular cartilage, seems to have little effect other than in its known analgesic properties. Aspirin and other anti-inflammatory agents are most likely to be helpful in osteoarthritis but have little or no effect on the malalignment syndromes.

Orthotics may be helpful for certain athletes but are not appropriate for other conditions.

Category 3—not advised. The use of casts and splints is not recommended because of the rapid muscle atrophy produced. One of the objectives of treatment is to preserve good muscle tone, and immobilization has no place in the management of patellar pain. The use of crutches is to a lesser degree open to the same objection and very rarely is indicated. Intra-articular injections with steriods may be helpful for patellofemoral arthritis, and judicious use in such patients is acceptable. However, steroid injections are to be condemned in the malalignment syndromes and for athletes.

SURGICAL TREATMENT

The indications for surgical treatment also vary according to the cause of the patellar pain. Surgery is more effective for malalignment syndromes than for any other causes.

Malalignment syndromes and patellar incongruence. An operation should not be considered with the sole objective of returning the patient to sports. Instead, all kinds of athletic activity should be discontinued, and if this is sufficient to relieve symptoms, the situation must be accepted. An operation can be considered when the patient has had constant symptoms for 6 months or more and has not responded to the type of conservative treatment previously described. Surgery is only indicated for unremitting pain that interferes with everyday activity and where there is sufficient intensity so that the patient cannot live comfortably. The other indication is frequent instability with associated pain and swelling. The most effective conservative measure is a patellar restraining brace, and often this will succeed in lessening pain and controlling instability.

The underlying fault in these cases is malalignment and patellar incongruence. There is often a family history of similar problems and the malalignment may be considered as a dysplasia of the extensor mechanism. Most patients will have (1) an increased quadriceps angle or (2) a high-riding patella or (3) a combination of both. Anatomic abnormalities can be diagnosed from physical examination and by study of lateral radiographs and incongruence confirmed by the Merchant technique. Sometimes incongruence is observed in the absence of abnormal anatomy (as when there is severe atrophy of the vastus medialis after medial meniscectomy). Surgical approaches therefore are aimed at correcting patellar incongruence. Three methods may be used: (1) lateral release of the extensor retinaculum, (2) proximal realignment, and (3) distal realignment.

Lateral release. This may be considered as a "halfway" measure in that it is indicated for milder cases for which a more extensive operation would not be justified. The operation is performed through a small vertical lateral incision, and in addition to the lateral retinaculum, the lower fibers of the vastus lateralis (about 2 inches) are cut. It is usually possible to perform an extra synovial release, though if the synovium is entered it is not important. The blood vessels that cross the region about an inch or more distal to the vastus lateralis can bleed profusely if not coagulated. Motion can begin a few days after surgery and recovery occurs in about 3 weeks. It is also possible to perform the procedure through the arthroscope, and some surgeons prefer this method. However, coagulation of potential bleeding points cannot be achieved, and thus the risk of hemarthrosis is greater. It is also impossible to adequately divide the vastus lateralis through the arthroscope.

The results of lateral release are somewhat unpredictable. Thirty-two operations have been done at The Hospital for Special Surgery, and for about half of these patients there was some improvement. Of the remainder, seven knees have had a subsequent and successful proximal realignment.

Proximal realignment. This is the definitive procedure for patellar symptoms secondary to malalignment, malposition, and incongruence.

Surgical technique of proximal realignment[15] (Figs. 15-5 to 15-9). The operation is done under tourniquet exsanguinating the limb either by elevation or with a bandage. A midline skin incision is made extending proximally from the tibial tubercle for a distance of approximately 6 inches (15 cm). The skin edges are undermined sufficiently to expose the patella and quadriceps expansion: the incision should be sufficiently extensive so that the components of the quadriceps tendon are seen. Both the vastus medialis and the vastus lateralis are clearly exposed, as well as the proximal extent of the quadriceps tendon with the insertion of the fibers from rectus femoris. Arthrotomy is performed by an incision beginning proximally at the apex of the quadriceps tendon and placed within the tendon close to the border of vastus medialis. The incision is continued distally to the patella and extended across the medial third of this bone and then distally medial to the patellar ligament. The incision described is therefore straight. The fibers of the quadriceps

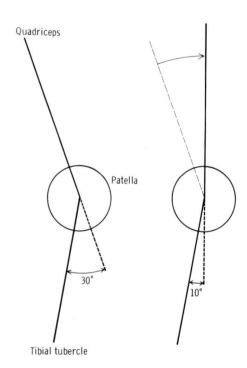

Fig. 15-5. The objective of proximal realignment is to make the quadriceps muscle pull medially. As shown in the diagram this will result in a functional reduction of the quadriceps angle (though the surface measurement of the Q angle will be unchanged and may even be slightly increased because the patella is returned to a normal relationship within the femoral sulcus).

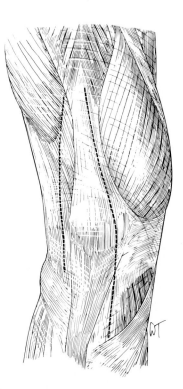

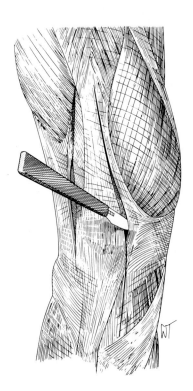

Fig. 15-6. Capsular incisions made for proximal patella realignment. The medial incision is almost straight and crosses over the medial edge of the patella. It extends proximally to the apex of the quadriceps tendon. The lateral capsular incision extends as far proximally as the medial incision dividing the lower fibers of the vastus lateralis.

Fig. 15-7. The medial capsular incision is developed when one separates the medial quadriceps expansion from the surface of the patella by sharp dissection.

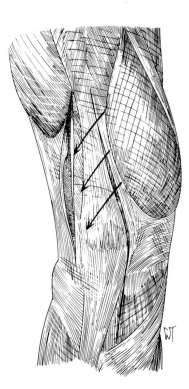

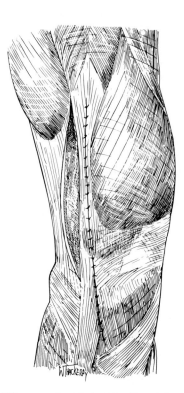

Fig. 15-8. Realignment is achieved by overlapping of the medial flap "over and down."

Fig. 15-9. The completed closure shows that the vastus medialis has been brought laterally and distally across the patella. It is virtually impossible to overdo the amount of overlap, and in fact the usual error is an inadequate release of the vastus lateralis and insufficient overlap.

expansion medial to the incision are dissected from the patella with a scalpel. Because of the vertical ridges on the anterior surface of the patella, this can present difficulty and should be done with deliberation and care so that the quadriceps expansion is preserved intact and without lacerations. This is necessary to obtain a secure closure when the quadriceps repair is completed. The fibers of the expansion can be easily separated from the bone if one dissects from above to below alternately leaving the thinnest central part until last, thereby forming a V. When done in this manner, the central portion separates from the bone easily and can be fully preserved. At the medial border of the patella the synovial covering is incised and distally the fat pad is divided in the line of the capsular incision sufficiently to allow the joint to be explored with the patella everted.

A second capsular incision is now made on the lateral side, beginning proximally in the fibers of the vastus lateralis 1 cm from the apex of the quadriceps tendon. The incision is continued distally with the same relationship to the quadriceps tendon being maintained to a point corresponding to the lower pole of the patella. It is desirable, but not essential, to maintain the integrity of the synovial cavity. Sometimes this is not possible because of fibrous bands that appear to be in the substance of the synovium itself, but if holes are made no harm is done. There are a number of substantial vessels that cross to the patella in the lateral retinaculum. There is a group of vessels, two or three in number as a rule, at the level of the upper pole of the patella, usually the largest, that will bleed profusely if not coagulated or ligated. A second group of vessels runs in the fat pad more distally at the lower pole of the patella, usually one or two in number. These also should be identified and coagulated.

The interior of the knee is thoroughly explored and may often appear to be normal. However, in those knees in which the patella is high riding, "chondromalacic" changes may be present. When these are seen, they are usually as described by Owre in the region of the patellar crest extending for a variable distance onto the medial and lateral facets. The distribution of these changes is fairly symmetric and may extend to the medial and lateral margins of the patella forming an elliptic area of softening in the middle third of the patellar articular surface. Only rarely is the cartilage on either the upper or lower part involved.

The articular cartilage abnormalities may consist entirely of swelling and softening, but deep fissures, which usually run roughly parallel to the crest, are also common and may extend through the full thickness of the cartilage. In the more severe cases, the cartilage may have a jelly-like consistency and can be moved a few millimeters from side to side.

Occasionally two other lesions may be seen:

1. *Blisters.* A circular eruption rarely more than 7 mm in diameter sometimes occurs usually situated just medial to the patellar crest and more distal than proximal. The remaining articular cartilage usually appears almost normal. Sometimes the surface of the blister is intact, though protruding from the surface of the adjoining more normal cartilage. At other times the surface may have broken and quite long fronds can be present.

2. *"Crab meat" lesions.* Almost the entire articular surface may have degenerated (saving the most proximal and distal articular rim of cartilage) giving rise to an appearance characteristic of the name. Crab meat lesions are seen almost exclusively with a high-riding patella, though not necessarily with a history of patellar dislocation.

In the malignment syndromes, regardless of the extent of the patellar lesions, the femoral groove is normal. (The only exception is occasional evidence of an osteochondral fracture at the lateral border of the femoral sulcus caused by a patellar dislocation.) In older individuals erosive changes may be seen, together with a similar appearance on the patella itself, and this kind of appearance should be characterized as a degenerative arthritis. Usually some other type of surgical management is required.

Chondroplasty. Shaving or excision of articular lesions must be considered. Although no definitive evidence exists as to the best management of these, it is true that no repair is possible unless the entire thickness of articular cartilage is removed followed by curettage, or drilling of the underlying bone. In these circumstances, however, only an imperfect repair of fibrocartilage occurs; often the surface is no better than what existed before excision, and sometimes it is worse. If the area of chondromalacia is small and circumscribed (for example, blister lesions), excision may be the best course, but crab meat lesions covering a large area should not be excised because it is unlikely that subsequent formation of fibrocartilage will provide an adequate surface. A conservative shaving is better, with projecting fronds being removed so that the surface becomes more or less smooth. Shaving creates a depression so that a portion of the patellar articular surface is removed from the articulation and it is no longer making contact with the opposing surface of the femur.

The third method, which is preferred in most cases, is simply to leave the patellar surface as it is. This is the course that should be followed when the surface is grossly smooth even though extensive softening and fissuring may be present. As discussed later, it is highly likely that the mechanism of pain is largely independent from the integrity of the articular surface so that a conservative approach to chondroplasty, if this is done at all, seems the best course.

Quadriceps reconstruction. At this stage of the operation the tourniquet should be released to enable any bleeding points not previously identified to be coagulated. The tourniquet is reinflated and a thorough irrigation performed. Then the quadriceps must be reconstructed in such a manner that the subsequent line of pull will be more medial. This is the purpose of the entire operative procedure, and it is by altering the direction of quadriceps action that patellar congruence is restored and patellar instability prevented. The first suture is placed in such a manner that the most distal part of the vastus medialis is brought as far as possible laterally and distally, overlapping the upper pole of the patella and adjoining the quadriceps tendon. Before performing this overlap, the synovium should be removed from the deep surface of the medial flap, which comprises the vastus medialis, the medial part of the quadriceps expansion and, distally, the medial capsule of the knee. The amount of overlap that can be achieved depends on the preoperative laxity of the tissues. In some knees the vastus medialis will be sutured to the lateral border of the patella, but the more usual amount of overlap is 10 to 15 mm. The second suture is inserted at the lower pole of the patella also bringing across the medial flap as tightly as the tissues will allow. The type of suture material used is not important and may be absorbable or nonabsorbably according to the surgeon's preference. The two initial sutures determine the remainder of the closure. On the patella and distally, the sutures are placed so that the medial flap is tight. Proximally the vastus medialis is brought over the quadriceps tendon and sutured to the

distal stump of vastus lateralis at the lateral border of the quadriceps tendon. The suture line is straight and in the midline and when completed should be tested by flexion of the knee to at least 90 degrees. If any sutures are broken that portion of the repair is too tight and should be loosened appropriately.

Two features of the repair should be emphasized:

1. The incision into vastus lateralis extends proximally as far as the medial incision. The most common error is a reluctance to make and adequate division of the vastus lateralis; unless this is done, a proximal rearrangement of the quadriceps is not possible. One might expect that an extensive division of the muscle would cause quadriceps weakness, but in practice this does not seem to be the case.

2. The more distal part of the closure (over the patella and distal to the patella) must be tight. It is impossible to overdo the overlapping because this is prevented by soft-tissue tension and the anatomy of the femoral sulcus. Medial dislocation as a result of excessively tight closure has not been seen. At the completion of an adequate repair, it will be seen that the lateral facet of the patella rides off the corresponding surface of the femoral sulcus (though this can only be clearly seen if the synovium has been opened).

The most common mistake is to perform an insufficient operation with too little overlap of the medial flap and insufficient division of the vastus lateralis.

After a routine closure of the skin a compression dressing is applied. A suction drain is not normally needed.

Aftercare. The patient is allowed to get out of bed on the second postoperative day and from the beginning is allowed full weight-bearing as tolerated. Crutches are usually needed for a few days, and the patient can go home within a week. The compression dressing is left in place for 2 full weeks, at which time the sutures are removed. Straight-leg raises are then begun (if the quadriceps is not working by this time, side raises are done initially). Flexion is also allowed and encouraged. With normal progress, 90 degrees of flexion is reached approximately 4 to 6 weeks after surgery, and at this time the gait has returned to normal. Three hundred straight-leg raises each day are continued by the patient, and my preference is to avoid weights completely because it has not proved necessary to rehabilitate quadriceps strength and may provoke patellar pain if used too vigorously.

RESULTS OF PROXIMAL REALIGNMENT

The results from 65 patients (10 bilateral) were recently studied.[28] There were 25 males and 40 females. The malalignment was manifest as an increase in the quadriceps angle in 36 knees, a high-riding patella in 21 knees, and a combination of high-riding and increased quadriceps angle in 18 knees. The follow-up time was from 2 to 10 years. The results were excellent in 37%, good in 54% fair in 5%, and poor in 4%. Postoperative Merchant views were taken in 55 knees. There were 50 knees in the excellent and good categories, and in these the average congruence angle was normal (−11 degrees). Five knees, in the fair and poor categories, showed an abnormal congruence angle (average +5 degrees), suggesting that adequate correction of incongruence is necessary to obtain a good result. Twenty-one of the 75 knees also had a chondroplasty. (Most were done early in the series when excision of damaged cartilage was the rule, whereas later a more selective approach was adopted.) The results of the chondroplasty were almost identical with the group as a whole. The current policy is to reserve chondroplasty for blister and crab meat lesions (grade III) and to leave alone softening and fissuring (grades I and II). Whether it is better to excise en bloc or to more superficially shave damaged cartilage is still not determined. It is true that theoretically en bloc excision is preferred, as only this allows any degree of healing. However, such healing as does occur is often imperfect in a large proportion of cases (some estimates put this as high as 40%). Our experience has demonstrated this at subsequent arthrotomy in unsuccessful cases, and even a good fibrocartilaginous repair does not produce a normal articular surface. With this in mind, it is a good principle to leave the articular surface alone when it seems probable that the expected repair would be no better, or possibly worse, except for excision of only the areas that are so damaged that even a poor reconstitution would be an improvement. Using the same principle, shaving of some areas may be preferable to en bloc excision, depending on the depth of cartilage degeneration.

DISTAL REALIGNMENT

Under this heading come all procedures in which the attachment of the patellar ligament to the tibial tubercle is detached and transferred in a medial and distal direction, thereby reducing the quadriceps angle and, to some extent, correcting patella alta. Many variations exist and the exact technique may consist of removal of a block of bone, which is then locked into a slot cut distally and medially (the Hauser operation), or more simply by removal of the ligament insertion together with a sliver of bone, which is then reattached with staples. The latter method not only is simpler, but allows greater precision in placement. A lateral release is usually combined with a distal transfer and sometimes an advancement of the vastus medialis obliquus.

In an earlier series of cases published in 1976[13] the results of distal realignment were excellent and good in 23 of 34 knees (68%). This compares with 53 cases of proximal realignment done over the same period of time in which the excellent and good proportion was 81%. In another study[6] at The Hospital for Special Surgery, the results of the Hauser operation were studied retrospectively in 69 additional knees with an average follow-up time of 8 years. Significant complications occurred, and largely because of this, 19 subsequent operations of 14 knees have been done. (Five of these were revisions for further dislocation, and five were tibial osteotomies for deformity secondary to arrest of the proximal tibial epiphysis.) After revision excellent and good results were obtained in 72%. To compare these results to the results without surgery, we reviewed 26 knees with patellar dislocations that were seen during the same period of time, but in which surgery was not done (an operation either was not recommended or was refused by the patient). In this group dislocation was generally less frequent, but the follow-up time was longer than for the surgical cases (average 16 years). Excellent and good results were seen in 18 of the 26 knees (69%) or about the same proportion as in the surgical group. The major reason for an unsatisfactory result after operation was pain, whereas for the nonsurgical cases it was continued instability though very few became painful. A study of the postoperative roentgenographs revealed the reason. Evidence of osteoarthritis was seen in the majority of the surgical cases, whereas it was rare in those managed conservatively. These findings are in agreement with Hampson and Hill[11] (1975), who found that 70% of knees followed for more than 10 years after the Hauser operation had roentgenologic evidence of osteoarthritis.

In our study we were not able to correlate excessive distal transfer of the patellar tendon with the degree of osteoarthritis; rather it appeared that medial transfer was the factor most responsible. Medial transfer causes an excessive external rotation of the tibia, but more importantly because of the triangular shape of the upper tibia, it is also a posterior transfer.[10] The effect of moving the ligament insertion posteriorly produces a relative increase in articular pressure because the quadriceps muscle is now working at a mechanical disadvantage. This situation is the reverse of the tibial tubercle elevation that is proposed by Maquet[23] to reduce patellofemoral contact pressure.

Techniques of distal transfer that mitigate the unfavorable effect described do exist. It will be less, for example, when only half of the patellar ligament is transferred medially. The Elmslie and Trillat method,[29] especially when combined with a bone graft, results in a pure medial transfer without any posterior displacement. The results of proximal realignment for this condition have been consistently good so that it seems reasonable to make this the routine operation of choice, with distal realignment being reserved only for failure of the proximal operation or the infrequent cases in which there is such severe abnormality of the extensor mechanism that the patella cannot be repositioned by proximal realignment alone.

Operative treatment should be reserved for those with very frequent dislocations or for those in whom pain is a disabling symptom. It does not seem necessary to recommend any type of realignment for patellar instability on the grounds that the operation is necessary to prevent osteoarthritis. Possibly with longer experience of proximal realignment this advice may change since it would seem that correction of patellar incongruence can only be beneficial. At present there is no evidence that proximal realignment is associated with the late development of osteoarthritis.

PATELLAR PAIN CAUSED BY OTHER SYNDROMES

In the treatment of patellar pain from overuse osteoarthritis, idiopathic cartilage degeneration,

direct trauma, or any other cause, surgery is not nearly so satisfactory. In these situations it is recommended that conservative treatment should be followed if possible.

There are a number of surgical procedures to be considered: débridement, decompression by tibial tubercle elevation, patellar replacement, and patellectomy.

Débridement. Débridement alone, not associated with realignment, has a mixed reputation. Some authors have reported success with this method particularly when the subchondral bone is drilled, whereas others have found the procedure unpredictable and unreliable. Our experience[14] would suggest that the later view is correct (unless the case is also suitable for a realignment procedure). Otherwise, about two-thirds of the patients may be expected to show some improvement, whereas the remaining third will not and some of these will be worse. The major indication is for active middle-aged people with early degenerative arthritis who have not responded well to conservative management. Posttraumatic chondromalacia may also be treated by débridement, though the results are often unsatisfactory and patellectomy is usually a better choice. The other indications for excision are the Goodfellow cartilage lesion at the junction of medial and odd facets and the Outerbridge bony ridge on the femur.

Patellar resurfacing. Previous reports for patellar replacement have not been very encouraging.[19] In 1974[2] we described the design of a new patellar prosthesis that because of its dome shape did not require a rotatory realignment. The fixation was made by cement, and we believed from our early experience that the design change might give improved results.

Recently the results of 29 patellar prostheses of this type were studied.[16] The diagnosis was osteoarthritis in 22 knees, chondromalacia occurring after a Hauser procedure in five knees, and habitual dislocation with severe osteoarthritis in two knees. The follow-up time was from 3 to 6 years. Seven patients were male, and 21 females with an average age of 47 years (range, 17 to 73 years). In 12 knees there was also evidence of femoral tibial arthritis. Six knees were associated with high tibial osteotomy.

The results were excellent in two knees; good, in 14 knees; fair, in three knees; and poor, in 10 knees. In five of the 10 poor cases the patella together with the implant was later removed. Of the remainder, four knees had persistent pain and crepitus, and one knee had a postoperative dislocation that although repaired resulted in persistent quadriceps weakness. In the 12 knees with degenerative arthritis (without femoral tibial narrowing), the result was good in eight (67%). The results in chondromalacia were surprisingly no better than in osteoarthritis, though in these cases the femoral groove initially had normal articular cartilage.

Except in one case the poor results were all attributable to persistent pain, which seemed to be caused by the well-known unpredictability of a metallic partial joint replacement. No doubt the results could be improved if the patellar groove were also resurfaced with polyethylene. We are unwilling to accept this solution for isolated patellar femoral arthritis, however, because salvage cannot then be obtained by patellectomy alone. We believe instead that patients who might be candidates for this type of prosthesis would be better treated by total knee replacement. Likewise, it seems unwise to combine patellar replacement with tibial osteotomy because these cases also are better managed by total knee replacement.

Patellar replacement in the younger patients with patellar disorders and who had already failed to respond to a previous surgical procedure such as realignment was disappointing.

Tibial tubercle elevation. This procedure advocated by Maquet[23] is based upon the biomechanic principle that increasing the lever arm reduces the pressure across the patellar femoral joint. It can also be used to enhance quadriceps action after patellectomy.[18] Reports in the literature have mostly been favorable, but our experience has not confirmed this.[27] Thirty knees were studied after the procedure. The diagnosis was chondromalacia in 15 knees and patellar femoral osteoarthritis in 14 knees, and two cases followed a patellectomy. The average age was 34 years (range, 16 to 38 years). The patients were followed from 1 to 5 years. Seventeen knees had various prior procedures (including five Hauser procedures and eight meniscectomies).

The operative technique was similar to that described by Maquet. An anterior longitudinal approach to the tibial tubercle was made and the crest of the tibia elevated by a long tonguelike os-

teotomy extending some 10 cm distally. The tibial tubercle and crest were then elevated anteriorly with the distal attachment being left intact, and bone graft was placed proximally to maintain the advancement. The graft was obtained from the adjoining proximal tibia in 15 cases, the iliac crest in 12, and the excised patella in four knees (when done in conjunction with patellectomy). Usually the graft was securely locked in place by mechanical means, but in three knees a screw was also needed. The initial amount of elevation averaged 1.75 cm, but some settling usually occurred; therefore, the average elevation at the time of follow-up was 1.37 cm.

The operation was combined with tibial osteotomy (eight knees), proximal realignment (six knees), and patellectomy (four knees). In the remaining 12 knees the tibial tubercle elevation was done as a solitary procedure.

There were a significant number of complications. Skin necrosis occurred in the region of the tibial tubercle in four knees, which in one case led to a subsequent deep infection ultimately requiring débridement and skin grafting before healing. A stress fracture through the tibial tubercle proximal to the graft occurred in three knees, resulting in the formation of a separate small ossicle. In all of these, there was some residual tenderness and slight extension weakness. The ossicle was excised in one knee because of local tenderness. A fracture through the proximal tibia occurred in one case: an obese female who fell 6 weeks after the operation. The fracture resulted in a nonunion that has to date not healed despite two bone-grafting procedures. There were two deep infections, one, as mentioned before, occurred after a skin necrosis.

Evaluation of the results in these cases is complicated by varying causes and additional procedures done at the same time. However, these variables will be found in any comparable series for which the indications exist.

The major preoperative complaint was pain, and a subsidiary complaint, in some cases, was weakness and buckling. The success or failure of the procedure thus depended largely on relief of pain with the element of subjectivity that this implies. Complications previously noted were not taken into account, except insofar as they affected the result at the time of evaluation.

Because of the number of associated procedures, it was decided to divide the knees into two groups for evaluation:

Maquet alone—12 knees: The results were good in eight knees, fair in two knees, and poor in two knees.

Maquet combined—18 knees: The results in this group were good in 10 knees, fair in seven knees, and poor in one knee.

From this it can be seen that about two thirds of the patients gained satisfactory pain relief whether the Maquet was done by itself or combined with another operation. The remaining two thirds were not improved, and three knees were actually worse. The poor rating in two knees was directly attributable to a complication: in one, a persistent nonunion of a tibial fracture and, in the other, an osteomyelitis after deep infection.

Our conclusion concerning the merits of the operation was although the procedure did relieve pain in the majority of cases, the significant number of serious complications and the unpredictability of the result must limit the indications to a few severely disabled cases.

Patellectomy. Patellectomy has been the subject of controversy for many years, and although some authors claim good results, the majority opinion is that excision of the patella should be a end-of-the-road solution to the problem of patellar pain. Most published series have contained a mixed group of patients, and the indications have included rheumatoid arthritis, osteoarthritis, chondromalacia, and patellar fractures. This and the association of arthritis in the femoral tibial joint has made evaluation difficult. Our experience is probably representative. In a recent retrospective study of a 100 cases of patellectomies,[20] the result was considered good in 72 knees. Failure was nearly always attributable to unrelieved pain with, in some cases, additional complaints of weakness and instability. The age of the patient, range of motion, extension lag, and cosmesis were not important factors. Calcification in the patellar tendon was not related to complaints of pain, and the type of surgical technique also did not seem to influence the outcome.

With regard to technique, a recently published method of patellectomy is worthy of consideration.[5] After enucleation of the patella through a longitudinal incision, the patellar tendon is "tubed" so that the original anterior surface (originally subcutaneous) now articulates in the femoral groove. The rationale is that any ossification in the tendon now lies within the tube and hence will not be a source of irritation. Excellent and good results were claimed in 90% of cases using this technique, which is better than any other published series.

In our experience the results of débridement, patellar replacement, tibial tubercle elevation, and patellectomy are similar. For all these procedures roughly two thirds of the patients improve and one third do not. The choice between them must thus be based upon individual experience, a consideration of the possible complications, and the options that remain should the procedure fail. With the latter in mind, patellar débridement and patellar replacement offer a clear advantage in that the option of patellectomy still remains. The much greater incidents of serious complications are a disadvantage to tibial tubercle elevation. Patellectomy is a relatively simple procedure, gives results comparable to any of the others, and possibly by use of the "tube" technique may emerge as the preferred choice for these difficult cases.

SUMMARY

Patellar pain must be separated from other causes of internal derangement of the knee by a careful history and precise examination followed by appropriate investigations. Once the cause of the pain is determined, malalignment or malposition of the patella must be sought. The Merchant view of the patellar femoral joint is recommended in this regard to demonstrate patellar incongruence. The malalignment syndrome may or may not show the pathologic changes described as "chondromalacia" and respond particularly well after proximal patellar realignment.

In the remaining cases, pain may be caused by overuse, trauma, the odd-facet syndrome, an abnormal femoral ridge, or degenerative arthritis. This group of cases should be managed conservatively if possible because the results of surgical treatment are often disappointing. In selected cases some improvement may occur after excision of abnormal cartilage, tibial tubercle elevation, patellar replacement, or patellectomy

REFERENCES

1. Aglietti, P.: Personal communication, New York, 1980.
2. Aglietti, P., Insall, J., Walker, P.S., and Trent, P.: A new patella prosthesis: design and application, Clin. Orthop. **107:**175-187, 1975.
3. Bennett, G.A., Waine, H., and Bauer, W.: Changes in the knee joint at various ages. New York, 1942, The Commonwealth Fund.
4. Büdinger, K.: Über Ablösung von Gelenkteilen und verwandte Prozesse, Dtsch. Z. für Chir. **84:**311-365, 1906.
5. Compere, C.L., Hill, J.A., Lewinnek, G.E., and Thompson, R.G.: A new method of patellectomy for patellofemoral arthritis, J. Bone Joint Surg. **61A:**714-719, 1979.
6. Crosby, E.B., and Insall, J.: Recurrent dislocation of the patella: relation of treatment to osteoarthritis, J. Bone Joint Surg. **58A:**9-13, 1976.
7. Ficat, R.P., and Hungerford, D.S.: Disorders of the patellofemoral joint, Baltimore, 1977, The Williams & Wilkins Co.
8. Goodfellow, J.W., and Bullough, P.G.: The pattern of ageing of the articular cartilage of the elbow joint, J. Bone Joint Surg. **49B:**175-181, 1967.
9. Goodfellow, J., Hungerford, D.S., and Woods, C.: Patellofemoral joint mechanics and pathology. 2. Chondromalacia patellae, J. Bone Joint Surg. **58B:**291-299, 1976.
10. Goutallier, D., and DeBeyre, J.: Le recentrate rotulien dans les arthroses fémoro-patellaires latéralisées, Rev. Chir. Orthop. **60:**377-386, 1974.
11. Hampson, W.G.J., and Hill, P.: Late results of transfer of the tibial tubercle for recurrent dislocation of the patella, J. Bone Joint Surg. **57B:**209-213, 1975.
12. Harrison, M.H.M., Schajowicz, F., and Trueta, J.: Osteoarthritis of the hip: a study of the nature and evolution of the disease, J. Bone Joint Surg. **35B:**598-626, 1953.
13. Insall, J., Falvo, K.A., and Wise, D.W.: Chondromalacia patellae: a prospective study, J. Bone Joint Surg. **58A:**1-8, 1976.
14. Insall, J.:, The Pridie debridement operation for osteoarthritis of the knee, Clin. Orthop. **101:**61-67, 1974.
15. Insall, J., Bullough, P.G., and Burstein, A.H.: Proximal "tube" realignment of the patella for chondromalacia patellae, Clin. Orthop. **144:**63-69, 1979.
16. Insall, J., Tria, A.F., and Aglietti, P.: Resurfacing of the patella, J. Bone Joint Surg. **62A:**933-936, 1980.
17. Karlson, S.: Chondromalacia patellae, Acta Chir. Scand. **83:**374-381, 1939.
18. Kaufer, H.: Mechanical function of the patella, J. Bone Joint Surg. **53A:**1551, 1971.
19. Levitt, R.L.: A long-term evaluation of patellar prostheses, Clin. Orthop. **97:**153-157, 1973.
20. Lewis, M.M., Fitzgerald, P., Jacobs, B., and Insall, J.: Patellectomy: an analysis of one hundred cases, J. Bone Joint Surg. **58A:**736, 1976.
21. Macnab, I.: Recurrent dislocation of the patella, J. Bone Joint Surg. **34A:**957-976, 1952.
22. Marshall, J.: Personal communication, 1979.
23. Maquet, P.G.: Biomechanics of the knee, Heidelberg, 1976, Springer-Verlag.
24. Merchant, A.C., Mercer, R.L., Jacobsen, R.H., and Cool, C.R.: Roentgenographic analysis of patellofemoral congruence, J. Bone Joint Surg. **56A:**1391-1396, 1974.
25. Outerbridge, R.E.: The etiology of chondromalacia patellae, J. Bone Joint Surg. **43B:**752-757, 1961.
26. Owre, A.: Chondromalacia patellae, Acta Chir. Scand., Suppl. 41, 1936.
27. Rozbruch, J., Campbell, R.D., and Insall, J.: Tibial tubercle elevation (the Maquet operation): a clinical study of thirty-one cases, Orthop. Trans. **3:**291-292, 1979.
28. Tria, A.J., Insall, J., and Aglietti, P.: Anatomic basis of patellar pain. Presented at the American Academy of Orthopaedic Surgeons Meeting, Atlanta, Georgia, 1980.
29. Trillat, A., Dejour, H., and Coutette, A.: Diagnostic et traitement des subluxations récidivantes de la rotule, Rev. Chir. Orthop. **50:**813-824, 1964.
30. Wiberg, G.: Roentgenographic and anatomic studies on the femoropatellar joint, with special reference to chondromalacia patellae, Acta Orthop. Scand. **12:**319-410, 1941.
31. Wiles, P., Andrews, P.S., and Bremner, R.A.: Chondromalacia of the patella: a study of later results of excision of articular cartilage, J. Bone Joint Surg. **42B:**65-70, 1960.
32. Wiles, P., Andrews, P.S., and Devas, M.B.: Chondromalacia of the patella, J. Bone Joint Surg. **38B:**95-113, 1956.

Chapter 16

Operative arthroscopy of the knee

ROBERT W. METCALF, M.D.
Salt Lake City, Utah

BACKGROUND AND HISTORY

Nearly every surgical specialty now has an "-oscopy" of some type that allows the conversion of certain "open" operations to "closed" endoscopic techniques. Many of these new procedures would have been considered impossible to do just a few years ago. This general advance in endoscopic practice and technology is attributable to two main factors: first, the great improvement in instruments, lenses, and fiberoptics and, second, the willingness of surgeons to explore the possibilities that this technology permits.

The results in each specialty have been similar. There has been general skepticism at first, followed by many surgeons wanting to do endoscopic surgery but finding the techniques completely foreign to any prior experience they have had, thus making the learning process a self-taught endeavor requiring much patience and persistence.

Orthopedic surgery is no exception in the expansion of this new endoscopic technology. In the past 4 years, arthroscopic surgery of the knee has become a feasible alternative to arthrotomy for certain types of knee disorders.

The origins of surgical arthroscopy are entwined with the developmental history of diagnostic arthroscopy. The Japanese, so innovative in looking into the knee joint and photographing it, also began doing limited meniscal resections as early as 1962.[24,25,59] In North America, O'Connor[49] designed the first operating arthroscope (Fig. 16-1) in 1975 and also pioneered the concept that significant surgery can be done for certain knee problems using arthroscopic techniques.

Knee surgery through an endoscope is appealing because of the benefits to patients, which include the following:

1. Reduced initial morbidity (outpatient surgery, decreased pain, immediate ambulation, tiny incisions, and so on)
2. More rapid knee rehabilitation
3. Significant reduction in postoperative complications
4. Minimal intervention with almost no disruption of normal surrounding knee muscles and fascial layers
5. Accurate evaluation of the knee disorder with potential for more accurate surgery
6. Possible reduction in degenerative sequelae, such as those seen after total meniscectomy
7. As a net result of all the above factors, a reduction in the need for further or repeated surgeries to correct the original problem.

However, the technique can be difficult and frustrating to learn and will probably not appeal to every orthopedic surgeon. Technologic advances in instruments and standardization of surgery methods and instruction are making operative arthroscopy easier to master. The learning process is still longer than many busy orthopedic surgeons have time for. It is based on a desire to learn an entirely new skill. There is a step-by-step building of experience based first on proficiency in diagnostic arthroscopy.

Despite the disadvantages associated with the learning of operative arthroscopy, there is currently (1980) much interest in this new knee surgery method among orthopedic surgeons. It is entirely possible that arthroscopic knee surgery will become the standard of care for some types of

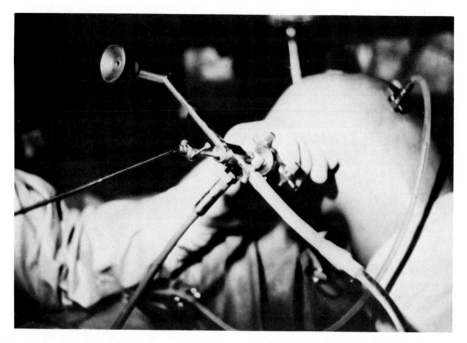

Fig. 16-1. O'Connor-design operating arthroscope inserted into the posteromedial compartment of the left knee. A 3 mm instrument is about to be passed through the central operating channel. Note the offset viewing eyepiece and the attached fiberoptic light cable and tubing for continuous inflow of irrigating fluid.

knee disorders. It should be stressed that this is presently not the case. Traditional methods of open-knee surgery that have given good results should not be abandoned too quickly. Long-term results are not yet available for arthroscopic procedures such as patellar shaving and partial meniscectomy. Although 3 and 4-year arthroscopic results can now be tabulated, this is not enough time to compare with the long-term results in the literature for similar procedures done by arthrotomy.[2,4,8,15,20,26,27,35,36,39,48,50,56,58]

A SELF-TAUGHT TECHNIQUE

Arthroscopic surgery involves a different type of surgical skill. Small (3 to 5 mm diameter) instruments are used that are manipulated in a tight, closed compartment (Fig. 16-2). Everything is greatly magnified. Because of the monocular lens system, everything is two-dimensional, making depth perception a matter of experience rather than observation.

As orthopedic surgeons we have no prior training that gives a background for endoscopic work. It takes time and patience to learn the techniques. The training process is not difficult unless it is

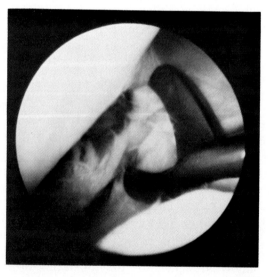

Fig. 16-2. Arthroscopic view of the tip of a 3 mm scissors inserted to begin resection of a posterior horn tear of the medial meniscus. This amount of magnification can be difficult to get accustomed to.

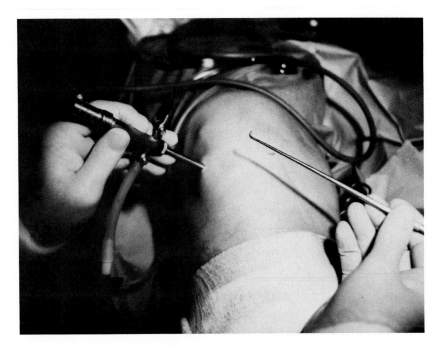

Fig. 16-3. Probe used to palpate menisci and other parts of the knee joint. Probe is inserted directly percutaneously without the use of a sleeve.

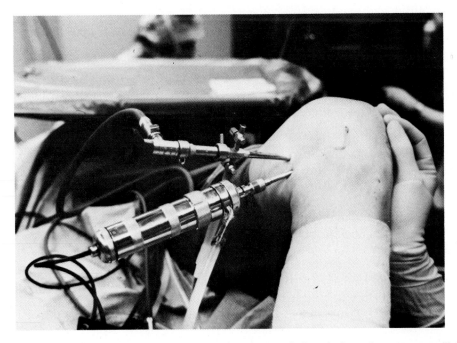

Fig. 16-4. Motorized meniscal cutter has been inserted directly into the posteromedial compartment for removal of a posterior horn flap tear. The 5 mm arthroscope is used here for observation. This is an example of the use of "triangulation" techniques for meniscal surgery.

rushed. It is mostly a self-taught learning process. There is a graduated step-by-step progression of skills that develops, but not overnight. The following is a suggested list and order of development of these arthroscopic skills:

1. Diagnostic arthroscopy—managing the basic exam.[1,5,7,10-12,16,37,42,49,53,54]
2. Use of a probe (Fig. 16-3).
3. Learning to triangulate so as to be able to position an instrument to a desired place inside the joint. This is a stereoscopic "sixth sense" that develops.[60]
4. Facility in changing easily from use of small scopes to larger scopes and vice versa, to enable exploration of all parts of the joint.
5. The ability to solve all problems of visualization, for example, fat pad in the way, bleeding, and keeping adequate flow rate. Not being able to see clearly is one of the primary roadblocks to doing good posterior intra-articular surgery.
6. Posterior compartment puncture—becoming familiar with the anatomy and being able to insert smaller and larger scopes and other instruments into the posterior recesses (Fig. 16-4).
7. Use of motorized equipment.
8. Positioning of drills and curettes within the joint; drilling defects in the femoral condyles and patella.
9. Placement of threaded pins across an osteochondritic fragment using triangulation and arthroscopic control.

TYPES OF LESIONS TREATED

There is also an order of difficulty with the types of knee lesions that can be managed by arthroscopic surgery. The easier procedures can be done earlier in one's experience. More difficult procedures, such as resection of a complicated posterior horn meniscal tear, should not be attempted until confidence is gained in the managing of the simple knee lesions. If a more complicated problem is encountered during diagnostic arthroscopy than had been anticipated from a clinical exam, it is much better to proceed with standard, open-knee surgery rather than struggling with an endoscopic procedure. The question is often asked, How many diagnostic cases should be done before arthroscopic surgery is attempted? This question cannot be answered in terms of an exact number of cases. It is entirely an individual

matter. The point is that you must have adequate experience with diagnostic work before starting operative work.

The following list is a suggested progressive order of difficulty with various types of arthroscopic procedures and knee lesions:

1. Excision of a medial synovial shelf
2. Removal of a loose body in the suprapatellar pouch
3. Patellar shaving using a motorized shaver
4. Lateral retinacular release
5. Excision of a "flap" tear, middle third, either meniscus
6. Bucket handle tear, either meniscus
7. Loose body or foreign body, posteromedial compartment
8. Curettage and drilling chondral defect femoral condyle
9. Posterior and anterior horn tears, lateral meniscus
10. Posterior and anterior horn tears, medial meniscus
11. Synovectomy
12. Placement of pins in an osteochondritis dissecans fragment, femoral condyles
13. "Total" meniscectomy

INSTRUMENTS

The number and types of arthroscopic surgery instruments are changing and expanding rapidly. The type of operating technique that is used will also help dictate which instruments will be given in this course, with acknowlegment that there will likely be further advances and changes in the year's time involved from writing to publication.

Arthroscopes

I routinely use both a larger diameter (5 mm) arthroscope and a smaller diameter (2.7 mm) arthroscope for diagnostic and operative work. The larger diameter is used for the majority of cases because it gives a wider angle of vision, which helps in orientation. The larger size is also better for photography and television because of greater light transmission. The smaller diameter arthroscope is helpful for looking into the "tighter" areas of the knee, such as under the medial femoral condyle to inspect the superior or inferior surfaces of the posterior horn of the meniscus. A 30-degree angle at the tip of the arthroscope gives the ability to see a wider area as the scope is rotated. A 70 or 90 degree–angled scope is occa-

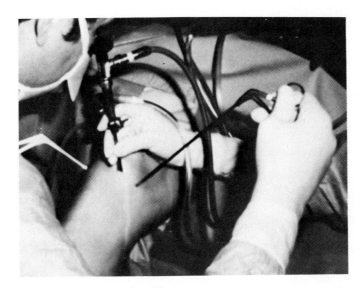

Fig. 16-5. Another example of "triangulation" of an instrument into the joint while the arthroscope is being viewed through. Here the arthroscope is positioned just medial to the patellar tendon. Two instruments are being used, one laterally for grasping and one medially for cutting. This "three-portal" technique is a variation of the central patellar tendon method of Gillquist and Oretorp.

sionally helpful for "looking around the corner" such as in the inspection of the posterior attachments of the menisci through the intercondylar notch. Arthroscopes are inserted into the joint through a sleeve that allows a continuous flow of irrigation fluid (saline) through the sleeve, exiting the knee through an outflow cannula in the suprapatellar pouch. This continuous irrigation system is most important for clear visualization during surgery. All the current arthroscopes use a fiberoptic light source for illumination within the knee joint.

Most operative work is done when one views through an arthroscope inserted through one incision and then resects or cuts with a second or third instrument inserted through other incisions. We often call this positioning of instruments *triangulation* (Fig. 16-5). The operating instrument might be a hand-controlled or a motorized device. The principle is still the same. The ability to accurately place an instrument within the knee joint by this triangulation method while viewing through an arthroscope is a skill that is gradually developed.

There are times when it is helpful to have small scissors or a knife or a single-jaw cutting forceps passed into the joint in direct line with the viewing arthroscope. This would be cumbersome if done through one or two closely approximated incisions. Therefore an operation arthroscope was developed by O'Connor (Fig. 16-1) that allows the passage of the operating instrument through a central channel in the arthroscope. There is an offset eyepiece to facilitate passage of the instrument. The operating arthroscope is very helpful in 20% to 30% of meniscal tears. Although meniscal surgery can be done without an operating arthroscope, its use greatly facilitates work in hard-to-reach areas such as a posterior-based flap tear of the medial meniscus or the posterior detachment of a bucket-handle tear.

The probe

This should be the first "instrument" that is purchased along with diagnostic arthroscopes. Although needles, crochet hooks, and the tips of other instruments can be used as probes, the best probe design has a tip with a right angle 4 mm long and has a smooth, round end that will not scratch the joint (Fig. 16-6). The shaft of the probe should be rigid so that there is no flex occurring while the probe is used.

The probe is inserted on the side of the knee opposite from where the arthroscope is inserted. A small skin incision is made 1 cm above the joint-line level, the capsule is pierced with a sharp trochar, and the synovial cavity is entered with a blunt obturator. The probe is then passed into the joint percutaneously without a sleeve. Usually, the arthroscope is lateral and the probe medial, but the two can be reversed if needed to get another angle of approach to a particular spot in the joint.

The value of routine probing cannot be overemphasized. Diagnostic accuracy is improved and the skill of triangulation is developed. There are

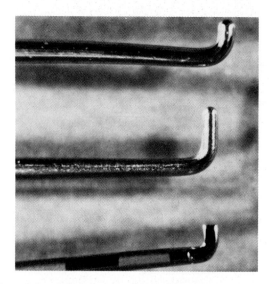

Fig. 16-6. Close-up view of the tips of three different probes. The upper probe tip is too short, making it difficult to palpate some meniscal tears. The lower tip is too sharp and can easily scratch the articular cartilage. The middle tip seems just right—smooth, right angle, 4 mm long, and rigid with no malleability.

some meniscal tears that are not obvious to observation alone (for example, an incomplete vertical tear on the inferior or superior surface of the posterior horn, medial meniscus). The integrity of the anterior cruciate ligament can also be better evaluated when observation is combined with the manipulation and stretching possible with a probe. During the course of a meniscectomy, the probe helps to delineate how much meniscus should be removed. There soon develops a tactile sensation as to what is normal and what is abnormal within the knee joint. It is better to "see and feel" rather than just "see" alone.

Hand-operated instruments

Scissors, knives, single- and double-jaw biopsy forceps, single-jaw cutting forceps, curettes, and grasping forceps are basic tools now used in arthroscopic surgery. Their size ranges from 3 to 5 mm in diameter at the tip. Their shaft may be straight or curved (Fig. 16-7). There has been a recent proliferation of both manufacturers and instruments to stay sharp longer. There are also some disposable blades available.

The ability to use these hand instruments is still the first and basic skill to be learned in operative arthroscopy.

It is easy to scratch or score articular cartilage as these instruments are moved about in the joint. This danger is greater when knives are used and so I generally prefer to use a scissors or a cutting forceps for meniscal resection because there is less chance of articular damage.

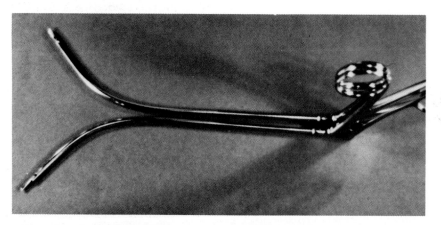

Fig. 16-7. Two cutting single-jaw meniscal forceps placed side by side showing right and left curved shafts. This curved design facilitates placement of the instrument into extreme anterior or posterior meniscal horns.

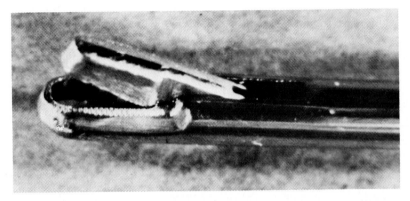

Fig. 16-8. Magnified view of tip of single-jaw meniscal cutting forceps. It is used for trimming and recontouring of the meniscal rim.

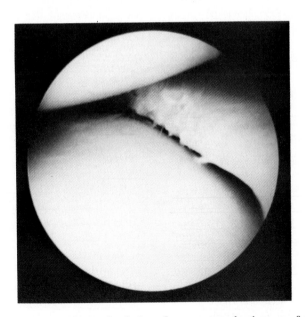

Fig. 16-9. Appearance of the meniscal rim after a parrot beak type of tear is trimmed away by use of a single-jaw forceps. Note that the undamaged meniscus has been left with no disturbance of the capsular support to the knee.

The single-jaw cutting forcep (Fig. 16-8) is still the "workhorse" of meniscal surgery in my hands. I use it extensively for trimming and recontouring the meniscal rim (Fig. 16-9). The design of this forceps provides a shearing action as the upper jaw passes the lower jaw. This gives a clean and crisp cutting action. A sensation is developed of knowing what type of meniscal tissue is being cut by the texture of it. For example, soft degenerative fibrocartilage can be differentiated from firm normal cartilage as it is being cut. Also, the width of the piece being cut can be determined by how wide the jaws open. I don't recommend using this instrument blindly, but this tactile sensation is very helpful.

Use the *tip* of the single-jaw forceps to cut with, and don't take large bites or there may be problems with breakage of these small instruments. Once the instrument is inserted, multiple bites of the meniscus are taken and the pieces are allowed to float free in the joint. These pieces are removed by irrigation. Using the instrument in this manner avoids multiple passes in and out of the joint and thus decreases the chance of joint trauma and skin-incision irritation.

There are a large variety of arthroscopic knives currently available. The meniscus is tough and fibrous to cut if the knife is at all dull. Knives dull easily. Just autoclaving them a few times will destroy the razor blade–like edge needed to cut the meniscus. If a knife is dull, you have to push harder, with less control and more likelihood of damage to adjacent articular surfaces. There are surgery methods using knives with curves[6] and specialized tip designs, such as a retrograde configuration, that make meniscal surgery easier. Gillquist and Oretorp of Sweden designed a sheath blade[19] that retracts in and out of a slot at the rounded end of the outer cannula. The blade can be exposed to a varying degree and locked with a special button.

In using knives, it is most important to always have the knife in good view whenever it is within the joint. There should never be a blind insertion into the joint of a knife or cutting without visual arthroscopic control. It is easy to have the cut being made into the meniscus wander out into or near the capsular portion of the meniscus. If this capsular junction is cut, a total meniscectomy must be done because otherwise an unstable meniscal rim will be left.

Motorized instruments

The first intra-articular motorized device was designed by Johnson[32] (Fig. 16-10). Its introduction was a significant advance in the technology associated with arthroscopic surgery. There are now several motorized systems available, but all use Johnson's original design of an outer sheath with a window and an inner sheath with matching window (Fig. 16-11). Suction power is generated down the center of these two sheaths, and the tissue is cut by the rotating action of the inner sheath window against the outer sheath window. There are designs for shaving of articular cartilage and other cutting tips for meniscus or joint débridement.

At the present state of development, all these instruments are a help and an adjunct to operative arthroscopy, but they should not be regarded as primary instruments for doing all endoscopic surgery. The day may come when meniscal cutters, for example, will be efficient enough to do all the trimming and resection required. That day is not here yet, and it is still necessary to use hand-operated cutting instruments for portions of the meniscal resection.

These motorized devices are used for patellar shaving, joint débridement of synovium, resection of medial synovial shelves and synovectomies, removal of small loose bodies, and meniscal resection and also for a "vacuum-cleaner" type of action to remove the small bits of debris from the joint after the surgery is completed. Irrigation inflow rate and pressure must be increased to operate these instruments efficiently. This is usually done by elevation of the inflow bottle of saline at least 4 to 5 feet above the level of the knee and also by the use of an extra inflow cannula if needed. If this irrigation flow is not adequate, tissue to be cut wil not be drawn into the window system.

Use of television

Small television cameras can be attached either directly to the viewing arthroscope or to an articulated optical device. The color image can then be transmitted to television monitor at the side of the operating table. This gives an even further magnification of the inside of the knee joint but with some loss of clarity. The use of television during arthroscopic surgery has the advantage of allowing others to observe what is being done, which

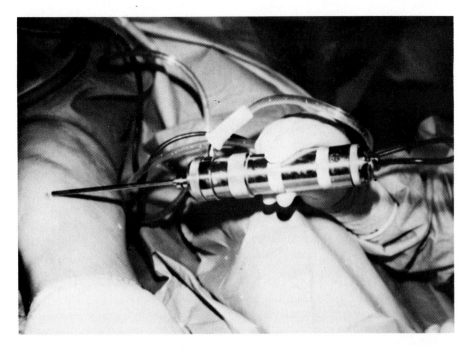

Fig. 16-10. Motorized intra-articular device first designed by Johnson. Suction draws fragments out of the joint as they are trimmed away by the rotating blades.

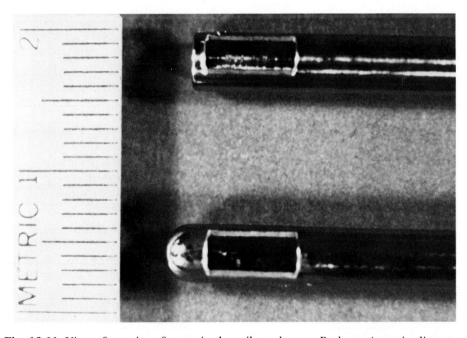

Fig. 16-11. View of two tips of motorized cartilage shavers. Both are 4 mm in diameter. The upper unit has the cutting window placed nearer the tip allowing débridement down into articular defects or craters.

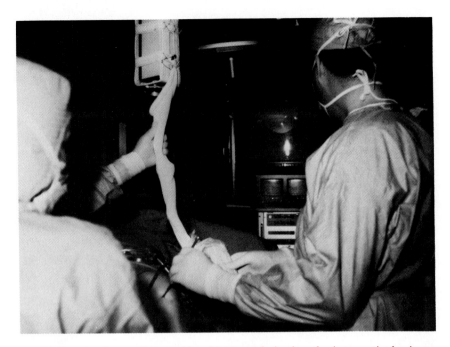

Fig. 16-12. Surgeon is standing at side of knee and viewing the intra-articular image on the television monitor at the head of the table. This image is transmitted from the eyepiece of the arthroscope through an articulated optical arm to a television camera suspended overhead. The articulated device is covered with sterile draping and allows good mobility of the television system to avoid encumbering the surgeon during the procedure.

can be a great help in training other orthopaedic surgeons and in keeping the operating room personnel interested and involved in the case. The surgeon can stand or sit while viewing the monitor (Fig. 16-12). A videotape record can be made of interesting cases, preserving a dynamic rather than a static documentation that might be valuable in studying the tracking alignment of the patellofemoral joint or the motions of a meniscal tear as it is probed.

There are several disadvantages to television. Expense is a major objection. Although the hospital may purchase equipment, this cost is passed on to the patient. This expense is not practical unless a fairly large volume of knee work is done. The view through television is not so clear and sharp as looking through an arthroscope directly. The use of television adds time to each case. There is a tendency to get engrossed in the television presentation rather than concentrating on developing one's basic operative skills. I believe that operative skills are developed faster at first without television. It is another thing to worry about and takes precious time, which is often critical at first.

BASIC TECHNIQUES
Preoperative instruction and management

For the past 3 years I have been doing all my arthroscopic knee surgery in a free-standing outpatient surgical center. The advantages of outpatient surgery are similar to the advantages for arthroscopic surgery and include the following:

1. Cost savings.
2. Patients having a positive attitude and a faster rehabilitation.
3. Less anesthetic problems.
4. Scheduling easier.
5. Immediate ambulation.
6. Fewer complications.

There are only two disadvantages that I am aware of:

1. If an arthrotomy is necessary, the patient may need to be admitted to a hospital afterwards.
2. There are a few insurance companies that still will not cover ambulatory surgery.

A successful outpatient surgery unit, either hospital based or free standing, requires the interest and cooperation of an anesthesiologist who likes the concept of the outpatient type of anesthesia.

I routinely explain to each patient in some detail the nature of arthroscopic surgery. I try to stress the following points:

1. This is a relatively new method of surgery that allows a patient to ambulate almost immediately with minimal discomfort and a more rapid recovery time.
2. An arthroscope is a telescopic device. It allows accurate visualization of the interior of the knee joint. Light is provided by fiberoptics. The instrument is approximately the diameter of an ordinary pencil. It is inserted into the knee joint through tiny incisions.
3. Diagnostic arthroscopy is first done to thoroughly examine the knee and try to find the source of the symptoms.
4. Once a diagnosis has been established, surgery is done as indicated. All surgery cannot be done through the arthroscope, and it may be necessary to open the knee in the way that has been traditionally done for many years. The patient should understand this and be willing to have surgery done by an arthrotomy if necessary.
5. One knee problem can mimic another and sometimes a type of surgery is done differently from what was originally anticipated. There is also the possibility that only a diagnostic procedure will be done and surgery will not be indicated. This will avoid an unnecessary operation.

I have found that patients accept these explanations very well and particularly the idea that arthroscopic surgery is a new technique and that it may be necessary to open the knee joint. If a patient insists that a guarantee be given that the surgery will be done arthroscopically, I would not do the surgery or allow myself to be restricted. It is possible to manage this type of patient by scheduling only for a diagnostic arthroscopy. The patient then returns at a later date for either arthroscopic surgery or an arthrotomy. This of course adds to the expense.

Patients are asked to refrain from the use of salicylates or any salicylate-containing medications for 1 week before surgery to help reduce postoperative bleeding. Prophylactic antibiotics are not used. To date I have had no deep infections in over 3500 diagnostic and operative cases. One of the contraindications to doing arthroscopic surgery would be sepsis in some other part of the body. I also prefer that arthroscopic knee surgery not be done concurrent with any other operation such as herniorrhaphy.

Anesthesia

Although local anesthesia is preferred by some for diagnostic arthroscopy,[22,43] I prefer general anesthesia (for arthroscopic surgery) because thigh muscles are more relaxed and the knee joint can be opened up much better. There is also no tourniquet discomfort. Under local anesthesia, the patient often becomes apprehensive and this adds a feeling of needing to hurry, which can then make arthroscopic surgery frustrating and strained. We have found that general anesthesia takes less time than local anesthesia and therefore the costs work out about the same. No preanesthetic medication is given in our ambulatory surgery setting. Another advantage to general anesthesia is the ability to go right ahead with an arthrotomy (after reprepping and draping the knee) if needed. If only local anesthesia is used, it would be necessary to reschedule the arthrotomy for another day.

Instrument sterilization

Some arthroscopes and other equipment cannot be steam autoclaved. Gas sterilization is good overnight for a onetime use but is not practical for several cases in one day. We have routinely used activated dialdehyde (Cidex) as a bactericidal soaking agent for over 6 years. Telescopes and light cables are soaked for 10 minutes and then rinsed in sterile water. There has been no damage to any equipment. The accumulated experience of other surgeons has produced a similar large number of cases where chemical sterilization has been used safely[33] (Fig. 16-13).

The remarkably low incidence of infections is probably not related so much to sterilization methods but rather is a result of the high volume of fluid that is used to bathe the knee joint during the procedure. This continual irrigation with several liters of saline is more thorough than any other orthopedic procedure that I know of.

Methods of positioning and holding the knee during endoscopic surgery

There are now at least three methods of holding and maneuvering the knee during surgery, and it is important that the beginning arthroscopist choose one of these methods and become proficient with it. It is important to be able to stress

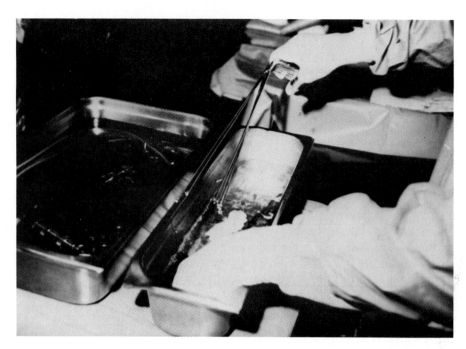

Fig. 16-13. Instruments are sterilized between cases by being soaked in Cidex for 10 minutes. The larger pan is for the soak, and the smaller pan contains sterile water for rinsing.

the joint open adequately and also to maintain a position of varus or valgus stress while doing the surgery.

This manipulation of the joint can be done by the surgeon himself (Fig. 16-14, *A*). The medial compartment of the knee is opened by placement of the knee in a valgus external rotation position with the hip in abduction. Force can be applied against the abducted hip and thigh. The surgeon can be sitting at the side of the table with the foot resting in his lap or standing with his own foot resting on a stationary stool, and the foot of the patient resting on his flexed thigh. An assistant may help by pushing against the side of the patient's knee joint.

For viewing the lateral joint compartment the foot is brought across and placed on the opposite limb, and then a downward pressure is applied on the medial side of the knee to produce a varus internal rotation stress.

The addition of a simple padded post to the edge of the operating table can provide a fulcrum to push against to open the medial joint compartment.

Another variation of this is to have an assistant hold and maneuver the knee (Fig. 16-14, *B*). The fulcrum for leverage is applied by the hand of the assistant at the jointline level. This allows a comfortable sitting position for the surgeon, and the assistant can apply a variety of maneuvers to the joint to help expose the knee. The assistant soon becomes an integral part of the procedure and can open various parts of the joint almost automatically. However, this is tiring, requires considerable stamina and is somewhat difficult for females.

In both of the above methods, the table is kept flat. If the knee needs to be flexed, it is either brought up on the table by flexion of the hip or over the side of the table with the hip in abduction. This "table-flat" method allows easier access into the suprapatellar area, and also, with the hip and knee flexed, posterior compartment punctures are easier (Fig. 16-15).

A third method involves the use of a thigh-holding device, which securely encircles the middle of the thigh. This method has been advocated by Johnson[32] (Fig. 16-16), who has devised a very sturdy holding device that controls rotation and allows either the surgeon or an assistant to maneuver against this mechanical device. The advantages to these devices include the ability to hold the joint in a maximum varus or valgus position for exposure of the posterior meniscal horns and

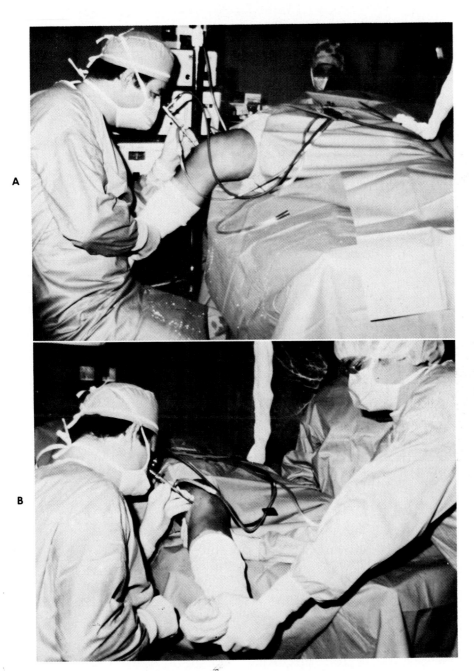

Fig. 16-14. Two methods for manipulation of the knee joint to obtain exposure for arthroscopic surgery. **A,** The surgeon is stressing the joint himself. Here the hip is abducted and a valgus stress is applied by pressure against the lower leg. **B,** The assistant is applying stress using his hand as a fulcrum laterally and using external rotation and valgus pressure to open the medial compartment.

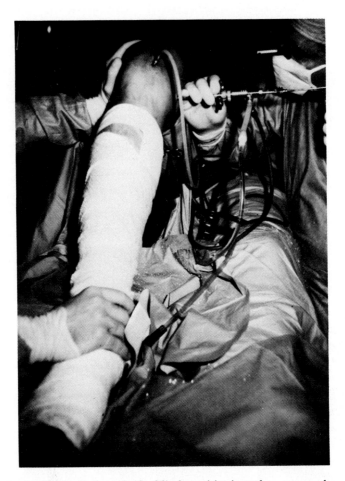

Fig. 16-15. In the "table-flat" method of limb positioning, the surgeon has more room for work in the posterior compartment. Here the knee is flexed to 90 degrees and the operating arthroscope is inserted posteromedially. Note how the assistant can hold or maneuver the limb as needed during the surgery.

also the ease with which the surgeon or assistant can maintain this joint exposure.

The thigh-holding device can get in the way of suprapatellar approaches. They also can cause a tourniquet effect and are only used with a regular tourniquet inflated superior to the thigh holder. If the tourniquet is released, the pressure of the holding device should also be released. Great force can be applied to the knee joint with these devices, and it is possible to stretch or even tear collateral ligaments.

Irrigation system

Although clear visualization for diagnostic arthroscopy is important, it is absolutely essential for good endoscopic surgery. There must be sufficient inflow pressure and flow rate. This is accomplished by raising the inflow bottles of saline at least 4 to 5 feet above the level of the knee (Fig. 16-17). A large-diameter outflow cannula having multiple perforations should be used. This reduces clogging. The outflow cannula is connected by tubing for gravity flow to a bucket at the side of the table. We use saline for irrigation. Distilled water and even half-normal saline can cause a mild synovitis in the knee joint postoperatively.

Use of a tourniquet

As mentioned above, if an encircling thigh-holding device is used, there is a venous tourni-

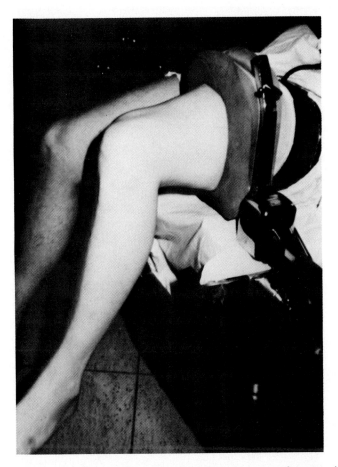

Fig. 16-16. Johnson leg-holding device placed just inferior to the tourniquet on the upper part of the thigh. This device holds the thigh firmly and serves as a fulcrum against which great leverage can be applied to open up the knee joint.

quet effect and so a regular tourniquet is placed superior to the thigh-holding device.

If this type of thigh holder is not used, use of a tourniquet can be optional. The tourniquet should always be in place on the upper thigh for use if needed. There is often some bleeding that occurs with meniscal resection, with resultant poor visualization. This slows the operative case considerably. A tourniquet inflated on the upper thigh in the standard manner can greatly improve visualization by eliminating bleeding. When one does a lateral retinacular release, the tourniquet is essential and should not be deflated until after a compressive dressing is applied. The tourniquet should not be left inflated in any case longer than

90 minutes. All operative arthroscopy cases can be completed within this time limit with current methods.

Operating room personnel

We routinely have *two* operating room personnel scrubbed in surgery *besides* the surgeon. One individual (the scrub nurse) has the responsibility for organizing, caring for, and passing instruments. This individual may also occasionally help hold an instrument or "freeze" an arthroscope in a certain position. The second individual (the surgical assistant) has the responsibility of helping with the prepping and draping, holding the limb during the surgery, and then assisting with the

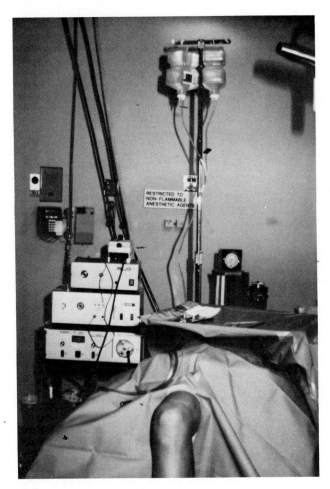

Fig. 16-17. Bottles containing irrigating saline solution are placed at least 4 to 5 feet above the level of the knee assuring adequate inflow pressure and flow rate so essential for good irrigation and visualization during surgery.

thorough irrigation of the joint after the surgery and application of dressings. This assistant can also help with holding the television camera when used. Residents, interns, referring physicians and partners do not make very good assistants, because they naturally want to see through the arthroscope or otherwise be involved in the case and often do not hold the knee so steadily as is desirable. Development of this team approach really helps both the beginning and more experienced arthroscopist.

Time limits and scheduling considerations

It is easy to use excessive time in doing arthroscopic surgery. Rigid time limits should be set and adhered to. I recommend that if the case is not progressing toward a conclusion at 60 minutes it is better to reprep and drape and proceed with an arthrotomy. The key word in this rule is "progress." It is usually quite clear at 60 minutes whether the case can be completed arthroscopically or not. I am not recommending that cases should be prematurely stopped, but only that common sense be used. Surgeons should never feel that the case must be completed arthroscopically no matter what the time involved.

Because arthroscopic surgery does require so much concentration, it is important to have a reasonably tranquil atmosphere. Cases should not be sandwiched into a busy schedule or in a situation where other surgeons are anxiously waiting to start their cases to follow. I recommend that, where possible, arthroscopic surgery cases be done at a separate unhurried time in the operating room schedule and not intermixed with general orthopedic open cases.

BASIC TECHNIQUE
Using leg-holding device

The following description of our basic operating technique is currently used for all cases except lateral retinacular release or those where we strongly suspect a pathologic condition in the suprapatellar pouch, such as a medial synovial shelf or synovitis. In these types of cases, the leg-holding device is not used.

The patient is lying supine on the operating table under a light general anesthetic. The tourniquet is placed on the thigh as far superiorly as possible. The limb is wrapped from toe to tourniquet with an Esmark rubber bandage for devascularization and the tourniquet inflated. The thigh is then placed in a leg-holding device and the device tightened securely and positioned as high on the thigh as possible to give clearance for work in the suprapatellar area. The table is flexed 90 degrees at the knee level, allowing both legs to hang in a 90-degree dependent position. Padding is used for the nonoperative limb to assure that there are no pressure points against it. The nonoperative limb is wrapped with an elastic bandage if the patient has a history of varicose veins or phlebitis problems. The knee is prepped from the leg holder to the ankle with a 2% tincture of iodine paint. This is left to dry and is not removed before drapes are applied. Hair about the knee has been previously removed with a depilatory cream (Surgex). A cotton stockinette encases the foot and ankle and is then covered with a plastic adhesive drape to make it waterproof. A single large drape is then used to isolate the knee covering the leg holder and the rest of the body. This drape has a central elasticized section that fits the upper part of the thigh snugly.

The scrub nurse has a large back table for instruments. This is positioned for her convenience usually at the side opposite the knee having surgery. A Mayo stand is placed over the operating table at the level of the upper part of the thighs and the more commonly used instruments are placed on this. Power cords and light cable are attached to the appropriate sources placed on a side table. The irrigation bottles are suspended from an intravenous stand at the head of the table, and the bottles are raised at least 4 to 5 feet above the level of the knee. The surgeon sits at the foot of the table on a stool with wheels (Fig. 16-18). The assistant can either sit or stand just in back of the surgeon and to the side so that he can maneuver

the knee against the thigh holder by pushing against and controlling the limb at ankle level. In addition to regular sterile gowns, the surgeon fashions an apron from waist to floor level with a waterproof drape to avoid contaminating the foot when sitting. A diagnostic arthroscopy is first done. A 5 mm scope and its sleeve are inserted into an anterolateral joint-line incision. A probe is inserted routinely directly percutaneously through a medial anterior joint-line incision. If necessary, the viewing arthroscope is switched to the medial incision (portal) and the probe to the lateral portal. If the posterior horn of the medial meniscus is not seen clearly and thoroughly, two additional methods may be used. I first will substitute a 2.7 mm telescope for the 5 mm telescope. This smaller diameter scope can then be used to look between the femoral condyle and tibial plateau onto the superior or under the inferior surfaces of the posterior horns of the menisci.

Posterior puncture technique

A posterior medial puncture can also be done and should be done if there is any question about seeing the entire posterior horn of the meniscus. This posterior puncture is done as follows:

The knee is flexed to 90 degrees. The outflow cannula is removed and is now used as an inflow cannula when it is inserted into the posterior compartment by the intercondylar notch through either the anteromedial or anterolateral incision already made. This takes a little practice to feel it slip into the back of the joint past the cruciate ligaments.

A syringe filled with 60 ml of saline solution is then attached to this cannula, but the saline is not injected yet. A small skin incision is made over the small triangular soft spot formed by the posteromedial edge of the femur and the posteromedial edge of the tibia. Any-sized arthroscope can be inserted with this technique. I usually use the 5 mm 170-degree telescope. The sleeve of this scope is positioned with a sharp trochar just under the skin but not yet piercing the capsule. The capsule is then distended when the surgeon has the assistant inject the 60 ml of saline. It is now very easy to pierce the distended capsule, aiming the tip of the trocanter slightly anteriorly (Fig. 16-19).

The sharp obturator is removed and the saline, under pressure in the posterior compartment, flows out through the sleeve. The arthroscope is then inserted. The anatomy of the posterior com-

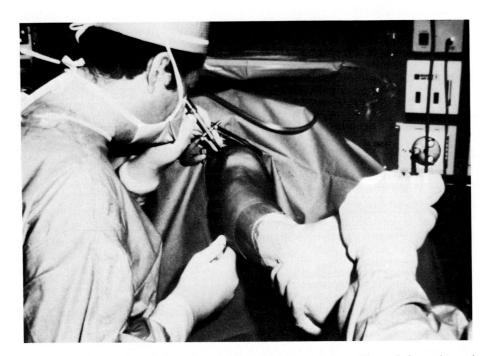

Fig. 16-18. The surgeon is seated at the foot of the operative table and the assistant is maneuvering the limb against the thigh-holding device. Most operative arthroscopy is done with the knee extended or slightly flexed.

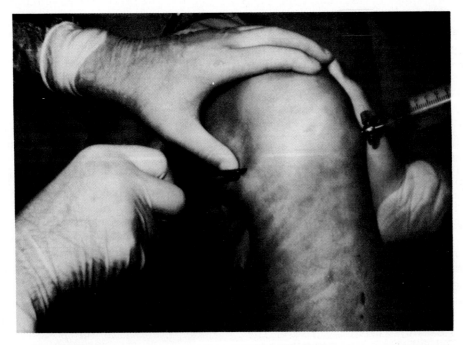

Fig. 16-19. Posteromedial puncture technique. The knee is flexed to nearly 90 degrees, and the arthroscope sleeve is inserted by use of a sharp trochar.

partment can then be examined. Have the assistant maneuver the leg into internal and external rotation, flexion, and extension to visualize as much as possible this compartment.

It is possible to probe the posteromedial compartment. One can do this by passing the probe through the intercondylar notch, using the anterolateral incision if the posteromedial compartment and the anteromedial incision for the posterolateral compartment are being examined.

Once the diagnostic examination has been completed, the surgery then proceeds according to the type of knee lesion encountered, and these techniques will be discussed with each knee lesion.

Number and sites of incisions

The number of incisions made does not seem to alter the postoperative morbidity. Incisions are merely punctures in the skin and capsule and as such do not require stitches and have minimal pain associated with them. For this reason, the surgeon should be willing and ready to make a puncture wherever it is needed to better approach a particular area of the knee. It is important to mention this because some believe that there has to be a set number or routine of incisions. The

addition of extra incisions (a suprapatellar portal for example) should always be done if another angle of approach is needed.

Gillquist and Oretorp[19] report arthroscopic surgery done using a three-portal technique. The central portal is made through the patellar tendon (Fig. 16-20). They report an extremely low incidence of irritation of the patellar tendon or other complications. The method allows an arthroscope in the central portal to view instruments passed through medial and lateral anterior joint-line portals. A 30-degree telescope is most often used, but a 70-degree telescope can be helpful in viewing either the medial or lateral posterior compartments through the intercondylar notch.[18] A modified triple puncture approach can be done if you do not want to pierce the patellar tendon. In this instance, the central incision is made as close as possible to either the medial or lateral border of the patellar tendon. The other two incisions are then made as widely apart as possible, usually just in front of the collateral ligaments.

The main advantage to this method seems to be the ability to look on either side of the joint without moving the arthroscope from one portal to another. The disadvantages include an increased

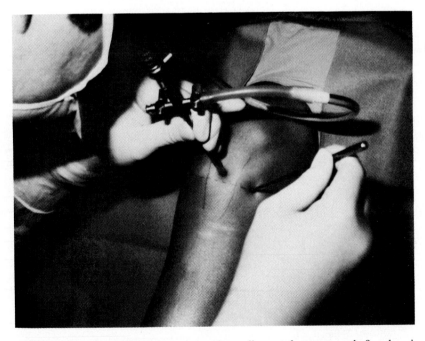

Fig. 16-20. Swedish technique uses a central patellar tendon approach for the viewing arthroscope. The patellar tendon borders and the joint-line level have been outlined to show the position of the scope and insertion of the probe.

difficulty at first in the manipulation of instruments from one side to the other of the joint, with the arthroscope centrally tending to get in the way of these other instruments. This can be overcome with practice. A 70-degree telescope takes time to become familiar with, and it is easy to get lost in the joint with this right-angle orientation. It is recommended that you try this approach a few times and if it feels comfortable then use it all the time. I still prefer the "double-puncture" technique already described. Erickson has done a cadaver study showing no advantage to the patellar tendon approach versus a standard anterolateral approach.[13]

Patel has recommended insertion of a 30-degree mm telescope in the lateral suprapatellar pouch.[51] The incision is made just adjacent to the superolateral border of the patella. With the arthroscope tip placed in the intercondylar notch area, both menisci can be visualized. This method is particularly helpful for viewing the anterior horns of the menisci.

Method of joint irrigation to remove loose fragments

During partial meniscectomy, there are numerous loose pieces that collect in the joint, particularly when using the single-jaw cutting forceps. It is too traumatic on the articular cartilage to remove the forceps after each bite of meniscus is taken; so these pieces are allowed to float about in the joint until later removal.

It is important to remove all this debris. At the conclusion of the procedure the assistant inserts the sleeve to the 5 mm arthroscope into the suprapatellar pouch. The knee joint is extended to help open up the suprapatellar pouch. A large syringe is used to forcefully irrigate 60 to 80 ml of saline into the joint.

The syringe is then removed and the saline allowed to flow back out the arthroscope sleeve into a basin by gravity (Fig. 16-21). The outflow fluid is inspected to see how many pieces are removed, and then this fluid is emptied into another pan so that the outflow can be inspected each time to see that it is getting clearer of any debris.

Once the outflow has been clear for three or four times, you can be quite certain that the joint is also clear.

It also helps to flex and extend the knee a few times or milk the back and front of the joint as the irrigation takes place. This seems to help work any pieces up in the suprapatellar pouch where they can be washed out.

The use of the intra-articular shaving devices also can help clean out the joint by acting much

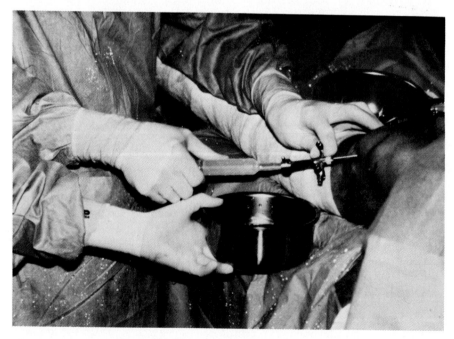

Fig. 16-21. The knee joint is thoroughly irrigated at the conclusion of the arthroscopic surgery to remove small, loose pieces of cartilage or synovium.

like a vacuum cleaner to grind up and suction out small pieces of synovium and cartilage.

Postoperative care

After arthroscopic meniscectomies a fluffy cotton compressive dressing is used for 24 hours for hemostasis. Other procedures, such as lateral retinacular release, require a localized sponge pad compressive dressing, which is usually worn for 7 to 10 days.

Immediate ambulation is encouraged, and crutches are seldom used except in osteochondritis dissecans or a chondral defect where articular loading is not desirable. Vigorous isometric exercises are begun in the recovery room and range-of-motion exercise is encouraged within the first 24 to 48 hours. The patient is encouraged to walk as normally as possible. More vigorous isotonic exercises are begin at 7 to 10 days, sometimes with the help of a physical therapist. Non–weight bearing range-of-motion exercises such as swimming and bicycling are encouraged. Return to sedentary jobs is often possible within 2 to 7 days.[9] Return to vigorous athletics is not permitted until there is absence of joint effusion, complete return of the thigh muscle strength and size, full range of knee motion, and absence of pain. These are the same criteria that would be used after an arthrotomy type of procedure.

POSTOPERATIVE PROBLEMS AND MANAGEMENT

Fat pad syndrome. An occasional patient will develop a puffiness and tenderness of the infrapatellar fat pad. This will be persistent and painful when the area is bumped or when the patient kneels. This minor complication will usually develop at about 3 to 6 weeks after surgery. If a 5 to 7-day treatment with an anti-inflammatory systemic medication does not help, inject the fat pad with corticosteroids, which take care of the problem rapidly.

Hemarthrosis. Postoperative bleeding will occasionally occur after a lateral retinacular release or partial meniscectomy. If the meniscal resection has gone out to the capsular level, there will invariably be some hemarthrosis. I have not aspirated the hemarthrosis unless extremely large and painful. It is preferable to let the hemarthrosis gradually absorb. Repeated isometric quadriceps exercises seem to speed up this absorption process. Aspiration should be done under strict sterile technique. I have not seen any long-term problems or complications resulting from hemarthrosis. Initial morbidity is increased, and return to work and other activities may be prolonged, but the results seem the same. Having patients refrain from using salicylates both before and after the surgical procedure helps to reduce the incidence of hemarthrosis.

Joint effusions. After partial meniscectomies the development of joint effusions is related to two factors: first, quadriceps atrophy and weakness and, second, the extent of chondromalacia of the articular surfaces of the joint. Posterior horn tears that are complex and require resection out to the capsule level often cause more effusion and bleeding.

Usually the initial effusion will subside in 10 to 14 days, particularly if the patient will concentrate on isometric quadriceps exercises. Effusions that persist beyond 14 days are related to overuse of the knee with associated quadriceps weakness, and this may require the services of a physical therapist.

Phlebitis. The ability of patients to ambulate the same day as surgery seems to be the reason that postoperative phlebitis or thrombophlebitis rarely occur. Patients are encouraged to walk normally as soon as possible and avoid limping.

Infections. To date I have not had any patient develop a deep infection after either diagnostic arthroscopic examination or arthroscopic surgery. A few patients have developed a superficial inflammation around one of the incisions, occasionally occurring 3 to 4 weeks after surgery. This minor problem responds well to hot moist soaks and occasionally a systemic antibiotic, though cultures from the area always show negative findings. This cellulitis is likely related to use of subcutaneous skin stitches.

Joint scuffing. Some scuffing seems to occur in most meniscal cases. The scuffed areas of articular cartilage are greatly magnified, and so they look worse than they actually are. Those cases where we have been able to look back several months later show these small scratches to have healed over with a fibrocartilage. You can still see the mark, but it is smooth and there is no evidence of further deterioration. There is experimental evidence that the body has some ability to heal minor articular surface damage.[57] However, deep articular cuts and scratches will not heal and great care should be taken at all times to watch the position (inside the joint) of an instrument that has a sharp edge such as a knife or scissors. The power meniscal cutters will take out little chunks of articular cartilage if the cutting window is turned against a femoral condyle or tibial plateau.

SUMMARY OF BASIC TECHNIQUES

A very important concept in arthroscopic surgery is that there are a variety of techniques and skills that should be at one's command for various operative situations within the knee joint. Sometimes one method or technique will succeed where another will not. Some examples of ways that helpful changes can be made are as follows:

1. *Change the viewing scope to a different portal.* This can give a different angle of view that may be helpful.
2. *Change the type of stress on the knee joint.* For example, you may change from a varus to a valgus or internal to external rotation.
3. *Change the type of instrument being used.* A scissors may not be making progress, and so a basket forceps or a knife is used or perhaps a power instrument.
4. *Change the size of the viewing arthroscope.* Going from a larger to a smaller or vice versa or to an operating arthroscope may give a different perspective that will be helpful.
5. *Remove the instrument being used and reprobe.* This reevaluation by probing may indicate another approach that could be used to solve the particular problem that is causing difficulty.
6. *Add an additional portal.* A grasping instrument can be inserted or perhaps a probe from another angle. Don't be afraid to make an incision (portal) wherever it would be helpful.

TECHNIQUES FOR SPECIFIC LESIONS
Synovial biopsy

A single- or double-jaw biopsy forceps can be inserted into the suprapatellar pouch to obtain synovial biopsies. The incision for inserting the biopsy instrument is usually made in the suprapatellar pouch either medially or laterally. The arthroscope is inserted through one of the anterior joint-line incisions used for the diagnostic arthroscopy. There are no particular problems associated with this procedure. Three to five specimens are usually taken to ensure enough tis-

sue for the pathologist. A compressive fluffy cotton dressing is worn for 24 hours, and the patient is allowed immediate ambulation.

Medial synovial shelf

Resection of a medial shelf is a simple procedure. The only difficulty is knowing which shelf to resect. The incidence of a normal synovial plica or shelf is in the 20% to 50% range.[23] This longitudinal medial fold of synovium is usually 2 to 5 mm in width and quite thin and pliable. When this shelf becomes thickened, fibrotic, and wider than 5 mm, it will become forced between the patella and the femur, sometimes causing patellar chondromalacia or grooving or erosion along the medial edge of the femoral condyle.

This lesion is a great imitator of other types of knee problems.[52] It can exactly simulate a torn medial meniscus, producing locking, catching, and giving way of the knee joint. It can also mimic chondromalacia and subluxation of the patella where the patient will describe a parapatellar aching pain, aggravated by bent-knee activities such as going up and down stairs. It is therefore difficult to establish the diagnosis of a pathologic medial synovial shelf before arthroscopy examination. Sometimes there is localized tenderness along the medial patellar border about an inch above the joint-line. A ridge may be palpated over the femoral condyle that can be felt to flip back and forth as the knee is flexed and extended.

The best arthroscopic approach to see the medial synovial shelf is from the lateral superior suprapatellar incision. The shelf is usually divided by insertion of a scissors or basket forceps into the superolateral portal while one views from the inferolateral portal. A 4 or 5 mm single-jaw cutting forceps can be used to remove the shelf. I also use a motorized shaving device to do a partial synovectomy, removing the shelf entirely and also a segment of the synovial wall about 2 to 3 cm anterior and posterior to the shelf. I believe this reduces the chances of the shelf reforming. There may be an associated fringe of synovitis around the medial patellar border, and this is removed. If necessary, I change the viewing arthroscope to the superior incision and the resting instrument to the inferior incision to get a better angle for doing the partial synovectomy.

There will be postoperative bleeding from the area of the medial synovial wall where the shelf was resected. To control this bleeding a compres-

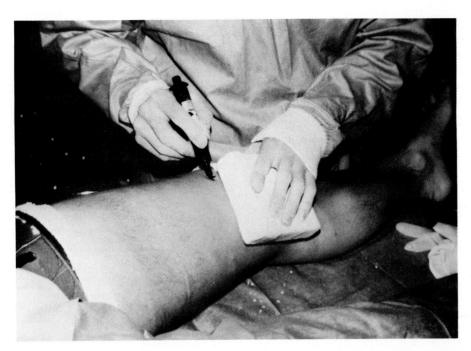

Fig. 16-22. Sponge pad is used for compression to prevent postoperative bleeding after resection of the medial synovial shelf. Note corner marks drawn on the skin to guide the patient in proper placement of pad when dressings are changed at home. A similar pad is used laterally after a lateral patellar release.

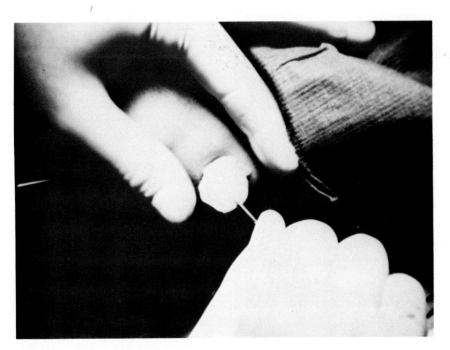

Fig. 16-23. Large loose body being removed from small suprapatellar incision. This fragment was located with the arthroscope and then grasped, with a triangulation technique being used.

sion pad is used over the medial side of the joint for 3 to 5 days. This pad is made from a firm foam rubber and measures 4 × 4 × 1 inch (Fig. 16-22). It is covered with a cotton stockinette. The patient is instructed to change the compression pad daily and reposition the pad if necessary according to corner marks that are drawn on the skin as a guide.

Loose bodies

The majority of loose bodies are cartilaginous. The usual sites of origin are from the articular cartilage of the medial femoral condyle and the patella, often related to trauma. Osteochondritis dissecans can be the source of loose pieces, and these are usually osteochondral. Loose bodies tend to gravitate to the posterior compartments of the knee joint, and they can be difficult to find. The lateral femoral gutter is also a common location. It is not so common to find these in the suprapatellar pouch initially unless they are of very large size (greater than 1.5 cm). Sometimes a loose body will be hidden in the area of the fat pad beneath the patellar tendon.

Technique of removal is not difficult. A grasping forceps is triangulated to the loose body. The

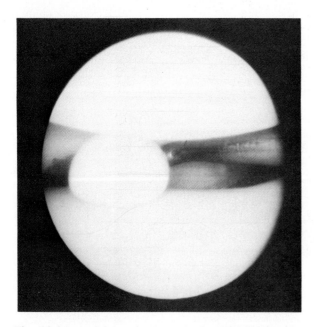

Fig. 16-24. Arthroscopic view of a loose body that has been located beneath the lateral meniscus and down into the popliteus tendon sleeve. A probe is used to pull this piece of cartilage out into the joint where it can be grasped and removed.

piece is then pulled out through the same incision as the grasping forceps (Fig. 16-23). The incision may have to be enlarged slightly. Another technique suggested by McGinty[41] is to grasp the loose body and then push it out into the suprapatellar pouch and make a small skin incision over the palpable fragment. The fragment is then pushed out through this incision and removed. This is probably safer where the loose body is large or where it cannot be firmly grasped.

Loose bodies can be very elusive and difficult to find. They have a way of staying ahead of the viewing arthroscope. The important principle in removing these loose fragments is that once the loose body is seen, it is kept under observation until removed. This may seem obvious, but many times just looking away from the arthroscope to obtain a grasping instrument or a minor shift of the knee position will cause the loose body to move out of sight and be difficult to find again. Be prepared to turn off the irrigation system once the loose body is sighted. A needle can also be passed percutaneously to pierce the loose body and hold it until a grasping forceps can secure it.

For loose bodies that are hiding in the lateral posterior compartment, take a probe and lift up the lateral meniscus (Fig. 16-24). The loose body is often lodged in the sleeve of the popliteus tendon. By manipulation of the meniscus, it will pop into the lateral joint compartment where it can be removed.

Loose bodies in the posterior medial compartment are usually easily identified with a posteromedial puncture. Grasping instruments can then be triangulated directly into the posteromedial compartment or across the intercondylar notch. Sometimes a motorized device is triangulated into the posterior compartment and the loose body ground up and removed by suction.

Foreign bodies

Everything that has been said about loose bodies could also be said about foreign bodies. Probably the most common "foreign body" that is encountered is a broken instrument within the joint. Once the foreign body is sighted, the irrigation flow is immediately turned off and the foreign body is kept in view and secured with a grasping instrument. There is presently available a small suction tube that has a magnet incorporated at its tip that can be helpful in removing metallic foreign bodies.

PATELLAR SURGERY

The term "patellar compression syndrome"[38,50] emphasizes the forces that can produce chondromalacia of the patellar articular cartilage. This syndrome has also been called "subluxation syndrome," "lateral overpull syndrome," and "excessive lateral facet syndrome".[14,46] All these terms indicate an abnormal lateral tracking pattern and subluxation of the patella that produces increased compressive forces between the patella and the femur. These stress forces produce a characteristic central and centromedial pattern of breakdown of the articular cartilage.[26] (Fig. 16-25). These shearing and compressive forces cause a bursting action in the articular cartilage just at the edge of where the compressive force is located. This is the reason why we see chondromalacic changes more medially than laterally. The lateral facet articular cartilage is nourished by the pressure of the lateral femoral condyle and so it does not break down until much later. The medial patellar facet has very little, if any, pressure against it and therefore is poorly nourished and easily broken down by the shearing forces. The shaggy fibrillated crab meat–like appearance that we see arthroscopically is the result of the chronically malaligned patella.

Although there are other etiologic factors in chondromalacia patellae this malalignment syndrome seems to be the most common. For this reason I very seldom do an arthroscopic patellar shaving without an accompanying release of the tightened and overpulling lateral structures.

My indications for an arthroscopic lateral retinacular release are as follows:

1. Typical history of peripatellar, intermittent pain related to bent-knee type of activities
2. Clinical and roentgenographic evidence of patellar malalignment
3. Failure to respond to nonsurgical management, including rest, salicylates, and isometric exercises
4. Arthroscopic confirmation of the malalignment with typical lateral subluxation seen while the knee is flexed and extended (Fig. 16-26).

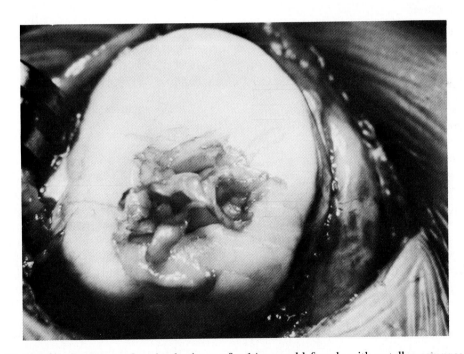

Fig. 16-25. Patellar surface in the knee of a 14-year-old female with patellar compression syndrome. Note the severe disruption of the central articular surface, which has broken down at an early age because of constant shearing and pressure over the lateral femoral condyle. This photograph was taken during an open lateral release. This type of lesion can now be managed arthroscopically as discussed in text.

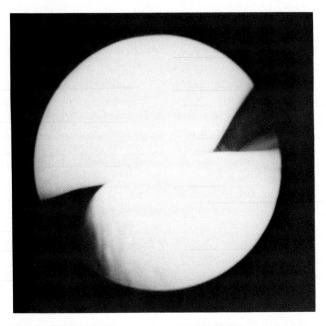

Fig. 16-26. Arthroscopic view of lateral tilting and subluxation of the patella. The knee is flexed 30 degrees. The arthroscope is inserted into the lateral suprapatellar pouch. Although there is no breakdown of the articular cartilage yet, it will not be long before this type of malalignment produces chondromalacia of the patella (see Fig. 16-25).

Dynamic realignment

Lateral retinacular release has been advocated by others for patellar realignment, with reported good results.[14,44,46] The main advantage in doing this type of releasing procedure with arthroscopic control is that the tiny incisions that are used allow the patient immediate ambulation and active range of motion. There is no time spent with the limb immobilized. Early active motion keeps the lateral structures from reattaching themselves or forming a new fibrotic lateral contracture. The patient is able to realign the patella by building up the remaining central and medial quadriceps musculature, which has been left untouched by surgery. A dynamic realignment of the patellofemoral joint occurs. Once the release is done, the quadriceps mechanism seems to be able to track the patella properly and there is no need to worry about exactly where to transfer the patellar tendon or how much to tighten the medial retinaculum, as is often the dilemma with open patellar alignment surgery.

It is essential that a thorough release be done. The synovium is fibrotic and should be cut. The vastus lateralis must be divided at its insertion and the incision extended well above the level of the patella as mentioned. By attention to these details, this procedure offers an alternative to major patellar realignment surgery that is cosmetically pleasing and involves significant reduction in morbidity.

Technique of lateral release

A routine diagnostic arthroscopy is first done from the anterolateral approach. The center of the patella will be seen gliding over the lateral femoral condyle rather than down into the patellofemoral groove. The overhand of the lateral facet of the patella past the edge of the lateral femoral condyle is usually best demonstrated at 30 to 45 degrees of flexion. Occasionally it helps to use a superolateral suprapatellar incision for the diagnostic arthroscopy to look at the patellofemoral tracking from a different angle. Twenty milliliters of 0.5% Marcaine with Epinephrine (bupivacaine HCl with epinephrine) is infiltrated into the subcutaneous fascia and retinaculum along the line of intended release. A heavy Mayo type of scissors is then used to create a subcutaneous tunnel along the edge of the patellar tendon. The synovium and thickened retinaculum are then divided with the scissors from the level

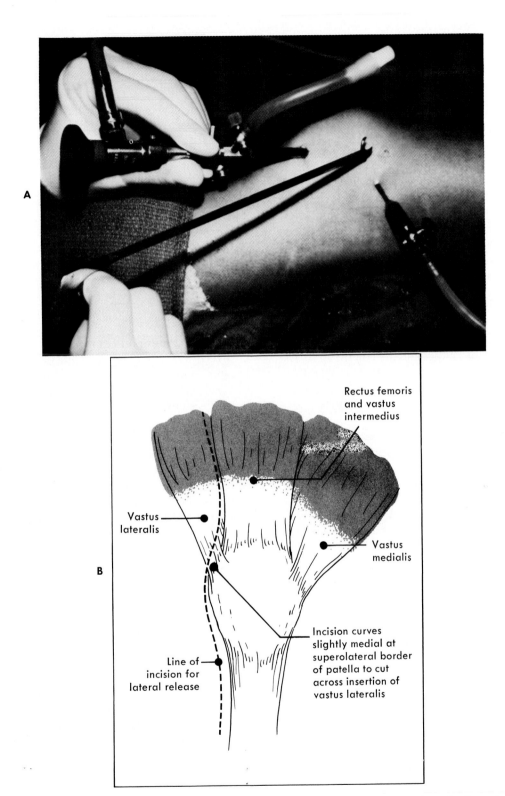

Fig. 16-27. A, A 5 mm intra-articular scissors being inserted to complete the lateral release. **B,** Diagram of line of incision for a lateral patellar release of the right knee.

of the patellar tendon insertion to the superolateral border of the patella. This maneuver is usually just done percutaneously without using arthroscopic control. Be sure to cut all strands of synovium. If it hasn't been done previously, a superolateral-suprapatellar incision is made just adjacent to the superolateral border of the patella. The lateral release is completed with arthroscopic control by inserting a 5 mm telescope in the inferolateral incision and a 4 or 5 mm intra-articular scissors in the superolateral incision (Fig. 16-27, *A*). A specially designed knife shaped much like a meniscotome can also be used instead of the scissors. Continue the release superiorly by curving slightly medially to detach the insertion of the vastus lateralis muscle (Fig. 16-27, *B*). The incision is then continued superiorly well up into the vastus lateralis muscle. This involves going at least 8 to 10 cm above the superior border of the patella. The advantage to using the arthroscope for this upper part of the release is to be more certain that all the tight lateral structures are completely divided. It is most important to cut through the insertion of the vastus lateralis so that lateral overpull will not reoccur. The patellofemoral joint is again inspected with the arthroscope to be sure the patella now glides congruously in the patellofemoral groove as the knee is flexed and extended. The joint is then thoroughly irrigated to remove any loose debris.

Bleeding is controlled by use of a compression pad. The tourniquet is not released until this pad is applied. The pad is made of 1-inch thick firm foam rubber measuring 1 × 4 × 8 inches and is covered with cotton stockinette. The corners where the pad is supposed to go are marked on the skin with a felt-tip pen as a guide to the patient for replacing and rewrapping the pad. The patient is given strict instructions about rewrapping this pad, starting 24 hours after the surgery. The pad is kept rewrapped night and day for 7 to 10 days. I often have the patients come into the office the next morning to be sure they understand how to do this dressing change and the importance of it.

The patients are also instructed to refrain from taking any salicylates before or after the surgery for 2 to 3 weeks. Postoperative exercises are begun in the recovery room with isometric quadriceps tightening and straight-leg lifts. The bupivacaine (Marcaine) allows the patient to do this without pain for 6 to 8 hours postoperatively. Range-of-motion exercise is begun in 2 to 3 days.

Immediate weight-bearing is allowed, though crutches may be used if desired. If a patellar shave has been done, isotonic exercises are not allowed. Patients are encouraged to use a stationary bicycle and swim, and they are not permitted to go back to any running or jumping activities until they have achieved full muscle strength and there is no pain or swelling, which usually takes 6 to 8 weeks at a minimum.

Contraindications to lateral release

A patient with severe patella alta will continue to have subluxation of the patella after a lateral release. The problem is that the patella will still tend to subluxate superiorly and then it slides off laterally in the characteristic inverted J pattern. These patients will gain relief of pain, and a lateral release alone may be worthwhile if the patient understands that a medial reefing or patellar tendon transfer may have to be done later if the subluxation becomes bothersome.

Severe chondromalacia with involvement of greater than 50% of the area of the patella down to subchondral bone may better be managed with a patellectomy.

Technique of patellar shaving

A motorized intra-articular shaver is used to trim off the fragmented and fibrillated areas of chondromalacic cartilage. Johnson[33] emphasizes that it is not necessary to remove this chondromalacic cartilage down to subchondral bone. One advantage that he stresses to this technique is that the normal contour of the articular cartilage is not changed as it often is when a scalpel is used to plane down the acticular surface in an open proceedure. The cartilage "débridement" can be done either before or after the retinacular release, but I prefer to do it before because the patella is not quite so mobile and it is therefore easier to push up against it with the tip of the shaving device. There is also less bleeding and better visualization. The shaving head is triangulated from either the superolateral or inferolateral portal (or from medial portals if preferred). It takes time for the shaving device to do its work, and one must be patient with it and not feel rushed. The rotating direction of the inner cutting sleeve is alternated repeatedly to facilitate the cutting action. Also trim away the hypertrophied synovium from around the edges of the patella. This seems to help in postoperative pain relief. The shaving device will suction out the pieces that it cuts, but it is still a good idea to irrigate the joint to remove any pieces of cartilage that might have escaped going into the suction apparatus. I usually start with the shaver in the superolateral portal and the arthroscope inferolaterally but will often switch these around.

MENISCAL SURGERY
Principles of partial meniscectomy

The primary goal of arthroscopic meniscal surgery is to leave the capsular portion of the meniscus intact. Even though the remaining cartilaginous rim may look ragged and somewhat uneven

(Fig. 16-28) the capsule is still present, and it is the preservation of this cuff of fibroelastic tissue around the joint that adds to its overall stability, possibly preventing the late sequelae of degenerative changes often seen after a total meniscectomy.

Another goal is to remove all meniscal tissue that is offending the joint, which includes anything that can get caught in the joint interface by the shearing, gliding action of the femur against the tibia.

There is also no disruption of surrounding muscle and fascial layers. Meniscal tears can be approached from within the joint at the inner

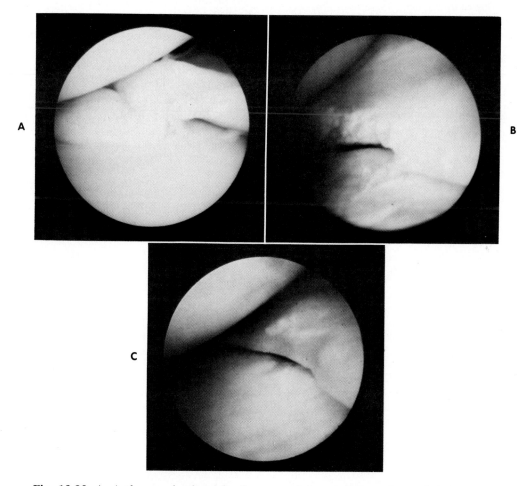

Fig. 16-28. A, Arthroscopic view of a flap tear of the medial meniscus, right knee. **B,** Immediate postoperative view showing the remaining meniscal rim. The area of meniscal resection looks uneven and somewhat ragged. **C,** Second look taken 9 months later (when patient had torn the opposite meniscus playing basketball) shows the meniscal rim to have become smooth and retriangulated. The line of meniscal resection can still be seen. The darker-looking tissue appears to have been "added on" to fill in the meniscus to a nearly normal contour.

margin of the meniscus where the tears begin. It makes good sense to start the resection at the most damaged area (the inner margin) and work toward the normal meniscal cartilage. This would be difficult to do as well with an arthrotomy. Arthroscopic surgery is thus more accurate because of the magnification and illumination possible with modern optical and fiberoptic technology.

Classification of meniscal tears

If a total meniscectomy is done, classification of tear patterns is unnecessary. With partial menis-

Table 16-1. Classification of 258 meniscal tears

Vertical longitudinal tears (bucket handle)	92
Oblique tears (flap)	117
Multiple-plane tears (fragmented or degenerative)	30
Miscellaneous tears (vertical transverse, horizontal, discoid, complex)	19
	258

cectomy however, it is important to know exactly the type of tear to be dealt with. The method of resection and amount of meniscus removed will depend upon the particular tear.

Table 16-1 shows the types of tears classified in a series of 258 partial meniscectomies. Fig. 16-29 shows an anatomic representation of the four basic types of tear patterns. Probing helps delineate these tear planes and define the amount of damaged cartilage that will have to be removed to obtain an even remaining rim. The majority of meniscal tears occur in the posterior horns and medial meniscal tears are more common than lateral ones.

Technique for excision of bucket-handle tears

During diagnostic arthroscopy, the displaced meniscal fragment may be jammed so tightly into the intercondylar notch that it obscures all views of the medial joint compartment and will have to be reduced back to its rim origin with a probe or even removed before the joint can be seen very

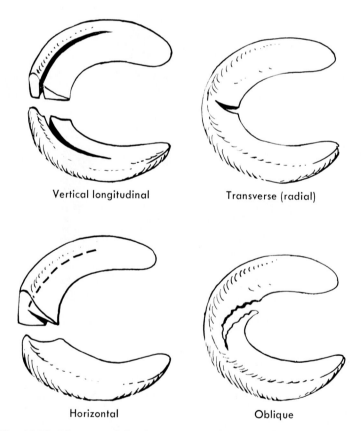

Vertical longitudinal   Transverse (radial)

Horizontal   Oblique

Fig. 16-29. Diagram of the four basic types of meniscal tear patterns.

well. The femoral condyle may have localized areas of chondromalacia at the joint interface where the patient has been walking on the meniscal fragment. Secondary tears of the posterior peripheral rim are more common in the chronic tear than with fresh tears. Associated tears of the opposite meniscus are also common. Sixty percent of patients with a bucket-handle tear will also have a tear of the anterior cruciate ligament.

A step-by-step approach is helpful[45] for this particular tear. The following description is for a bucket-handle tear of the medial meniscus. The same steps are used for a similar tear of the lateral meniscus except that the portals would be reversed.

Step 1. Probing. The diagnostic arthroscope is inserted anterolaterally and a probe anteromedially. The places where cuts are to be made are carefully delineated before any cut is made. Hypertrophied synovium or fat pad that might obstruct a good view of the anterior horn is removed with a motorized shaver inserted anteromedially.

Step 2. Cutting the anterior horn. Cut the anterior attachment of the bucket-handle fragment as close as possible to the countour of the remaining rim to avoid leaving a remnant. The cut is usually made with a scissors, but a meniscal knife works well also. If a tag of meniscus is left attached to the anterior rim, it should be later trimmed.

Step 3. Grasping the fragment (Fig. 16-30). Change the 5 mm scope to the medial anterior portal and grasp the cut end of the bucket-handle fragment with a grasping forceps inserted lateral anteriorly. Be sure to have a secure grip on this fragment as tested by applying traction on the fragment into the intercondylar notch.

Step 4. Cutting the posterior horn. The diagnostic arthroscope is removed and the operating arthroscope is inserted into the medial anterior portal. The bucket-handle fragment is then placed on tension by being pulled into the intercondylar notch. It may help to visualize the posterior attachment by rotating this fragment 180 degrees. A 3 mm scissors is inserted through the operating arthroscope, and under direct vision the fragment is cut free right at its posterior attachment on the tibia. Do not cut blindly in this area. Have the scrub nurse hold the operating arthroscope while you maneuver the grasping instrument in one hand and scissors in the other hand.

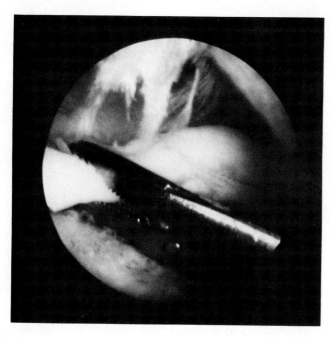

Fig. 16-30. Arthroscopic view of a bucket-handle fragment being firmly grasped and pulled into the intercondylar notch.

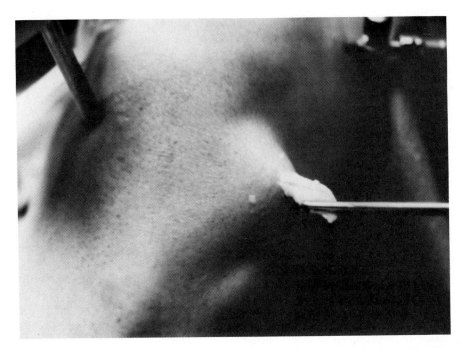

Fig. 16-31. Fragment of meniscus from a bucket-handle type of tear is being removed from the lateral incision. A large fragment can be twisted and teased out of a small incision.

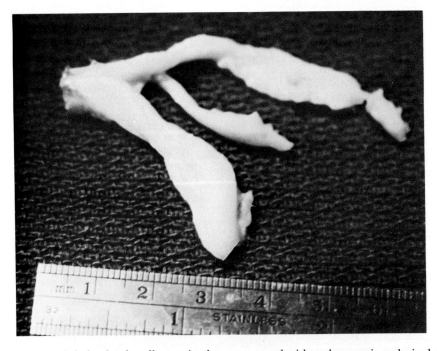

Fig. 16-32. Triple bucket-handle meniscal tear removed with arthroscopic technic demonstrating that this method of knee surgery can be just as thorough as open surgery. It is important to always inspect for further tears once the primary torn fragment has been resected.

Step 5. Removing the fragment. It can be easy to lose the fragment with this maneuver. Be sure there is a good grip near the end of the fragment. Twist and tease the fragment carefully out through the lateral anterior portal (Fig. 16-31). It helps to watch with a 5 mm arthroscope inserted in the medial anterior portal while removing the fragment. If the fragment does become dislodged, it can usually be found in the suprapatellar pouch or lying just under the infrapatellar fat pad.

Step 6. Inspecting and trimming the remaining rim. This is the most important step of all. The rim should be probed and also inspected from a posterior medial puncture. Most trimming is done with a 3 mm single-jaw forceps. A power meniscal cutter may also help. Don't stop until convinced that the remaining rim contains no further tears. If secondary bucket-handle tears are found in the remaining rim, these are removed with the same steps as outlined (Fig. 16-32).

Technique for removal of flap tears

The "flap" tear is the most common type of meniscal tear that occurs. The tear usually starts in an oblique plane and produces a small tag off the inner margin of the meniscus that can then get caught into the more central part of the joint. As the tear extends, the "flap" gets larger and may eventually become a firm, rounded pedunculated mass that catches and locks into the joint interface, producing localized joint-line pain.

Although the patterns of these flap tears are quite variable, their arthroscopic resection has a common technique (Fig. 16-33).

The base of the flap is cut with a knife, scissors, or single-jaw forceps. This can be facilitated if the flap is grasped and put on a stretch. If the flap itself is soft and fibrillated, it can be easily removed with a power meniscal cutter and no other instruments are required. A firm lobulated flap can be cut into several segments and then fed into the meniscal cutter. Fig. 16-33 represents some of the common patterns and the amount of meniscus that is resected. As with the bucket handle tear, always inspect the remaining peripheral rim after resecting the damaged meniscus. Usually only a little fibrillated area is left and this can be trimmed. Be careful that this trimming does not go too deeply into the normal meniscus. If the capsular junction is cut into, the remaining peripheral rim is unstable and a total meniscectomy will be necessary. It is better to resect just a little meniscus at a time and then reprobe. Repeat this process carefully until satisfied that just the right amount of meniscus has been removed.

Technique for horizontal cleavage tears

This type of tear runs longitudinally but in a transverse rather than a vertical plane. In other words, it is at right angles to a bucket-handle tear (Fig. 16-34). It is not common. It is seen in the remaining peripheral rim of a bucket-handle tear and sometimes as a primary tear. Probing will help determine if there is a segment of the torn portion that is protruding out into the joint or feels unstable. This is often a stable type of tear and needs very little trimming.

The resection is done of both superior and inferior "leaves" of the tear, going as deep into the body of the meniscus as needed so that any meniscus that may get caught in the joint is removed. Sometimes the cleavage plane extends out into the capsule, but it may not be necessary to resect the entire meniscus, if the remaining rim is stable. This is determined by repeated probing. Use a 3 or 4 mm single-jaw forceps to do the trimming. Resect 2 or 3 mm of the inner margin all along the extent of the tear and then reprobe. Then resect another strip of 2 mm depth along the margin and probe again, and so on. By careful resection in this manner, an end point will be reached where all damaged meniscus is removed and the capsular support is preserved.

Technique for transverse (radial) tears

This tear rarely extends out into the capsule. It is often associated with a tear of the opposite meniscus and the anterior cruciate ligament. The tear is easy to see, even in the posterior horn. Internal and external rotation maneuvers of the tibia will help open up the tear as it is probed. The important point in the resection of this tear is to remove only enough meniscus to get around the tear without going into the capsule. This is done using a single-jaw forceps and a triangulation technique as already explained. Scallop out on either side of the tear to give a good contour to the remaining rim (Fig. 16-35).

"Total" meniscectomy

The goal of doing arthroscopic resection of these various meniscal tears is to avoid doing a so-

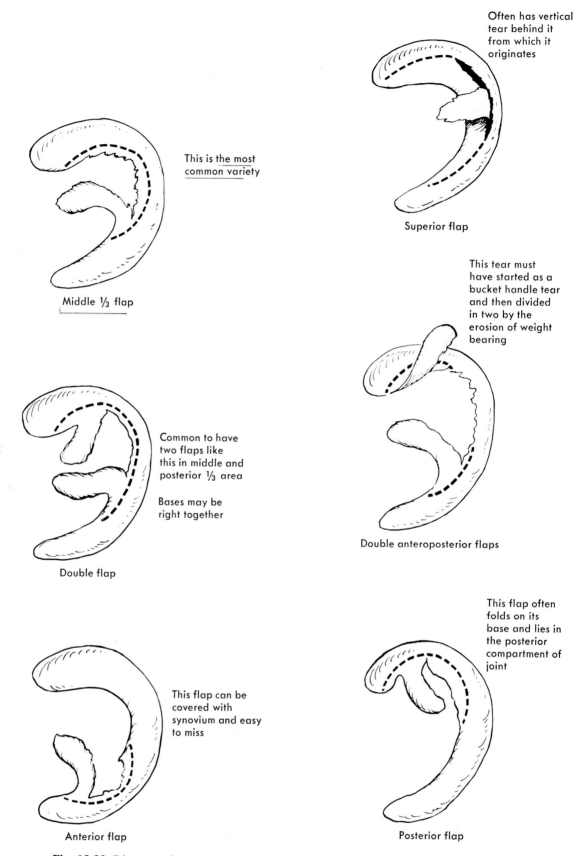

This is the most common variety

Often has vertical tear behind it from which it originates

Superior flap

Middle ⅓ flap

This tear must have started as a bucket handle tear and then divided in two by the erosion of weight bearing

Common to have two flaps like this in middle and posterior ⅓ area

Bases may be right together

Double flap

Double anteroposterior flaps

This flap often folds on its base and lies in the posterior compartment of joint

This flap can be covered with synovium and easy to miss

Anterior flap

Posterior flap

Fig. 16-33. Diagram of some of the common patterns of flap tears. *Dotted line,* Amount of meniscus that is resected.

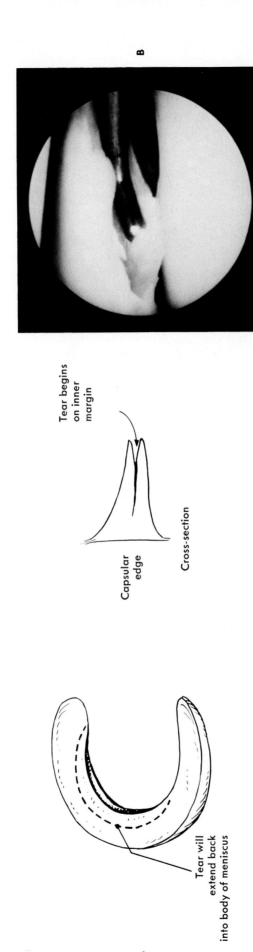

Fig. 16-34. A, Diagram of the horizontal meniscal tear. **B,** Arthroscopic appearance of horizontal meniscal tear.

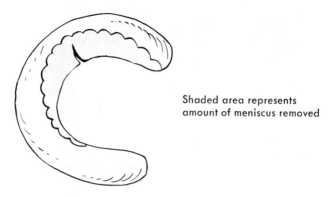

Shaded area represents
amount of meniscus removed

Fig. 16-35. *Shaded area,* Amount of meniscal tissue removed in a radial (transverse vertical) type of tear.

called "total" meniscectomy. By leaving the capsular support to the knee intact, the future sequelae of instability and degenerative changes may be reduced or avoided.

But occasionally, it is necessary to completely excise the meniscus, particularly the posterior horn. These instances include tears that extend out into the capsule and also situations where the capsular rim that is left is so small and unstable that it will likely continue to subluxate into the joint and cause symptoms.

The anterior horn almost never needs to be completely resected, but only tapered slightly to join the resection of the posterior and middle thirds. I have not seen any problems from leaving this anterior segment, and it may continue to have some function in cushioning the anterior joint interface in extension.

Usually the posterior and middle portions are removed in a piecemeal fashion with a single-jaw cutting forceps, augmented by the power meniscal cutter. Using a knife along the peripheral edge of the meniscus, as described by Oretorp and Gillquist[21] can be helpful, especially in the areas of the junction of the middle and posterior thirds. The cutting forceps or power cutter can be used directly in the posterior compartment by triangulation to finish removing the posterior segment of meniscus.

The lateral meniscus is the easier of the two menisci to resect the complete posterior horn, because the lateral compartment opens up wider and allows the use of a larger cutting forceps (4 or 5 mm). Be cautious not to get so vigorous with the cutting forceps that you take out the popliteus tendon as well.

Synovectomy

It is possible to do a relatively thorough synovectomy with endoscopic technique using a motorized cutting instrument (Fig. 16-36). The reduced morbidity is of great benefit to the patient with rheumatoid arthritis. The absence of a long skin incision and the rapid regaining of strength, knee motion, and ambulation are dramatic in comparison to the results of open synovectomy.

Synovectomies are done using a rotary motorized chondral shaver. A tourniquet must be used. Medial and lateral suprapatellar incisions are used in addition to the routine anterior joint-line incisions. A high flow rate or irrigation saline solution must be maintained to enhance the cutting action of the motorized device. Rheumatoid synovium dissects quite easily away from its underlying fascial tissue. A plane can be started inferiorly near the fat pad and then the tip of the motorized shaver used to help dissect away the synovium as the edges are also trimmed and suctioned out of the joint. Once the suprapatellar synovium has been removed, the intercondylar notch is cleaned out. Finally, posterolateral and posteromedial punctures are done (if there is enough tourniquet time left) and as much synovium is removed posteriorly as possible. Let the motorized device do its work and try not to rush its action. I have not liked to go over 90 minutes of tourniquet time, but this has been adequate in the cases I have done.

We have used a padded cotton compression dressing for 48 hours and allowed patients to bear full weight as able, which is usually the day of surgery. Active range-of-motion exercise is begun immediately, even with the bulky dressing after

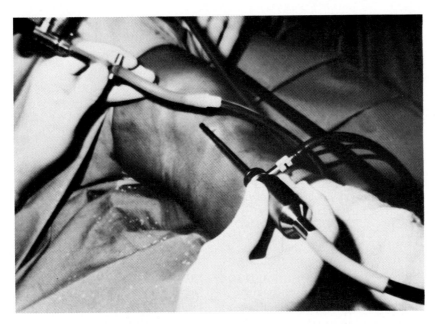

Fig. 16-36. Another type of motorized intra-articular cutter used for patellar shaving, synovectomy, and meniscal resection.

48 hours. An Ace bandage wrap is then used until all swelling has subsided. Postoperative swelling and bleeding is surprisingly minimal. No patient has yet required postoperative aspiration of fluid from the knee. Isometric exercises are stressed, both preoperatively and postoperatively.

Currently, there are being developed new types of motorized devices that show promise of being able to do a synovectomy much faster. They have a reciprocating cutting action and an increased suction power. Their guillotine type of action cuts synovium very rapidly and cleanly.

Joint adhesions

Arthroscopic resection of joint adhesions is a beneficial procedure (Fig. 16-37). By elimination of another arthrotomy, in the case of postoperative adhesions, there is a much better chance of regaining and maintaining active motion in the knee. Motion can also be started immediately after surgery, which is an advantage over excision of adhesions with an arthrotomy. The arthroscope also aids in establishing an exact location and extent of the adhesions. Dense adhesions can be gradually broken by use of a blunt obturator. Thickened bands of fibrous tissue may have to be cut with scissors and sometimes removed with the motorized shaver. Occasionally single bands of fi-

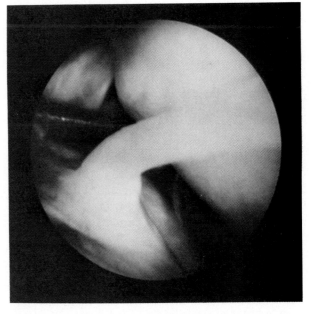

Fig. 16-37. Arthroscopic view of a dense, fibrous adhesion that was found to be bowstringing across the medial femoral condyle and simulating a meniscal tear. It was a result of an episode of direct blunt trauma to the knee. This type of lesion can be easily resected with arthroscopic technique.

brous tissue are found that will catch or pop along some part of the knee joint, usually in the suprapatellar pouch or the medial and lateral gutters.

Chondral defects

Chondral fractures do occur with injuries to the knee and are often overlooked as a cause of hemarthrosis. They occur with blunt trauma and also in association with tears of the anterior cruciate ligament where the anterior tibial spine rotates and impinges against the femoral condyle (usually medial) producing a circumscribed type of chondral defect and associated loose body. There are three types of defects that are commonly encountered:

1. *Stellate or linear fractures.* This type of lesion occurs with blunt trauma and may be a single longitudinal cleft or furrow in either the femoral or tibial articular cartilage. There may be some undermining of one side of the cleft so that a flap of articular cartilage is created that can be lifted up with a probe. The stellate type has multiple clefts radiating out from a central area.

2. *Crater.* This type of chondral defect comes from trauma. It is seen on the femoral condyles and occasionally in the patellofemoral groove area. A dislocation of the patella will sometimes cause a craterlike defect on the lateral edge of the lateral femoral condyle, though this is more often an osteochondral fracture shearing off the edge of the condyle. When these craters are seen arthroscopically, there has to be a loose body somewhere within the knee joint and it must be searched for thoroughly.

3. *Shaggy fibrillated chondromalacia.* This type of chondral defect comes from excessive pressure, shearing force, and wear and is usually associated with an aging process. However it can occur in younger patients and is seen after total meniscectomy, sometimes within 2 or 3 years after surgery. Large flap tears of the menisci will often produce a localized area of chondromalacia and erosion of the adjacent femoral condyle and tibial plateau.

There is a tendency in doing diagnostic arthroscopy to skip over the femoral condyles and concentrate on the menisci and suprapatellar and patellar areas. Injection of diluted methylene blue dye into the joint will show a differential staining of abnormal articular cartilage, which takes on a more bluish tint. Probing is helpful and also switching the arthroscope to different portals for another angle of view will assist in finding these cartilaginous defects.

Arthroscopic curettage and drilling is done to stimulate proliferation of a fibrocartilage-healing process.[47] A smooth, 0.064 or 0.045 Kirschner wire is used for a drill, eliminating problems of small bone fragments getting into the joint or soft tissue winding up on the drill as encountered when a regular twist drill is used. The holes are placed as nearly perpendicular to the convexity of the condyle as possible. This may necessitate approaching the defect from several angles. Piercing the skin from the desired angle does not add to the morbidity of the case, even if several punctures are used. A ring curette can also be used to scarify hard subchondral bone at the base of the crater. High-speed dental burrs have also been used to help with the curettage.

Postoperative care includes nonweight-bearing using crutches for 3 to 6 weeks and immediate active range-of-motion exercise, which is pursued vigorously. Once weight-bearing has begun, the knee is further protected from any running or jumping activities for 6 to 12 months after surgery.

Clinically these patients do better than might be expected with relief of the aching pain they had preoperatively and elimination of recurrent joint effusions in most cases. The few knees that I have been able to reexamine arthroscopically have shown a definite covering of the defect with fibrocartilage. Johnson has coined the term "abrasion chondroplasty"[34] for the arthroscopic management of these patients and has routinely reexamined a series of knees arthroscopically at various postoperative time intervals. His observations show a sealing over of the chondral defect with fibrocartilage. This technique may have some application in the osteoarthritic knee.

Osteochondritis dissecans. Guhl[21] has shown that it is possible to treat all phases of osteochondritis dissecans of the knee joint with arthroscopic technique. Intact lesions on the femoral condyle that have not responded to nonsurgical treatment can be concentrically drilled. Craters with a salvageable loose body are treated by curettage and drilling of the base of the crater followed by fixation of the loose fragment with dual threaded Kirschner wires. Large avascular fragments can be bone grafted by a technique done with arthroscopic control. These techniques are technically difficult and should not be attempted until the surgeon has gained much experience in arthroscopic surgery.

CONCLUSION

Looking to future developments in arthroscopic surgery, it seems certain that these techniques will be used by more and more orthopedic surgeons. Applications of endoscopic surgery may be found for other joints.[55] Improvements in instruments and technology should make the surgery easier. Research is being done on the use of a laser beam to remove damaged or degenerative tissues from the knee joint. Mechanically operated instruments will also become more efficient. Diagnostic arthroscopy can be helpful for follow-up in other types of knee surgery.[40]

It should be stressed again that these endoscopic knee-surgery techniques take time and patience to learn and must be done carefully. But once learned by an interested orthopedic surgeon, this new method of knee surgery can be offered to patients with confidence that results will be at least equal to those achieved by traditional arthrotomy methods, with a dramatic reduction in postoperative morbidity and complications.

REFERENCES

1. Alm, A., Gillquist, J. and Liljedahl, S.: The diagnostic value of arthroscopy of the knee joint, Injury **5:**319-324, May 1974
2. Appel, H.: Late results after meniscectomy in the knee joint: a clinical and roentgenologic follow-up investigation, Acta Orthop. Scand. 133 (Suppl.):1, 1970.
3. Aritomi, H., and Yamamoto, M.: A method of arthroscopic surgery: clinical evaluation of synovectomy with the electric resectoscope and removal of loose bodies in the knee joint, Orthop. Clin. North Am. **10**(3):565, July 1979.
4. Bentley, G.: The surgical treatment of chondromalacia patellae, J. Bone Joint Surg. **60B:**74-81, 1978.
5. Carruthers, C.C., and Kennedy, M.: Knee arthroscopy: a follow-up of patients initially not recommended for further surgery, Clin. Orthop. **147:**275-277, 1980.
6. Carson, R.W.: Arthroscopic meniscectomy, Orthop. Clin. North Am. **10**(3):619-628, July 1979.
7. Casscells, S.W.: Arthroscopy of the knee joint, J. Bone Joint Surg. **53A:**287-298, 1971.
8. Cullen, J.C.: Meniscectomy, NZ Med. J. **89:**138-140, 1979.
9. Dandy, D.J., and Hodge, G.J.: Closed partial meniscectomy, Physiotherapy **64:**367-368, 1978.
10. Dandy, D.J., and Jackson, R.W.: The impact of arthroscopy on the management of disorders of the knee, J. Bone Joint Surg. **57B:**346-348, 1975.
11. DeHaven, K.E., and Collins, H.R.: Diagnosis of internal derangements of the knee: the role of arthroscopy, J. Bone Joint Surg. **57A:**801-810, 1975.
12. Edgar, M.A., and Lowy, M.: Arthroscopy of the knee: a preliminary review of fifty cases, Proc. R. Soc. Med. **66:**512-515, 1973.
13. Eriksson, E., and Sebik, A.: A comparison between the transpatellar tendon and the lateral approach to the knee joint during arthroscopy: a cadaver study, Am. J. Sports Med. **8:**103-105, 1980.
14. Ficat, R.P., and Hungerford, M.D.: Disorders of the patellofemoral joint, Baltimore, Md., 1977, The Williams & Wilkins Co.
15. Fox, J.M., Blazina, M.E., and Carlson, G.J.: Multiphasic view of medial meniscectomy, Am. J. Sports Med. **7:**161-164, 1979.
16. Funk, F.J., Jr.: A color atlas of arthroscopy, J. Sports Med. **1:**24-26, 1972.
17. Gilley, J.S., Gelman, M.I., Edson, M.V., and Metcalf, R.W.: Chondral fractures of the knee: arthrographic, arthroscopic, and clinical manifestations, Radiology **138:**51-54, 1981.
18. Gillquist, J., Hagberg, G., and Oretorp, N.: Therapeutic arthroscopy of the knee, Injury **10:**128-132, 1978.
19. Gillquist, J., Hagberg, G., and Oretorp, N.: Arthroscopic visualization of the posteromedial compartment of the knee joint, Orthop. Clin. North Am. **10:**545-547, 1979.
20. Goodfellow, J., Hungerford, D.S., and Woods, C.: Patellofemoral mechanics and pathology, J. Bone Joint Surg. **58B:**291-299, 1979.
21. Guhl, J.F.: Arthroscopic treatment of osteochondritis dissecans: preliminary report, Orthop. Clin. North Am. **10:**671-684, July 1979.
22. Halperin, N., Axer, A., Hirschberg, E., and Agasi, M.: Arthroscopy of the knee under local anesthesia and controlled pressure-irrigation, Clin. Orthop. **134:**176-179, 1978.
23. Hughston, J.C., Whatley, G.S., Dodelin, R.A., and Stone, M.M.: The role of the suprapatellar plica in internal derangement of the knee, Am. J. Orthop. **5:**25-27, 1963.
24. Ikeuchi, H.: Total meniscectomy of the complete discoid meniscus under arthroscopic control: a case report, J. Jpn. Orthop. Assoc. **44:**374, 1970. (In Japanese.)
25. Ikeuchi, H.: Surgery under arthroscopic control, Rheumatologie **33:**57-64, 1976.
26. Insall, J., Bullough, P.G., and Burstein, A.H.: Proximal realignment of the patella for chondromalacia patellae, Clin. Orthop. **144:**63-69, 1979.
27. Insall, J. Falvo, K.A., and Wise, D.W.: Chondromalacia patellae: a prospective study, J. Bone Joint Surg. **58A:**1-8, 1976.
28. Jackson, R.W.: Etiology of chondromalacia patellae, AAOS: Instructional course lectures **25:**39-40, St. Louis, 1976, The C.V. Mosby Co.
29. Jackson, R.W., and Abe, I.: The role of arthroscopy in the management of disorders of the knee: an analysis of 200 consecutive cases, J. Bone Joint Surg. **54B:**310-322, 1972.
30. Jackson, R.W., and DeHaven, K.E.: Arthroscopy of the knee, Clin. Orthop. **107:**87-92, 1974.
31. Johnson, L.L.: Comprehensive arthroscopic examination of the knee joint, St. Louis, 1978, The C.V. Mosby Co.
32. Johnson, L.L.: Arthroscopic surgery of the knee and other joints, St. Louis, 1981, The C.V. Mosby Co.
33. Johnson, L.L.: Schneider, D., Goodwin, F.G., and Bullock, J.M.: A sterilization method for arthroscopes using activated dialdehyde, Orthop. Rev. **VI**(9):75-77, Sept. 1977.

34. Johnson, L.L.: Abrasion chondroplasty, personal communication, East Lansing, Mich., 1980.

35. Johnson, R.J., and Kettelkamp, D.B., et al.: Factors affecting late results after meniscectomy, J. Bone Joint Surg. **56A:**719-729, 1974.

36. Jones, R.E., Smith, E.C., and Reisch, J.S.: Effects of medial meniscectomy in patients older than forty years, J. Bone Joint Surg. **60A:**783-786, 1978.

37. Kreft, E.: Arthroscopy: its place in the diagnosis of knee lesions, J. Bone Joint Surg. **57B:**255, 1975.

38. Larson, R.L., Cabaub, E., Slocum, D.B., et al.: Patellar compression syndrome: treatment with lateral retinacular release, Clin. Orthop. **134:**158-166, July 1978.

39. Lauttamas, L., Haikara, J., and Korkala, O.: Late results of meniscectomy of the knee: a follow-up study of 41 patients, Ann. Chir. Gynaecol. **68:**169-171, 1979.

40. Matsui, N., Moriya, H., and Kitahara, H.: The use of arthroscopy for follow-up in knee joint surgery, Orthop. Clin. North Am. **10**(3):713-723, July 1979.

41. McGinty, J.B.: Method of loose body removal, personal communication, Newton Lower Falls, Mass., 1980.

42. McGinty, J.B., and Freedman, P.A.: Arthroscopy of the knee, Clin. Orthop. **121:**173-180, 1976.

43. McGinty, J.B., and Matza, R.A.: Arthroscopy of the knee: evaluation of an out-patient procedure under local anesthesia, J. Bone Joint Surgery **60A:**787-789, 1978.

44. McGinty, J.B., and McCarthy, J.C.: Lateral retinacular release: an endoscopic procedure, presentation at annual meeting of the American Academy of Orthopaedic Surgeons, Atlanta, 1980.

45. Metcalf, R.W.: Instructional manual of arthroscopic surgery, Salt Lake City, 1980, Press Publishing Ltd.

46. Merchant, A., and Mercer, R.: Lateral release of the patella: a preliminary report, Clin. Orthop. **103:**40-45, 1974.

47. Murray, D.G.: Patellar revision resurfacing and removal, AAOS: Instructional course lectures **25:**54-60, St. Louis, 1976, The C.V. Mosby Co.

48. Noble, J., and Erat, K.: In defense of the meniscus: a prospective study of 200 meniscectomy patients, J. Bone Joint Surg. **62B:**7-11, 1980.

49. O'Connor, R.L.: Arthroscopy, Philadelphia, 1977, J.B. Lippincott Co.

50. Outerbridge, R.E., and Dunlop, J.A.: The problem of chondromalacia patellae, Clin. Orthop. **110:**177-196, 1975.

51. Patel, D.: Proximal approach to intraarticular closed endoscopic knee surgery, presentation at the International Arthroscopy Association, Philadelphia, 1980.

52. Pipkin, G.: Lesions of the suprapatellar plica, J. Bone Joint Surg. **32A:**363-369, 1950.

53. Poehling, G.G., Bassett, F.H., and Goldner, J.L.: Arthroscopy: its role in treating non-traumatic and traumatic lesions of the knee, South. Med. J. **70:**465-469, 1977.

54. Schoenholtz, G.J.: Arthroscopy of the knee joint, South. Med. J. **69**(11):1493-1495, 1976.

55. Shifrin, L.Z., and Reis, N.D.: Arthroscopy of a dislocated hip replacement: case report, Clin. Orthop. **146:**213-214, 1980.

56. Tapper, E.M., and Hoover, N.W.: Late results after meniscectomy, J. Bone Joint Surg. **51A:**517-526, 1969.

57. Thompson, R.C., Jr.: An experimental study of surface injury to articular cartilage and enzyme responses within the joint, Clin. Orthop. **107:**239-248, 1975.

58. Vahvanen, V., and Aalto, K.: Meniscectomy in children, Acta Orthop. Scand. **50:**791-795, 1979.

59. Watanabe, M., Takeda, S., and Ikeuchi, H.: Atlas of arthroscopy, ed. 2, Tokyo, 1969, Igakushoin.

60. Whipple, T.L., and Bassett, F.H.: Arthroscopic examination of the knee: polypuncture technique with percutaneous intra-articular manipulation, J. Bone Joint Surg. **60A:**444-453, 1978.

Chapter 17

Fixation failure of tibial component: causes and prevention

CHITRANJAN S. RANAWAT, M.D.
New York, New York

The most feared complication of total knee arthroplasty has been failure of fixation of the tibial component with the condylar type of prosthesis. The incidence of mechanical failure of the tibial component of the condylar prosthesis has been reported between 0 to 25% at 2-year follow-up.[7] A long-term follow-up of total knee arthroplasty from the point of fixation failure is not available in the current literature. The fixation failure or loosening of the component is defined as (1) loss of position of the component, (2) increase or recurrence of deformity at the knee, or (3) progressive radiolucency at the cement-bone interface of 2 mm or more. These criteria of loosening should be differentiated from cement bone–interface radiolucency, which is often present. In this report factors that are responsible for fixation failure of the tibial component are presented.

MATERIAL AND METHOD

The presence of radiolucency at the cement-bone interface as seen on a routine roentgenogram is compatible with a good knee arthroplasty. When this interface becomes progressively wider and exceeds 2 mm or more, severe symptoms with disability may appear because of loosening. To assess the radiolucency, one should obtain a proper roentgenogram. The x-ray beam should be parallel to the cement-bone interface. A slight obliquity may mask this radiolucency. The radiolucency at the interface can be divided into three zones: the outer half of the medial and lateral condyles as *zone I*, the medial half as *zone II*, and that along

the peg as *zone III*. A radiolucency in all the three zones indicates a loose component. The other diagnostic tests to assess the loose tibial component are bone scan and arthrography. Both of these tests are usually diagnostic only when there is obvious loosening as can be detected from serial plain roentgenogram.

Factors that are responsible for loosening can be divided into (1) prosthetic design, (2) surgical technique, which includes alignment, cement technique, and stability of the joint, (3) quality of the bone, and (4) activity of the patient, body weight, age, and mobility of the joint above and below.

PROSTHETIC DESIGN

Three aspects of prosthetic design are (1) effect of confirmity, (2) stem, and (3) metal-backed tibial plateaus.

The effect of conformity has been studied by Greenwald et al.[3] They pointed out that the prosthesis with point contact between metal and polyethylene has the least torque and therefore would have the least amount of stress on the cement-bone interface. However, high concentration of pressure on the high-density polyethylene could cause fragmentation and failure in the long run.[2,9] The total conformity of the femoral and the tibial plateau will distribute the load broadly but produces high torque, which tends to loosen the tibial component as is seen with the Geometric design.[11] It appears that the optimum conformity is partial, but the exact amount of this is not yet defined.

397

The optimum thickness of the tibial plateau of high-density polyethylene has been shown to be 8 mm or more. Unsupported tibial plateaus that are 4 and 5 mm of thickness have been found to get loose very readily. Two separate tibial components, as in the Duocondylar type, have been shown to be inferior in terms of fixation as compared to a one-piece unit with a short stem.[12] The clinical study of Duocondylar prostheses showed the incidence of radiolucency under the tibial plateau to be 80% as against 22% of the Total Condylar.[5,6] Both studies were carried out at The Hospital for Special Surgery. On these data it can be inferred that placement of a short stem or two pegs on either side under the condyle provides better fixation. The forces in the knee joint are compressive and tensile associated with a large tilting moment, especially if the joint is unstable and the point of contact shifts from the center of the dish to the periphery. The stem or pegs obviously will resist tilting forces.

Controversy still exists in terms of metal-backed components versus high-density polyethylene components. If thick-enough high-density polyethylene components (such as 1 cm or more) are used, the plastic deformation is minimum. A metal-backed component obviously will give better support to the high-density polyethylene, but the technical difficulties of mounting the tibial plateau properly on the metal dish to eliminate the dead space and achieve secure fixation have not been solved. Furthermore, revision, when necessary, will be technically more difficult with a metal-backed component than those with high-density polyethylene because metal-backed ones cannot be cut through. Another drawback of the metal-backed tibial plateau is that the radiolucent zone is difficult to assess under the metal tray. Two recent studies[1,13] point out that the metal-backed component would provide better load distribution over the cement and therefore be more durable. However, at the present time there are no long-term clinical studies available to confirm or refute the above concept.

SURGICAL TECHNIQUE

The following are the important criteria for a proper knee arthroplasty:

1. Alignment in the frontal plane should restore 5 to 8 degrees of valgus to the knee.
2. There should be proper soft-tissue balance and tension in full extension and 90 degrees of flexion.
3. The cement-bone interface cuts should be 90 degrees to the mechanical axis of the femur and tibia. The mechanical axis passes from the center of the femoral head to the center of the ankle joint.
4. Proper orientation of the quadriceps mechanism is necessary.
5. Proper cement technique is necessary.

Alignment

Five to 8 degrees of valgus alignment is desirable. This valgus alignment is in the femoral side. The tibial plateau should be 90 degrees to the long axis of the tibia. The femoral component is 5 to 8 degrees in valgus position, which is 90 degrees to the mechanical axis of the femur. In the lateral plane, both the components should be at 90 degrees to the long axis. It is desirable to have 0 to 8 degrees of posterior slope in the tibial plateau. It has been shown quite clearly that those knee arthroplasties that have malalignment, especially toward the neutral or varus position are overloaded and are subject to loosening.[4,9,11] If the femoral implant is not put in neutral alignment in the coronal plane, there will be malalignment of the patellofemoral joint and improper tracking of the femoral component into the tibial dish. The neutral alignment is best judged by removal of equal amounts of condyles of the femur posterior to the femoral jig. This obviously has to be modified if there is unusual loss of bone.

Stability

The static stability of the joint is provided by the congruence of the femoral and tibial components, medial and lateral collateral ligaments, and the remaining soft-tissue sleeve. The dynamic stability is provided by active muscle control and the body weight. It is important that the medial or lateral ligaments along with the capsule should be released when there is fixed deformity of varus or valgus, respectively. The release of the fixed medial or lateral soft-tissue structures allows the knee to be brought into neutral position and the knee becomes balanced. Additional soft-tissue stability is achieved by selection of the proper size of the implant for a given knee. It is best judged by flexion of the knee and measurement of the height of the femoral condyles from front to back. An attempt should be made to match this size to the available sizes of the femoral prosthesis.

Cement technique

One of the most important causes of poor penetration of cement into the cancellous bone is residual bone debris, fat and blood. Fortunately, the knee arthroplasty is done under tourniquet and blood can be effectively controlled. The remaining fat, some blood and debris can be cleaned by a water lavage. Soft doughy cement does penetrate better than firm doughy cement. The pressurization of the cement can be done by special syringes or by pressure on the implant. The un-

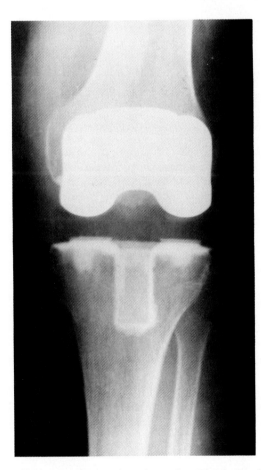

Fig. 17-1. Anteroposterior view of a Total Condylar knee arthroplasty. The cement penetration into the cancellous bone of 5 mm is achieved by use of soft doughy Simplex cement. Pressurization is obtained by the undersurface of the tibial plateau.

dersurface of the tibial plateau along with the peg allows the cement to be pressurized. The cement can easily penetrate up to 4 or 5 mm into the cancellous bone (Fig. 17-1). While the cement is hardening, pressure should be maintained and the excess cement removed. It is obvious that to maintain a steady pressure a vertical compression is essential. To achieve this, one should mobilize the tibia enough to bring it in front of the femur when possible for vertical compression. Using these techniques, one is able to achieve a high-quality mechanical bondage between the implant, cement, and bone.[8] In patients with rheumatoid arthritis who have osteoporotic bone, at times the trabecular system is so weak that a secure fixation is technically not possible. The bony cut of the tibia must be made within 0.5 to 1 cm from the articular surface of the condyle to preserve strong bone to achieve fixation with cement. It has been shown that the strength of the trabecular bone is superior in the subchondral region, and therefore attempts should be made to stay within this zone of good-quality bone.

MANAGEMENT OF LARGE BONE DEFECTS

Severe varus deformity of the knee causes loss of bone from the medial tibial condyle. There are several options available to handle such bone defects. The bone can be cut to the level of the defect in the bone and achieve a flat surface. In doing so, good-quality bone from the opposite side is lost and the width of the tibia is reduced and therefore a proper seating of the tibial plateau may be difficult. At times this may also reach at or below the level of the tibial tubercle. The second option available is to have a step-cut tibial plateau to fit such a defect. To perform the operation properly, one must have available many sizes of the implants. The pressurization of the cement will be uneven. The last method of handling this situation is to reduce the depth of the defect by 50% or less and to fill the remaining defect with cement in combination with a screw and mesh (Fig. 17-2). This does reinforce the cement. Occasionally, bone graft may be necessary to provide support when the defect is large. Alternatively, a metal-backed tibial component with a longer stem can be utilized and the load can be transmitted more into the stem and less on the condyle.

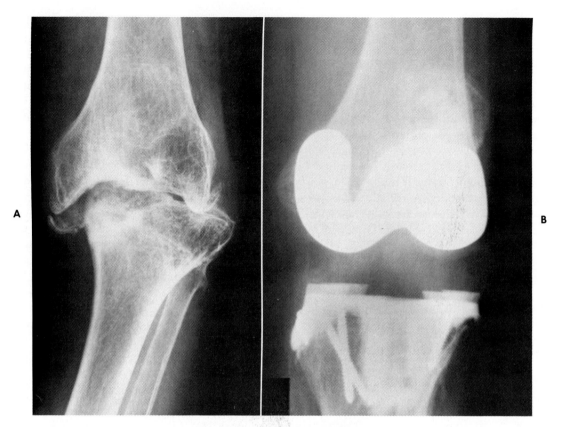

Fig. 17-2. A, Anteroposterior view of a knee preoperatively with 35 degrees of varus deformity. Loss of bone is present in the tibia and the femur. **B,** Same knee after Total Condylar knee arthroplasty. The tibial plateau fixation was achieved with bone cement, screws, and mesh. This combination is used to build up the defect of the medial plateau and reinforce the cement.

DISCUSSION

To the exclusion of infection, the loosening of the tibial plateau with loss of fixation appears to be the most important complication of knee arthroplasty in long-term follow-up. The reported incidence is 0 to 25%[7] for condylar prostheses and higher for hinged prostheses. The various factors responsible for loosening include design of the prosthesis, accurate surgical technique, and appropriate cement technique. With proper utilization of the above measures, the incidence of loosening can be significantly reduced. Since March 1974, I have performed over 400 total knee arthroplasties using total condylar prostheses with 1 to 6 years follow-up. Revision surgery for mechanical loosening has not been necessary to this date. The loosening has been defined as a shift of the component, recurrence or progression of deformity, and 2 mm of radiolucent zone at the cement-bone interface in and around the stem with progressive symptoms. In my experience it is possible to achieve good-to-excellent results in 95% to 98% of the patients with a carefully done knee arthroplasty and results should be durable at least for 5 years or so. I should point out that one third of the patients do show incomplete and nonprogressive radiolucency at the cement-bone interface in zones I and II. Rarely does one see radiolucency in zone III or along the stem. There are several factors, beyond the control of the operating surgeon, that include the status of the cancellous bone as in rheumatoid patients.

REFERENCES

1. Bartel, D.L., Santavicca, E.A., and Burstein, A.H.: The effects of pegs with trays on stresses associated with loosening of knee prostheses, Proceedings of the Orthopedic Research Society, Atlanta, Ga., **5:**165, 1980.
2. Ducheyne, P., Kagen, A., II, and Lacey, J.A.: Failure of total knee arthroplasty due to loosening and deformation of the tibial component, J. Bone Joint Surg. **60A:**384, 1978.
3. Greenwald, A.S., Black, J.D., and Matejczyk, M.B.: Rotational characteristics of non-hinged total knee replacements, Orthop. Trans. **1**(2):213, 1977.
4. Gunston, F.H., and MacKenzie, R.I.: Complications of Polycentric knee arthroplasty, Clin. Orthop. **120:**11-17, 1976.
5. Insall, J., Ranawat, C., Aglietti, P., and Shine, J.: A comparison of four models of total knee replacement prostheses, J. Bone Joint Surg. **58A:**754-765, 1976.
6. Insall, J., Scott, N., and Ranawat, C.S.: The Total Condylar knee prosthesis: a report of two hundred and twenty cases, J. Bone Joint Surg. **61A:**173-180, 1979.
7. Kettelkamp, D.B.: Knee implants: review of current status, J. Continuing Educ. in Orthopedics, p. 21, 1976.
8. Lee, A.J.C., Ling, R.S.M., and Vangala, S.S.: Some clinically relevant variables affecting the mechanical behavior of bone cement, Arch. Orthop. Traumat. Surg. **92:**1-18, 1978.
9. Marmor, L.: Marmor modular knee in unicompartmental disease, J. Bone Joint Surg. **61A:**347, 1979.
10. Ranawat, C.S., and Shine, J.: Duo Condylar total knee arthroplasty, Clin. Orthop. **94:**185, 1973.
11. Skolnick, M.D., Coventry, M.D., and Ilstrup, D.M.: Geometric total knee arthroplasty, J. Bone Joint Surg. **58A:**749-753, 1976.
12. Walker, P., Ranawat, C., and Insall, J.: Fixation of the tibial component of condylar replacement knee prostheses, J. Biomechanics **9:**269-275, 1976.
13. Walker, P., Greene, D., Ben Dov, M., Thatcher, J., and Ewald, F.: Fixation of tibial components of knee prosthesis, Orthop. Trans. **3**(2):188, 1979.

TECHNIQUES OF REVISION SURGERY AND CONTROVERSIES IN TOTAL HIP

Chapter 18

Indications for surface replacement of hip

MARK B. COVENTRY, M.D.
Rochester, Minnesota

Why surface replacement? What is the advantage, if any, over total hip arthroplasty? It has been said that surface replacement is more "physiologic."[1] Does it actually function better? It more closely resembles the normal anatomy of the hip. Does this necessarily imply a better hip? The very basic advantage of surface replacement lies in the fact that *it does not invade the femoral canal.* The upper portion of the medullary cavity is not violated, that is, curetted, packed with methyl methacrylate, and fitted with a stem of metal several inches long. By not doing so, one can assure that surface replacement destroys less tissue and saves bone stock. The chance of infection is lessened, the incidence of fat embolism is lower, and the long-term complication of loosening of the femoral component is avoided. Salvage, if complications including infection should occur, is made easier.

What disadvantages of surface replacement are emerging? Our number one complication at the Mayo Clinic is fracture of the femoral neck under, or just adjacent to, the rim of the femoral unit. During our first year's experience with surface replacement (1978), we used the THARIES (total hip articular replacement with internal eccentric shells) system exclusively. Seven of 66 hips suffered a fracture of the femoral neck 2 to 30 months postoperatively. In 1979, however, with a follow-up of a maximum of 16 months and a minimum of 4 months, no neck fractures occurred in 38 hip resurfacings. Surely this emphasizes the importance of experience in the selection of patients and with the detailed and exacting surgical technique of surface replacement.

Will the ultimate functional results of the surface replacement be superior to those of total hip

arthroplasty? The Harris hip score in patients with minimal 1-year follow-up averaged 91.33; this result compares favorably with our previously computed score of 89 for total hip replacement.[2]

With these considerations in mind, what, then, are the indications for surface replacement *at this time?* The diagnoses in the patients during our first year of experience were as follows: osteoarthritis 25, traumatic arthritis 8, avascular necrosis 8, rheumatoid arthritis 7, dysplasia 6, rheumatoid spondylitis 5, protrusio acetabuli 2, and a problem caused by a previous operation 5 (a failed cup 1, a [pinned] slipped capital femoral epiphysis 1, [pinned] fracture 2, and a Chiari osteotomy 1). In essence, the indications for surface replacement are the same as those for total hip arthroplasty, provided that there is enough bone stock to perform surface replacement. This means an adequate length of the femoral neck and strong, viable bone of the femoral head on which to cement the femoral component. At least two thirds of the head must be of normal bone. Bone of the acetabulum must be adequate centrally and peripherally for the rather large polyethylene acetabular unit. As is the case in total hip arthroplasty, the acetabulum can be "shored up" with a bone graft if necessary. Deformity of the existing bone should be minimal. A substantial coxa vara or an intertrochanteric fracture healed with substantial deformity creates a poor mechanical base for surface replacement.

Because the femoral stem of the prosthesis is excluded, the potential for complications is minimal, and patients in a younger age group can be considered for the operation. Patients in their twenties, thirties, and forties who have posttrau-

405

matic residuals or postdevelopmental arthrosis from Legg-Calvé-Perthes disease, slipped capital femoral epiphysis, or acetabular dysplasia are perhaps the ideal candidates for resurfacing—and so is the conventional osteoarthritic patient in any age group, provided that excessive deformity has not developed. Osteoporosis will potentiate a femoral neck fracture, and such patients must be observed for a prolonged period and be managed with a postoperative program of graduated weight bearing.

What of the acetabular component? It is considerably thinner than any of the conventional units for total hip arthroplasty. Does this mean a less stress-absorbing effect before the thrust is placed on the bone-cement junction, and thus more instances of acetabular component loosening? There is some evidence emerging that this is, indeed, happening. Will the relative thinness of the acetabular unit result in wear rather early after implantation and thus vitiate the apparent advantage of using surface replacement in the younger patient? If infection or mechanical loosening occurs, necessitating removal of the component, will it be difficult to replace with another component or even a conventional total hip unit because of the lack of bone stock of the acetabulum? The relative sacrifice of acetabular bone stock by this operation is a concern, and one that will be resolved only as we gain more experience with the operation and its complications.

Today the four surface prostheses most commonly used in the United States and Canada are the THARIES, the ICLH (Freeman-Swanson), the Wagner, and the Indianapolis (Capello). In summary, they are indicated when a total hip replacement would be in order, provided that femoral and acetabular bone stock is adequate and there is relative freedom from deformity. Because of the lack of potential for complications related to the upper end of the femur and the femoral canal, surface replacement is used to best advantage in the younger person. It can be converted readily to conventional replacement if failure occurs. Infection, if it occurs, can be handled more easily because the femoral canal will not have been involved.

REFERENCES

1. Cabanela, M.E., Campbell, D.C., II, and Henderson, E.D.: Total joint arthroplasty: the hip, Mayo Clin. Proc. **54:**559, 1979.
2. Ilstrup, D.M., Nolan, D.R., Beckenbaugh, R.D., and Coventry, M.B.: Factors influencing the results in 2,012 total hip arthroplasties, Clin. Orthop. **95:**250, 1973.

Chapter 19

Improved cementing techniques

A.J.C. LEE, B.Sc., Ph.D.

R.S.M. LING, M.A., B.M., F.R.C.S.
Exeter, United Kingdom

The work to be described in this paper was carried out in Exeter, England, at the University of Exeter and at the Princess Elizabeth Orthopaedic Hospital, Exeter, by us and a number of our colleagues.

There is no doubt that clinical success of joint replacement depends on sound fixation of the implant to the bony skeleton. Failure of fixation will usually lead to failure of function. Fixation is thus of paramount importance in implant surgery and can be achieved in a number of ways. This paper will discuss the most widely used and accepted fixation method—fixation by cement and, in particular, fixation by self-curing polymethylmethacrylate bone cement.

The paper will be split into two parts. The first will deal with the mechanical properties of bone cement and, in particular, how the surgeon can affect the mechanical properties by the way in which he handles the cement. The second part will deal with the development of a surgical technique designed to enable the surgeon to obtain the best possible fixation of the implant with maximum-strength cement.

MECHANICAL STRENGTH

Turning first to mechanical strength, a number of properties of cement were assessed in the laboratory. The majority of tests were on the compressive strength of the material, which also gave values of Young's modulus and 0.1% proof strength. Some tests were carried out in the tensile, shear, and bending modes. It was realized that cement has properties that like those of any other material, vary according to the way the ma-

terial is made. In the case of bone cement, the surgeon and his team carry out the final manufacturing process of the material, and so the way the material behaves is influenced by the surgeon and can be classified under three headings: aspects totally under the surgeon's control, aspects partially under the surgeon's control, and aspects totally outside the surgeon's control. The mechanical properties to be described are, unless otherwise stated, average values for all cements.

Aspects under surgeon's control

The first of these aspects is the choice of cement. The eventual polymerized strength of all cements is very similar; however, the handling characteristics of each cement can vary considerably. Palacos, for example, becomes "rubbery" and can be handled very early; CMW also becomes stiff quite quickly, whereas Sulfix is runny for a comparatively long time. Most cements set at ambient temperatures of about 70° F (21° C) in 9 to 12 minutes.

The second aspect under the surgeon's control is the inclusion of a radiopacifier. If included, there is a nonsignificant loss in strength of about 5%. Next, the surgeon can choose whether or not to include an antibiotic. Various antibiotic cements are commercially available in Europe, and these are about 4% weaker in ultimate compressive stress than nonantibiotic cements. A number of surgeons have produced antibiotic cements by adding antibiotic powder to the cement in the operating room. Adding even small amounts of antibiotic by hand will produce a cement with variable properties, because of mixing difficulties.

407

Adding large amounts, say 6 gm of antibiotic to 40 gm of polymer powder, will significantly change the handling characteristics and reduce the mechanical strength of the cement by about 25%. Liquid antibiotics have a disastrous effect on cement and should never be used.

Coloring, which is included in Palacos cement, has a negligible effect on strength.

The mixing method is concerned with two effects: mixing speed and mixing duration. With Simplex cement, mixing with a very fast stirring rate of about 260 beats per minutes (4.3 Hz) produces a cement that is 10% less strong than a cement mixed at a gentle rate of 60 beats per minute (1 Hz). Mixing at a constant speed for 2.5 minutes produces a cement that is about 11% less strong than a cement mixed for 1.5 minutes.

After the cement has been mixed, it has to be inserted into the patient. With Simplex, late insertion at 7.5 minutes gave a cement that was 43% less strong than a cement inserted at 2.5 minutes.

Finally, applying pressure to the cement greatly improves its strength. De Wijn found that the application of 2 atmospheres of pressure before and during curing increased the ultimate compressive stress by 30%. In our laboratory, we found that applying 2 atmospheres of pressure for 15 seconds before curing increased the strength of the cured cement by 11%.

Aspects partially under surgeon's control

The first of these is the inclusion of blood and tissue debris in the cement. Cement specimens prepared to contain inclusions showed an average reduction in UCS of about 12%. T. Gruen in California has shown a 77% reduction in tensile strength and 69% reduction in shear strength for specimens containing blood. The high standard deviations show the unpredictable behavior of these specimens, some of which fractured spontaneously on being taken out of the molds.

The second aspect that is partially under the surgeon's control is the exposure of cement to sharp edges or corners on implant or bone. Cement is very sensitive to the stress concentration produced by sharp edges, especially under tensile conditions and at high strain rates. The effect can be demonstrated in the laboratory. Two cylinders of bone cement were prepared (Fig. 19-1). The first had a circular-section taper driven into it, the other a triangular-section taper. The metal tapers were forced down into the cement. The cement containing the triangular-section taper failed im-

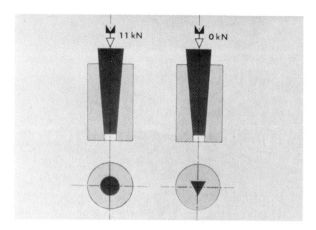

Fig 19-1. Cement cylinders with tapers: circular and triangular. *kN*, Kilonewton.

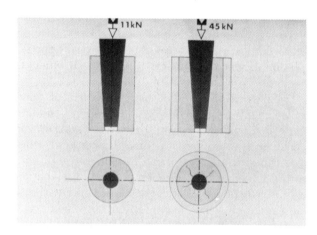

Fig. 19-2. Cement cylinders with taper: constrained and nonconstrained.

mediately because of the stress-concentrating effect of the sharp corners. The circular taper did not fail until a load of 11 kilonewtons (kN) was placed on it.

The third aspect is the very important effect of constraint *for* the cement and the support given to the implant *by* cement. The effect of constraint can be shown both in the laboratory and in clinical practice. In the laboratory, if the cement cylinder previously described containing a circular taper has a thin metal shell put all around it and is again put under compression, the cement will crack but the system will not fail (Fig. 19-2). It still takes load because the cracked cement transfers load into the constraining cylinder. In the body the constraint to the cement has to be provided by good-quality cancellous bone or by cortical bone. Two roentgenograms can show what happens to

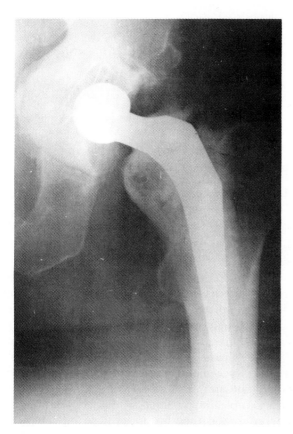

Fig. 19-3. Roentgenogram of Exeter stem showing unconstrained buttress of cement. (From Lee, A.J.C., Ling, R.S.M., and Vangala, S.S.: Arch. Orthop. Traumat. Surg. **92:**1, 1978.)

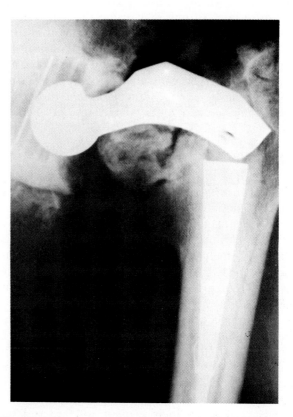

Fig. 19-4. Roentgenogram from stem in Fig. 19-3 showing that it failed. (From Lee, A.J.C., Ling, R.S.M., and Vangala, S.S.: Arch. Orthop. Traumat. Surg. **92:**1, 1978.)

unconstrained cement in the body. Fig. 19-3 shows an Exeter stem with a large, unconstrained buttress of cement above the cut surface of the neck of the femur. The outcome of this technical failure was predictable, the unconstrained cement failed, and the implant, in turn, failed through lack of support (Fig. 19-4). Support must always be given to an implant by constrained cement; otherwise failures like this will occur.

Optimal cement thickness is not yet defined. Generally a thin layer of cement requires less energy for crack propagation, and the effects of stress concentration, polymerization shrinkage, and viscoelastic behavior are more pronounced. A thick layer may deform excessively and thermal effects will be greater. It seems likely from unpublished work done in our laboratory that optimal thickness may be around 4 mm.

Bone cement is sensitive to ambient temperature as far as dough time and set time are concerned (Fig. 19-5). The mechanical strength of

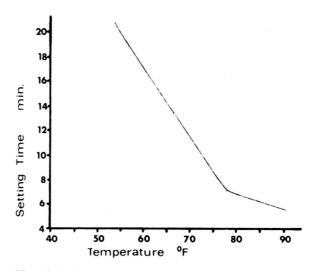

Fig. 19-5. Temperature sensitivity of bone cement.

the cement will not be affected by ambient temperature, and so one may argue that this aspect should not be discussed here. However, the clinical implications of a change in setting characteristics are obvious to all surgeons, and so this is an effect that has to be controlled. Luckily it is easily controllable by storage of the cement in a controlled-temperature environment until just before use.

Aspects outside surgeon's control

Although these aspects are outside the surgeon's control, he has to be aware of them if he is to understand the behavior of the material properly. Cement polymerizes and works in the body at a temperature of 98.6° F (37° C). This means that (1) cement will polymerize more quickly inside the body than it will in air, and (2) it will have at body temperature about 90% of its strength at 68° F (20° C, that is, room temperature).

Cement will take up body fluids in vivo. Wet cement is about 3% less strong than dry cement.

Cement in the body is loaded at high strain rates. The stiffness and failure stress will go up, and this is probably beneficial, but against this the stress concentration effect also gets larger.

Surgeons hope their cement will last a long time, probably 15 to 20 years. During this time it will age: laboratory tests predict a 10% loss in strength over 10 years, but some tests of cement recovered from patients who have had their cement in use for about 7.5 years indicate that the decline in strength may be somewhat less.

The cement is always loaded by cyclic loads and is thus under fatiguing conditions. Not much is known about the fatigue strength of cement, but to date it is probable that fatigue failures of *properly implanted* cement are not of clinical significance.

Surgical guidelines: best cement

Having looked at the various ways in which a surgeon can influence the mechanical strength of bone cement, we can review them and produce a set of guidelines for the surgeon to enable him to obtain the best possible cement:

1. He should mix cement with a low beating frequency.
2. The bony cavity must be clean to avoid blood and tissue debris becoming intermixed with the cement dough.
3. Cement should be pressurized before insertion.

4. Cement should be placed early at low viscosity.
5. Cement should be pressurized after insertion.
6. Cement should be fully constrained by good-quality bone.
7. There should be no stress risers in the cement.

If the surgeon obeys these guidelines, he will obtain good-quality cement of high strength.

SURGICAL TECHNIQUE

The second part of this paper is concerned with the design of good surgical technique to enable the surgeon to gain maximum fixation with bone cement.

A basic fact about cement is that it obtains fixation by mechanical interlocking of the cement with the implant or host tissue. It is *not* an adhesive. One may achieve interlocking with an implant by grooving the implant component—for example, most acetabular components have grooves for cement interlocking; or by taking advantage of the overall shape of the component—for example, many femoral components have a tapered shape that produces a strong interlock under a compressive load. To get fixation into bone, one has to force clean cement into open bony spaces or make it interlock with rough corticocancellous bone. To expose open trabecular bone we recommend the use of gouges rather than power tools. Power reamers, especially, have a cutting action that tends to drive debris into the bony spaces. Gouges, on the other hand, split bone away from the substructure and therefore tend to preserve open bony spaces.

Cleaning the bone

When the bone has been exposed, it has to be cleaned. The technique we use differs between open and closed cavities. In open cavities, such as the acetabulum, a lavage instrument is used (Fig. 19-6). In closed cavities, such as medullary canals, a combination of the lavage and an intramedullary brush is used.

The effectiveness of the procedure can be judged from the following pictures. Fig. 19-7 shows an uncleaned acetabulum. Fig. 19-8 shows the lavage in use in the acetabulum. Note the cleaning action of the lavage jet. Fig. 19-9 shows the clean acetabulum. The blood is welling up into the trabecular spaces, but the open nature of the bone can be seen.

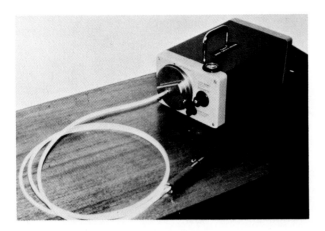

Fig. 19-6. Lavage instrument.

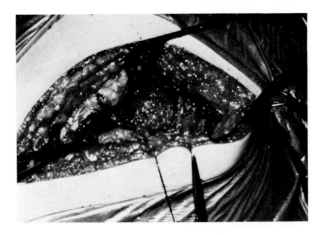

Fig. 19-7. Unclean acetabulum.

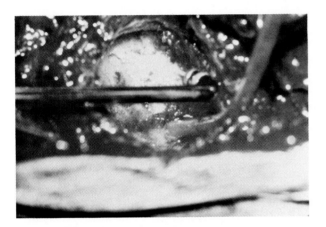

Fig. 19-8. Lavage in use in acetabulum.

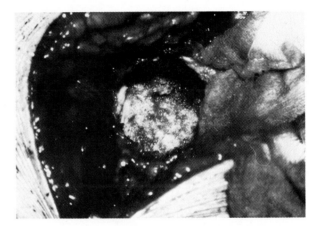

Fig. 19-9. Clean acetabulum.

Insertion and pressurization of cement

After the trabecular spaces have been cleaned, clean cement at low viscosity must be inserted and pressurized into the open spaces. Again the technique varies between the open acetabulum and the closed-cavity medullary canal. The open cavity, the acetabulum, is considered first. For the acetabulum, bone cement can be mixed in the conventional manner in a bowl. It is taken into the gloved hand as soon as possible and inserted into the clean acetabulum in a single bolus, without contamination by blood or tissue debris. Once the cement is in the acetabular cavity, it has to be forced into the open bony spaces. Finger pressure should be supplemented by a pressurizing instrument. The one we use is shown in Fig. 19-10. Its action is to form a seal around the lip of the acetabulum, with the cement inside the closed space

so formed. By pushing on the instrument, one forces the cement into the bony spaces. An early version of the pressurizer is seen in use in the operating room in Fig. 19-11. Note the rubber sheet between the instrument and the cement; this is needed to prevent the cement from sticking to the instrument. The latest technique uses a short length of gauze bandage between the rubber sheet and the instrument; pulling on it helps to break the seal between the acetabular lip and the pressurizer after pressurization. Some laboratory experiments were performed to test the effectiveness of the pressurizer. Cadaveric half pelvi were prepared in identical ways for the reception of cement. One half pelvis had cement inserted and packed by hand, the other half had cement inserted and then pressurized with the pressurizer. After the tests the acetabulums were sectioned.

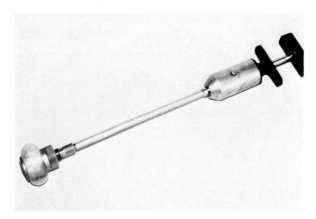

Fig. 19-10. Pressurizer. (From Poal-Manresa Caña, J., editor: Reemplazos articulares en las enfermedades reumáticas, Barcelona, 1979, Salvat Editores, SA.)

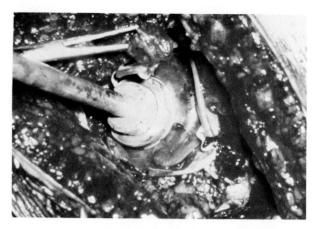

Fig. 19-11. Pressurizer in use in the operating room.

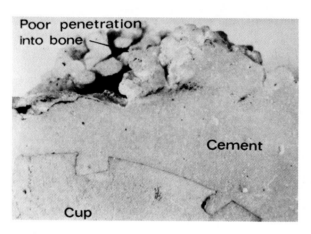

Fig. 19-12. Poor penetration of cement into bone.

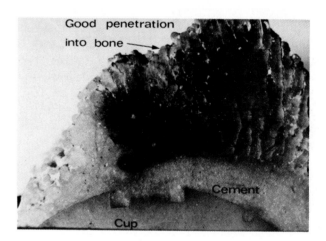

Fig. 19-13. Good penetration of cement into bone.

Fig. 19-12 shows the result of finger pressure—poor penetration into bone. Fig. 19-13 shows the result of the application of the pressurizer—excellent penetration into bone.

Having dealt with the insertion and pressurization of cement into the acetabulum, let us now turn to the femur. Since cement is going to be pressurized in the medullary canal, the canal has to be closed at its distal end, otherwise the cement will be forced down the canal to the knee. Many surgeons use a bone plug or a cement plug to achieve the seal. We use a high-density polyethylene plug designed by Seidel of Hamburg, Germany. The plug is available in diameters from 8 to 18 mm; the appropriate size is selected, and the plug is simply pushed down the femur.

Having blocked the distal end of the femur,

clean cement must now be inserted. If the cement is inserted by hand, it is bound to form laminations and to pick up blood and tissue debris. In medullary canals it is believed that a cement gun should be used. With our cement gun the plastic parts are disposable, and the cement is acually mixed within the barrel of the gun. To do this, we push the piston into the bottom of the barrel and place a funnel on top of the barrel. The polymer powder is poured into the barrel, followed by the liquid monomer. A second powder and liquid are poured on top of this, and the cement dough is mixed inside the barrel. Fig. 19-14 shows the mixing taking place in the operating room, and Fig. 19-15 the cement being injected into the femur. This gun is intended for use with cement at low viscosity. With Simplex at about 65° F (18° C) the

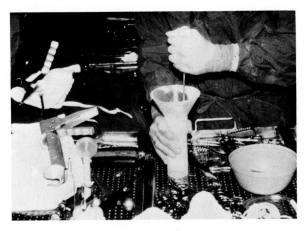

Fig. 19-14. Cement being mixed in the operating room.

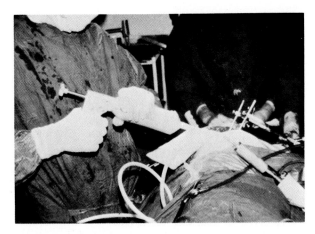

Fig. 19-15. Cement being injected into the femur.

cement is mixed for 2 minutes, the nozzle is put on, and the cement is injected immediately. Having inserted the cement by retrograde filling from the plug upward, we must now pressurize it into the bone. We use a plug of previously polymerized cement to seal the top of the femur. The plug has a hole in it through which the nozzle of the gun protrudes. With this method, cement continues to be injected by the gun into the closed space so formed; this forces the cement into the trabeculas, particularly at the proximal end where it is most important.

Insertion of implant components

When the cement has been placed in the acetabulum and pressurized, the acetabular cup is inserted. Similarly, when the cement has been placed in the medullary canal and pressurized, the femoral component is inserted. Both are pushed into their correct position by hand pressure and the appropriate insertion tools. It should never be necessary to hammer implants into place.

SUMMARY

To obtain good-quality cement, one should follow seven steps:
1. Mix with low frequency.
2. Clean bony cavity to avoid contamination of cement.
3. Pressurize cement before insertion.
4. Insert early, at low viscosity.
5. Pressurize cement after insertion.
6. Fully constrain cement.
7. Use no stress risers.

To obtain maximum fixation strength, one should follow four steps:
1. Use gouges to expose trabecular bone.
2. Use brush and lavage to clean bone.
3. Insert cement early at low viscosity.
4. Pressurize cement to force it into open trabeculas.

It is fortunate that the steps overlap; they are not mutually exclusive. Both require cleanliness. Both require the use of cement at low viscosity. Both require pressurization of the cement. If the steps are followed it is our belief that the best possible fixation with the best possible cement will be obtained.

SUGGESTED READINGS

De Wijn, J.R., Sloof, T.J.J.H., and Driessens, F.C.M.: Mechanical properties of bone cements in vitro and in vivo. In The knee joint, proceedings of the International Congress on the Knee Joint, Amsterdam, 1974, Excerpta Medica.

Gruen, T.A., Markolf, K.L., and Amstutz, H.C.: Effects of lamination and blood entrapment on the strength of acrylic bone cement, Clin. Orthop. **119**:250, 1976.

Howmedica Inc.: Surgical Simplex P bone cement technical monograph, Rutherford, N.J., 1977, Howmedica Inc.

Lee, A.J.C.: Exeter cement security system technical monograph, Rutherford, N.J., 1980, Howmedica Inc.

Lee, A.J.C., and Ling, R.S.M.: A device to improve the extrusion of bone cement into the bone of the acetabulum in the replacement of the hip joint, Biomed. Eng., p. 522, Nov. 1974.

Lee, A.J.C., and Ling, R.S.M.: Handling dependent properties of self-curing polymethylmethacrylate bone cement, Proceedings of the Third International Conference on Plastics in Medicine and Surgery, Enschede, Netherlands, June 1979.

Lee, A.J.C., Ling, R.S.M., and Vangala, S.S.: Some clinically relevant variables affecting the mechanical behavior of bone cement, Arch. Orthop. Traumat. Surg. **92**:1-18, 1978.

Chapter 20

Fixation failure and techniques of revision surgery in total hip replacement

HARLAN C. AMSTUTZ, M.D.
Los Angeles, California

Failure of cement fixation is the major cause of failure in total hip replacement. The quality of the fixation achieved at surgery is the single most important factor in the determination of long-term durability, and the optimal time for achieving durable fixation is at the initial surgery. Revision surgery is difficult, and there are growing numbers of patients who have had failed total hip replacements caused by loosening that have undergone revision and are again loose. Once again, the quality of fixation achieved at surgery determines the durability, but as the bone quality diminishes, so do the chances of good fixation. A loose prosthesis may contribute to massive osteolysis and loss of bone stock, making revision surgery even more difficult. Furthermore, the removal of acrylic cement rigidly fixed in bone around a fractured stem is difficult and can result in loss of bone stock. With each successive attempt at surgery, bone-stock loss occurs, and a Girdlestone resection may be the only salvage operation available. It is the purpose of this article to review the incidence of loosening, along with methods for identification, and to focus on techniques for prevention and revision surgery.

IDENTIFICATION INCIDENCE AND SIGNIFICANCE OF LOOSENING

At UCLA we have focused on methods to identify incipient loosening by carefully analyzing the prosthesis-cement and bone-cement interfaces by serial high-contrast roentgenograms using a chariot-like device to ensure consistent positioning.[2] This device facilitates obtaining roetgenograms at follow-up examinations that can be superimposed over previous roentgenograms to study the progression in extent and width of radiologic zones at the interface.

"Loosening" has been defined variously, but most observers believe that the demonstration of cement cracks or progressive radiolucent zones at either the bone-cement or the cement-prosthesis interface suggest looseness that can be associated with symptons. Femoral component subsidence and acetabular migration are gross signs of looseness. Beckenbaugh and Ilstrup reported a 24% incidence of loosening and a 1% acetabular and 1.7% femoral incidence of revision in a series of 301 hips followed for a mean of 5.7 years.[3] Charnley's series as reported by Cupic had a 0.9% acetabular and a 0.9% femoral incidence of revision (combining stem fracture with loosening) in a series of 222 hips with a mean follow-up of 11.5 years.[5] The average age of his patients at surgery was 68 years. Salvati reported a 3% incidence of femoral revision, none acetabular, in his series of 67 hips with Charnley replacement after a mean follow-up of 10 years.[10] There were six patients in whom there was gross loosening of the femoral prosthesis that "stabilized." There were two hips with gross socket migration that also did not require a revision. The average age of these patients was 67 years.

It is also clear from the recent literature that there is an increasing incidence of socket loosening. Mueller, reporting on 81 total hips with a 10- to 12-year follow-up, found an overall incidence of 17% requiring revision.[9] However, loose sockets comprised 13.5% and femoral components 7.4%. Both components were loose in 3.7%. In Charnley's 12 to 15 year results, 47% of his sockets showed no loosening, though his definition allowed a radiolucent zone up to 1 mm, which apparently could encompass the entire interface. Thirty-four showed "slight" radiolucent lines up to approximately 1.5 mm. Fourteen percent showed severe demarcation, with radiolucencies greater than 1.5 mm, and 11% showed actual migration of the socket. The incidence of those with severe demarcation or migration at 4 to 5 years was 4.5% and progressed to 25% at 12 to 15 years.[5] In assessing these results, one must bear in mind that there was minimal attempt to clean the trabeculas with either pulsatile or nonpulsatile lavage, and a rather quick-setting high-viscosity CMW cement was utilized. On the other hand, the patients averaged 67 years at the time of surgery. Chandler et al. reported a failure rate of 54% fixation after 5 years in patients under 30 years of age.[4] Our UCLA conventional-hip major-complication rate in this younger group with a 5-year follow-up was 35% and was primarily attributable to loosening. It is true that many of these patients have severe bone-stock deficiencies and complex problems, but the relationship of loosening to age and activity is apparent.

We have recently critically analyzed 444 hip replacements with a follow-up of 2 to 9 years and a 4-year mean.[8] A complete line of radiolucency was observed at the acetabular bone-cement interface in 47.3%. Complete absence of interface radiolucency was uncommon (4.3%). A statistically increased incidence of complete radiolucent zones greater than 2 mm in width was found surrounding the acetabular component in younger patients and those with longer follow-up. There was a trend toward increased radiolucent zones in men and heavier patients. There was a 1.1% incidence of patients requiring revision for acetabular prosthesis loosening.

On the femoral side, 12 patients required revisions for loosening of the femoral component (2.7%). Five of the 12 also had fractures of the femoral prosthesis, a 1.1% incidence. Complete zones of radiolucency around the femoral cement were less commonly observed than around the acetabular cement, with 60% having no cement-bone radiolucency at all. However, subsidence was observed in 5% of patients. A very thin radiolucent zone between the cement and prostheses in the proximal lateral femur often preceded more apparent signs of loosening, such as subsidence of the prostheses, and cracks in the acrylic cement. There was significantly increased incidence of femoral loosening in younger, heavier patients, men, those with osteonecrosis, those having previous hemiarthroplasty, and those with unsatisfactory cement technique. Inadequate fixation or loosening of the proximal femoral component has been classified as a cantilever fatigue mode (mode IV) and may lead to stem fracture.[6] Hypertrophy of the cortex around the tip of the stem, on the other hand, was not associated with progressive loosening. Both calcar resorption and distal cortical hypertrophy have been associated with signs of a well-fixed stem and not a loose one.

In a study of patients who had failed hemiarthroplasty and underwent total hip replacements, a few hips showed no interface change with follow-up and had no radiologic signs of loosening. In general, those were patients who had exceptionally good cementing technique initially or were elderly, or patients with considerable built-in restraint, and so the interface was not stressed heavily. Women and patients of light weight were more likely to fall into this group. A second group of patients developed progression of the radiolucent zones in width and extent on either the femoral or acetabular side with no deterioration in function or in symptoms, and with time the changes on the roentenograms have "stabilized." Again, they were patients who were older or who were limited in activity. A third group of patients had progressive signs of loosening, most of whom became symptomatic. Therefore, it is clear that there are multiple factors, all of considerable importance, that affect the durability of fixation, including surgical technique, body habitus, cause of hip disorder, bone stock, and activity level.

Since the longer the follow-up of a series of patients, the more frequent the radiologic loosening signs, the ultimate prognosis cannot be precisely determined. Many patients remain asymptomatic, and the progression of radiologic loosening signs may cease when the activity level of the patient declines because of age or other infirmity. A younger, more vigorous group of patients is likely to have a higher revision rate.

Loosening can be largely prevented by improved bone preparation, dry interface, elimination of cement voids, and good trabecular penetration. We would like to endorse wholeheartedly the compression containment procedures of fixation first recommended by Ling[7] for the acetabulum[7] and by our UCLA Biomechanics Section[2] for the femur.

Mild osteoporosis appears to favor fixation, since we have had no failures of fixation in cases with rheumatoid arthritis, or in patients who have had solid arthrodeses revised to prosthetic hip replacement where osteoporosis has been present in the area where a new socket has been implanted. It is helpful to select prosthetic components that are designed for the bone cavities, and hence wide selection of component size is important. Although extended postoperative nonweight-bearing has not been definitively shown as improving the long-term durability, we favor applying a graduated increasing stress to the interface while it heals and become remodeled. Currently this calls for a 2-month period of nonweight-bearing and then graduated weight-bearing over the subsequent 2 months.

DIAGNOSIS OF LOOSE TOTAL HIP REPLACEMENT

It is important to carefully assess the patient who presents with pain after total hip replacement. Femoral component loosening may produce pain in the groin, radiating to the knee. Pain from acetabular origin generally presents as buttock pain but may also present in the groin. Tenderness, when present, is usually located posteriorly along the ilium. The patient's emotional status must be carefully evaluated, especially if there are no signs of gross loosening or sepsis. In patients in whom we have not established a definitive diagnosis preoperatively, removal of suspected but not definitely loose components has not improved the patients's symptoms.

Differentiating between aseptic and septic loosening is crucial. In addition to careful history, physical examination, and high-contrast roentgenograms, we recommend that one determine the sedimentation rate and take an aspiration arthrogram. It has been our practice to aspirate the hip in the clinic, carefully prepping the inguinal area, sealing with a small Vidrape, and inserting a no. 22 spinal needle down to the prosthesis. One can palpate the metallic prosthetic component easily with the tip of the needle. The no. 22 needle is flexible enough that is can be passed around the ball or the neck and increase the opportunity of aspirating fluid, which is sent for aerobic and anaerobic culture after its character and color are

carefully noted. The needle is generally directed superiorly from a position about 2 cm medial to the femoral artery and 3 cm inferior to the inguinal ligament. If no free fluid is obtained, a small amount of saline solution is injected, though we have found that results are not as satisfactory when fluid cannot be directly aspirated. If the culture is negative, we repeat the aspiration, verifying it with a radiopaque contrast material at the time of arthrography. Although arthrography may give misleading information, we find it useful to identify gross prosthetic loosening, presence of sinus tracts, and sometimes abscess cavities. In addition, dye may track distally down the femoral intramedullary canal. We always have the patient exercise for 15 to 20 minutes after dye injection because this may improve the sensitivity of the arthrogram. Some observers believe that black-and-white and color-subtraction techniques also improve the sensitivity of the test. If sepsis or loosening cannot be positively confirmed, we recommend careful observation and repeat studies at 6 months or a year, rather than surgery without a definite diagnosis.

In general, we have found that, unless the radiolucent zone at the bone-cement interface extends completely around the prosthetic component, it will not be loose at surgery. However, since the interface is three-dimensional, care should be taken when one interprets two-dimensional studies. On the socket side, the degree of interface irregularity determines to a certain extent whether gross loosening can be identified. Sockets with less than a 1.5 mm interface lucency maximally have usually not been obviously loose at operation. Between 1.5 and 2.5 mm the detection of gross loosening at operation may depend on the interface area, which means the number and irregularity of fixation holes and other factors. To assess movement, the bone-prothesis interface has to be carefully identified by removal of excrescent cement.

GENERAL PREPARATIONS FOR REVISION SURGERY

The patient should have careful medical evaluation because the magnitude of revision surgery is considerable. If the patient's condition warrants, we recommend autologous blood banking of 6 units. This can be done at weekly intervals, but it is wise to start at least 2 months in advance of surgery. Oral iron and ascorbic acid are prescribed. If the patient is medically sound, hypotensive anesthesia is preferable to minimize blood loss. Before surgery, the hip is again aspirated and fluid sent for Gram stain, culture, and sensitivity. At the time of surgery, one should rule out infection by taking specimens from tissue that appears to be granulomatous or inflammatory and evaluating it by frozen section; additional tissue is sent for culture. Even though infection is not apparent, we recommend thorough débridement of all abnormal tissue. Prophylactic antibiotics are begun before surgery and continued throughout the postoperative course until the cultures are negative at 7 days and the tissue has been examined histologically for signs of infection.

Preoperative planning is most important for selection of the proper components. One can determine the magnification factor of the roentgenogram by measuring the femoral head of the ball of the prosthetic component, which has a known diameter. In this way, the diameter of the socket needed for revision surgery can be fairly accurately determined. Templates are useful to be certain that the correct size is available. However, it is also important to determine the anteroposterior size, and this is more difficult. We have had some success with a computerized axial tomographic scan, though scatter caused by metal prostheses may be considerable with early generation scanners. We recommend protrusio sockets when there is a central protrusion, and eccentric sockets with increased wall thickness superiorly for those cases where there has been erosion superiorly.

We have found a wide-stem component most useful for filling the void occupied by failed hemiarthroplasty or total hip replacement, just as the eccentric sockets fill the void caused by the erosive process of loosening on the socket side.

We strongly recommend surgery in the lateral decubitus position with removal of the greater trochanter. The capsule is often exceptionally thick and trochanteric removal may be difficult using our preferred Gigli saw technique. Under these circumstances we recommend using a 2-inch osteotome, beginning distal to the vastus tubercle and cutting the trochanter in such a way as to avoid fragmentation.

The hip is dislocated by flexion, external rotation, and abduction with the leg carefully placed into a sterile Mayo stand cover. A large hook facilitates dislocation. If the femoral component is grossly loose, it is removed easily. If it is rigid within bone, the area of cement that is holding the prosthesis is osteotomized so that the prosthe-

sis may be removed. Bone stock is preserved in the trochanteric base if possible. The socket is removed carefully so that the bone stock is preserved. Curved gouges shaped to conform to the radius of the component should be carefully inserted at the interface. The gouge should be used all around the circumference of the acetabular component, osteotomizing the fixation studs to sllow the socket to be removed easily without wedging the gouges against the bone. If the socket is well fixed, the tendency is to attempt to pry the socket out against the bone margins. This may result in fracture of valuable bone stock (Fig. 20-1). If the bony rim is so thin that there is insufficient bone stock, it is preferable to bisect the acetabular component with a high-speed cutting burr (Fig. 20-2). Care should be taken when one approaches the area of the wire marker, since this will dull the cutting tip. Once free, the cup can be removed with pliers or Kocher clamps. The prosthesis can then be more readily removed. The remaining cement is then removed with an osteotome, which divides and removes it. The underlying membrane is first removed with a curette and then a high-speed burr.

We advise removing as much of the cement as possible from the femur by dividing it with sharp osteotomes and removing it piece by piece. A series of removal gouges and osteotomes, one with a small prominence to prevent migration into bone, is most helpful* (Fig. 20-3). Although time consuming, cement can often be removed to a

---

*DePuy Manufacturing Co., Warsaw, Indiana.

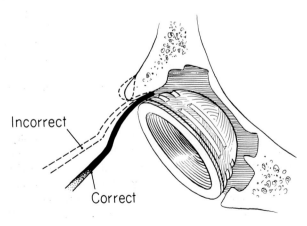

Fig. 20-1. Proper use of curved gouge to remove socket. Avoid wedging against acetabular bone.

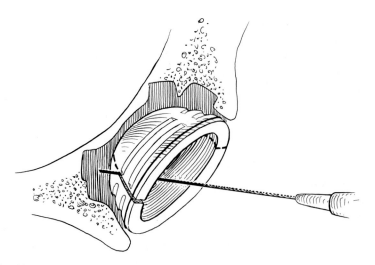

Fig. 20-2. Bisection of polyethylene socket with high-speed cutting scalpel.

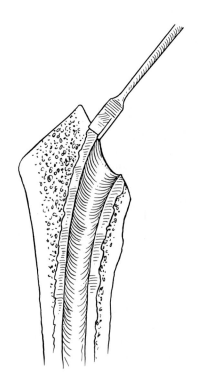

Fig. 20-3. The use of sharp gouge with blunt protruding tip for division of cement.

depth of 10 to 11 cm without too much difficulty, though it is essential to use a fiberoptic headlamp for visualization. When the canal narrows to the point that further use of the osteotomes is impossible, a high-speed pneumatic drill is utilized. It is important to assess the curvature of the femoral canal. Once a distance of 15 cm are reached, or if

there is any curve to the femoral canal, an image intensifier is essential to prevent bone destruction with the burr. Irrigation by means of pulsating lavage and drying with folded-out 4 by 8–inch gauze sponges is important.

The technique for removing the distal portion of a fractured stem is more complex. Once the cement has been removed down to the level of the fracture, a hole is drilled into the stem fragment with a carbide-tipped, high speed burr. This hole is slightly eccentric to allow insertion of the Midas Rex remover, which can then be tightened to fill the eccentric undermined hole. The stem can then be removed rather easily, and the remainder of the cement can be removed as described. We do not recommend windowing the femur because durable fixation will be more difficult to achieve.

BONE PREPARATION AND REVISION IMPLANTATION

After all the cement has been removed and débridement of the soft tissues carried out, the wound is thoroughly irrigated with pulsating lavage. The bone surfaces are then prepared for revision-component implantation. The first objective is to obtain a trabecular bone interface for the acetabulum. Usually much of the interface is thin sclerotic bone. This sclerotic bone should be removed carefully from the old fixation holes using a high-speed burr so that low-viscosity cement can be injected into fresh trabecular bone. New fixation holes are placed about 1 cm in diameter wherever there is sufficient bone stock to insert a hole 0.5 to 1 cm in depth. To avoid penetration, the acetabular walls are palpated digitally externally. It is preferable to have four-quadrant fixation. It has been our experience that the best areas for obtaining fixation are in the ischium and ilium. The remaining sclerotic cortical bone can be reamed carefully with the debris-retaining or Mira reamers, but often this is inadvisable because of the loss of bone stock. If the bone is relatively thin, it is our practice to use a high-speed burr to make ridges in the cortical bone. The advantage of increasing the surface area of the cortical bone has to be carefully weighed against the disadvantage of creating an oozing surface. Bone defects should be filled, preferably with autologous bone taken from the ilium. A large bone graft may be anchored into the remaining acetabulum. It is our preference to avoid where possible the use of metallic meshes and protrusio rings because they may interfere with optimal drying and penetration of the bone for good cement interdigitation. Small holes may be filled with a "top-hat" mesh, but the mesh should be trimmed so that it does not interfere with fixation. The appropriate-sized socket and femoral component is inserted for a trial reduction to evaluate limb-length restoration

and to make certain that the socket is covered by the bony acetabulum. If a bone graft is needed, it is performed at this time.

The acetabulum is then prepared for socket insertion. It is often our practice to mix cement in two separate batches if the bone has a predominately sclerotic base. Since fixation holes that have trabecular bone should be filled with low-viscosity cement, cement should be injected shortly after mixing. On the other hand, there is little to be gained from the use of low-viscosity cement when there is no trabecular bone to penetrate, and the cement will just take longer to polymerize, permitting more blood to enter the interface. With sclerotic bone, the objective is to insert cement in a higher viscosity state so that the oozing surface can be effectively tamponed. Therefore we mix sufficient cement for the sclerotic acetabulum several minutes before one mixes a batch that can be placed into a syringe gun and pressurized into the fixation holes.[1] Two suctions must be available, and team speed and coordination are essential. After the fixation holes have been filled under pressure, the bone is dried as carefully as possible with sponge sticks, and the first batch of cement, which is now in the dough stage, is inserted. Cement can then be further pressurized with a flexible compressor. Additional finger-packing is performed to pressurize the cement into the fixation holes for several minutes. The socket is then inserted, and all excess cement is trimmed from around the periphery, so that there is no cement outside the socket. The prosthetic socket should be covered by bone.

FEMORAL INSERTION TECHNIQUE

Once all the cement has been removed, there is rarely any remaining cancellous bone, and one is faced with obtaining fixation in a cortical tube. A cement plug is placed 2 cm distal to the prosthetic stem tip in the rubbery stage of polymerization. Be careful so that the cement does not stick to the cortical intramedullary canal walls and make it difficult to insert the prosthesis. After the canal has been thoroughly sealed by cement, it is dried. If there are small, oozing vessels, the area can be packed off or an attempt made to seal them with bone wax applied on the end of a spatula.

It is important to fill the canal with cement from distal to proximal by means of a syringe gun with a sufficiently long nozzle to carry it out rapidly. We experimented with returning to late insertion of cement in the shape of a sausage in an attempt to tampon the oozing surface more effectively. However, we found that it was difficult to eliminate small cement voids. If the canal can be dried sufficiently, it is preferable to use a syringe injection technique and then finger-pack for several minutes to make certain that there are no voids. The prosthesis is then inserted to the appropriate level, with care taken not to move it while the acrylic polymer is setting.

Before insertion of the femoral component, insert the trochanteric wires carefully gauging the site of reattachment. We utilize our standard two-wire cross-interlocking technique, and occasionally add a third wire if there is bone deficiency, or if the trochanter is placed down against the lateral shaft.

Case study (Fig. 20-4)

B.F. is a 62-year-old white female who underwent revision of a failed left Charnley-Mueller total hip replacement. She had two previous surgical procedures on the hip, including internal fixation for neck fracture and a hemiarthroplasty before the hip replacement.

The patient had an aspiration and arthrogram that showed gross loosening of both components. All the components were removed, and a thorough débridement was carried out. A wide-stem TR-28 and an eccentric acetabulum +10 mm superiorly were inserted.

Her preoperative ratings were pain 4, walking 5, and function 4. At 5 months the postoperative ratings were correspondingly 9, 6, and 4. Preoperative range of motion revealed a flexion arc of 105 degrees and an arc of rotation of 60 degrees, with a postoperative flexion arc of 110 degrees and an arc of rotation unchanged.

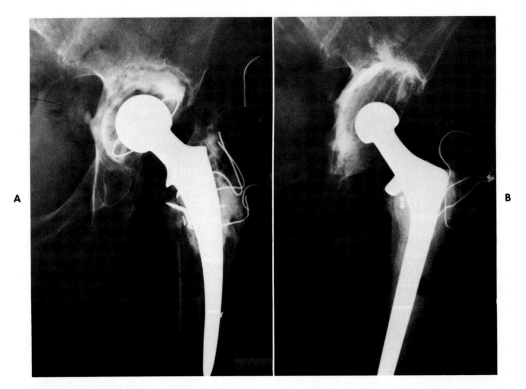

Fig. 20-4. A, A 62-year-old female with loose total hip replacement. There is gross loosening of both components, superior acetabular migration, and erosion. Note the wide femoral canal. **B,** Revision total hip replacement, with eccentric socket and wide-stem TR-28 prosthesis.

Examination of preoperative and postoperative roentgenograms reveals a completely radiolucent zone preoperatively, with a maximum width of 4 mm superiorly and with a 5 mm shift of the proximal aspect of the femoral component, along with broken trochanteric fixation wires. The 5-month postoperative roentgenograms reveal adequate fixation of the femoral component and a 100% acetabular radiolucent zone, with the maximum width of 1 mm in zone 2.

SUMMARY

Revision of the loose total hip replacement is complex and considerably more difficult than initial surgery. The surgeon who undertakes the surgery must be prepared to spend sufficient time in preoperative planning and obtaining appropriate-sized components. In addition, he must be apprised of the latest techniques for optimal fixation. Finally, he must gather a team that has sufficient numbers and experience to facilitate the operation.

REFERENCES

1. Amstutz, H.C.: Surface replacement of the hip. In The Hip, St. Louis, 1980, The C.V. Mosby Co.
2. Amstutz, H.C., Clarke, I.C., Christie, J., and Graff-Radford, A.: Total hip articular replacement by internal eccentric shells—the "THARIES" approach to total surface replacement arthroplasty, Clin. Orthop. **128:**261-284, 1977.
3. Beckenbaugh, R.D., and Ilstrup, D.M.: Total hip arthroplasty: a review of 333 cases with long follow-up, J. Bone Joint Surg. **60A:**306, 1978.
4. Chandler, H.P., Reineck, F.T., and Wixson, R.C.: A five-year review of THR's in patients under the age of 30 with emphasis on loosening, Orthop. Trans. **3**(3):303, 1979.
5. Cupic, Z.: Long-term follow-up of Charnley arthroplasty of the hip, Clin. Orthop. **141:**28, 1979.
6. Gruen, T.A., McNeice, G.M., and Amstutz, H.C.: "Modes of failure" of cemented stem-type femoral components: a radiographical analysis of loosening, Clin. Orthop.**141:**17, 1979.
7. Ling, R.: Prevention of loosening of total hip components. In The hip, St. Louis, 1976, The C.V. Mosby Co.
8. Moreland, J.: Loosening of total hip replacement: incidence and significance, In The hip, St. Louis, 1980, The C.V. Mosby Co.
9. Mueller, M.E.: Ten to twelve year follow-up of total hip replacements. Presented to the International Hip Society Meeting, Berne, Switzerland, 1980.
10. Salvati, E.A., et al.: A ten-year follow-up study of our first one hundred consecutive Charnley Total Hip replacements, J. Bone Joint Surg. **63A:**753, 1981.

Chapter 21

THARIES approach to surface replacement of hip

HARLAN C. AMSTUTZ, M.D.

ADRIAN GRAFF-RADFORD, M.D.
Los Angeles, California

The increasing incidence of complications with conventional stem type of total hip replacements, such as prosthetic loosening, stem fractures, and inherent difficulties of adequate revision, reawakened the basic need in the early seventies for an alternative approach to existing stem designs. These complications occur in a higher incidence in the younger, more active, or heavier patient and accentuate the need for improved durability.[8] The THARIES (total hip articular replacement with internally eccentric shells) surface replacement hip system was the result of collaboration of the Biomechanics Research Section and Joint Replacement Service of UCLA Orthopedic Surgical Division. The developmental work began in 1973 and led to the first clinical procedure in June 1975.[3]

DESIGN AND DEVELOPMENT

The design and development of the THARIES surface replacement was based on five main objectives[10]:

1. Use of eccentric shells to optimize component durability and fixation.
2. Optimal femoral head and acetabular reaming using specialized reamers and other instruments in a way to provide a reproducible safe technique.
3. Adequate range of components providing interchangeability and custom-fitting abilities for improved fixation with minimal loss of bone stock.

4. Positioning of the femoral and acetabular components in as anatomic a configuration as possible.
5. Use of a transtrochanteric approach for optimal visualization of the acetabulum and femoral head for both careful reaming and component orientation, and to facilitate trochanteric advancement when the neck requires shortening.

It was obvious from our anthropometric studies that *space is at a premium* in optimizing the design to provide good custom fitting of the patient range, with adequate mechanical strength and fixation ability.[9]

Based on these data, eccentric shell designs were proposed for the surface replacement to minimize bone resection and to put the bulk of the material where it was most required, on the superior load-bearing areas.[2] The eccentric metal cup has a minimum wall thickness of 1.25 mm, approximately 50% greater than that of the earlier Smith-Petersen cup.[18] The superior wall of the cup is 2.5 mm thick and provides strength and deep fixation channels of 1.5 mm in depth, tapering to 0.75 mm in the thin section.

Reaming the femoral head with the new cylindric reamers, trimming off the end portion, and further chamfer reaming allow space for additional metal bulk and fixation channels. All corners are well-rounded to minimize stress-concentration areas in both the sell of the cement. The interior of the metal shell is rough-cast for enhanced fixation and allows 3 mm (1.5 mm all around) for the cement layer on bone. The seven sizes at 3 to 4 mm increments now available provide the surgeon maximum flexibility in custom fitting the device with minimal loss of bone stock.

The ultrahigh molecular weight polyethylene shell is also eccentric. To aid the surgeon in this custom fitting, each of the seven sizes of femoral cups has three polyethylene sockets of varying superior wall thicknesses: small (5 mm), medium (6 mm), and large (7 mm). Each size relates to those above or below for maximum fitting selection, that is, an SR4 large liner has the same outside diameter as an SR5 small socket shell. The smallest shell size throughout the range is designed so that it fits the patient's acetabulum with minimal reaming, thereby assuring a fit except in the smallest dysplastic acetabulums. If more bone stock is available, the correspondingly thicker shells can be used. Alternatively, if the acetabulum can take an SR3 metal cup, the SR3 large shell can be substituted, thereby still keeping the cement volume to the required minimum.

In our early clinical experience we seldom used the large-socket component to preserve acetabular stock, and so only the small and medium-sized sockets were manufactured in the regular line. However, the large components are useful in some revision cases, should there be loss of femoral bone stock requiring the use of a smaller femoral component or larger socket shell.

The initial THARIES sockets were designed to a depth of 1 mm over a hemisphere, but these have been sequentially reduced to 3 mm under a hemisphere without loss of stability.

Since the head-neck ratios directly influence the obtainable in vitro range of motion,[21] one would like to insert the largest possible surface replacement on the femoral side, with minimal reaming, but this is not always possible because of either acetabular restrictions or the need to ream down to good femoral bone stock.

The range of motion of the THARIES surface replacement is very close to the anatomic range when its head-neck ratio is one decimal point less than that for the natural head-neck ratio, for example, 1.4 versus 1.3 for natural and prosthesis, respectively, as determined by in vitro range of motion studies.[11]

By reducing the overall depth of the socket shell to 3 mm under a hemisphere, a total of 4 mm from the original design, it has been much

easier to permit full implantation of the socket shell within the bony pelvis, resulting in a much improved range of motion, as determined at surgery, before neck pelvic impingement.

Clinically, we have observed no significant difference in the range of motion of patients who have had a THARIES and contralateral T-28 total hip prothesis indicating that underlying tissue and individual patient joint motion characteristics are the most important parameters in postoperative range of motion. This resulted in our current practice of downsizing component size to preserve acetabular stock. The result of reducing the head-neck ratio may be a slight loss of range of motion but, we believe, with a positive trade-off. However, to avoid possible socket distortion and impact during motion, which could lead to loosening, impingement of either component at the extremes of motion should be avoided by full socket containment. Any impingement should optimally be bone against bone. A further cushion is interposed by the reformed capsule.

OPERATIVE TECHNIQUE

With more than 6 years of clinical experience we have come to realize that a proper technique is critical if neck fractures and loosening are to be prevented. We recommend the lateral transtrochanteric approach to provide wide access. The trochanteric osteotomy is performed with a Gigli saw placed extracapsularly, using a saw-passer guide to ensure that the amount of trochanter removed is "smallish." It should be based below the vastus tubercle so that the vastus lateralis origin can be subsequently repaired and can enhance trochanteric reattachment (Fig. 21-1). A Gelfoam paste made from a small quantity of Gelfoam powder and a few milliliters of saline solution is smeared over the trochanteric base with a tongue blade to promote hemostasis. The greater trochanter is then reflected proximally onto the ilium and held in position with three 4-inch Steinman pins driven 2 to 3 cm apart and at least 1 cm proximal to the acetabular rim. The pin that is placed posteriorly to the other two should be placed more proximally into the ilium so that it will not interfere with application of the pin-centering guide to the femoral neck.

The length of the extremity is then referenced by measurement from the base of the trochanteric osteotomy to each of the three pins, and therefore the relative length of the extremity after trial re-

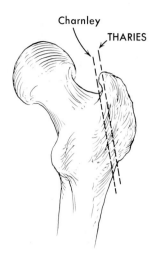

Fig. 21-1. Trochanteric osteotomy site.

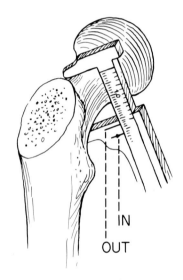

Fig. 21-2. Measurement of maximum neck width with caliper. (Modified from Amstutz, H.C., and Clarke, I.C.: Total hip articular replacement by internal eccentric shells—the THARIES technique for surface replacement, Warsaw, Ind., 1979, Zimmer USA.)

duction and after implantation can be assessed by comparison of these same measurements once the hip has been reduced.[2] If a true limb shortness is present, we do not recommend equalization except where the shortening is attributable to a protrusio acetabuli. In this situation a protrusio socket can be used to pull the socket shell out to the acetabular opening.

The capsule is incised circumferentially near the base, and the hip is dislocated by flexion, ad-

duction, and external rotation. This is facilitated by a curved ligamentum teres sectioner and a large dislocation hook. A subtotal capsulectomy is performed to thoroughly visualize the entire rim of the acetabulum.

The maximum width of the femoral neck is carefully determined with a caliper (Fig. 21-2). This dimension should be less than the internal dimension of the smallest reamer to be used for femoral component insertion. It is the surgeon's option to begin reaming on the femoral or acetabular side. If femoral reaming is performed first, one must carefully protect the reamed head during acetabular reaming so as not to compress exposed soft bone. Generally, one begins the acetabular preparation by reaming, using debris-retaining reamers, with the reamer just under the femoral head size and expanded so as to permit at least 1.5 to 2 mm of acrylic cement all around. We prefer to ream so that approximately 50% of the bed is cancellous. The socket gauge is used to assess the depth so that when the socket shell is pressed in, the shell will not "bottom out" during acrylic insertion (Fig. 21-3). We now recommend making four holes into the superior ilium and one each into the ischium and pubis. The holes should be about 6 mm in diameter, approximately the same size as the tip of the nozzle of a syringe gun, so that the acrylic resin can be contained when injected. The area is thoroughly cleansed of bone and clot by a pulsating lavage and dried as completely as possible. Acrylic polymer in a low-vicosity state is poured into a syringe and then injected under pressure into each of the fixation holes (Fig. 21-4). Additional acrylic polymer is then placed into the acetabulum and a flexible acrylic compressor (whose outside diameter is slightly larger than the acetabular opening) is applied, thereby causing the acrylic polymer to be forced into the cancellous bone (Fig. 21-5). Generally the acetabular ligament is left intact, but this does not ensure a seal. Low-viscosity acrylic extravasation may be prevented by use of a compressor designed to occlude the acetabular fossa opening.

At about 4 to 5 minutes before setting (Zimmer Bone Cement with a setting time in our operating room of 9 to 10 minutes), additional finger-packing of the fixation holes is performed. Acrylic resin is uniformly spread all around the acetabulum and the socket is inserted carefully. The acetabular margin is noted so as to avoid a "bottom-out" position with too thin an acrylic layer sur-

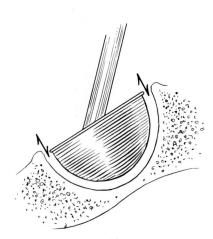

Fig. 21-3. In the use of socket gauge to assess depth of component insertion. (Modified from Amstutz, H.C., and Clarke, I.C.: Total hip articular replacement by internal eccentric shells—the THARIES technique for surface replacement, Warsaw, Ind., 1979, Zimmer USA.)

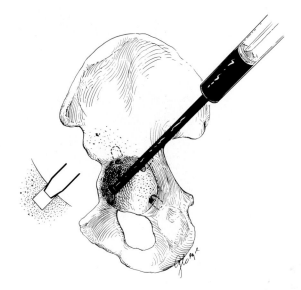

Fig. 21-4. Pressurization of low-vicosity acrylic polymer into fixation holes by use of syringe.

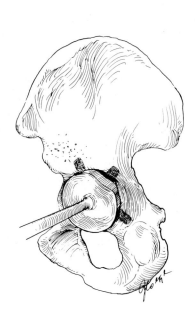

Fig. 21-5. Compression of acrylic polymer contained by flexible compressor.

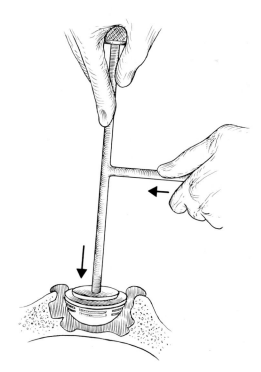

Fig. 21-6. Use of force couple with socket pusher handles to guide acrylic polymer extrusion all around.

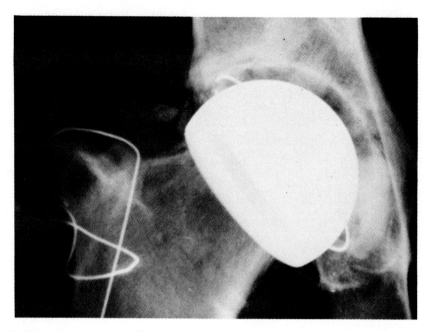

Fig. 21-7. Penetration of acrylic polymer by use of compression containment techniques. A 2-year follow-up.

rounding the cup. Recently we have been using 2 to 4 mm acrylic spacers to ensure a more uniform acrylic layer. The triangulation provided by the THARIES pusher helps to press the shell inward so that acrylic polymer exudes all around the periphery (Fig. 21-6). The acrylic polymer is then trimmed with a blunt spatula or sharp knife, with use of a curette being avoided because it may pull out acrylic polymer from the margins. In order to assist in preservation of acetabular bone stock the THARIES socket depth has been successively diminished from 1 mm over a hemisphere in depth to 1 mm under a hemisphere and then to 3 mm under a hemisphere without risking dislocation. This permits insertion of the socket fully within the bony pelvis to prevent neck-socket impingement. Combining the pulsating lavage, drying, and compression injection techniques, our recent postoperative roentgenograms show a much improved acrylic interdigitation with the trabeculas (Fig. 21-7).

To aid the surgeon in preserving neck integrity, the pin-centering guide was designed to assist in the insertion of a 4-inch Steinman pin down the central axis of the neck relative to its widest dimension (Fig. 21-8). It is important to realize that the central neck axis is located more superoanteriorly with respect to the head; that is, the head

will tend to overhang the neck inferoposteriorly. Osteophytes may tend to exaggerate the offset. Since the major axis of the neck lies close to the coronal plane, it is the integrity of the inferior and superior cortices that will be at risk during reaming of the head. In particular, we wish to avoid notching the much thinner superior cortex, where the maximum tensile stresses can be anticipated. The jaws of the pin-centering guide are generally attached to the neck across the major axis, which, though not precisely mediolateral, generally runs from superior and slightly anterior to inferior and slightly posterior toward the lesser trochanter. Osteophytes that may prevent a snug fit of the pin-centering guide should be rongeured away so that the device is tight. One should position the centering device itself by setting the same number of notches on the B scale as is indicated on the A scale.

It is also suggested that one drive the guide pin in a minimal amount, just enough to hold it stable while the cylindric reamer gauge is rotated, to check where the reamer will exit on the margins of the head inferiorly (Fig. 21-9). If positioning is not optimal, the pin can be repositioned before being driven into a depth of 5 to 15 mm, depending on bone density, before reaming. If the pin is off center by several millimeters, it is easy to re-

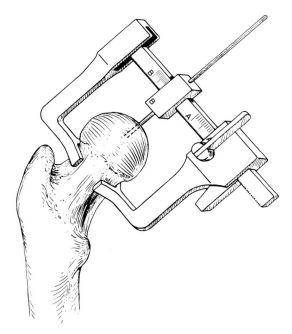

Fig. 21-8. Application of pin-centering guide. (From Amstutz, H.C.: Orthop. Rev. **9**[5]:51-56, 1980.)

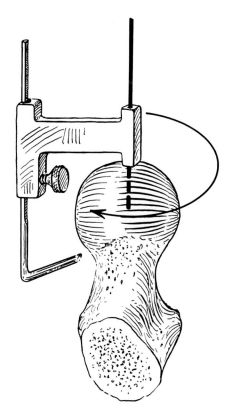

Fig. 21-9. Rotation of cylindric reamer gauge to check exit point of reamer blade. (From Amstutz, H.C.: Orthop. Rev. **9**[5]:51-56, 1980.)

position. If it is only off a millimeter, replacement is impractical because it will follow the original track. The pin must be stable to guide the reamer.

An oversized reamer (generally 2 sizes) is selected initially to remove a minimal amount of bone, and successive reamings are made with appropriate smaller reamers to the final reamed head diameter. Before reaming, we recommend placing a polyethylene sheet around the neck of the femur to collect debris. It is desirable to accurately assess the reaming process both visually and by palpation to make certain that there are no positioning errors and that the reamer will not invade the neck as it is advanced. The final reamer should have a diameter larger than the largest dimension of the neck. In other words, if the femoral neck diameter measures 38 mm, the femoral head should not be reamed with an SR-3 cylindric reamer, which has a 36 mm internal diameter. Instead, an SR-4 should be used. It is helpful to place the THARIES working dimensions on the wall of the operating room for reference. Each of the reamers has an intrinsic stop so that the teeth will not cut into the intertrochanteric area (Fig. 21-10). These stops are designed to be effective so long as the largest cylindric reamer is two sizes or less over the final reamer size based on neck dimension. Occasionally, with malformed heads or those that have great eccentricity, the reamer will stop too soon before the head is completely reamed. Then a second dome cut will have to be made. In this situation, or where additional bone has been removed, such as in avascular necrosis, care must be taken with the final cylindric reaming, since the stop may not protect against cutting the base of the neck.

The THARIES components are designed so that the femoral head need not be reamed down to or within the femoral neck. In other words, the desired component fit can be obtained on both the femoral head and acetabulum without invasion of the neck. Therefore, with the aid of preoperative planning and knowledge of the initial size of the femoral neck at surgery, we can closely predict the optimal THARIES size for any hip. We then progressively ream out the acetabulum, continuously feeling the extent of remaining bone and paying particular attention to the anterior and posterior wall thicknesses of the acetabulum. If acetabular bone stock is severely deficient, the decision may be made to ream the femoral head further for a smaller-sized femoral shell. Initially

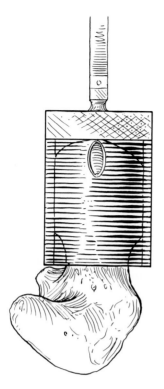

Fig. 21-10. Cylindric reamer with intrinsic stop. (Modified from Amstutz, H.C., and Clarke, I.C.: Total hip articular replacement by internal eccentric shells—the THARIES technique for surface replacement, Warsaw, Ind., 1979, Zimmer USA.)

we were concerned that neck fractures might result from this. However, we have identified some neck notches on our first cases before all the instruments were perfected, but *no* neck fractures resulted. So there may be a margin of safety wider than we initially anticipated, or the protection from weight-bearing advised for our patients postoperatively may have prevented them from "overstress." However, care must still be taken, since femoral neck fractures from THARIES procedures have been reported.

Most of the other published surface-replacement series are emphasizing valgus cup positioning as the method of choice.[7,15-17] However, they have experienced a considerable incidence of neck fracture. Both valgus and varus reaming run a greater risk of notching the neck and therefore should be avoided. Until definitive long-term results are in, we see no reason to change our goals of anatomic femoral component positioning. This philosophy has been supported by our mechanical testing and the studies of Shybut.[22,25]

After reaming, the saw guide is applied and positioned so that the inferior margin will *cover* the reamed portion of the head. The dome of the head is removed with a saber saw (Fig. 21-11). Sectioning the dome of the head at this level will

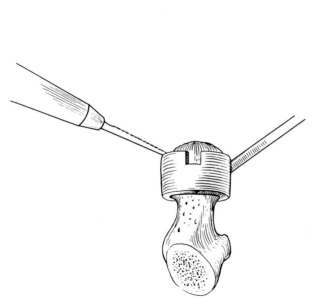

Fig. 21-11. The saw cut-off guide is positioned so that the inferior edge covers the reamed surface.

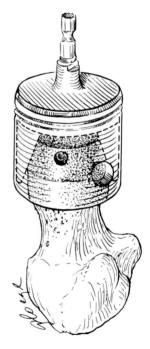

Fig. 21-12. New precision chamfer reamer with intrinsic stop.

ensure that the femoral component will cover the reamed surface and minimize the risk of a head-neck junction stress riser. This is especially important if there is severe osteoporosis. The next step is chamfering or beveling the margins of the proximally cut femoral head.

The new chamfer reamers have been designed to add a new dimension of precision to the procedure (Fig. 21-12). The final shape of the reamed femoral head is checked with a template that corresponds to the internal dimensions of the cup. If there are remaining cysts, the cyst linings should be carefully curretted. We have found a high-speed burr very effective in removing tenacious fibrous tissue.

Drill holes are placed into zones of relative avascularity down to areas of good bleeding bone, using a ¹/₈- to ¹/₄-inch drill. Healthy vascular bone throughout is desirable, but it may be feasible to leave small, relatively dense areas of sclerotic bone as long as drill holes are placed into vascular bone. In some hips with osteonecrosis it may be necessary to shorten the head as much as 1.5 cm to have sufficient healthy bone before final implantation. Trial reduction is performed to ensure that there is no neck-pelvic impingement. The femoral head is thoroughly cleaned and dried. This may require trimming of the trochanteric base, anterior or posterior. A small gas-sterilized balloon is filled with low-viscosity acrylic polymer (Fig. 21-13) and applied over the femoral head and then a wire is twisted at the neck base for containment (Fig. 21-14). The acrylic polymer is finger compressed into the interstices for several

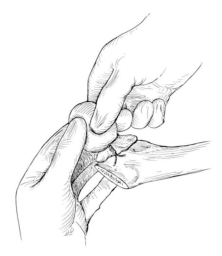

Fig. 21-14. Compression of acrylic polymer into trabeculas contained by twisted wire around balloon and femoral neck.

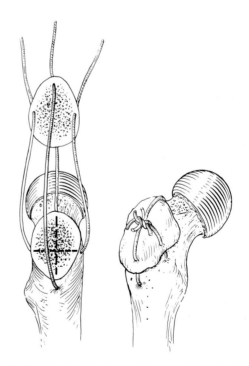

Fig. 21-15. Greater trochanteric reattachment with two cross-wire interlocking technique. (Modified from Amstutz, H.C., and Clarke, I.C.: Total hip articular replacement by internal eccentric shells—the THARIES technique for surface replacement, Warsaw, Ind., 1979, Zimmer USA.)

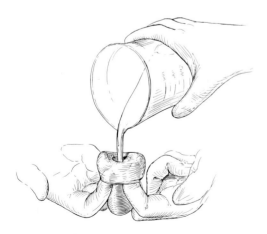

Fig. 21-13. Fill stretched balloon with low-vicosity acrylic polymer.

minutes. The balloon is then cut free and additional acrylic polymer is further compressed by finger-packing. The component is filled circumferentially with remaining acrylic polymer to avoid air spaces and is pressed onto the femoral head. Trimming of acrylic is performed, preferably with a blunt spatula. The femoral cup is inserted in a neutral position.

The greater trochanter is reattached with two cross wires placed approximately 5 to 10 mm under the trochanteric base (10 mm are required if the bone is osteoporotic) (Fig. 21-15). The wire ends should be pulled and tested to ensure that they will not cut out of the bone on being tightened. A single drill hole placed at the base of the neck has not been a significant stress riser, but it should be placed more distally or, if possible, in the trochanteric fossa. The use of the self-capturing drill-wire guide is helpful. The vertical wires are marked with curved clamps and the horizontal wires with straight clamps to obviate any confusion. The vertical wire is then passed over the top of the trochanter through the abductor muscle mass. Three drill holes are placed in the trochanter, with the trochanter holder being used as a guide. The distal hole is 1 to 2 cm from the distal tip, depending on the degree of advancement. The anterior and posterior holes are drilled as close to the bone margin as possible, so that there is a minimal tendency to cause separation of the trochanter when the knots are pulled tight. The vertical wire is pulled tight to advance the trochanter over the vastus ridge after the vastus has been stripped with a periosteal elevator. A lap sponge is applied to the slightly advanced trochanter and is impacted with a mallet against the bed, and the no. 18-gauge wires are tightened with interlocked square knots. The wires are cut about 1 cm long, bent at a right angle, and impacted into the bone base. The trochanter must be rigidly fixed at the time of closure. Closure is routine using suction drainage. Antibiotic irrigation is used.

Postoperatively, prophylactic cefazolin sodium, one gm every 6 hours for 24 hours and 1 hour before surgery is given intravenously, and then cephalexin monohydrate (Keflex) for 3 days. Warfarin anticoagulation is routine with 10 mg given the night of surgery and subsequent doses adjusted to maintain $1\frac{1}{2}$ times the control prothrombin time. The suction drainage tubes are removed at 24 hours if two successive 8-hour periods have less than a 50 ml output. Antiembolism stockings are used.

The limb is placed in balanced suspension for 3 days for leg elevation and to assist in bedpan transfer. Sling suspension is used for the remainder of hospitalization to assist gentle active assisted exercises. Physical therapy is limited to sitting exercises and hip flexion. The patient is mobilized on crutches, with no weight-bearing for 2 months, and then allowed to partially bear weight in the third month. Swimming and bicycling are encouraged, usually beginning with the third month.

We now believe that it is important not to overstress the freshly reamed bone interface during the early postoperative period in order to minimize the cellular response and promote long-term durability. Light nonimpact sports, such as golf, are permitted at about 6 months, depending on the quality of socket-bone acrylic interfaces. Very active sports, such as tennis, skiing, and horseback riding, are not advised for any patient under 50 years. For those older individuals these sports may be undertaken with some risk, though less than with a conventional replacement. For older individuals a revision or conversion to conventional replacement could be sufficiently durable for a reduced activity level.

Sample case with options for component insertion

We recommend the following method of assessment for THARIES replacement: standard AP and Johnson lateral roentgenograms to assess bone stock. For conventional roentgenograms (40-inch tube-to-subject distance), the 20% magnified templates are helpful in preoperative assessment. These are accurate to ±6% for 2 standard deviation, depending on the thickness of the patient. Since the mediolateral neck dimension is generally the widest, superimposition of the template will give the surgeon an idea of the smallest femoral component size possible. The acetabular stock can then be assessed. If one has concern about sizing, a 6-foot film can be obtained. Using the 10% magnification templates, the 2-standard-diviation error is reduced to ±3%. Oblique views are helpful to assess dysplastic hips. CAT scan reconstructions are now our preferred method of evaluating dysplastic hips and those with osteonecrosis. Precise mensuration is possible.

The dimensions contained on the THARIES

worksheet will help in planning and at surgery (Table 21-1). We recommend that this chart be accessible in the operating room. For example, a 44 mm diameter head on a 29 mm neck can be reamed safely to an SR-2 (Fig. 21-16). The THARIES SR-2 femoral component has an outside diameter of 39 mm. One should ream the acetabulum to a diameter of 50 mm to accommodate an SR-2 small socket shell, allowing for 1.5 mm of acrylic polymer all around. If more acetab-

Table 21-1. Working dimensions of the THARIES system for surface replacement

THARIES component	*Neck width (mm)*	*Reamed head diameter (mm)*	*Femoral shell (ID/OD mm)*	*Acetabular shell (OD mm)*	*Reamed acetabulum (ID mm)*	*Mira reamer code*	*Mira reamer (OD mm)*
*SR-0	26	26	29/33	41-s	44	6A	44
				43-m	46	4A	48
SR-1	29	29	32/36	44-s	47	4A	48
				46-m	49	AA	51
SR-2	32	32	35/39	47-s	50	AA	51
				49-m	52	AB	52
SR-3	36	36	39/43	51-s	54	AC	54
				53-m	56	A	56
SR-4	40	40	43/47	55-s	58	C	59
				57-m	60	D	60
SR-5	44	44	47/51	59-s	62	DE	62
				61-m	64	E	64
*SR-6	47	47	50/54	62-s	65	E	64
				64-m	68	F	67

*Available on a custom-order basis

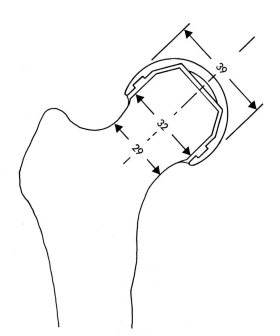

Fig. 21-16. Example of SR-2 implantation.

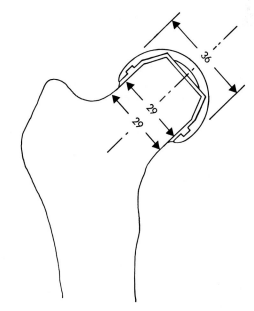

Fig. 21-17. SR-1 implantation for similar anatomy.

ular stock is available, a medium or large socket may be used with 2 to 4 mm or more of reaming, and correspondingly thicker polyethylene can be provided. If the acetabular stock is deficient and full coverage of the socket cannot be accomplished without unnecessary thinning of the acetabular walls anteriorly or posteriorly, or deepening too much, it is possible to come down one size. Reaming the femoral head to 29 mm is sufficient to accommodate SR-1 components (Fig. 21-17). Care must be taken not to notch the neck. This degree of precision is possible with the instrumentation and careful scrutiny and palpation during final reaming. If the pin guiding the reamer is not centered down the neck axis, it is suggested that it be removed and the final reaming be guided by application of appropriate pressure on the reamer away from the neck, which is in jeopardy of notching. With SR-1 implantation considerable stock may be preserved, though in dysplastic cases an iliac graft may be necessary to provide full coverage.

INDICATIONS AND CONTRAINDICATIONS

Our initial selection of patients for THARIES was designed for those whose lifestyle or hip problem might prejudice the fatigue life of conventional stem type of femoral prostheses or component fixation. Included were patients with varying combinations of characteristics such as heavy build, younger age group, potentially high activity level (either socially in sports or in heavy-duty work), and other physiologic factors known to contribute to prosthetic stem loosening, such as the following:

1. Young active individuals who developed osteoarthritis secondary to slipped capital femoral epiphysis, congenital hip dysplasia, Legg-Calvé-Perthes disease or a posttraumatic condition with significant symptoms and functional loss.
2. Patients with multiple joint arthropathy, that is, juvenile and rheumatoid patients and those with other arthritides who have increased risk of postoperative sepsis caused by steroids or other immunosuppressive drugs and general debility. Management of infection and salvage, if necessary, are much simpler and require less traumatic procedures than conventional system total hip replacements.
3. Patients with traumatic or nontraumatic os-

teonecrosis: Patients with nontraumatic osteonecrosis often (30% to 50%) have bilateral disease and are generally young or middle-aged adults.
4. Dwarf patients: Like the patients with juvenile rheumatoid arthritis, dwarf patients have congenital dysplastic intramedullary canals that could only accept small femoral stems, which may be inadequate on the basis of strength for long years of service.

As we improved our technique and confidence in the procedure and obtainable results, we extended our indications to patients in their sixties and occasionally seventies at their option, after carefully explaining the risks, advantages, and disadvantages of both THARIES and conventional replacement. We believe that this older group with lower activity level is likely to have fewer complications than the younger group, and this has been true to date. The procedure offers a distinct advantage over the conventional replacement because of the ease of revision even if the hip should become septic. However, we are concerned about recommending the procedure for the older patient with significant osteoporosis. Should these patients fall, they would have at least the same hazard of neck fracture as they would without a replacement, and fractures in the neck area that had been resurfaced would require a total hip replacement. It is probably true that this same population could sustain fractures below conventional total-hip-replacement prosthetic stems or precipitate loosening of the femoral component; so there may well be a positive trade-off in favor of the surface replacement.

There are few absolute contraindications. They include active sepsis with high virulent gram-negative organisms and open epiphyseal plates. There are many relative contraindications, including active sepsis with low virulent gram-positive organisms, pronounced loss of bone stock, and severe leg-length discrepancy.

In the event of a neck fracture, we have designed a series of conversion conventional stem replacements, which are available on custom order. These would be indicated in situations where the socket shell was tight within bone. It would be desirable to utilize an optimal stem and neck length, and we have available combinations in a micrograin high-strength cobalt-chrome stems to match SR-0 to SR-6 anthropometrically. However, any combination of neck length can be obtained.

RESULTS

The first 350 THARIES includes 12 from 1975, 36 from 1976, 75 from 1977, 96 from 1978, 90 from 1979, and 41 through 4½ months of 1980. The primary etiology reflects a preponderance of osteoarthritis, but with a high incidence of osteonecrosis and dysplasia, and contains nearly all diagnostic categories of hip disease (Table 21-2). The average age was 45.4 years. There were 21 patients with bilateral THARIES. An additional eight patients had contralateral conventional replacement.

The average operating time was 171 minutes. Although we have gradually reduced the operating time with experience, it is rare to complete a hip replacement in less than 2 hours. The average blood loss at the time of surgery plus the suction drainage postoperatively averaged 1352 ml. The majority of procedures have been performed following an autologous blood protocol whereby the patients bank 3 units preoperatively for use in the operative and postoperative periods. With greater use in later patients of hypotensive anesthesia to aid in achieving dryness at the interface for opti-

mal fixation, blood loss has decreased on an average of approximately 500 ml. Only those patients who have good general health without cardiac or renal medical problems were considered for hypotensive anesthesia. The hospital stay averaged 16.8 days, with a range of 10 to 49 days. The standard deviation was 5.3 days. The distribution of SR sizes was skewed slightly to the left with a mode of SR-4. However, the SR-6 did not become available until the 173rd THARIES hip (Table 21-3). The small-thickness acetabular component was used in 57% of patients. In the entire series, the first 73 patients had a socket depth of 1 mm over a hemisphere, the next 43 had 1 mm under a hemisphere, and all subsequent patients had 3 mm less than a hemisphere.

The preoperative and postoperative results in terms of pain, walking, function, and range of motion are shown in Table 21-4 for the group of 116 patients with 130 hips who have an actual follow-up of greater than 2 years, with a mean of 37 months.[4] Pain relief has been excellent, improving from an average of 4.2 to 8.5 on a 10.0 scale, and is comparable to results in our conventional hip replacement series. Further, results have not deteriorated from our early follow-up studies. The walking and function parameters both improved significantly from preoperative status. Although on the average the patients who underwent surface replacement were not so seriously disabled as in our early conventional hip replacement series, it is of interest to note a continued overall improvement with time in both parameters of function and walking.[1,4]

The arc of flexion improved from 82 to 106 degrees, and the rotation arc in extension from 24 to 61 degrees. These latest postoperative values demonstrate improvement over our short-term follow-up study, in which the average postopera-

Table 21-2. Etiologic factors in population of 350 hips

Cause	%
Primary osteoarthritis	41.8
Avascular necrosis	18.9
Rheumatoid arthritis	12.9
Congenitally dysplastic or dislocated hips	7.5
Condition after trauma	5.4
Slipped capital femoral epiphysis	2.6
Ankylosing spondylitis	2.6
Other	8.3

Table 21-3. Frequency of component size

SR size	1	2	3	4	5	6	Total
Surface—small	7	13	58	57	62	4	201 (57%)
Surface—medium	5	12	35	48	20	7	127 (36%)
Surface—large	2	3	0	1	1	0	7 (2%)
Protrusio	1	2	3	4	3	0	13 (4%)
Custom			2				2 (1%)
Total	15 (4%)	30 (9%)	98 (28%)	110 (32%)	86 (25%)	11 (3%)	350

Table 21-4. Clinical evaluation of 130 hips followed at least 2 years

	Preoperative	*Postoperative*
Pain	4.2 (1.5)	8.5 (1.7)
Walking	5.7 (1.5)	8.4 (1.9)
Function	5.6 (1.7)	8.1 (1.8)
Arc of flexion	82 (35)	106 (21)
Arc of rotation	24 (21)	61 (19)

tive flexion was 95 degrees and the rotation arc 52 degrees. In general, flexion contractures have been substantially reduced or eliminated. In the early series there was a tendency to develop a flexion contracture of 15 to 20 degrees, which was difficult to eliminate if therapy was not instituted until 2 months postoperatively. With the new protocol, which includes having the patient lie prone on about the fifth day, flexion contracture is no longer a problem except in an occasional patient who has a contralateral hip with a severe flexion contracture. There were nine hips in eight patients with less than 75 degrees of flexion at follow-up, but these occurred in hips that were stiff to begin with or that developed grade III or IV heterotopic bone.

RADIOGRAPHIC ANALYSIS

A shift of the femoral component occurred in six patients, four of whom have come to revision and are discussed in the section on complications. In two patients the component underwent a varus shift in the early postoperative period but did not progress, and the patients have remained asymptomatic up to 3 years postoperatively.

There have been two hips in which the trochanter migrated from its reattachment bed approximately 1 cm, and one hip in which migration was greater than 2 cm. This latter patient weighed approximately 250 pounds and returned to work as a professor 3 weeks postoperatively. Fibrous union was noted in six other hips. None of the patients have enough abductor muscle weakness to warrant reattachment of a migrant trochanter.

Both the AP and lateral postoperative roentgenograms were reviewed for the presence of heterotopic bone and rated as to severity.[5] Fifty-seven percent had no evidence of heterotopic ossification. Mild (grade I) formation (islands less than 1 cm) was noted in 28%, moderate (grade II)

(bone greater than 1 cm but less than 1 cm from the pelvis or trochanter) in 14%, and grade III (bone closer than 1 cm to the pelvis or trochanter) in 4.6%. No hips were ankylosed. Two of six patients with grade II had removal of heterotopic ossification, but there was subsequent recurrence.

Serial roentgenograms were critically evaluated at periods of approximately 6 months, 1 year, and greater than 2 years (mean 30 months) postoperatively for the presence, width, and extent of radiolucencies at the bone-cement interface. Ten percent had no radiolucent zone at the first interval, 6% had none at the second interval, and only 4% showed none after 2 years. The percentage of patients that had a 10% to 49% lucent zone decreased from 24% at the first period of 20% at the second period and 12% at the third period. Of those with 50% to 99% lucency, there was a similar decrease from 22% to 11%. As expected, the increase was in those with a 100% zone: 35% had a complete lucency initially, increasing to 57% at the second follow-up and 70% at the final followup. Of those having lucencies at first follow-up, 65% were of equal width in all zones,[13] 16% had maximum width in zone 1, 6% in zone 2 and 13% in zone 3. At last follow-up, 33% of the lucencies were of equal width in all zones, but there was an increase in the incidence of eccentric width in the other three zones, with zone 1 27%, zone 2 17% and zone 3 19%. At the first evaluation period there was less than 0.5 mm maximum radiolucent zone in 84%, 1 mm or less in 13%, and only 3% 1 to 2 mm. At last follow-up there was 49% less than 0.5 mm, 25% 0.5 to 1 mm, 18% 1 to 2 mm, and 7% greater than 2.5 mm.

There were no patients who required socket revision when the radiolucent zone remained equal, though some were greater than 2 mm. All patients requiring revision had some eccentricity of the lucent zones and seven had a wide zone in zone 3. It is also of interest that the width of the zone was not related to symptoms, with four sockets requiring revision having 2 mm or less and three having greater than 2.5 mm. The progression of patients with eccentric width of radiolucent zones is therefore of concern. However, many of these patients have shown stabilization of zone width and progression. Detailed multivariant analyses of age, sex, weight, cause, and activity levels are pending and may provide greater insight into the tissue response at the interface and provide prognostic information.

SYSTEMIC COMPLICATIONS

There have been relatively few systemic complications in this entire series. Two patients developed thrombophlebitis while in hospital on anticoagulation, and one developed a nonfatal pulmonary embolus. We have no documentation of those patients who returned at their 6-week follow-up with some residual swelling of the operated leg. One patient required hospital readmission for phlebitis. There have been 18 patients requiring catheterization and seven urinary tract infections. Six patients have had some cardiopulmonary complication, all of which resolved. Two patients with less than 1 year of follow-up died of causes unrelated to their surgery. There have been six patients who have developed postoperative peroneal nerve palsy, five in the first 200, and one in the most recent 150. In three, there was a complete recovery, but three are incomplete.

MINOR COMPLICATIONS REQUIRING SURGERY

Five patients had trochanteric bursitis temporarily relieved by injection but subsequently underwent trochanteric wire removal (Table 21-5). Three of the patients achieved complete relief and are functioning normally. Two of the patients continue to be symptomatic; both have complex psychosocial histories. Two patients have had heterotopic bone excised, and both recurred. Another "minor" complication we encountered was with a patient who developed a femoral neck cyst that required bone grafting at 33 months postoperatively. Seven months postoperatively this became filled in though she still has some pain.

Dislocation. We have had no dislocation in patients who have had normal or relatively normal bone stock and abductor musculature. Additionally, the large femoral component size selection has enhanced stability. Two dislocations have occurred in patients who have had major deficiencies of bone or muscle stock. Both have been reduced without further dislocation.

MAJOR COMPLICATIONS REQUIRING SURGERY

Loosening. In our first 350 THARIES there have been one septic and 10 aseptic loosenings of components that required revision surgery (Table 21-6). Five of the aseptic patients had socket loosenings, two had femoral loosenings, and three had loosened both the femoral and socket components. Of the 10 patients, four had congenitally dysplastic or dislocated hips, two had osteonecrosis, two osteoarthritis, one a slipped capital femoral epiphysis, and one a congenital coxa vara. The average age of patients with loosening was 37 years at the time of revision. Ninety percent of loosenings occured in patients under 50 years of age, who comprise 60% of our patient population. The time before revision averaged 24 months (range 10 to 45). Six of our loosenings occured in hips 1 to 50, none in 51 to 100, two in 101 to 150, and two in 151 to 200. There have been no loosenings in the last 150 patients who have a 3-month to 20-month follow-up.

One latent sepsis has been successfully debrided and revised. The patient is a 58-year-old man with bilateral osteonecrosis who developed some culture-positive drainage in the postoperative period. In retrospect, this should have been debrided at that time. However, the wound healed, but the drainage recurred at 9 months and was culture-positive for *Streptococcus*. At revision, the acetabular component was loose and was removed, and thorough débridement was performed. The femoral component was tight and was not disturbed. At 3 weeks after removal, an acetabular penetration was bone grafted and the socket was reinserted. The patient is now at 1 year after revision and is asymptomatic, though he has a complete lucent zone around his socket.

LOOSENING—COMPARISON OF WORLDWIDE RESULTS

Despite a 4.7% incidence of loosening in the first 168 cases (3.5% overall for 350), clinical results of THARIES procedures are indeed promising, especially when compared to the performance of conventional stem type of replacements in a young and active population and the worldwide results of other surface replacements. This is especially true, since we are including all our cases from initiation of the clinical trial in 1975, and we have been aggressive in advising reoperation once the patient becomes symptomatic, in order to preserve bone stock. Loosening in conventional total hips with up to 7 years of follow-up has shown rates as high as 24%. Furthermore, Chandler et al.[16] reported a failure rate of 54% after 5 years in patients under 30 years of age. Our own conventional-hip major-complication rate in this younger group with a 5-year follow-up was 35% and is primarily attributable to loosening. Al-

Table 21-5. THARIES minor complications requiring surgery*

THARIES number	Age	Cause	Sex	Problem	Operation to revision (months)	Revision procedure	Revision result (P-W-F = pain walking, function)	Current new follow-up (months)	Comments
12	21	CDH	F	Heterotopic bone formation (severe)	19	HBF excision; revision of acetabular component	4,6,6, Recurrence of HBF (moderate)	26	
43	16	SCFE	M	Trochanteric bursitis	14	Trochanteric wire removal	4,6,6	15	
41	29	Osteochondritis dissecans	F	Enigmatic pain HBF (moderate)	17	1. HBF excision; revision of acetabular component	5,5,5 Recurrent HBF	13	Rim bone formation
						2. Trochanteric wire removal	Still symptomatic		Possible socket loosening?
35	21	CDH	F	Trochanteric bursitis	22	Trochanteric wire removal	8,7,6 Asymptomatic	17	
14	33	CDH	F	Femoral neck cyst	36	Autogenous bone graft	8,7,6 Graft filling in	7	
124	25	Osteoarthritis after trauma	F	Trochanteric bursitis	12 24	Trochanteric wire removal	3,4,3 Still symptomatic	3	Subsequently reexplored; components tight
02	51	Osteoarthritis	F	Trochanteric bursitis	36	Trochanteric wire removal	9,10,10 Asymptomatic	14	
133	52	Osteoarthritis	F	Trochanteric bursitis	20	Trochanteric wire removal	9,9,9 Asymptomatic	14	
234	59	Arthrodesis	M	Dislocation	4	Open reduction	10,6,6	13	Open reduction at another hospital

*CDH, Congenitally dysplastic or dislocated hips; SCFE, slipped capital femoral epiphysis; HBF, heterotopic bone formation.

Table 21-6. THARIES major complications requiring surgery*

THARIES number	Age	Cause	Sex	Problem	Operation to revision (months)	Revision procedure	Revision result (P-W-F = pain, walking, function)	Current new follow-up (months)	Comments
04	24	CDH	F	Socket loose	10	Replacement of acetabular component	6,5,8	48	Socket uncovered initially
01	16	SCFE	M	Femoral component and socket loose	24	TR-28 THR	10,6,7	31	Incomplete seating Poor interdigitation
18	48	Osteonecrosis	M	Femoral loose	28	Replacement of femoral and acetabular components; SR4 to SR3	8,8,8	17	High stress
114	58	Osteonecrosis	M	Sepsis; socket loose	8	Débridement; removal of acetabular component; bone graft; acetabular insertion 1 month after débridement	9,8,8	23	Had culture positive with postoperative drainage
122	34	Congenital coxa vara	M	Femoral component and socket loose	10 / 12 (22)	1. Revision of acetabular component; 2. Conversion to TR-28	5,4,4	2	Poor PMMA interdigitation
47	33	CDH	F	Femoral component and socket loose	24	TR-28 THR with bone graft	8,5,3	13	Poor technique
139	20	CDH	F	Socket loose	20	Socket revision	8,7,8	8	High stress
46	50	Osteoarthritis	F	Socket loose	18	Socket revision	7,5,5	3	Not grossly loose
173	67	Osteoarthritis	M	Socket loose	18	Socket revision	7,9,7	4	High stress
19	47	CDH	F	Femoral component and socket loose	45	TR-28 THR	8,5,5	2	Poor PMMA interdigitation
182	35	Osteonecrosis	M	Femoral component loose	19	Femoral revision	6,6,6	2	Poor technique

*CDH, congenitally dysplastic or dislocated hips; SCFE, slipped capital femoral epiphysis; THR, total hip replacement; polymethylmethacrylate.

Table 21-7. Loosening—fracture

	Number	Follow-up (years)	Loose		Fracture		Fracture and loose	
			Number	%	Number	%	Number	%
UCLA	266	1-5	10	2.7	0	0	10	2.7
Early	168	2-5	8	4.8	0	0	8	4.8
Capello	110	0.5-4	7	6.4	2	1.8	9	8.2
Early	32	4	8	25	6	19	14	44
Freeman	107	2-4	11	10.2	2	1.9	13	12.1
Early	33	4	7	21	18	29	15	45
Trentani	140	1-7	22	16	5	3.6	27	19
Wagner	426	1-5	23	5.3	3	0.07	26	6

though those loosening results are unsatisfactory, we cannot predict as yet what our incidence will be at 5 years. The incidence of socket radio-lucencies is slightly higher than our conventional total hip group of patients followed from 2 to 9 years (average 4 years).[23] The same low incidence of absent radiolucency was noted in 4.3%; 31.7% had interface lucency up to 50%; 16.7% had 51% to 99%; and 47.3% had a complete zone compared to 61.9% of surface replacements. There was also a slightly greater incidence of wider zones, with 8% 2 mm or greater with surface replacement as opposed to 6.5% with conventional replacement. The socket revision rate was much higher: 4.8% compared to 1.1%. However, there were pronounced age, sex, cause, and activity-level differences. The conventional hips were 16 years older at surgery (57.6 years), and 65% were of women. A detailed comparative multivariant analysis will be necessary for true comparison.

Comparison of clinical results of surface replacement from other innovators is complex because there are many design and technique variables, and each has different indication, so that there are etiologic as well as six, age, and activity-level differences.[1] Capello,[6] who is carrying on the work of Eicher, and Freeman[17] have a preponderance of osteoarthritic patients. Trentani[27] and Wagner[28] have many more patients with dysplasias, whereas Freeman and Wagner have less patients with osteonecrosis. Capello and those at UCLA have been performing surface replacements primarily on younger, active patients who have a higher risk for loosening than do older, less active patients. Wagner frequently utilizes osteotomy for the treatment of younger patients, and therefore his patients and those of Freeman had a higher average age at surgery.

The major complications have been loosening and neck fracture (Table 21-7). Capello and Freeman have reported complication rates of 44% and 45% in their early experiences with the Indiana Conservation Hip (ICH) and Imperial College London Hospital (ICLH) protheses. Both have made design and technique changes, with significant lowering of complications in their more recent series. Of concern is the increasing loosening rate over time, as reported by Trentani.[27] His 1975 report included 140 hips having up to a 7-year follow-up with a 20% fracture and loosening rate. It is difficult to separate the fracture and loosening cases because of the long neck flange and method of reporting. In addition, other authors have not yet reported details on the extent and progression of socket radiolucencies, which may indicate future loosening problems, or details of other patients who derive less than optimal clinical results. Although Wagner has used a ceramic femoral component in selected cases, the femoral component otherwise obscures observation of the cement-bone interface, and changes in position must be carefully evaluated. It is important to note that Wanger, Freemen, Trentani, and Capello have relative contraindications to performing resurfacing patients with "inflammatory arthritis," in whom they have had a higher rate of loosening. Capello and Trentani include rheumatoid patients in that ill-defined group of inflammatory arthritis, but Wagner and Freeman have a special catagory.' We have had no loosening in these groups.

It is also necessary to assess the design variables that may have influenced the complication rates of other types of surface replacements. Trentani and Freeman basically use a cylindrically prepared femoral head. We have observed that the peripheral rim of bone left after cylindric reaming is often sclerotic or necrotic, depending on the cause, and that chamfering does not remove good viable bone stock in the majority of hips. Since removal of the peripheral rim enhances fixation, we have now developed a precision method of chamfering with a new reamer. Trentani's femoral component extends distally onto the neck, and although this may hold a loose component in place for a longer period, we believe that component impingement may be a significant factor for his increasing loosening rate.

The ICH and Wagner both use spheric reaming. Wagner's femoral component is cup shaped, with intrinsic ridges for internal fixation. These ridges are 0.5 mm, leave little margin for any technical error, and may compartmentalize the acrylic cement. The ICLH socket has 5 mm less than hemispheric coverage of the component and has a thicker medial wall. This could lead to instability when the vertical opening is excessive. The ICH has an area cut out from the socket inferiorly. However, our range-of-motion studies have shown very little benefit from this, and impingement in adduction is not a problem if the component is properly covered by the acetabulum. There are also numerous designs for socket fixation, but as yet there have been few problems reported at the socket–acrylic cement interface.

There are also differences in the operative approach, type of acrylic cement, and the technique of bone preparation and fixation utilized. Wagner uses an anterior approach, and Freeman a lateral without trochanteric removal. We have routinely removed the trochanter, whereas Capello and Trentani partially section the gluteus in some patients and use trochanteric osteotomy in patients with more difficult exposure problems. These factors, especially in the absence of detailed radiolucency x-ray analysis by the various authors, make comparisons difficult. However, we remain firmly convinced of the importance of good technique to obtain optimal results. Our current THARIES polyethylene sockets are 3 mm less than a hemisphere, permitting full containment within the acetabulum without sacrificing excessive bone stock. This serves to prevent neck socket impingement, which could deform or loosen the polyethylene socket.

In assessing fixation concepts, we opted to design for severe conditions. The keying of cement to the THARIES cup is enhanced by a circumferential groove, deepest in its superior aspect, and a polar groove for cement buttressing and torque resistance. These are complemented with additional cement keyholes on the facing dome of the femoral head.

For the socket, we elected to utilize the grooves in the range of 0.5 to 1 mm and place them so that in most situations they would be away from the wear axis.

Despite our detailed analysis that led to the THARIES design, component loosening, as observed with all acrylic fixed prostheses, remains the most frequent complication. Our loosenings have occurred, with one exception, in high-risk patients who were young, very active, or had some deficiency in bone stock. In six of the 10 patients we believe that there were obvious technical errors: one had incomplete socket coverage, one had incomplete seating of the femoral component, and four had poor acrylic interdigitation (shown by analysis of the acrylic cement remaining in situ in the femoral component or by roentgenographic evaluation of the acetabular cement-bone interface in the early postoperative period). Of the other four, high-activity stress coupled with more subtle technical deficiencies were noted. The hips of those patients might not have loosened if current techniques for improved fixation with containment and compression had been utilized. These techniques have gradually evolved and were not uniformly adopted by all five of the UCLA joint-replacement surgeons at the same time. Gradual evolution of improved techniques for acetabular fixation has resulted in a sharp improvement in the immediate and short-term follow-up, by fewer and thinner radiolucencies. We have had no actual or suspected loosenings in a group of 150 more recent THARIES with a 5- to 23-month follow-up. This is encouraging, since all our previous loosenings became symptomatic less than 18 months postoperatively. The acetabulum-radiolucent zones are thinner and less extensive than in the early cases.

In the canine model, good intrusion of acrylic resin into the trabeculas has routinely been followed by a thin membrane that is benign and stable.[20,24] On the other hand, when intrusion of acrylic resin is poor, immediate fixation is suboptimal. A thicker membrane forms, which, with further instability, is associated with osteoclasts and osteoclasis leading to gross loosening. When stress is high, as in a young, active patient, the process can be rapid. We therefore believe that technique is obviously critical for long-term durability.

We firmly believe that the socket should be well recessed within the pelvis, so that there is no real risk of impingement. Initially we opted to try for a large head-neck diameter ratio by implanting large femoral components and corresponding large acetabular sockets. This left many of the sockets uncovered. Reduction of the depth of the component of 3 mm enabled containment in all but a few dysplastic patients. Perhaps a few millimeters of uncovering is acceptable in different situations, since we have had no loosenings in a group that had up to 20% of the socket uncovered laterally. We do advise full containment anteriorly. However, we also observed, in analyzing patients who had bilateral replacements with different size components, that there was very little difference in the range of motion. We therefore have opted to place a smaller femoral component approaching the neck size in order to preserve acetabular stock. This has also enabled us to place a thicker acrylic layer on the socket side, which will, we hope, obviate cracking of thin acrylic cement that might lead to fragmentation and loosening.

Although we believe that significant long-term improvement can be achieved with newer techniques, the very young and active patient (under 40) remains at higher risk for loosening. For this reason we believe it is wise to consider other alternatives. For the osteonecrotic patient, stages 1 to 4, up to approximately 40 years of age, we now perform selective core decompression[14] and Sugioka[26] rotational osteotomies. We have recommended and performed arthrodesis in the young male and suggest that this procedure be utilized primarily in the healthy patient in his twenties. It is likely that for this group even the best of our arthroplasty techniques (circa 1980) will require revision, at a time when the patient is still young and active. Unless our revision technique greatly improves, especially on the acetabular side, there probably will be a progressive loss of bone stock, which would make a subsequent arthrodesis much more difficult to achieve. In addition, we and others have had excellent success with takedown of arthrodeses, even when performed initially with sacrifice of good bone and muscle stock. We believe that arthrodesis deserves more consideration in our present armamentarium of treatment methods.

OTHER COMPLICATIONS

We had two dislocations, one with gross muscle and bone stock deficiencies. Proper postoperative precautions, given the absence of an abductor mechanism in one patient and a very short neck in the other, might have prevented them. However, we do recommend trochanteric advancement in those patients who require shortening or who have osteonecrosis or other bone-stock deficiencies, or in whom abductor musculature is weak. We have revised two loose femoral components from our series and two others whose initial operation was performed at other hospitals, and had the femoral component placed on shortened necks in order to accomplish implantation on relatively good bone stock. These four patients had some restricted range of motion after reconstruction despite sculpturing to improve motion. In one patient we fashioned a neck by advancing the cylindric reamer distally through the base of the greater trochanter. The lesser trochanter was osteotomized and removed, but the medial calcar support was not violated. The greater trochanter was advanced to the lateral shaft. The total shortening was estimated to be 3 cm. He was placed on protective weight-bearing for 6 months while the freshly-exposed cancellous bone became remodeled laterally.

The incidence of sepsis recorded in the worldwide literature has not been greater than conventional rates, and perhaps lower. Freeman has reported four of 248 (1.6%),[17] Capello two of 110 (1.8%),[6] and other authors reported less than 1%. Our incidence of one in 350 shows a suggestive decrease, though not statistically significant over our recent conventional replacement series, particularly when one considers that the majority had no previous surgery and only a few had previous sepsis.

The overall incidence of heterotopic ossification was comparable to our conventional hip replacement series. There has been a 2% incidence of severe ossification (bone larger than 1 cm and closer than 1 cm to the pelvis or trochanter), though there has been no ankylosis. It is difficult to compare heterotopic bone incidence and severity from the various innovators because of the different population mix and method of evaluation. The anterior approach has been implicated as forming more bone in comparison with a similar operation performed transtrochanterically.[19] Wagner has reported an incidence of moderate formation as 12%, and severe formation as 4%.

His average postoperative flexion arc of only 76 degrees suggests restriction of motion, but his average preoperative flexion of 60 degrees was less than in another series. Freeman has reported higher bone formation rates than with conventional replacement, but he is now using a different approach for resurfacing. To date we have not observed any significant difference in conventional hip replacement versus THARIES using the same approach.

The cause of heterotopic ossification is unknown, but most high-risk male osteoarthritic patients are now placed on a diphosphonate protocol, which includes 20 mg/kg of Didronel* per day started at 2 weeks before surgery and for 3 months after surgery, in addition to careful removal of accumulated debris by thorough cleansing at operation. Radiotherapy using the Mayo Clinic protocol has been used once.[12]

The incidence of nerve palsy has been distressing, though most did recover. We believe this complication was attributable to stretching of the nerve during surgery, which was performed in a lateral decubitus position. This could occur because of inadequate support of the leg held by the assistant after dislocation of the hip. If the hip is dislocated over the side of the table, the proper method of support includes placing the foot on a bar of the fracture table for support or the assistant straddling and supporting the leg.[1] When the hip is further externally rotated to deliver the femoral head for reaming, the leg is supported by the assistant's leg and hands and the peroneal nerve at the knee is protected from pressure. Overzealous retraction could be implicated during bone preparation and component insertion and can be avoided by careful positioning of the Hohman retractors and prevention of unnecessary retraction.

Five patients have had trochanteric wires removed, and we believe this increase over our conventional series is attributable to the young, active patient population. We have been pleased at the low incidence of systemic and thromboembolic complications in comparison to conventional hip replacement rates, but perhaps this is more reflective of the overall youth of the patient population.

Although we have not had any fractures of our 350 THARIES patients to date, we have had an

*Proctor & Gamble, Cincinnati, Ohio.

opportunity to study a group of roentgenograms and in some cases histologic material from patients sent to us from other orthopaedic surgeons. In all but one we were able to identify one or more factors as probably responsible for contributing to fracture. Excessive femoral reaming or poor techniques of trochanteric osteotomy or attachment can predispose the neck to fracture, especially if there is osteoporosis. We strongly recommend that a small trochanteric osteotomy performed extracapsularly is important to obviate a stress riser and to prevent unnecessary vascular compromise.

Necrotic or weak bone should be removed, and we now generally shorten the neck in severe osteonecrosis or osteoporosis. In addition, the neck must be safeguarded by selection of the appropriate component size and by protection during preparation. The most obvious, and possibly the most important design aspect, is having an adequate range of sizes. The smaller the size increments between components, the better any hip joint can be effectively custom-fitted with minimal bone-stock removal. The THARIES system now has seven sizes available in 3 to 4 ml increments to fit any femoral head with a diameter of 35 to 65 mm, corresponding to a maximum neck size range of 25 to 46 mm.

SUMMARY

We have demonstrated that hip resurfacing can achieve results comparable to conventional total hip replacement in terms of pain relief, walking, function, and range of motion. Further, the enhanced stability and apparent lower risk of sepsis weigh in favor of its use for certain specific indications. There is and will continue to be a need to improve long-term interface stability to minimize, and hopefully eliminate, loosening. We will continue to explore other modes of fixation, though we do not believe the ultimate in materials and technique have been achieved using acrylic cement as the interface material. Whether or not sufficient lifetime durability can be achieved for the very young and very active patients remains uncertain.

We have included in our series the most difficult group of patients, the young and very active. The changes in component design, improvement in instrumentation, and, most importantly, in fixation technique, coupled with more discretion in recommending the procedure for patients in whom other surgical procedures (such as pelvic shelving, rotational osteotomy or arthrodeses) would be better, should result in improved long-term results.

The worldwide incidence of loosening with other types of surface replacement is of considerable concern. Although there are many contributing factors, including prosthetic design, instrumentation, and technique, fixation technique is the most important single factor in prevention of loosening. Socket fixation may be more critical than with conventional replacement because of the large ball size and increased frictional torque. The importance of these factors is under study. There have been no cases of dislocation in patients with reasonably normal muscle and bone stock, and our sepsis rate, 0.33%, is exceptionally low, with no cases of hematogenous origin. Other complications, such as nerve palsy, should be preventable. Although there is an increased difficulty of performing resurfacing surgery to optimize fixation in comparison with conventional replacement with the femoral head and neck present, judicious use of retraction and leg support should minimize or prevent this complication.

Each surgical team that engages in surface replacement of any kind must focus on each complication and strive for prevention. Since we have had no neck fractures to date, this complication is largely preventable. The THARIES range of components enables the surgeon to customize the prosthesis to the hip, rather than the hip to the prosthesis. The instrumentation provides a useful guide to protect the neck, but the surgical team must be thoroughly versed in its advantages and its shortcomings. When bone stock is poor, such as in severe osteoporosis or necrosis, it is preferable to shorten the neck.

Although we understand the surgeon's preference for using a different surgical approach to the hip joint, we feel that at the outset surgeons learning the technique should use a lateral transtrochanteric approach because of the wide exposure provided with a relatively low incidence of significant heterotopic bone formation. Surgeons should not compromise on bone preparation, and exposure is most helpful in utilizing the new techniques of compression and containment for acetabular fixation. If the surgeon wishes to explore another approach, he should do so only after he can demonstrate to himself a consistent optimal interface with no radiolucencies on a high-contrast postoperative reentenograms. The fear of

trochanteric migration can be minimized when one concentrates on a technique that is proved to produce reliable results.

We do agree that there is concern regarding excessive sacrifice of acetabular bone stock, and we believe that this can be minimized utilizing our current technique. Although we have had considerable initial success with our revision resurfacing techniques, we are not satisfied with our ability to obtain a quality interface on the socket side, which becomes sclerotic when loosening occurs. Improved techniques are needed to achieve better interface stability when there is minimal trabecular bone remaining.

There is no doubt that the best time for optimizing fixation is at the initial surgery, when maximal trabecular bone can be exposed by reaming. However, we believe that the hip should be protected from excess stress in the postoperative period. The length of protection or degree to which the surgeon and patient should strive to achieve this goal has not yet been carefully defined. We feel porous ingrowth may be the ultimate in achieving long-term fixation stability. In the equation of decision for surface or conventional replacement, it is wise to consider the age of the patient, anticipated activity levels, weight, limb-length discrepancy, need for restoration of bone mechanics, bone stock available, mechanical disabilities, risk of sepsis, and the possible need for revision. Our follow-up suggests that the THARIES procedure is an excellent method for the young or active patients, who are at greater risk for complications with the stem type of replacement. The quality of THARIES results will ultimately require critical long-term 10 year-minimum analysis such as is now becoming available with conventional replacements. In patients with conventional replacements we have also observed that once a painless replacement is installed it is more easy for the young to forget the precautions regarding avoiding impact and protecting the hip for long-term durability. For this reason, we must continue to evaluate the alternatives of osteotomy and arthrodesis for the very young active patient. We have experienced more complications and poorer results from unknown causes in patients who have had psycho-social abnormatlities. For most patients there is no urgency, and "buying time" until technologic improvements are available is sometimes the best choice for the very young.

REFERENCES

1. Amstutz, H.C.: Surface replacement of the hip. In The Hip, St. Louis, 1980, The C.V. Mosby Co.
2. Amstutz, H.C., and Clarke, I.C.: Total hip articular replacement by internal eccentric shells—the THARIES technique for surface replacement, Warsaw, Ind., 1979, Zimmer USA.
3. Amstutz, H.C., Clarke, I.C., Christie, J., and Graff-Radford, A.: Total hip articular replacement by internal eccentric shells—the "THARIES" approach to total surface replacement arthroplasty, Clin. Orthop. **128:**261-284, 1977.
4. Amstutz, H.C., Graff-Radford, A., Mai, L., and Thomas, B.: THARIES surface replacement of the hip, J. Bone Joint Surg. **63A:**1069-1077, 1981.
5. Brooker, A.F., Bowerman, J.W., Robinson, R.A., and Riley, L.H.: Ectopic ossification following total hip replacement, J. Bone Joint Surg. **55A:**1629-1632, 1973.
6. Capello, W.: Symposium on surface replacement of the hip, American Academy of Orthopaedic Surgeons, Atlanta, Georgia, Feb. 10, 1980.
7. Capello, N.W., Ireland, P.H., Trammel, T.R., and Eicher, P.: Conservative total hip arthroplasty: a procedure to conserve bone stock—parts I and II, Clin. Orthop. **134:**59-74, July-Aug. 1978.
8. Chandler, H.P., Reineck, F.T., and Wixson, R.C.: A five-year review of THR's in patients under the age of 30 with emphasis on loosening, Orthop. Trans. 3(3):303, 1979.
9. Clarke, I.C., and Amstutz, H.C.: Human hip joint geometry and hemiarthroplasty selection. In The hip, St. Louis, 1975, The C.V. Mosby Co.
10. Clarke, I., Amstutz, H., Christie, J., and Graff-Radford, A.: The John Charnley Award Paper: THARIES surface replacement arthroplasty for the arthritic hip: rebirth of an earlier concept? In The hip, St. Louis, 1977, The C.V. Mosby Co.
11. Clarke, I., Black, K., and Amstutz, H.: Range of motion in natural and surface-replacement types of hip joint, Trans. Twenty-third Annual Meeting of the Orthopaedic Research Society, Las Vegas, 1977, p. 155
12. Coventry, M.B., and Scanlon, P.W.: The use of radiation to discourage ectopic bone: a nine year study in surgery about the hip, J. Bone Joint Surg. **63A**(2):201-208, 1981.
13. DeLee, J.G., and Charnley, J.: Radiological demarcation of cemented sockets in total hip replacement, Clin. Orthop. **121:**20, 1976.
14. Ficot, P., and Arlet, J.: Arthrosis: new diagnostic procedures, Acta Orthop. Scand. **46:**329-337, 1975.
15. Freeman, M.A.R.: Some anatomical and mechanical considerations relevant to the surface replacement of the femoral head, Clin. Orthop. **134:**19-24, 1978.
16. Freeman, M.A.R.: Total surface replacement arthroplasty, Clin. Orthop. **134:**2-4, 1978.
17. Freeman, M.A.R.: Symposium on surface replacement of the hip, American Academy of Orthopaedic Surgeons, Atlanta, Georgia, Feb. 10, 1980.
18. Gibson, A.: Vitallium cup arthroplasty of the hip joint, J. Bone Joint Surg. **21A:**861-868, 1949.
19. Hamblen, D.L., Harris, W.H., and Rottger, J.: Myositis ossificans as a complication of hip arthroplasty, J. Bone Joint Surg. **53B:**764, 1971.
20. Hedley, A.K., Clarke, I., Moreland, J., et al.: Durability of acrylic cement fixation of femoral head prosthesis: a canine surface replacement model. (Submitted for publication, 1979.)
21. Amstutz, H.C., Lodwig, R.M., Schurman, D.J., and Hodgson, A.: Range of motion studies for total hip replacements: a comparative study with a new experimental apparatus, Clin. Orthop. **(111):**124-130, 1975.
22. Markolf, K.L., and Amstutz, H.C.: Mechanical strength of the femur following resurfacing and conventional total hip replacement procedures, Clin. Orthop. **147:**170-180,1980.
23. Moreland, J.: Loosening of total hip replacement: incidence and significance. In The hip, St. Louis, 1980, The C.V. Mosby Co.
24. Sew Hoy, A., Hedley, A., Clarke, I., Gruen, T., Amstutz, H., Coster, I., and Moreland, J.R.: The acetabular cement-bone interface—a canine study, Clin. Orthop. **155:**231-243, 1980.
25. Shybut, G.T., Askew, M.J., Hori, R.Y., and Stulberg, S.D.: Theoretical and experimental studies of femoral stresses following surface replacement hip arthroplasty. In The hip, St. Louis, 1980, The C.V. Mosby Co.
26. Sugioka, U.: Transtrochanteric anterior rotational anatomy of the femoral head in treatment of osteonecrosis affecting the hip, Clin. Orthop. **130:**191-201, Jan. 1978.
27. Trentani, C.: Personal communication, Feb. 1980.
28. Wagner, H.: Symposium on surface replacement of the hip, American Academy of Orthopaedic Surgeons, Atlanta, Georgia, Feb. 10, 1980.

Chapter 22

Complications of surface replacements

ANTHONY K. HEDLEY, M.B., B.Ch., F.R.C.S.
Los Angeles, California

Surface replacement of the hip is gaining popularity as a method of total hip replacement, which many believe is more suitable for use in the younger patient. It requires less removal of bone stock and allows the implantation of smaller, less invasive prosthetic devices, particularly the femoral component. It requires, however, a wide exposure of the hip joint so that the surgical procedure can be performed accurately. The postoperative management parallels that of conventional total hip replacement, and although the average age of the patient is considerably less than those undergoing conventional total hip replacement, many of the complications encountered in the immediate perioperative period are common to both procedures. It appears that the incidence of these complications is somewhat less in the surface replacement group, perhaps reflecting the younger average age of the patient undergoing this procedure.

The complications can be divided into systemic and local groups. Systemic complications such as phlebitis, pulmonary embolism, atelectasis, and cardiac and pulmonary problems are potential hazards common to both procedures. It is not my object to discuss these complications but rather to focus on some of the specific technical and biomechanical problems encountered with surface replacement. Therefore the following complications are discussed:

1. Heterotopic ossification
2. Trochanteric nonunion or migration
3. Vascular compromise to femoral head
4. Fracture of femoral neck
5. Dislocation
6. Loosening
7. Invasive cyst formation

HETEROTOPIC OSSIFICATION

Reports from many centers indicate that the incidence of heterotopic ossification associated with surface replacement appears to be higher than that occurring with conventional total hip replacement. The exact cause is obscure. The surgical approach has been implicated[3] in many cases. The UCLA experience with a transtrochanteric osteotomy has led to an incidence of heterotopic ossification that parallels the incidence occurring with conventional hip replacement. Freeman uses an extensive combined anterior and posterior approach without removal of the trochanter and reports a higher incidence with surface replacements than that with conventional total hip replacement.[2] Wagner's experience using an anterior approach, again without removal of the trochanter, has produced a somewhat higher incidence of about 12%.

We recognize clinically a group of so-called high-risk patients, which consists of cases who have had previous trauma to the affected hip, previous slipped capital femoral epiphysis, patients who develop exuberant osteophyte formation as part of the osteoarthritic process such as in Forrestier's disease, patients with ankylosing spondylitis, and those who have had previous surgery on the same hip.

The average age of the patient is somewhat lower in the surface replacement group which may have a significant influence on the formation of periarticular new bone, as many of these patients fall into the posttraumatic group.

Our current regimen is to place these patients on a therapeutic course of diphosphonate (Didronel). A dose of 20 mg/kg per day administered for a month before surgery and continued for 2 months after surgery has appeared to be beneficial. A multicenter placebo controlled double-blind study suggested that diphosphonate given at 20 mg/kg per day decreased the incidence and severity of heterotopic ossification after total hip replacement. There was an increased incidence of diarrhea and hyperphosphatemia in the drug-treated patients however.

The Mayo Clinic protocol of irradiation administered in a dose of 2000 rads over 10 days has been used in several of our higher risk cases with good results.[1] A cautionary note, however, is indicated if trochanteric osteotomy has been performed, since the irradiation may prevent or retard subsequent union of the trochanter.

TROCHANTERIC NONUNION OR MIGRATION

Problems relating to trochanteric osteotomy, both major and minor are not insignificant where trochanteric osteotomy has been performed as part of the surgical procedure. The following problems vary from asymptomatic fracture of the wires, which is a common incidental finding, to frank separation of the trochanteric fragment and resultant loss of abductor power.

Minor problems

Asymptomatic fractures of wires. Fracture of trochanteric wires without symptoms or related problems is frequent. Fatigue fracture or stress-corrosion fractures of trochanteric wires is a common finding and can occur from several weeks to several months after surgery. The majority of these are asymptomatic and present no problem.

Bursitis. Bursitis can occur over prominences produced by the wire-securing technique. These techniques vary from simple twisting of the wires to knot-tying. Where prominences occur over the lateral aspect of the trochanter, bursas will form. Occasionally a patient will present with persistent trochanteric bursitis with crepitus and discomfort that is felt immediately over the trochanteric wires. If this occurs and persists, we advocate removal of the wires provided that the trochanter is completely united.

Apparent fibrous union. Routine radiologic examination may reveal an apparent fibrous union of the trochanter. Fibrous union without separation of the fragment is seldom a problem and may in fact be an apparent finding rather than a real one. Tomography will often reveal actual union in certain areas of the trochanteric-femoral interface. We do not advocate active treatment for apparent fibrous union of the trochanter because most of these are asymptomatic at the time of discovery.

Major problems

Nonunion. Nonunion with slight separation of the fragments (up to 1 cm) may be slightly painful in the early postoperative period but tends to become asymptomatic if treated conservatively. Provided that the fixation device remains intact and there does not appear to be migration of the fragment away from the trochanteric bed, I believe that symptoms will eventually resolve despite an apparently wide fibrous union. Many of these patients may have a persistent Trendelenburg lurch, which too, given time, will resolve.

Trochanteric rip-off. Trochanteric rip-off represents the major problem related to trochanteric osteotomy. This can occur in several ways. In cases where the bone is severely osteoporotic the majority of trochanteric fixation techniques will not be adequate. For severely osteoporotic patients we have advocated the use of wire mesh as adjuvant fixation for the trochanter. Where wires have been used for trochanteric fixation, failure may occur in several ways. Wire fracture is not uncommon and meticulous care must be taken with placement of the wires to avoid knicks from drill points and kinks. Both of these will lead to "stress risers" in the wire, and fracture may occur with tension in the very early postoperative period. Care must be taken when one is securing the wires. This is usually done by twisting or knot-tying. I advocate the latter because I have encountered no failure of fixation from slippage or separation of knots. Careful placement of the wires is important to prevent the trochanter slipping between the wires with abductor pull. I use a cruciate fixation technique by placing one wire in the axis of the femoral shaft and one perpendicular to this. The wires are placed through the femur approximately 1 cm deep to the trochanteric bed. With trochanteric reattachment I advocate passing the superior wire through the abductor mass proximal to the trochanter and placing the remaining three wires through drill holes in the substance of the trochanter to prevent slippage of the trochanter at the time of fixation.

• • •

Despite the occurance of complications with trochanteric osteotomy, I advocate that surface replacement is done by the transtrochanteric approach because I believe that this offers the widest and the most accurate exposure to the proximal femur. It also affords the opportunity for trochanteric advancement. Furthermore, the exposure allows for meticulous protection of the retinacular blood supply to the femoral head. Further, with this wide approach to the proximal femur the full circumference of the femoral neck can be visualized at the time of femoral reaming and thus the possibility of notching the femoral neck can be avoided.

A further important factor in preventing trochanteric problems is prolonged protection from weight-bearing in the postoperative period. I advocate a minimum of 2 months on crutches subsequent to surface replacement. This has contributed significantly to lowering the problems from trochanteric osteotomy in our clinic.

VASCULAR COMPROMISE TO FEMORAL HEAD

Massive avascular necrosis after surface replacement was predicted by Charnley when surface replacement was still in its infancy. This has not been our experience either clinically or in our experimental models.

The normal femoral head has a diffuse blood supply originating from several following sources:

1. *Large vessels.* Medial and lateral circumflex vessels arise predominantly from the profounda femoris artery and form a circular anastomosis about the base of the femoral neck. Further anastomosis occurs from descending branches from the gluteal arteries and ascending branches from the deeper femoral perforating arteries creating the crucial anastomosis. The bulk of this rich blood supply is anastomotic and occurs around the piriformis fossa on the posterior aspect of the femoral neck. From this anastomosis are derived several perforating branches, which penetrate the piriformis fossa and the base of the femoral neck.

2. *Retinacular vessels.* These vessels originate from the circular anastomosis at the base of the femoral neck and travel subsynovially up the femoral neck to enter the femoral head just distal to the epiphysis. These vessels then travel through the substance of the femoral head and anastomose diffusely at the epiphyseal scar. In the adult situation, when the epiphysis is closed, several branches cross the epiphyseal scar to supply the epiphysis. The exact contribution of these vessels is debated, however, as the epiphysis tends to remain somewhat more avascular than the remainder of the femoral head and neck.

3. *Artery of ligamentum teres.* The artery of the ligamentum teres plays an important role in the immature individual. Once the epiphysis is closed, however, the exact contribution of the artery of the ligamentum teres is debatable. Some estimates are that this vessel supplies as little as 10% to 15% of the epiphysis.

4. *Intraosseous vessels.* The anastomosis between the retinacular vessels entering the femoral neck and the intraosseous vessels, which are extensions of the nutrient vessels traveling proximally in the intramedullary canal, is very diffuse. Furthermore, a diffuse anastomosis exists between those vessels and the vessels perforating the posterior aspect of the femoral neck in the area of the piriformis fossa. Many believe that the intraosseous blood supply represents the bulk of the blood supply to the femoral head in the adult.

Bearing in mind the fact that bone has the potential to shunt more than two thirds more blood through its substance than is necessary to maintain its viability, the potential of the intramedullary blood supply is enormous. This is seen particularly in pathologic states that cause an increase in the local blood supply to the femoral head as in the various arthritides. Freeman has suggested that in pathologic states the blood supply to the femoral head in fact is exaggerated and represents a far more hyperemic state than in the normal situation.[2] It must further be noted that many of the retinacular vessels that are originally subsynovial in the normal situation actually become intraosseous with increasing age as they are invested by the remodeling of the femoral neck in response to stress and are also covered by the formation of osteophytes.

It thus appears that the femoral head has a potentially diffuse blood supply, which is accentuated in certain pathologic conditions. An exception to this would obviously be the early stages of avascular necrosis.

Massive collapse of the femoral head after surface replacement has not occurred clinically or in our experimental model. Transient ischemia will result in a *normal* femoral head after destruction of the retinacular vessels. The brunt of this insult appears to occur in the epiphysis and is manifested by early ischemic changes occurring in the marrow.[4,6] The structural integrity of the bone, however, is maintained for a prolonged period of time and healing by the formation of appositional bone has been observed. Experimentally it has been shown that if fixation of the femoral component is secure, appositional bone formation will occur beneath the component.

Retrieved human specimens in whom subsidence of the femoral component has occurred have shown dense fibrous tissue between the component and the remainder of the bone. Histologically, there is no evidence to support the premise that this is attributable to massive avascular collapse, but rather it appears that continued erosion of the femoral head is caused by loosening of the components with massive progression of the fibrous membrane at the interface between the acrylic cement and bone.

FRACTURE OF FEMORAL NECK

Fracture of the femoral neck occurs because of mechanical failure of the neck to support the load on the femoral head. The exact site for initiation of the fracture varies and usually occurs in an area where a "stress riser" is present. The stress riser may be in the form of a notch inadvertently produced at the time of femoral head preparation, or at the junction between avascular and viable bone, or in an area of simple overload such as would occur with gross osteoporosis.[5]

Fractures of the femoral neck may result from the following:

1. Inferior notching of the femoral neck (Fig. 22-1)
2. Superior notching of the femoral neck (Fig. 22-2)
3. Fracture through the junction of viable and nonviable bone (such as with cases of avascular necrosis) (Fig. 22-3)
4. Fractures of the femoral neck resulting from a large trochanteric osteotomy (Fig. 22-4)
5. Fractures through stress risers such as screw holes or drill holes.

Notching and stress risers in the femoral neck are probably a fairly common surgical occurrence. Absolute attention to detail and meticulous preparation of the femoral head is necessary to avoid this. If a notch or a stress riser is introduced into the femoral neck inadvertently at the time of surgery, the surgeon should be cognizant of this. This would require strict adherence to an ex-

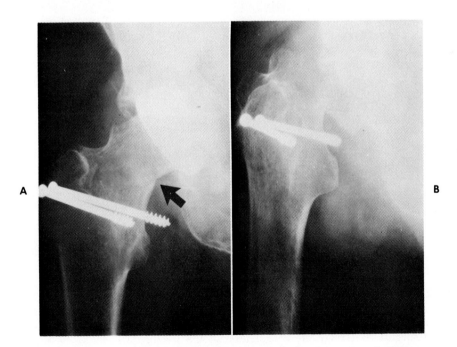

Fig. 22-1. A, *Arrow* indicates a large notch in the inferior femoral neck. This occurred at the time of cylindric reaming. **B,** Fracture occurred several months later and appeared to originate through the "stress riser" caused by the notch.

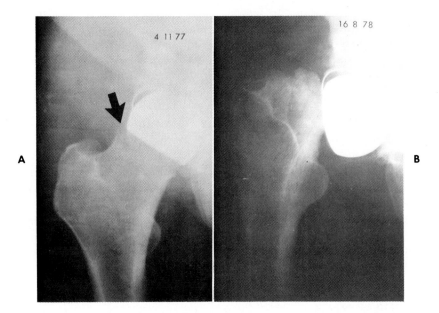

Fig. 22-2. A, *Arrow,* Large notch caused in the superior femoral neck at the time of femoral head preparation. **B,** Approximately 1 year later fracture of the femoral neck occurs and appears to originate through the area of weakness caused by the neck notching.

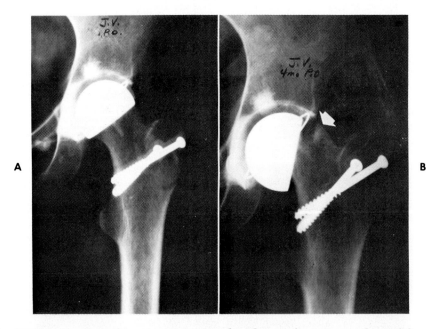

Fig. 22-3. A, Postoperative roentgenogram of surface replacement performed for avascular necrosis of the femoral head. The postoperative roentgenogram is satisfactory with the components in excellent orientation and no apparent technical problems at the time of surgery. **B,** *Arrow,* Site of initiation of the fracture, which can be seen as a slightly sclerotic area in the superior aspect of the femoral neck. Histologically, this was shown to be the junction between avascular and remodeling bone.

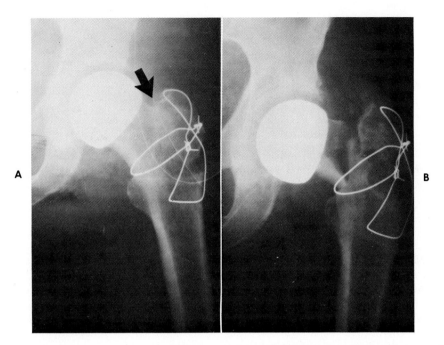

Fig. 22-4. A, *Arrow,* Position at which the trochanteric osteotomy transects the superior femoral neck. This is an unusually large trochanteric osteotomy. **B,** The fracture appears to occur through the weakened lateral femoral neck.

tended nonweightbearing protocol in the postoperative period. We have advocated a minimum of 2 months of nonweightbearing to allow such stress risers to remodel according to Wolff's law. Sudden impact loading as would occur with heel strike should be avoided, and the patient should be cautioned to continue for several months thereafter with crepe soles and a much reduced activity level. We believe that strict attention to the postoperative rehabilitation protocol is essential if these late complications are to be avoided.

DISLOCATION

Dislocation of surface replacement arthroplasty of the hip has not been a problem. The large component size appears to be inherently stable when compared with the dislocations occurring where smaller ball-socket ratios have been used.

The causes for dislocations are as follows:

1. *Absent or nonfunctioning abductors* (Fig. 22-5). This would happen where there has been actual loss of abductor muscle mass. This could occur with trauma or after excision in cases of myositis ossificans. Paralysis, as seen in polio or trochanteric rip-off associated with trochanteric osteotomy, may render the abductors similarly ineffec-

tive. It appears that actual loss of abductor muscle mass or muscle tone renders the patient more prone to dislocation.

2. *Impingement.* Impingement between the side wall of the pelvis and the femur, or between the components and bony parts, occurs in the following instances:

   a. *Short femoral head-neck segment where the femur impinges against the side wall of the pelvis in certain movements of the patient's normal range of motion.* This shortening may be caused by a resurfacing procedure having been performed on abnormal head-neck segments, or by excessive shortening of the head-neck segment at the time of femoral preparation.

   b. *Malalignment of acetabular components.* Care must be taken to avoid retroversion or excessive horizontalization of the acetabular component as this will tend to impinge on the femoral neck in flexion. When impingement of this nature occurs, the patient is often aware of a "clunking" sensation as the femoral component relocates in the acetabular component. Although a small degree of subluxation of the joint

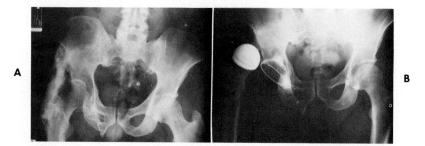

Fig. 22-5. A, The patient preoperatively. Massive heterotopic bone is present in the abductor muscle mass after trauma. **B,** A surface replacement was performed. At the time of surgery the heterotopic ossification was removed, and so the patient was left with virtually no abductor muscle mass. Dislocation in this case was reduced, and the patient was kept in an abduction splint for several months. Redislocation has not occurred.

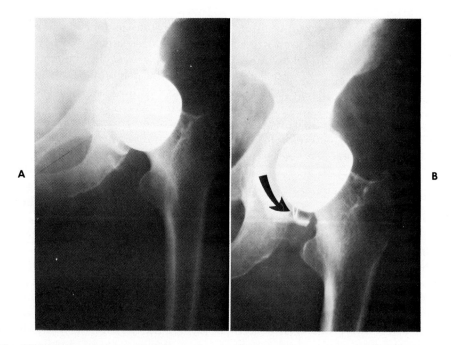

Fig. 22-6. A, Roentgenogram of a surface replacement seen at routine follow-up. Note the discernible marker wires of the acetabulum indicating good containment of the acetabulum within the bony pelvis. **B,** *Arrow,* Position that the acetabular component has adopted after loosening at the bone-cement interface. This is probably attributable to continual impingement between the femur and the margin of the acetabular component leading to loosening with gross movement of the acetabular component.

may be tolerable, the continual concentration of stress on the edge of the acetabular component may well contribute to its eventual loosening. (Fig. 22-6).

The fact that dislocation has not been a significant problem with surface replacement of the hip does not obviate the necessity, however, of not allowing the patient to abduct or internally rotate the leg in the immediate postoperative period. We feel that the abducted, externally rotated position should be maintained while the patient is supine and that sitting in low chairs should be discouraged for at least 6 to 8 weeks after surgery. This ensures the development of an adequate fibrous encapsulation of the hip joint, thus creating more stability.

A further factor that deserves attention is the maintenance of abductor muscle tension. Whenever the head-neck segment is shortened, I believe that it is mandatory to advance the trochanter in order to take up the slack in the abductor mechanism. Failure to do so will lead either to an increased risk of dislocation, a positive Trendelenburg gait, or a persistent "clunking" of the joint, of which the patient will be aware.

LOOSENING

Loosing is now recognized as the major complication of total joint replacements. It has been found that methyl methacrylate implanted into bone results in a foreign body response at the interface between the bone and cement having the potential to form a membrane between the acrylic cement and the bone.[4] With prosthetic instability that results from either poor prosthetic design or inadequate intrusion of the acrylic cement, micromovement occurs at this interface, which appears to be the initiating factor in the progression of this fibrous membrane. The membrane progresses until it becomes radiologically visible, at which time it appears as a radiolucent zone between the acrylic cement and the bone.

This radiolucent zone may either become stable (at a width of approximately 1 to 1.5 mm) or, if prosthetic instability persists or the patient's activity level is excessive, the width of this radiolucent zone may progress. Histologically, such progression is accompanied by osteoclasis and loss of bone with replacement by a fibrous membrane. This process when progressive may result in eventual failure of the joint replacement because of grossly loose prosthetic components.

I believe that subsidence or settling of the femoral component (Fig. 22-7) is caused by progressive loosening. Histologic analysis of retrieved specimens reveals a mass of fibrous tissue between the acrylic within the femoral component and the bone. Thus far no evidence of massive necrosis of the femoral head has been observed. The deeper layers of the membranous "stump" contain numerous osteoclasts. These appearances resemble those seen in analysis of the fibrous membrane obtained from progressively widening radiolucent zones.

The assessment of loosening is primarily based on accurate radiologic evaluation. Routine followup roentgenograms at regular intervals are necessary, and every attempt should be made to ensure that the rotation and alignment of the roentgenograms is consistent. This is achieved when the x-ray beam is centered directly over the prosthetic joint. Good quality roentgenograms are necessary for an accurate determination as to whether progression of a radiolucent zone is occurring or not.

The majority of grossly loose prosthetic devices are symptomatic. When a progressive radiolucent zone occurs and is accompanied by increasing discomfort or pain, loosening should be suspected. This can be confirmed by aspiration arthrography and radioisotope scanning.

A rapidly progressing radiolucent zone is diagnostic of gross loosening or rapid bone destruction at the interface caused by fragmentation of acrylic cement. I believe that under these circumstances revision should be undertaken at the earliest possible opportunity to preserve the remaining bone stock.

Aspiration is undertaken with each arthrogram or as a separate procedure so that the possibility of infection is ruled out. In all cases of loosening the possibility of infection should be excluded.

The occurrence of loosening with prosthetic devices is in many cases attributable to inadequate cement techniques. We have advocated the use of methyl methacrylate in a liquid or low viscosity phase, combined with pressurizing techniques. Acetabular cement is introduced in a liquid phase by pressure injection of the cement into the fixation holes and then further pressurization of the cement into the cancellous bone with a silicone rubber pressurizing device. Fixation of the femoral device is similarly achieved by pressurization of the acrylic cement into the femoral canal using

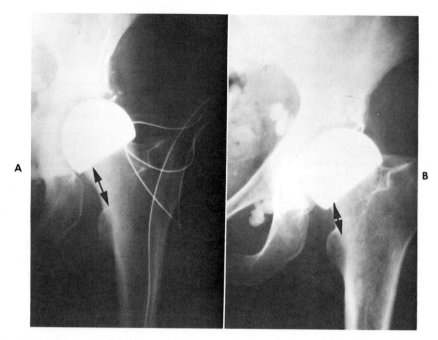

Fig. 22-7. A, Note the distance, *arrow,* between the lesser trochanter and the distal edge of the femoral component. **B,** This distance has narrowed greatly with the subsidence of the femoral component.

a balloon to contain the cement while it is forced into the cancellous bone.

Fixation is a function of the surface area exposed to the acrylic cement. Intrusion of the acrylic cement into the interstices of cancellous bone obviously increases the available surface area many times. The bond between acrylic cement and bone is a nonadhesive, interference fit and this is vastly improved by the use of pressurizing devices. I believe that by increasing the surface area of fixation greater prosthetic stability will be achieved.

Attention to these details has yielded interfaces that have a far better radiologic appearance with a reduced incidence of radiolucent zones. The long-term results of pressurization, however, are yet to be assessed, but it appears to be beneficial in the short term.

Containment of acetabular component. Containment of the acetabular component within the bony confines of the pelvis is essential to prevent loosening. If the resurfacing procedure is carried out for congenital hip dysplasia, careful preoperative planning is necessary. Pelvic bone stock should be assessed both with routine roentgeno-

grams and, in the majority of cases, with the help of a CT scan. This will indicate whether supplementary bone grafting will be necessary to cover the component. CT scanning and routine roentgenograms will also reveal the degree of femoral neck anteversion. This latter problem is encountered in many cases of congenital dysplasia and presents the potential for problems not encountered with conventional total hip replacement.

Excessive femoral neck anteversion. This problem is peculiar to resurfacing total hip replacement. With implantation of conventional hip replacement the femoral component can be placed in such a way as to correct the previously existing femoral neck anteversion. This is not possible with resurfacing procedures and should be taken into consideration with the preoperative planning.

If surface replacement is carried out in the face of excessive femoral neck anteversion, the risk of dislocation or loosening of the components is great. I therefore advise that if excessive femoral neck anteversion is present, consideration should be given to a derotation osteotomy of the femur.

This could be done either before or during the resurfacing procedure.

Invasive cyst formation. We have one patient, a female in her midthirties, who developed a painful surface replacement several months after surgery. All investigations at this time were non-contributory. Her pain and discomfort continued and she eventually underwent an aspiration arthrogram. The arthrogram indicated a large cystic defect within the femoral neck, which the lateral projection of the arthrogram was seen to fill approximately 40% of the anterior femoral neck. On the anteroposterior projection the cyst extended from the margin of the femoral component to approximately the intertrochanteric line.

This case was taken to the operating room with the intention of revision of the surface replacement to a conventional hip replacement. After dislocation of the hip joint, both surface replacement components were found to be stable. A window was made into the cyst and was subsequently curetted. A Wood's lamp indicated that a preoperatively administered tetracycline label had been taken up in all the bone surrounding the cyst. In view of the fact that both components were tight and the femoral head and neck appeared viable, it was decided to pack the lesion with cancellous bone. After meticulous curettage of the cyst, it was packed with cancellous bone and no revision was undertaken. Two years after surgery the patient remains asymptomatic and the cyst appears to be consolidating satisfactorily.

The histologic specimens obtained indicated that the cyst contained an invasive synovium strongly resembling villonodular synovitis. It is believed that this could have been debris-induced because abundant polyethylene debris particles could be demonstrated on polarized light microscopy.

ACKNOWLEDGMENTS

I would like to acknowledge all my co-workers in the Joint Replacement Unit at UCLA. These include Dr. Harlan Amstutz, Gerald Finerman, Andrea Cracchiolo III, and John Moreland.

I would also like to thank John Moreland for several of the illustrations. These were obtained during his sojourn as a joint replacement fellow with Mr. Michael Freeman, F.R.C.S., at the London Hospital. I would like to thank both these gentlemen for allowing me to include this material and, in particular, Mr. Michael Freeman for sharing with us some cautionary notes derived from his pioneering experiences.

REFERENCES

1. Conventry, M.B., and Scanlon, P.W.: The use of radiation to discourage ectopic bone. J. Bone Joint Surg. **63A:**201-208, 1981.
2. Freeman, M.A.R.: Symposium on surface replacement of the hip, American Academy of Orthopaedic Surgeons, Atlanta, Georgia, Feb. 10, 1980.
3. Hamblen, D.L., Harris, W.H., and Rottger, J.: Myositis ossificans as a complication of hip arthroplasty. J. Bone Joint Surg. **53B:**764, 1971.
4. Hedley, A.K., Clarke, I.C., Bloebaum, E.D., Moreland, J.R., Gruen, T.A.W., Coster, I., and Amstutz, H.C.: Viability and cement fixation of the femoral head on canine hip surface replacement. In the hip, St. Louis, 1979, The C.V. Mosby Co.
5. Markolf, K.L., and Amstutz, H.C.: Mechanical strength of the femur following resurfacing and conventional total hip replacement procedures, Clin. Orthop. **147:**170-180, 1980.
6. Whiteside, L.A., Ogata, K., Lesker, P., and Reynolds, F.C.: The acute effects of periosteal stripping and medullary reaming on regional bone blood flow, Clin. Orthop. **131:**266-272, March-April 1978.

SELECTED READINGS

Amstutz, H.C., and Clarke, I.C.: Total hip articular replacement by internal eccentric shells—the THARIES technique for surface replacement, Warsaw, Ind., 1979, Zimmer U.S.A.

Amstutz, H.C., Graff-Radford, A., Gruen, T.A., and Clarke, I.C.: THARIES surface replacements: a review of the first 100 cases, Clin. Orthop. **134:**87-101, 1978.

Capello, W.N., Ireland, P.H., Trammel, T.R., and Eicher, P.: Conservative total hip arthroplasty: a procedure to conserve bone stock—parts I and II, Clin. Orthop. **(134):**59-74, July-Aug. 1978.

Capello, W.H., Wilson, N.M., and Wellman, H.N.: Bone imaging: a means of evaluating hip surface replacement arthroplasty. In The Hip, St. Louis, 1980, The C.V. Mosby Co.

Chandler, H.P., Reineck, F.T., and Wixson, R.C.: A five-year review of THR's in patients under the age of 30 with emphasis on loosening, Orthop. Trans. **3(3):**303, 1979.

Charnley, J.: Tissue reactions to polytetrafluoroethylene, Lancet **1:**1379, 1963.

Clarke, I., Amstutz, H., Christie, J., and Graff-Radford, A.: The John Charnley Award paper: THARIES surface replacement arthroplasty for the arthritic hip: rebirth of an earlier concept? In The hip, St. Louis, 1977, The C.V. Mosby Co.

Freeman, M.A.R.: Total surface replacement arthroplasty, Clin. Orthop. **134:**2-4, 1978.

Freeman, M.A.R., Cameron, H.U., and Brown, G.C.: Cemented double cup arthroplasty of the hip: a five year experience with the ICLH prosthesis, Clin. Orthop. **134:**45-52, 1978.

Harris, W.H.: Treatment of traumatic arthritis of the hip by mould arthroplasty, J. Bone Joint Surg. **49A:**1484, 1967.

Harris, W.H.: Traumatic arthritis of the hip after dislocation and acetabular fractures: treatment by mould arthroplasty: an end-result study using a new method of result evaluation, J. Bone Joint Surg. **51A:**737-755, 1969.

Hedley, A.K., Clarke, I., Moreland, J., Coster, I., Gruen, T., Bloebaum, R. and Amstutz, H.C.: Durability of acrylic cement fixation of femoral head prostheses—a canine surface replacement model. (Submitted for publication, 1979.)

Sew Hoy, A.L., Hedley, A., Clarke, I., Gruen, T., Amstutz, H., Coster, I., and Moreland, J.R.: The acetabular cement-bone interface—a canine study, Clin. Orthop. **155:**231-243, 1980.

Wagner, H.: Surface replacement arthroplasty of the hip, Clin. Orthop. **134:**102-130, 1978.

Wagner, H.: Symposium on surface replacement of the hip. American Academy of Orthopaedic Surgeons, Atlanta, Georgia, Feb. 10, 1980.

Section VII

THE SPINE

Chapter 23

Spinal stability: evaluation and treatment

AUGUSTUS A. WHITE III, M.D., Dr. Med. Sc.
Boston, Massachusetts

MANOHAR M. PANJABI, Dr. Tech.
New Haven, Connecticut

IRA POSNER, M.D.
Boston, Massachusetts

W. THOMAS EDWARDS, M.S.
Boston, Massachusetts

WILSON C. HAYES, Ph.D.
Boston, Massachusetts

One of the challenging issues in orthopaedic surgery is represented by the following question: How do you determine when the injured spine is unstable? No one seems to have a clear and valid answer. Moreover, it is apparent that making such a crucial determination in the clinical situation is extremely difficult. In many instances, such a decision can very significantly affect patient care. Misjudgment of one type may result in death or major neurologic deficits. Misjudgment of another type may result in unnecessary surgery, again with death or other major complications. Evaluating a patient's condition erroneously can cause considerable needless inconvenience related to wearing complex encumbrances, such as Minerva casts or halo pelvic fixation devices. Correct judgment provides the patient with realization of the maximum recovery with an absolute minimum of risks and inconvenience. This chapter does not purport to provide physicians with ideal judgment and wisdom. It does, however, endeavor to present a systematic approach to the problem, based on current clinical and biomechanical knowledge.

DEFINITIONS

"Clinical instability" is defined as the loss of the ability of the spine under physiologic loads to maintain relationships between vertebrae in such a way that there is neither damage nor subsequent irritation to the spinal cord or nerve roots and, in addition, there is no development of incapacitating deformity or pain from structural changes.

This is the working definition. The complexity of the subject matter demands a few qualifiers. Physiologic loads are those that are incurred during normal activity of the particular patient being evaluated. Incapacitating deformity is defined as gross deformity that the patient finds intolerable. Incapacitating pain is defined as pain that cannot be controlled by nonnarcotic drugs. Clinical instability can occur from trauma, disease, surgery, or some combination of the three.

Unless the term "clinical instability" or "clinical stability" is used, we are not referring to the pre-

☐ Supported by National Institutes of Health Grant No. AM25601

ceding definition. Stability or instability alone is used when the term found in the literature is repeated and when other statements about it are reported. The term "instability" has rarely been defined in previous publications. Its connotation, in other works, occasionally overlaps to some extent, with the definition we have offered.

BACKGROUND AND ORGANIZATION

In the diagnosis of clinical instability in any region of the spine, several crucial factors are important. Anatomy is significant when it concerns space relationships between neural structures and potentially damaging structures. It is also important because various structures provide different magnitudes and types of forces that are helpful in preserving stability. Biomechanical studies and information on kinematics are presented whenever they are contributory. For each region of the spine, recommended methods of evaluation and management are discussed.

RADIOLOGIC INTERPRETATION

The major practical consideration in the determination of clinical instability is the evaluation of the patient's roentgenographs. A good deal of emphasis has been placed on roentgenographic measurements to determine abnormal displacements and the likelihood of encroachment upon neurologic structures. By adopting standard distances, more meaningful measurements may be made from roentgenographs. Roentgenographic examination is currently the only objective means of determining the relative positions of the vertebrae in a potentially unstable spine. Therefore it is important to give some consideration to the accurate interpretation of linear roentgenographic measurements.

Magnification of linear measurements. The parameters measured on roentgenographs are either linear, such as the distance between two points, or angular, such as the angle between two lines. The relative position of the roentgenographic source, the spine, and the film are the only factors that affect the magnification.

The formula that shows the dependency of magnification on source, object, and film positions is

$$M = \frac{100 \times D_2}{D_1 - D_2}\%$$

where D_1 is the distance between the roentgenographic source and the film, and D_2 is the distance of the object (spine) from the film.

Table 23-1. Percentage magnification of image associated with different spine-to-film distances

Source-to-film distance: 1.83 m (72 inches)

Spine-to-film distance, m (in)	0.15(6)	0.20(8)	0.25(10)	0.30(12)	0.36(14)
Magnification, %	9	12.5	16	20	24

(From White, A.A., III, and Panjabi, M.M.: Clinical biomechanics of the spine, Philadelphia, 1978, J.B. Lippincott Co.)

The most commonly used value for the distance D_2 is 1.83 m (72 inches). If the film is placed next to the shoulder, the object-to-film distance D_1 in a lateral roentgenogram is half the shoulder width. If one assumes 0.3 m (12 inches) for the "average" person, the magnification, using the above formula, is 20%.

This range of magnification is for the "average" person. However, there is considerable variation of shoulder widths among individuals. For a nominal value for D_1 of 1.83 m (72 inches), the magnification factors for different shoulder widths (D_2) can be calculated. The results are shown in Table 23-1.

There are several suggestions to help control this magnification problem. One is to use standard source–to–spine–to–film distances. The recommendation is to use 1.83 m (72 inches) from source to film, and 0.36 m (14 inches) as the spine-to-film distance. This gives a 24% magnification. Another is to measure the distances with each roentgenogram and calculate the magnification. Finally, we should begin to develop linear roentgenographic criteria that can be utilized as percentage of displacement that will eliminate the magnification problem. This advantage is already enjoyed in our angular measurements that are not affected by magnification.

MUSCLE FORCES

The role of the muscles in clinical stability remains obscure. Although an understanding would be useful, it is our view that the muscles offer a small amount of protection through splinting in the acute phases of injury. Furthermore, in the less acute situation and against the normal range of physiologic loading, the muscles do not play a significant role. For example, in polio patients with total paralysis of cervical muscles, there is no loss of clinical stability as long as the bony and ligamentous structures remain intact.[33] Based on such examples, we fell justified in our endeavor to analyze clinical instability without full knowledge of the exact role of the muscle forces exerted. The physician cannot rule out the possibility that in the acute phase, voluntary and reflex muscle activity in response to pain may be operative.

OCCIPITOATLANTAL JOINT

With the possible exception of the terminal coccygeal joint, the occipitoatlantal joint has received less attention than any of the articulations in the axial skeleton. This generalization seems to hold for anatomic as well as biomechanical and clinical studies.

Evaluation

Anatomy. The anatomic structures that provide stability for this articulation include the cup-shaped configuration of the occipitoatlantal joints and their capsules, along with the anterior and posterior atlanto-occipital membranes.

Additional anatomic stability is gained through the ligamentous connections between the occiput and the axis. This is achieved through the tectorial membrane, the alar ligaments, and the apical ligaments, which are of less mechanical significance.[18] We believe that, based on structural characteristics, the occipitoatlantal joint is relatively unstable, at least in the child. There may be some increase in stability in adult life because of a decrease in elasticity of the ligaments.

Biomechanics. Wiesel and Rothman have shown that the normal range of sagittal-plane translation in flexion-extension does not exceed 1 mm.[44] This measurement is made between the basion of the occiput and the tip of the odontoid. Hypermobility may be seen in association with a congenital legion of the C1-C2 and C3-C4. Based on our present evaluations of the anatomy of this point and the dangerous risks involved in its displacement, we suggest that any dislocation or subluxation be considered unstable. The finding of more than 5 mm between the tip of the dens and the basion of the occiput or more than 1 mm of translation in flexion-extension are important and useful criteria.

The presence of symptoms of weakness of the limbs with or without associated neck and occipital pain, provide additional indications of instability. The criteria are listed in Table 23-2 and the measurement is shown in Fig. 23-1.

Treatment

Treatment for clinical instability at this level consists of fusion from occiput to C2 with immobilization in a halo cast. The question will be

Table 23-2. Occiput-Cl instability

Dens (tip) to basion of occiput	4 to 5 mm
Flexion-extension translation	1 mm
Neurologic signs or symptoms	

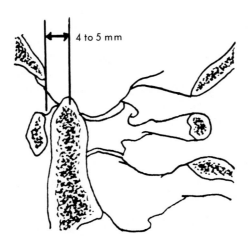

Fig. 23-1. Ocp-Cl lateral view. The distance between the basion of the occiput and the top of the dens is 4 to 5 mm. An increase of more than 1 mm in this distance with flexion-extension views is believed to indicate instability, if one assumes that the transverse ligament of the atlas is intact.

raised about the desirability of fusing to C3. This should not be necessary if the C1-C2 joint is normal. Although we may "feel" more secure extending to C3 a high price is paid, in that as much as 50% of axial rotation is lost.

ATLANTOAXIAL JOINT
Evaluation

Anatomy. The most important anatomic structures affecting the clinical stability of this articulation are transverse ligaments, dentate ligaments, and the apical and alar ligaments. The denate, alar, and apical ligaments are thought of as secondary stabilizers of the C1-C2 complex. The cruciate ligament, the most well developed portion of which is the transverse ligament, is the major stabilizing ligament of the atlanto-occipital membrane also play a role in the stabilization of these joints. The importance of the mutual dependence of these major ligaments, and an intact normal dens is apparent through a study of the anatomy of ligaments.[47] If the dens is hypoplastic, congenitally not intact, or fractured, the ligament cannot provide stability.

Biomechanics. The studies of horizontal translation showed that an anterior dislocation of C1 on C2 can occur with an insufficiency of the transverse ligament only. The alar ligaments and the tectorial membrane were not found to prevent dislocation after the transverse ligament was transected. If the alar ligaments happen to be short, as may be expected in persons over 25, they may possibly offer some restraint against gross dislocation. The tectorial membrane depends on an intact transverse ligament to offer resistance to anterior translation. The biomechanical studies by Fielding on the transverse ligament showed that although the structure was very weak in some subjects, when present it prevented more than 3 mm of anterior displacement of C1 on C2.[13] He also showed that the alar ligaments deform readily and are not capable of preventing additional displacement under loads that would rupture the transverse ligament.

Clinical considerations

Comminuted fracture of ring of C1 (Jefferson fracture). On the open-mouth view of the odontoid, with the head in neutral rotation, the normal roentgenograph does not show any overhang of the lateral masses of C1 in relation to the lateral border of the body of the second cervical verebra.

Table 23-3. Subluxations and dislocations of C1-C2

Translatory
Bilateral anterior
Bilateral posterior
Rotatory
Unilateral anterior
Unilateral posterior
Unilateral combined anterior and posterior

However, with a Jefferson fracture there is overhang on both sides. If the total overhand from the two sides is as great as 7 mm, there is presumably also a rupture of the transverse ligament. When these conditions are present, there is clinical instability.[39]

Subluxations and dislocations at atlantoaxial joint. Based on our review of the literature and our own analysis and evaluation, we submit the following five patterns of abnormal displacement at the C1-C2 joint. Two of the patterns are primarily translatory, and the other three are mainly rotatory (Table 23-3).

A summary of the clinical evaluation of these entities is given in Table 23-4. The criteria for evaluation of clinical instability are given in Table 23-5.

Treatment

Treatment of C1-C2 instability should be by fusion of C1-C2. One can do this by utilizing the Brook method or one of its modifications 9, 20 or by employing the Gallie technique or one of its modifications. In some instances where there is infected, hypoplastic, avascular, or absent posterior ring of C1, the surgeon may elect to fuse the occiput to C2 or consider one of the anterior C1-C2 procedures such as that described by Barbour[2] or Fang.[12] In general, we recommend the halo apparatus for postoperative fixation.

LOWER CERVICAL SPINE
Evaluation

Anatomy. The anatomy of the lower cervical spine of importance to clinical stability is depicted in Fig. 23-2. Going from front to back, we note that the most important anterior structure is the intact anulus fibrosus. Its strong attachments to the vertebral bodies by Sharpey's fibers embedded in the bone is a very important source of stability. Next, the posterior longitudinal ligament is a well-developed structure that provides considerable

Table 23-4. Summary of C1-C2 subluxations and dislocations

Type	Causes	Physical findings	Radiologic studies	Clinical stability	Treatment
I Bilateral anterior	Dysplastic dens, trauma, infection +z translation *(forward)*	Neutral or cock robin position of head	Lateral of C1, CT scan → anterior displacement of C1 on C2	Anterior displacement of 3 mm, neurologic deficit—clinically unstable	Fusion or trial of conservative therapy
II Bilateral posterior (very rare)	Fractured, absent, or destroyed dens −z translation *(backward)*	Patient may hold head in hands	Lateral of C1, CT scan → posterior displacement of C1 on C2	Clinically unstable	Fuse C1-C2
III Unilateral anterior (most common)	Arthritic conditions and infections ±y axis rotation Instantaneous axes of rotation at opposite joint *(axial rotation)*	Cock robin position of head; difficulty in rotating head away from direction in which it faces; not difficult to move farther in that direction; anterior tubercle of C1 may be shown to be displaced laterally by palpation of posterior pharynx	Lateral of C1, CT scan → anterior displacement of C1 on C2 AP open-mouth laminagrams, C1-C2 → lateral masses in different planes Ciné or several roentgenograms of axial rotation → no motion of C1 or C2	With no neurologic deficit, these are probably stable situations	Trial of reduction and conservative treatment; if symptoms require it, fuse C1-C2
IV Unilateral posterior (rare)	Usually associated with a deformed or fractured dens ±y axis rotation Instantaneous axes of rotation at opposite sides *(axial rotation)*	Cock robin position of head	Lateral of C1, CT scan → *no* anterior displacement of C1 on C1 AP open-mouth laminagrams, C1-C2 → lateral masses in different positions. Ciné or serial roentgenograms of axial rotation → no motion of C1 or C2	With no neurologic deficit, these are probably stable situations	Attempt reduction, and if symptoms require it, fuse C1-C2

Continued.

Table 23-4. Summary of C1-C2 subluxations and dislocations—cont'd

Type	Causes	Physical findings	Radiologic studies	Clinical stability	Treatment
V Unilateral combined (anterior and posterior)	Trauma ±y axis rotation Instantaneous axes of rotation at dens *(axial rotation)*	Cock robin position of head	Lateral of C1, CT scan → *no* anterior displacement of C1 on C2 AP open-mouth laminagrams, C1-C2 → lateral masses in different positions Ciné or several roentgenograms of axial rotation → no motion of C1 or C2	If no neurologic deficit, it may be clinically stable	Trial of reduction and conservative treatment; if not satisfactory, fuse C1-C2

Table 23-5. C1-C2 instability criteria

Spence's more than 7 mm total
Ring* (C1) ↔ Odontoid space more than 3 mm
Avulsed transverse ligament
Neurologic deficit

*At 3 to 5 mm displacement, transverse ligament is out, alar ligaments are intact. At more than 5 mm displacement, transverse and alar ligaments are out. (Modified from Fielding, J.W., et al.: Tears of the transverse ligament of the atlas: a clinical biomechanical study, J. Bone Joint Surg. **56A:**1683, 1974.)

stability. Regarding the posterior elements, the joint capsules and articulations are the most important source of stability. The yellow ligament is a well-developed structure that, although elastic, in the physiologic range, it provides some stability at the extremes of this range.

Biomechanics. Experiments have been carried out on cervical spine segments in high humidity chambers using physiologic loads to simulate flexion and extension. The experimental arrangement is shown in Fig. 23-3. The ligaments were cut in sequence from posterior to anterior in some motion segments and from anterior to posterior in others. The failure point was defined as the point at which the upper vertebra suddenly rotated 90 degrees or was displaced across the experimental table. The anterior elements were defined as the posterior longitudinal ligament and all structures anterior to it. The posterior elements were defined as all structures behind the posterior longitudinal ligament (Fig. 23-2). Based on these studies, we suggested that if a motion segment has all its anterior elements plus one additional structure, or all its posterior elements plus one additional structure, it will probably remain stable under physiologic loads. To provide some clinical margin of safety, we suggest that any motion segment in which all the anterior elements or all the posterior elements are either destroyed or are unable to function should be considered potentially unstable. Therefore these studies show that the important anatomic structures for maintaining clinical stability are either all the anterior elements plus one posterior, or all the posterior elements plus one anterior.

Clinical considerations

There are a number of important clinical studies that have considerable bearing on the analysis of clinical stability of the lower cervical spine. These studies are reviewed in more detail elsewhere. We shall report a few highlights here. The overall incidence of dislocations from non–surgically treated unstable cervical spine fractures is about 10%. Although there are exceptions, in general there is some correlation between neurologic deficit and the radiographic appearance of the spine after trauma. Bursting fractures are highly correlated with spinal cord injury. Usually, if the

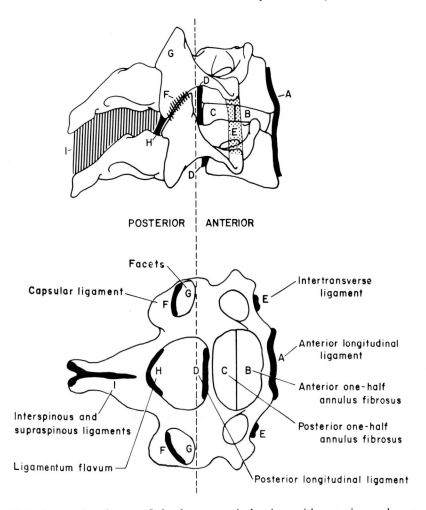

POSTERIOR | ANTERIOR

Facets

Capsular ligament

Intertransverse ligament

Anterior longitudinal ligament

Anterior one-half annulus fibrosus

Posterior one-half annulus fibrosus

Interspinous and supraspinous ligaments

Ligamentum flavum

Posterior longitudinal ligament

Fig. 23-2. Anatomic scheme of the lower cervical spine, with anterior and posterior elements being indicated. (From White, A.A., Southwick, W.O., and Panjabi, M.M.: Spine **1**:15, 1976.)

trauma is severe enough to cause a neurologic deficit, the structures of the spine have generally be altered enough such that they are unstable. Unilateral facet dislocations tend to be stable injuries and bilateral facet dislocations are unstable injuries. Multiple-level laminectomy with or without facetectomy may lead to instability in the lower cervical spine. When facetectomy has been performed or when laminectomy has been combined with discectomy, the probability is even greater.

Checklist evaluation. Although we believe that the following checklist evaluation system will allow the clinician to make the correct diagnosis, we would like to give warning about a very specific clinical instability complex that must be looked for. This type of instability was first pointed out to one of us (A.A.W.) by McSweeny of Oswestry,

England, who has subsequently published several cases.[43]

There is a history of a severe flexion injury in an athlete with or with out transient tetraparesis or dysesthesias in the limbs. X-rays show slight fanning or widening of the spinous processes and the posterior elements. There is subtle evidence of a compression fracture of the vertebral body of the lower vertebra. The intervertebral disc space at this same level is a bit narrowed and there is loss of normal cervical lordosis. There will most probably be a positive stretch test. The *stretch test* is described in Table 23-7.

One should consider this to be an unstable injury until proved otherwise. We think there should be a local posterior fusion at the interspace in question. An alternative treatment would be to protect the patient with an appropriate orthosis

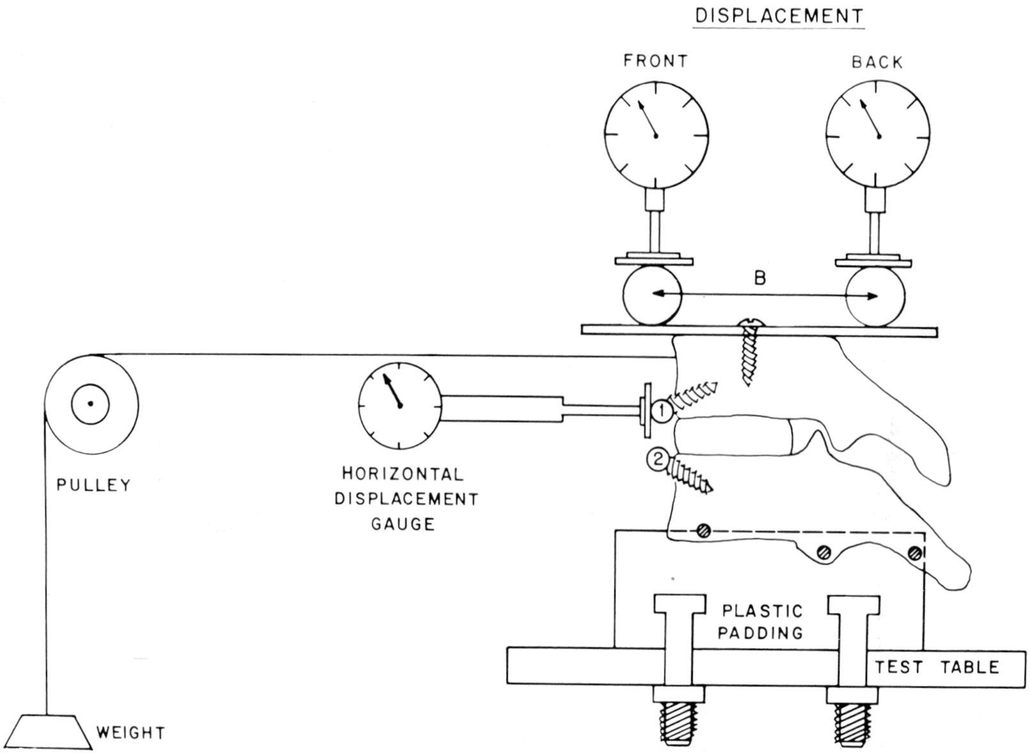

Fig. 23-3. Experimental setup to show motion segment on test stand. The vertical displacement of the balls at either end of line *B* measures angular displacement. This is the setup for testing flexion. When extension is tested, the motion segment is rotated 180 degrees on the vertical *(y)* axis. (From White, A.A., Johnson, R.M., Panjabi, M.M., and Southwick, W.O.: Clin. Orthop. **120:**85, 1975.)

and reevaluate according to the schedule outlined in Table 23-7.

A standard checklist for the diagnosis of clinical instability in the lower cervical spine is presented in Table 23-6. The rationale for the checklist is to ensure that all relevent considerations are taken into account, enhance reproducibility of results, and offer a basis for standard objective criteria for prospective clinical studies. The entities are weighted according to our best jugement about their relative importance. The list therefore is designed to ensure some checks and balances. There is the possibility of utilizing a partial weighting where a given criterion may be uncertain. The following paragraphs provide cogent information about the use of the checklist.

The patient is evaluated, and each item that applies is checked. If the numbers assigned to the checked items total five or more, the spine should be considered clinically unstable. It is not assumed that the information available on all patients will provide a definitive answer for each item on the list. It is recommended that when the evaluation of a given element leads the clinician to a borderline decision that cannot be resolved, the value for that entity should be divided by two and added to the other points.

The evaluation of the first two entities, that is, the status of the anterior and the posterior elements, is based on clinical history, evaluation of roentgenograms, and interpretation of flexion extension films, or the stretch test, if results are available. A history of disk removal does not necessarily indicate that all the anterior elements are destroyed, but the situation may be suspect, since there is a possibility of disruption and weakening of the posterior longitudinal ligament from either surgery or degenerative disease. A separation of the vertebral end plate after an extension injury, as described by Taylor,[41] or a transverse fracture

Table 23-6. Checklist for diagnosis of clinical instability in lower cervical spine

Elements	Point value	Individual clinical value
Anterior elements destroyed or unable to function	2	
Posterior elements destroyed or unable to function	2	
Relative sagittal-plane translation > 3.5 mm	2	
Relative sagittal-plane rotation > 11 degrees	2	
Positive stretch test	2	
Cord damage	2	
Root damage	1	
Abnormal disk narrowing	1	
Dangerous loading anticipated	1	

Total of 5 or more = unstable

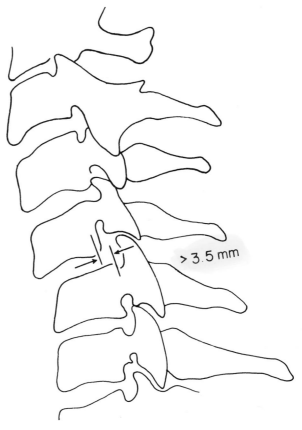

Fig. 23-4. The method of measuring translatory displacement. A point at the posteroinferior angle of the lateral projection of the vertebral body above the interspace in question is marked. A point at the posterosuperior angle of the projection of the vertebral body is also marked. The distance between the two in the sagittal plane is measured, *arrows.* A distance of 3.5 mm or greater is suggestive of clinical stability. (This distance is to be measured on a lateral roentgenogram. It is computed from experimentally obtained value of 2.7 mm and an assumed radiographic magnification of 30%.) (From White, A.A., Johnson, R.M., Panjabi, M.M., and Southwick, W.O.: Clin. Orthop. **120**:85, 1975.)

of the vertebral body, as described by Marar,[26] may result in either the destruction of, or the loss of the ability of, the anterior elements to function. Although the study by Beatson did not mention the yellow ligament, it showed that with bilateral facet dislocations virtually all the anterior elements and all the posterior elements may be destroyed.[4]

With regard to posterior elements, it is wise to assume that bilateral pedicle fractures or bilateral facet and lamina fractures have negated all functional supports provided by the posterior elements.

Roentgenographic measurements. The measurement of translation is shown in Fig. 23-4. This method takes into account variations in magnifications and should be useful when there is a tube-to-film distance of 1.83 m (72 inches).

The roentgenographic interpretation in general, especially for sagittal-plane translation, is decidedly different in children up to at least 7 years of age. It is risky to interpret roentgenograms of patients in this age group without a knowledge of

some of the normal findings that may appear to be pathologic to the uninitiated.

There is no magnification problem in measuring rotation. Note that 11 degrees of rotation means 11 degrees greater than the amount of rotation at the motion segment above or below the segment in question. This standard of comparison takes into account the normal rotation between motion segments. The angles between these vertebral bodies are dictated largely by the existing

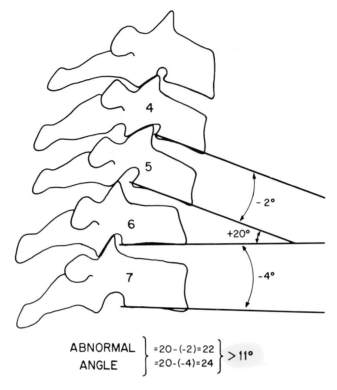

ABNORMAL ANGLE $\Big\}$ $\begin{array}{l} =20-(-2)=22 \\ =20-(-4)=24 \end{array}$ $\Big\}$ $> 11°$

Fig. 23-5. The angulation between C5 and C6 is 20 degrees, which is more than 11 degrees greater than that at either adjacent interspace. The angle at C4 and C5 measures −2 degrees, and the one at C6 and C7 measure −4 degrees. The finding of abnormal angulation is based on a comparison of the interspace in question with either adjacent interspace. This is to allow for the angulation that is present because of the normal lordosis of the cervical spine. We interpret a difference of 11 degrees or greater than that of either adjacent interspace as evidence of clinical instability. (From White, A.A., Johnson, R.M., Panjabi, M.M., and Southwick, W.O.: Clin. Orthop. **120**:85, 1975.)

lordosis and muscle spasm. Angular measurements are shown in Fig. 23-5. They are significant when measured on either flexion-extension or resting lateral roentgenograms. A discussion of roentgenographic standardization and analysis has already been presented.

Stretch test. The validity of the concept has been supported by laboratory studies and clinical observations.[32,46,47] The basic idea of the test is to measure the displacement patterns of the test spine under carefully controlled conditions and to identify any abnormalities in these patterns, which may be indicative of ruptured ligaments. Biomechanically the spinal cord can tolerate considerable displacement in the axial direction. Thus, in the acute clinical situation, we believe that a test employing displacement in the axial direction is safer than the less physiologic and potentially hazardous horizontal-plane displacement.

Case report

L.C. is a 23-year-old female who was involved in an automobile accident. She was unconscious for several minutes after the accident. When awake, she had neck and arm pain. However, the neurologic examination was within normal limits. Fig. 23-6 shows a subluxation of C4 on C5. Fig. 23-7 is a laminagram taken with only 17 pounds of axial traction. When the amount of axial displacement was noted, the traction was reduced. The patient's neurologic status remained normal.

This case report illustrates several important points. The diagnostic value of axially directed traction to establish the presence of ligament disruption is demonstrated. Traction revealed that there was total disruption of all the anterior and posterior ligaments, which rendered the spine grossly unstable. The roentgenogram in Fig. 23-7 exhibits dramatically the observations of Brieg, who found that the cord can withstand considerable axial displacement without structural damage and neurologic deficit.[8] The case report also shows the

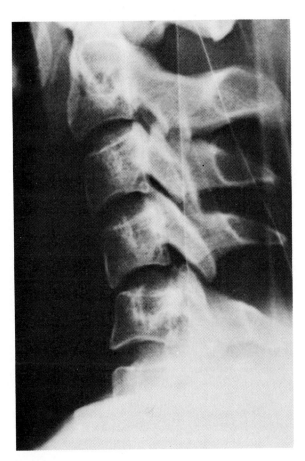

Fig. 23-6. Roentgenogram of a patient with disruption of all ligaments between C5 and C6. The spine in the resting position. (From White, A.A., III, and Panjabi, M.M.: Clinical biomechanics of the spine, Philadelphia, 1978, J.B. Lippincott Co.)

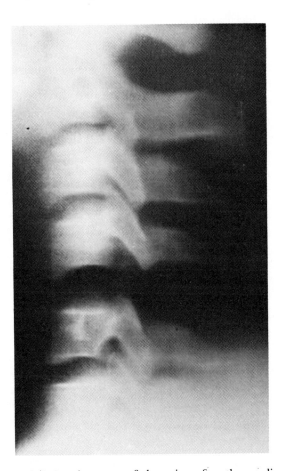

Østretch test

Fig. 23-7. Laminagram of the spine after the application of 17 pounds of traction. There was no neurologic damage or irritation. (From White, A.A., III, and Panjabi, M.M.: Clinical biomechanics of the spine, Philadelphia, 1978, J.B. Lippincott Co.)

necessity of careful application of axial traction with close monitoring. The research background for this particular test is described in detail elsewhere. Here in Table 23-7 we will present the procedures and precautions. Fig. 23-8 shows the method. The important points are (1) have a physician in attendance, (2) monitor the neurologic status with the patient awake, and (3) study each film before adding additional weight.

Cord or nerve-root damage. Clinical evidence of cord damage indicates probable spinal instability, as discussed previously. Evidence of root involvement is, however, a less strong indicator of clinical instability. For example, a unilateral facet dislocation may cause enough foraminal encroachment to result in root symptoms but not enough ligamentous damage to render the motion segment unstable.

Disk space narrowing. Bailey remarked, and we have observed, that in the traumatized spine there

may be a narrowing of the disk space at the level of the damaged functional spinal unit.[1] We submit that in a young person where the other disk are normal, this finding is suggestive of disruption of the anulus fibrosus and of possible instability.

The final consideration involves the important individual variation in physiologic load requirements, especially with regard to differences in habitual activities. The clinician employs judgment in an attempt to anticipate the magnitude of loads that the particular patient's spine is expected to sustain after injury. Easy examples include an interior lineman on a professional football team and a sedentary retired seamstress.

Anticipating dangerous loads can be especially helpful when other available criteria are inconclusive. In situations where a particular life style obviously exposes the patient to large physiologic loading, the desirability of surgical fusion is

Table 23-7. Procedure for stretch test to evaluate clinical stability in lower cervical spine*

1. It is recommended that the test be done under the supervision of an attending physician.
2. Traction is applied through secure skeletal fixation or a head halter. If the latter is used, a small portion of gauze sponge between the molars improves comfort.
3. A roller is placed under the patient's head to reduce frictional forces.
4. Place the film a standard distance from the patient's neck. The tube-film distance is 1.82 m (72 inches).
5. Take an initial lateral roentgenogram.
6. Add weight up to 15 pounds. If initial weight was 15 pounds, omit this step.
7. Increase traction by 10-pound increments. Take a lateral film and measure it as shown.
8. Continue by repeating step 7 until either one third of body weight or 65 pounds are reached.
9. After each additional weight application, the patient is checked for any change in neurologic status. The test is stopped and *considered positive* should this occur. The roentgenograms are developed and read after each weight increment. Any abnormal separation of the anterior or posterior elements of the vertebrae is the typical indication of a positive test. There should be at least 5 minutes between incremental weight applications; this will allow for the developing of the film, necessary neurologic checks, and creep of the viscoelastic structures involved.

*The test is unnecessary and contraindicated in an obviously unstable spine.

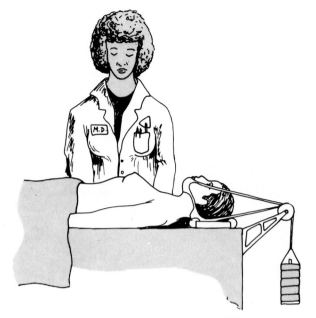

Fig. 23-8. Diagrammatic synopsis of stretch test. A physician who is knowledgeable about the test is in attendance. The neurologic status is monitored by following signs and symptoms. Incremental loads up to 33% of body weight or 65 pounds are applied. Each lateral roentgenogram is checked before augmentation of the axial load. Note the neurologic hammer to symbolize a neurologic exam and the roller platform bed under the head to reduce friction. Despite the cartoonlike presentation, this is a serious test. (From White, A.A., III, and Panjabi, M.M.: Clinical biomechanics of the spine, Philadelphia, 1978, J.B. Lippincott Co.)

greatly increased. The strength of ligamentous healing in the human spine is not known. It is reasonable to assume that arthrodesis provides better stability than healed ligaments do. The fusion may be thought of as protection against large anticipated loads. An active patient would be better off with a fusion rather than depending on ligamentous healing to withstand the anticipated loads.

Treatment

A schematic organization of the management of clinical instability is presented in Fig. 23-9.

Starting with patients with cervical spine trauma, note that initial treatment consists of bed rest for 1 to 7 days and skeletal traction if there is evidence of severe injury. Patients with spinal cord involvement, with and without fractures or fracture dislocations, are considered to have major injuries. The patients without evidence of neurologic deficit who have either no fracture or only a minor compression fracture, without evidence of other damage, may be treated with head-halter traction. Minor injuries, such as strains, sprains, and muscle pulls, may be treated for symptoms and observed with subsequent roentgenographic examinations as indicated.

During the first week of traction, patients are given a thorough clinical evaluation and whatever supportive care is required. After the patient is stabilized physiologically and evaluated for decompression, closed reduction with traction may be attempted, and, if necessary, the various tests and maneuvers to rule out clinical instability may be performed.

It would be worthwhile to have a checklist to make a determination about decompression; however, at present, only the previously presented guidelines are available. Appropriate decompressions are carried out where indicated, and the pa-

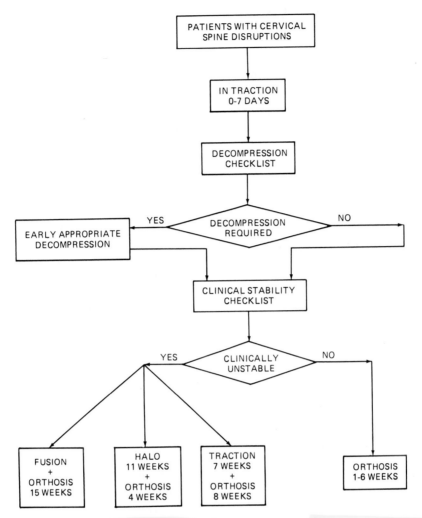

Fig. 23-9. Recommended flow diagram for the management of patients with disruptions of the lower cervical spine. (From White, A.A., III, and Panjabi, M.M.: Clinical biomechanics of the spine, Philadelphia, 1978, J.B. Lippincott Co.)

tient is then evaluated for clinical stability by use of the checklist provided. If the decompression itself renders the spine clinically unstable, reconstruction, and fusion may be carried out at the time of decompression.

All patients who are diagnosed as clinically stable can be treated with some modification of the following regimen. The assumption is that in 3 to 6 weeks, these patients will be comfortable and whatever damage they sustained will be healing. A four-poster cervical collar with a thoracic attachment is desirable for adequate support and an effective intermediate range of control of movement. Such a device, along with the intrinsic stability of the spine, should be adequate to protect the patient from neurologic damage and allow in-

jured structures to heal. It is possible that clinical instability may develop at a later time.

We have recommended in Table 23-8 a basic schedule for follow-up of patients treated for problems of clinical instability in all regions of the spine. This schedule should allow cases of delayed instability to be recognized and treated before any complications occur. The visits are primarily for radiologic and neurologic evaluation. The frequency of the schedule is altered according to the individual patient's progress and prognosis.

Treatment of clinically unstable conditions. The three alternatives suggested provide clinical stability in the majority of patients. There is no convincing evidence in the literature that any of the three approaches is superior. The considera-

Table 23-8. Suggested follow-up schedule for management of clinically stable and unstable spine problems

1. Schedule begins after the termination of initial treatment, surgical or nonsurgical, that is, after removal of brace, cast, completion of bed rest, and initial physical therapy.
2. Patient is to be seen approximately
   - 3 weeks
   - 6 weeks
   - 3 months
   - 6 months
   - 1 year

   after termination of initial treatment.
3. If the appropriate clinical evaluation is carried out on this time schedule, all early and late complications should be recognized in time for treatment. Whenever possible, techniques should be standardized for purposes of comparison.

tions are complex and have not been thoroughly studied. A successful fusion constitutes the strongest reconstruction for the unstable motion segment. However, it carries all the risks of spinal surgery in a seriously ill patient. Munro considered the risks to be significant.[28]

More recently, the halo apparatus has been used in the treatment of spinal trauma, with or without fusion.[23] This apparatus has an important place in the therapeutic armamentarium for this disease. The use of the halo apparatus (a halo attached to an outrigger stabilized on the body) may serve effectively as the primary treatment for some of these injuries. This method has promise and merits careful study in the management of clinical instability in the lower cervical spine.

The halo apparatus offers the best immobilization for the facilitation of ligamentous healing, and it may shorten hospitalization for the patient who has no major neurologic deficit. However, there has been no extensive experience with it as a primary treatment for clinical instability. The halo apparatus has its own complications. In addition, there is the unanswered question of whether ligamentous healing in any given case of spinal trauma is of satisfactory strength to withstand physiologic loads. The use of skeletal traction for a total of 7 weeks, followed by an orthosis of intermediate control for 8 weeks, is probably a more conservative approach and can be expected to be effective. We recommend 7 weeks of traction because Brav and colleagues showed that pa-

tients treated for 6 weeks or more had a redislocation rate of only 2.3%.[7]

All these regimens include careful clinical follow-up evaluations. Lateral views of flexion-extension films are helpful for recognizing failed treatment or delayed or progressive subluxation or deformity. There are, of course, other regimens. Some surgeons prefer early or late Minerva casts. We believe that the halo apparatus gives better immobilization and that in most cases after 8 weeks of healing an orthosis of intermediate control is all that is required.

Each surgeon must choose from the various alternatives. The ideal would be to have some well-controlled prospective clinical studies comparing the effectiveness of the different regimens. It would, of course, be essential to evaluate the various treatment levels in terms of effect on clinical stability. In addition, patient attitude, cost benefits, complications, rehabilitation, nursing care, and hospitalization time are all crucial variables to be evaluated before the best treatment regimen can be determined.

Based on our experience with successful surgical fusions for unstable spines, we recommend this procedure.

THORACIC AND THORACOLUMBAR SPINE

There are several unique considerations in the evaluation of clinical stability in the thoracic and thoracolumbar spine. This region of the spine is mechanically stiffer and less mobile than any of the other regions. There is less free space and a more precarious blood supply for the spinal cord in this region of the spine. It is well stabilized by the articulations and the rib-cage structure.

Evaluation

Anatomy. With the wedged configuration of the disks and the vertebra in the thoracic spine there is a normal kyphosis that makes this region of the spine relatively more unstable in flexion. The anatomy of this region that is important to clinical stability is shown in Figs. 23-10 and 23-11.

The anterior longitudinal ligament is a distinct well-developed structure in this region of the spine. The anulus fibrosus and the posterior longitudinal ligaments also play an important role in stabilizing the thoracic spine. The attachments of the ribs to adjacent vertebral bodies through the costotransverse and radiate ligaments also provide

Fig. 23-10. Diagram of the major ligament involved in the thoracic spine. Ligaments are numbered according to the order in which they were cut. *Anterior elements: 1,* anterior longitudinal ligament; *2,* anterior half of the anulus fibrosus; *3,* radiate and costovertebral ligaments; *4,* posterior half of the anulus fibrosus; *5,* posterior longitudinal ligament, *Posterior elements: 6,* costotransverse and intertransverse ligaments; *7,* capsular ligaments; *8,* facet articulation; *9,* ligamentum flavum; *10,* supraspinous and interspinous ligaments. (From White A.A., III, and Panjabi, M.M.: Clinical biomechanics of the spine, Philadelphia, 1978, J.B. Lippincott Co.)

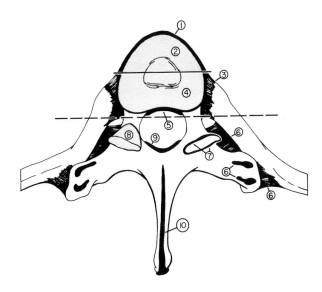

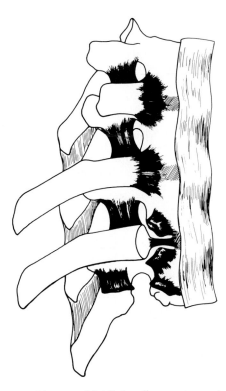

Fig. 23-11. Diagram highlights ligamentous structures in the costovertebral articulation that make some contribution to the clinical stability of the thoracic spine. Note the radiate ligaments attaching to the head of the rib and both adjacent vertebral bodies. There are also the costotransverse ligaments, which may offer some secondary stability. (From White, A.A., III, and Panjabi, M.M.: Clinical biomechanics of the spine, Philadelphia, 1978, J.B. Lippincott Co.)

important stabilizing influences on this region of the spine.

As regards the posterior ligaments, the facet joints and their capsules provide the major posterior stabilizing structures. The yellow ligament is thick, well developed, and also a contributor to posterior stability. The supraspinous and interspinous ligaments probably play a less vital role in the stability.

Biomechanics. In addition to the previously mentioned anatomic factor of the attachment of the ribs to the adjacent vertebrae, there is another factor. This has to do with the inertia produced by the rib cage. This results in added resistance or increaed stiffness to flexion extension, lateral bending, and axial rotation.

From a series of biomechanical studies of the thoracic spine similar to those done in the cervical region it was possible to make some observations that are helpful in the evaluation of clinical stability. The results are as follows. With all posterior elements cut, the segment remains stable in flexion until the costovertebral articulation is destroyed; all anterior ligaments plus at least one posterior component must be destroyed to cause failure; with the motion segment loaded to simulate extension, stability can be maintained with just the anterior longitudinal ligament intact; with the motion segment loaded to simulate flexion, stability can be maintained with just the posterior longitudinal ligament and the other anterior elements intact. The maximum physiologic sagittal-plan translation was 2.5 mm, and the maximum sagittal plane rotation was 5 degrees.[17,48]

Clinical considerations

A detailed review of the clinical literature is published elsewhere.[47] To follow is a synopsis of some of the most cogent material. Bedbrook and Edibaum indicated that if the ititial observed displacement was one half the anteroposterior diameter of the vertebral body the situation was unstable.[5] Other authors reported that wedge-shaped fractures with the interspinous ligament disrupted were unstable.[30] Holdsworth emphasized the gross instability of rotational fracture dislocations of the thoracolumbar juncture.[19] Roberts and Curtiss offered a classification based on evaluation of the lateral roentgenogram.[37]

These classifications may be summarized in the following manner. Anterior wedge, lateral wedge, and bursting compression fractures are generally stable unless the posterior interspinous ligaments are destroyed. The bursting fracture is likely to undergo spontaneous fusion. Dislocations and fracture dislocations are generally considered unstable, especially the classical fracture dislocation of Holdsworth.

Other clinical studies by Riggins and others show a distinct tendency for structural damage of the traumatized thoracic spine to be associated with neurologic deficits.[35] It is also important to point out that kyphotic deformities of 30 degrees or more were not associated with deterioration of neurologic function.[25]

In the thoracic and thoracolumbar spine we generally assume that most injuries that produce neurologic deficits are unstable. The rationale for such an assumption is as follows. If there is enough deformation at the time of injury to produce neural damage, there must also be sufficient structural damage to the vertebral column to render it clinically unstable. In the majority of cases this is true. However, there can be a neurologic deficit in situations in which there is either no structural damage or no recognizable damage.[15,26] The canal size in the thoracic region is relatively smaller in relation to the spinal cord size than that in other regions. Therefore deformation of ligaments within the elastic range can allow enough displacement to deliver a detrimental impact to the neural structures. Although the majority of cases with neural deficit in the thoracolumbar spine are clinically unstable, it is important to

keep in mind the possibility of exceptions to the rule, as well as the presence of unrecognized structural damage.

Checklist. A checklist for the evaluation of clinical instability in the thoracic and thoracolumbar spine is presented in Table 23-9. The rationale for this checklist is the same as was previously described for the cervical spine.

We suggest that injuries in this region be evaluated by use of laminagrams in the anteroposterior and lateral planes, in addition to the regular anteroposterior and lateral roentgenograms. Here it is appropriate to emphasize the importance of, and the difficulty in, obtaining a good lateral roentgenogram of the C6-T1 area of the spine when one is evaluating a patient with spinal trauma. This issue has been well presented by Lauritzen, who recommends the use of lateral tomograms.[24] The swimmer's view can also provide a satisfactory lateral roentgenogram of this region.

It is desirable to review some information that will be helpful in utilization of the checklist. In the evaluation of the status of the anterior elements, special attention should be paid to the articula-

Table 23-9. Checklist for diagnosis of clinical instability in thoracic and thoracolumbar spine

Elements	Point value	Individual clinical value
Anterior elements destroyed or unable to function	2	
Posterior elements destroyed or unable to function	2	
Relative sagittal-plane translation > 2.5 mm	2	
Relative sagittal-plane rotation > 5 degrees	2	
Spinal cord or cauda equina damage	2	
Disruption of costovertebral articulations	1	
Dangerous loading anticipated	2	

Total of 5 or more = unstable

tions of the ribs and vertebral bodies in a lamina-graphic studies. These articulations, through the linkages of vertebra, ligaments, and rib, provide considerable stability to the motion segments.

Key factors in making this determination are the physical examination and the evaluation of the position of the spinous processes on the anteroposterior roentgenogram. When there is extensive destruction of the posterior elements, there may be localized swelling, tenderness, edema, and a palpable defect under the skin. Wide separation of the spinous processes may be discernible. The anteroposterior roentgenogram shows wide separation of the spinous processes at the level involved. If there is a Holdsworth rotary dislocation, there will be an offset of the spinous processes, showing axial rotation at the level of the injury. More subtle fractures, subluxations, and dislocations of the posterior elements are seen on the usual lateral films or laminagrams.

A relative sagittal-plane translation of greater than 2.5 mm is highly suggestive of thoracic-spine clinical instability. A relative sagittal-plane rotation of more than 5 degrees is strongly indicative of clinical instability in the thoracic spine.

One might consider giving spinal cord damage a full 5 points on this checklist. However, there are situations in which there is no recognizable stjuctural damage and yet there is a neurologic deficit. Some of these may be overlooked structural lesions, but it is also possible to have cord damage with a truly intact column. This, of course, would not be a clinically unstable situation. Thus, spinal cord damage is given a high value, but in such a manner that some other evidence of instability must also be present in order to make the diagnosis. Neural damage is also assigned a high value because in the thoracic region, the space occupied by the cord is such that there is minimal opportunity for any abnormal displacement to occur without damaging the neural structures. Therefore, once the structural integrity has been altered enough to cause damage, the risk of subsequent damage is very high, and the patient should be protected against this.

Concerning the magnitude of future stress, the evaluation is the same as that recommended in the evaluation of the cervical spine. However, it is even more crucial in this region. The forces applied to this region are likely to be greater because the superincumbent weight is greater and the moment arms are greater.

Treatment

The flow chart given in Fig. 23-12 may be helpful as an outline of the major considerations in managing patients with disruption of the thoracic and thoracolumbar spine.

The patients may be placed in bed or on a turning frame. The latter should be used if there is significant neurologic deficit. The patient is given the necessary supportive therapy and thoroughly evaluated through various neurologic and roentgenographic examinations and base-line laboratory studies. Within the first 48 hours, a decision about the indications for operative decompression is made and carried out as soon as the patient's condition permits. (The evidence suggests that laminectomies should rarely be performed.) Decompression, which is preferably carried out anteriorly, is indicated when there is an incomplete neurologic deficit, with roentgenographic evidence of spinal cord compression. The patient, with or without decompression, is then evaluated according to the clinical stability checklist.

Treatment of clinically stable condition. Patients who have been evaluated and determined to be clinically stable are treated with 1 to 6 weeks of bed rest.[30] After termination of bed rest, they are then followed by roentgenographic and clinical evaluation, according to the schedule in Table 23-10. The length of initial bed rest is determined by patient response and the severity of the injury. Once the patient can tolerate it, physical therapy may be instituted. The patients are given a series of treatments until they can stand erect. They are then taught to walk and are given exercises to strengthen the spinal and abdominal muscles. If there is prolonged or excessive pain or conditions suggestive of a possible increase in deformity, we suggest a Milwaukee brace. The brace is prescribed by use of the three-point system, as in the treatment of adolescent kyphosis. This is the most effective orthosis for the treatment of these conditions. This brace offers support comparable to a cast and has the advantage of being readily adjustable.

Treatment of clinically unstable condition. There is no definitive study that convincingly shows the superiority of either operative or nonoperative therapy. Therefore, based on currently available information, we suggest that both approaches are justified. Clearly, we do not advocate any protocol that assumes that a diagnosis of instability is equal to an indication for surgery.

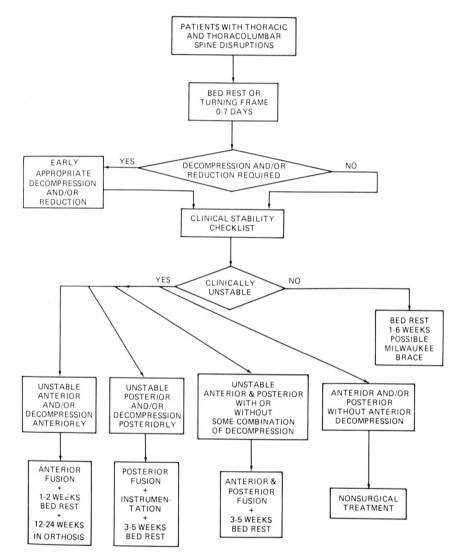

Fig. 23-12. A recommended flow diagram for the management of patients with disruption of the lower cervical spine. (From White, A.A., III, and Panjabi, M.M.: Clinical biomechanics of the spine, Philadelphia, 1978, J.B. Lippincott Co.)

There are, however, certain situations in which we strongly favor operative stabilization of an unstable spine. They are (1) the conditions occurring after anterior decompression with removal of a complete vertebral body and (2) compelling conditions that demand rapid and immediate rehabilitation activity.

Thoracic-spine clinical instability may be the result of anterior or posterior structural damage resulting from anterior or posterior surgical decompression. Let us discuss some of the various possibilities.

In the presence of anterior clinical instability (structural damage mainly in the anterior elements) with or without anterior decompression we suggest anterior fusion, followed by 1 to 2 weeks bed rest and rehabilitation as tolerated. A plaster jacket with chin and occipital support or a Milwaukee brace is recommended. If there is instability at T6 or above, chin support is important. The individual is ambulatory in the orthosis for 12 to 24 weeks. The patient is then managed by the guidelines suggested in the follow-up schedule.

In the presence of posterior clinical instability (structural damage mainly in the posterior elements) with or without posterior decompression we suggest the following. When instability is primarily posterior because of disruption of the posterior elements from natural or iatrogenic disease, posterior fusion with instrumentation is indicated. Appropriate wiring or Harrington instrumentation is the best available method. There is room for additional improvement in instrumentation and techniques for open reduction and internal fixation of fractures in this region. We suggest that the patient be kept in bed for 3 to 5 weeks in a plaster jacket (including chin support if T6 or above), or a Milwaukee brace. The recumbency time will permit some degree of soft-tissue healing and allow reduction of cord edema. After this, if possible, the patient is then treated with ambulation in the same device for 12 to 24 weeks. The rehabilitation and follow-up schedule is the same as that described in Table 23-8.

In the presence of anterior and posterior instability with or without anterior or posterior decompression we suggest the following. In some situations, posterior fusion alone is satisfactory, even when there is anterior and posterior instability. However, when there is a need for vertebral body removal, it is generally better to operate posteriorly first. Instrumentation or wiring can be used to provide some immediate postoperative stability, and posterior fusion can be done with no additional loss of stability. Then the spine may be approached anteriorly, allowing decompression and fusion to be carried out with the assurance of some stability from posterior instrumentation. The regimen is carried out as follows. Posterior instrumentation and fusion is followed immediately or in 3 to 7 days by anterior decompression or fusion, as indicated. The postoperative regimen is the same as that for patients with posterior instability.

In situations where there is clinical instability anteriorly or posteriorly without anterior decompression there is also a place for nonsurgical treatment. These nonsurgical methods offer several justifiable alternatives. One may elect to proceed with postural reduction followed by additional best rest and then some orthotic device.[16] Another approach is to simply have the patient rest in bed, or if there is significant sensory deficit, the patient may us a turning frame. After 6 weeks the patient is then given rehabilitation and activity as tolerated, and followed according to the suggested schedule.

Several nonsurgical options have been offered here. There are a number of other regimens to be considered. Bedbrook and Edibaum, for example, suggested that possibly there should be trials of mobilization of some patients with neurologically involved spines after 3 weeks.[5] If such a series were shown to be successful, a number of the surgical "advantages" would be eliminated. The nonoperative regimens offered by us are all based on well-documented experience and sound clinical biomechanics and rehabilitation. They all seem to be equally appropriate, and the nonsurgical regimens selected might well be determined by some equilibrium between the individual patient's and physician's needs and preferences, as well as the local practices and available facilities.

LUMBAR SPINE L1-L5

The problem of clinical instability in the lumbar spine has some unique considerations, related to both aspects of the definition of clinical instability. The associated neurologic deficits are relatively rare, less disabling, and more likely to recover. A large epidemiologic series of all spine injuries reported that only 3% of patients with lumbar spine dislocations and fracture dislocations had neurologic deficits.[35] The second consideration is related to the phenomena of subsequent pain, deformity, disability, and the very high loads that must be borne by this region of the spine.

Evaluation

Anatomy. The major anatomic structures are shown in Fig. 23-13. The anterior longitudinal ligament is a well-developed structure in the lumbar spine. The anulus fibrosus, which has been studied extensively, contributes in a major way to the ligament in this region of the spine. The posterior longitudinal ligament is less important than the anterior longitudinal to the stability of these lumbar functional units. The facet joints in the lumbar region play a critical role in its stability. In dislocations and fracture dislocations of the facet articulations of the lumbar spine there is a great tendency for instability to be present. The interspinous ligaments appear not to be very important, and in fact they are often absent in the normal situation.[36] The loss of useful function of the posterior elements in spondylolisthesis shows that at least in some cases this can result in instability.

Biomechanics. The role of the muscles in clinical stability, as previously discussed, is difficult to evaluate. Certainly the lumbar region is well endowed with active muscles. The erector spinae, the abdominal muscles, and the psoas are all actively involved in maintaining the functional upright and sitting stability of the lumbar spine.[3,27,29] They also contribute to the very high loads to which the lumbar spine is subjected. In this region, these well-developed muscles and their characteristic loading patterns may render the lumbar spine less vulnerable to clinical instability.

There have been some biomechanical studies designed specifically to evaluate lumbar-spine clinical stability. The data from these works are currently under analysis and are not yet fully ready for clinical application.

Clinical considerations

Little has been written specifically on the problem of lumbar dislocation and fracture dislocation. There has been some observed gross, but not entirely consistent, correlation between structural damage and neurologic deficit as observed in the lumbar spine.[35]

There is a relatively large margin of safety in the lumbar spine because the space available for the neural elements amply exceeds the space occupied by them. Therefore the presence of neurologic deficit is very likely to be the indicator of clinical instability. In other words, if there is enough displacement to cause neural damage, one must assume that enough displacement has occurred to cause significant ligamentous or bony failure. The pure vertically loaded compression fracture is an exception to this principle. The clin-

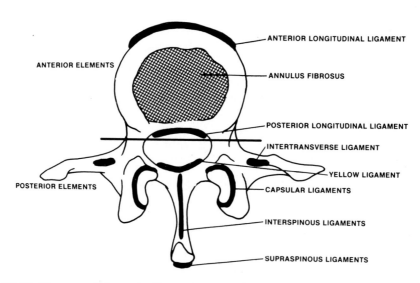

Fig. 23-13. Diagram of the major ligaments operative in the lumbar spine. (From White, A.A., III, and Panjabi, M.M.: Clinical biomechanics of the spine, Philadelphia, 1978, J.B. Lippincott Co.)

ical observation of the study by Kaufer and Hayes,[22] in which two patients progressed from mild to severe neurologic deficit between the time of injury and definitive treatment, supports this contention. These changes did not occur in transport but while the patients were hospitalized, during bed rest in Foster frames.

Checklist There are comparatively very few biomechanical studies or clinical studies that can provide a solid basis for the systematic approach to the problem of clinical instability in the lumbar spine. The guidelines suggested here are as vigorously proposed as are those for other regions of the spine (Tables 23-10 and 23-11). For the proper use of Tables 23-10 and 23-11, Fig. 23-14 should be studied. The checklist and Fig. 23-14 are derived from the work of Posner et al.[34] Basically, we want to take full advantage of the recuperative power of the cauda equina and minimize the possibility of prolonged disability associated with low back pain.

The specific question has been raised concern-

Table 23-10. Checklist for diagnosis of clinical instability in lumbar spine (Ll-L5)

Elements	Point value	Individual clinical value
Cauda equina damage	3	
Relative flexion sagittal-plane translation >16% or extension sagittal-plane translation >12%	2	
Relative flexion sagittal-plane rotation > 11 degrees	2	
Anterior elements destroyed	2	
Posterior elements destroyed or unable to function	2	
Dangerous loading anticipated	1	

Total of 5 or more = clinically unstable

In part from Posner, I., et al.: Spine. (In press.)

Table 23-11. Situations in which anterior elements are destroyed or unable to function

Failure of anterior ligamentous structures
  Increased forces
  Infection, tumor, disease
  Surgery
Failure of vertebral body
  Slice fracture
  Excessively comminuted fracture
  Aseptic necrosis
  Infection, tumor, disease
  Surgery

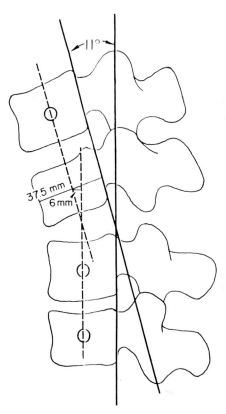

Fig. 23-14. The angular displacement of a fracture can be determined from roentgenograms when a line is drawn along the posterior surfaces of the vertical bodies above and below the fracture and the angle of the intersected lines (11 degrees in the drawing) is measured. The percentage of horizontal displacement is the distance that the center of the vertebral body above the fracture has moved forward (6 mm) divided by the width of the same vertebral body (37.5 mm), and so 6 mm divided by 37.5 mm multiplied by 100 equals 16% horizontal displacement. (From Posner, I., et al.: Spine. [In press.])

ing when the lumbar spine is clinically unstable after the various procedures for disk surgery. We recommend this checklist to make that determination. The use of this checklist will not indicate fusion of the lumbar spine purely as a treatment of pain.

We have presented a checklist that is a preliminary representation of some experiments on the lumbar-spine Functional Spinal Unit. The data has been separated for flexion and extension as seen in the checklist. A sagittal-plane rotation criterion is also included in the checklist.

Anterior elements destroyed or unable to function. This situation occurs most frequently when there has been failure of the anulus fibrosus or a slice (shear) failure through the vertebral body, either of which may be part of the classic fracture of Holdsworth.[19] There are other specific instances in which the anterior elements may be unable to function. The vertically loaded vertebral body fracture may be a bursting fracture with multiple fragmentation, which excessively compromises the mechanical function of the structure in resisting compressive loads. There is the obvious loss of normal mechanical function caused by infection, tumor, or surgery (see Table 23-11).

Status of posterior elements. It is important to evaluate the status of the posterior elements. A key factor in the evaluation of lumbar spine trauma is the relative position of the spinous processes. The position of these structures indicates the relationships of the posterior elements. Abnormal separation along the *y* axis or the *x* axis represents flexion and axial rotatory deformity, respectively.

The work of Kaufer and Hayes pointed out the importance of the status of the posterior elements when they documented in the classification the major patterns of structural failure that are associated with abnormal displacements of the facet joints.[22] Evaluation of the posterior elements fits very well with the observations of Holdsworth, who also pointed out the significance of malalignment of the spinous processes.[19]

In the evaluation of the status of the posterior elements after trauma, there may be certain findings on physical examination that are helpful. There may be a painful, palpable defect in the midline, with a large hematoma between two widely separated spinous processes. A subcutaneous hematoma that extended directly to the

dura in 85% of the cases was observed in the series of patients studied by Kaufer and Hayes.[22]

Nature has provided an interesting experimental model that allows us to make some assumptions about the role of the posterior elements in the clinical stability of the lumbar spine. Spondylolisthesis is an example of the loss of support function of the posterior elements caused by a defect of the pars interarticularis. Obviously, other patterns in this area, such as different combinations of pedicle and laminar fractures, can result in similar structural failures. With this problem, there may be associated clinical instability.

Finally, we must consider the variable of anticipated loads. This is an attempt to take into consideration the fact that there will be some variation in the physiologic loads, depending on the individual patient.

Treatment

For the clinically stable spine the patient is treated according to clinical judgment, that is, the patient may be left on bedrest until the symptoms allow the gradual ambulation and exercise. Severe pain or fear of increasing deformity may lead the surgeon to prescribe an appropriate spinal orthosis. This could be a cast, a Jewett three-point brace, or one of the several varieties of a lumbar spine brace, including the Williams brace, McAusland brace, and the Norton-Brown brace.

The time for bedrest should for 3 weeks with encouragement of the patient to get up but certainly not to be forced to ambulate if uncomfortable. When the patient is deemed to be stable after a careful checklist evaluation, one should take full advantage of the observed stability. We avoid any type of cast, brace, or encumberance and try to get the patient to progress as rapidly as he or she will tolerate. In this situation it is important to follow the schedule that has been recommended (Table 23-8). This is a safe approach that will allow any unrecognized instability to be picked up at an appropriate time and will allow alteration of the treatment if needed.

In treating the clinically unstable situation, the spines are separated into two groups based on whether or not there is clinical evidence of cauda equina damage and evidence of nerve impingment on myelographic examination. If there is cauda equina damage or evidence of nerve root impingement, exploration and appropriate relief of the impingement with reduction and internal fixation of the arthrodesis is recommended. In view of the good prognosis for recuperation of the peripheral nerves of the cauda equina we are in favor of this approach.

It has been clinically documented that in some instances reduction through instrumentation and realignment of the canal can provide an appropriate decompression. Attempts of closed reduction of these injuries is not recommended because such attempts are sometimes associated with additional neurologic damage.

In those situations where there is a diagnosis of clinical instability and the absence of any neurologic deficit, the need for surgical intervention is less urgent. When the spine is unstable without a neurologic deficit, several alternatives seem appropriate to consider. One is to go ahead with arthrodesis external fixation as an elective procedure within the first 7 to 21 days or even later if one wants to observe the patient for a longer period of time to determine whether there is any tendency for progression of deformity. This option in delaying the procedure for several months seems to be justified on the basis that there is no catastrophic risk involved in the possibility of additional neuroirritation and one has an excellent clinical trial of the appropriateness of nonoperative treatment. Another much more conservative option is to decide that even though the spine is believed to be unstable one wishes to commit the patient to a nonoperative treatment. This patient may be treated with bedrest for 6 weeks with gradual ambulation, physical therapy, and protected activity for another 6 to 12 weeks. This regimen may include the use of a lumbar orthosis after the first 6 weeks of bedrest.

Although we are not necessarily suggesting this as a preferred treatment, we think that it has a place and it is justified in the lumbar spine. There are several reasons for this opinion. In the lumbar spine the relative amount of free space in the cauda equina region in most patients allows some accommodation for displaced structural elements, which prevents additional neurologic deficit. Also, we believe that the large powerful muscles immediately adjacent to the vertebrae in the lumbar spine lessens the risk of catastrophic displacement causing gross irreparable nerve damage. Moreover, we recognize that the recuperative power of the cauda equina to injury is greater than the thoracic and the cervical spine.

In summary, cauda equina damage in an unsta-ble spine is probably best treated by surgical intervention. Unstable lumbar spine without cauda equina damage may be treated with either early surgical intervention or delayed surgical intervention, or nonoperatively.

LUMBOSACRAL SPINE L5-S1
Evaluation

A separate checklist is provided for assessing the stability of the lumbosacral articulation because the experimental findings indicate that its behavior is significantly different (Table 23-12). This checklist, also derived from the work of Posner et al.,[34] requires a study of Fig. 23-14. All other considerations apply here as were discussed for the lumbar spine.

Treatment

The flow diagram for management of these problems is shown in Fig. 23-15. Patients are treated in bed if there is no neurologic deficit; otherwise, they are treated on a turning frame. The patient is thoroughly evaluated clinically, and the necessary supportive and specific care is provided. Regular anteroposterior and lateral roentgenograms are taken. The clinical stability check-

Table 23-12. Checklist for diagnosis of clinical instability in lumbosacral spine (L5-S1)

Element	Point value	Individual clinical value
Cauda equina damage	3	
Relative flexion sagittal-plane translation >25% or extension sagittal-plane translation >12%	2	
Relative flexion sagittal-plane rotation >19 degrees	2	
Anterior elements destroyed	2	
Posterior elements destroyed or unable to function	2	
Dangerous loading anticipated	1	

Total of 5 or more = clinically unstable

In part from Posner, I., et al.: Spine. (In press.)

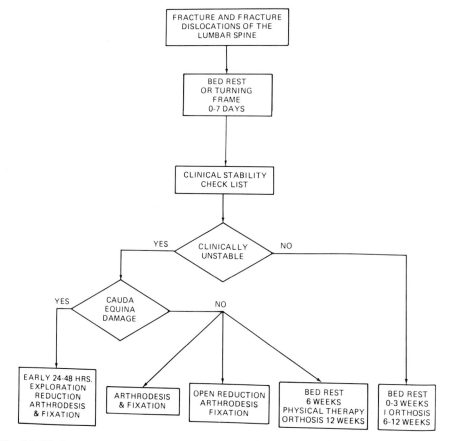

Fig. 23-15. A recommended flow diagram for the management of patients with disruptions of the lumbar spine. All treatment regimens include occupational and physical therapy, as tolerated, and follow-up schedule. (From White, A.A., III, and Panjabi, M.M.: Clinical biomechanics of the spine, Philadelphia, 1978, J.B. Lippincott Co.)

list is applied. In difficult cases, anteroposterior and lateral laminagrams are recommended for a detailed analysis of the status of the various anatomic elements.

Patients that are found to be stable may be treated with bed rest until their symptoms allow initiation of gradual ambulation and exercises. Pain or fear of increasing deformity may lead the surgeon to prescribe an appropriate spinal orthosis. The schedule for follow-up of all the patients allows any progression of deformity to be recognized.

Conditions determined to be clinically unstable are separated into two groups, based on whether there is clinical evidence of cauda equina damage and evidence of a defect on a lumbar myelogram.

If there is evidence of impingement upon the cauda equina or nerve roots, there should be early exploration, appropriate relief of the impingement, reduction, internal fixation, and arthrode-

sis. In view of the excellent recuperative potential of the cauda equina, we do not think that nonoperative treatment is justifiable in the presence of documented cauda equina impingement. Closed reduction of injuries in this group is not recommended because there have been reports of additional neurologic damage with such attempts.[6,21,40] Laminectomy is generally a less effective means of decompression than open reduction. Kaufer and Hayes reported a situation in which laminectomy of four levels failed to relieve a block in a patient who subsequently recovered 1 week after open reduction and stabilization.[22]

If there is a diagnosis of clinical instability without neurologic deficit, the need for surgery is less urgent. The available objective evidence does not lead to the conclusion that all clinically unstable lumbar spines must be treated with surgery. We suggest that there are at least three currently justifiable alternatives. The first involves performing arthrodesis, with internal fixation as an elective procedure at a later time. This is done relatively early (7 to 21 days) or at a later time (several months to years) based on the patient's symptoms and the judgment of the surgeon. Both approaches seem justified by available objective information. Note that these two options do not include reduction of dislocations. The delayed approach to the fixation of these injuries is believed to be justified by the fact that the risk of initial neurologic damage is less in this region. This factor allows time for prolonged observation to determine whether pain will be a problem. In other words, the urgency for the establishment of early or immediate clinical stability is not so great in the lumbar spine as in other regions.

The second alternative is to combine open reduction with internal fixation and fusion. This option should be exercised relatively early, at 7 to 14 days. In the opinion of some physicians, spondylolisthesis falls into this category. The necessity or desirability of reduction in spondylolisthesis is controversial. However, this can be surgically reduced months or years after its occurrence.

The nonsurgical alternative is also justified in this group of clinically unstable lumbar spine injuries. Patients are treated with bed rest for 6 weeks, followed by gradual ambulation, physical therapy, and protected activity for another 6 to 12 weeks. A lumbar orthosis of intermediate control may be useful if symptoms of pain demand it. Even though this is contrary to the recommendation of Kaufer and Hayes,[22] we believe that it is a justifiable alternative for several reasons. First, their study includes a modest number of cases, and there is no controlled study that advocates surgery. Second, there is a generous portion of free space in the lumbar spine to accommodate the cauda equina.

Thus, with adequate postinjury follow-up of the patient, surgical stabilization can always be done later for pain, deformity, or neural irritation if indicated. The large powerful muscle mass lessens the risk of a sudden catastrophic displacement in the lumbar spine. Moreover, the resistance to, and the recuperative power from, injury to the cauda equina is significantly greater than that of the thoracic or cervical spinal cord.

Sacroiliac joints

The sacroiliac joints, which have probably been overemphasized in the past, may now suffer some inappropriate neglect. The large gravitational and muscle forces associated with the erect trunk are ultimately transported to the lower limbs through these joints.

Previous studies of these joints have yielded widely disparate information on their kinematics. Movement between the sacrum and the ilium has been variably described as being from 5 to 26 mm, a little over an inch.[11,14,44] Recent studies by Walheim and Olerud using an electromagnetic measuring technique with transducers fixed to pins inserted into the pubic bone on either side of the symphysis pubis have been reported.[42] This unique experiment recorded motion between the two pins with active straight leg raising, hip abduction, and one leg standing. Fresh autopsy studies demonstrated very small motion at these points. There was a 0.5 mm motion in young people and no motion in older individuals.

Clinical considerations

Chronic pelvic sacroiliac instability can be difficult to diagnose. The nerve supply is such that one can readily explain low back pain with radiation into the leg without assuming that there is a herniated disk.[38]

Because of hormone-related changes during pregnancy and possibly even during menstruation, there is a ligamentous laxity at the pubic symphysis and particularly in the sacroiliac ligaments and the interosseous ligaments; hence obvious sacroiliac instability is more likely to be present in female patients.

Walheim and Olerud reported on two female patients believed to have pelvic instability.[42] One patient had the condition even many years after delivery, and the other had it 3 years after trauma. These patients were treated by skeletal immobilization of the pelvis by a Hoffman fixation technique. While the pelvis was fixed for 4 to 5 days, the symptoms subsided, but when the device was removed, the symptoms returned immediately. The authors suggested that temporary skeletal fixation might be an appropriate clinical test for instability of the pelvis. This is an intriguing idea meriting further consideration.

There is much work to be done in order to develop good clinical criteria for sacroiliac instability. At present, we have the guidelines of 1.5 to 10 mm displacement as abnormal or indicative of instability. This does not indicate how this distance is to be measured. Localized "clicking" sensations and a positive Trendelenburg test when present may be helpful in making the diagnosis.

Treatment

When the diagnosis can be made with certainty and the disability is significant, sacroiliac fusion is believed to be the procedure of choice.

DISCUSSIONS AND CONCLUSIONS

Our basic approach has been to take what is known of anatomy, biomechanics, and documented clinical experiment and to analyze it in a manner that is clinically useful. A major anatomic consideration is the clinical significance of regional variations of several structural characteristics. Examples include the anterior longitudinal ligament, the yellow ligament, and the spatial orientation of the facet articulations and the disk in the standing posture. The relative size of the neural elements to the space in which they are enclosed is an important consideration. Regional variations also exist in mechanical properties, such as kinematics, stiffness, and physiologic loads. We have emphasized the importance of a proper interpretation of the significance of neurologic deficit in the determination of clinical stability. Generally, when a deficit is associated with significant structural damage, clinical instability should be suspected. The importance of standardization of roentgenographic techniques for more precise interpretation cannot be overemphasized.

The bony architecture and the ligamentous elements comprise the structural components of the spine. With all components intact the biomechanical function is normal. When sufficient anatomic disruption causes or threatens to produce an inability to function normally, we recommend that the spine be considered clinically unstable.

The goal of good patient management is to gain maximal recovery as rapidly as possible and avoid unnecessary treatment (surgical or nonsurgical) and at the same time prevent the unhappy situation of initial or subsequent neurologic damage. There is no convincing evidence that the diagnosis of clinical instability demands that the treatment should surgical reduction, fusion, or fixation. However, the management of a patient with such a diagnosis should definitely differ from that of clinically stable patients, and modern trends appear to be in the direction of surgical management of the unstable spine.

The role of laminectomy in management of spine trauma should be diminished and is indicated in only a few very special situations. The indications for decompression need considerable elucidation.

Checklists, flow charts, and follow-up schedules have been presented to conveniently organize and summarize the information, to stimulate others to criticize and improve upon them, and to provide clinical protocols for systematic evaluation, management, and study. The concluding principle is that it is only through clear prospective clinical protocols that we can ever really improve our knowledge and base our decisions more on solid scientific evidence and less on well-meaning speculation.

Without theory, practice is but a routine bore of habit. Theory alone can bring forth and develop the spirit of invention.

PASTEUR

ACKNOWLEDGMENT

Thanks to Kashine Dolan for her diligent work in the preparation of this manuscript.

REFERENCES

1. Bailey, R.W.: Observations of cervical intervertebral disc lesions in fractures and dislocations, J. Bone Joint Surg. **45A**:461, 1963.
2. Barbour, J.R.: Screw fixation in fracture of the odontoid process, South Aust. Clin. **5**:20, 1971.
3. Bartelink, D.L.: The role of abdominal pressure in relieving the pressure of the lumbar intervertebral discs, J. Bone Joint Surg. **39B**:718, 1957.
4. Beatson, T.R.: Fractures and dislocations of the cervical spine, J. Bone Joint Surg. **45B**:21, 1963.
5. Bedbrook, G.M., and Edibaum, R.C.: The study of spinal deformity in traumatic spinal paralysis, Paraplegia **10**:321, 1973.
6. Böhler, L.: The treatment of fractures, ed. 5, New York, 1956, Grune & Stratton, Inc.
7. Brav, E.A., Miller, J.A., and Bouzard, W.C.: Traumatic dislocation of the cervical spine: army experience and results, J. Trauma **3**:569, 1963.
8. Breig, A.: Biomechanics of the central nervous system: some basic normal and pathological phenomena, Stockholm, 1960, Almquist & Wiskell.
9. Brooks, A.L., and Jenkings, E.G.: Atlanto-axial arthrodesis by the wedge compression method, J. Bone Joint Surg. **60A**:279, 1978.
10. Catell, H.S., and Filtzer, D.L.: Pseudo-subluxation and other normal variations of the cervical spine in children, J. Bone Joint Surg. **47A**:1295, 1965.
11. Colachis, S.C., Warden, R.E., Bechtol, C.O., and Strohm, B.R.: Movement of the sacro-iliac joint in the adult male, Arch. Phys. Med. Rehab. **44**:490, 1963.
12. Fang, H.S.Y., Ong, G.B., and Hodgson, A.R.: Anterior spinal fusion: the operative approaches, Clin. Orthop. **35**:16, 1964.

13. Fielding, J.W., Cochran, G.V.B., Lansing, J.F., and Hohl, M.: Tears of the transverse ligament of the atlas: a clinical biomechanical study, J. Bone Joint Surg. **56A:**1683, 1974.

14. Frigerio, N.A., Stowe, R.R., and Howe, J.W.: Movement of the sacro-iliac joint, Clin. Orthop. **100:**370, 1974.

15. Gosch, H.H., Gooding, E., and Schneider, R.C.: An experimental study of cervical spine and cord injuries, J. Trauma **12:**570, 1972.

16. Guttmann, L.: Management of spinal fractures. In Spinal cord injuries: comprehensive management and research, Oxford, 1973, Blackwell Scientific Publications.

17. Hausfeld, J.N.: A biomechanical analysis of clinical stability in the thoracic and thoracolumbar spine (thesis), Yale University School of Medicine, New Haven, 1977.

18. Hecker, P.: Appareil ligamenteux occipito-atloïdo-axoïdien: étude d'anatomie comparée, Arch. Anat. Hist. Embryol. **2:**57-95, 1923.

19. Holdsworth, F.W.: Fractures, dislocations and fracture dislocations of the spine, J. Bone Joint Surg. **45B:**6, 1963.

20. Johnson, R.M., and Southwick, W.O.: Surgical approaches to the spine. Rothmann, R.H., and Simone, F.A., editors: The spine, Philadelphia, 1975, W.B. Saunders Co.

21. Kallio, E.: Injuries of the thoraco-lumbar spine with paraplegia, Acta Orthop. Scand. Suppl. 60:1, 1963.

22. Kaufer, H., and Hayes J.T.: Lumbar fracture-dislocation: a study of twenty-one cases, J. Bone Joint Surg. **48A:**712, 1966.

23. Keim, H.A.: Spinal stabilization following trauma, Clin. Orthop. **81:**53, 1971.

24. Lauritzen, J.: Diagnostic difficulties in lower cervical spine dislocations, Acta Orthop. Scand. **39:**439, 1968.

25. Leidholdt, J.D., et al.: Evaluation of late spinal deformitites with fracture dislocations of the dorsal and lumbar spine in paraplegias, Paraplegia **7:**16, 1969.

26. Marar, B.C.: Hyperextension injuries of the cervical spine: the pathogenesis of damage to the spinal cord, J. Bone Joint Surg. **56A:**1655, 1974.

27. Morris, J.M., Lucas, D.B., and Bresler, B.: The role of the trunk in stability of the spine, J. Bone Joint Surg. **42A:**327, 1961.

28. Munro, D.: Treatment of fractures and dislocations of the cervical spine complicated by cervical cord and root injuries: a comparative study of fusion vs. no fusion therapy, N. Engl. J. Med. **264:**573, 1961.

29. Nachemson, A.: Electromyographic studies on the vertebral portion of the psoas muscle, with special reference to the stabilizing function of the lumbar spine, Acta Orthop. Scand. **37:**177, 1966.

30. Nicoll, E.A.: Fractures of the dorso-lumbar spine, J. Bone Joint Surg. **31B:**376, 1949.

31. Panjabi, M.M., White, A.A., and Johnson R.M.: Cervical spine mechanics as a function of transaction of components, J. Biomech. **8:**327, 1975.

32. Panjabi, M.M., White, A.A., Keller, D., Southwick, W.O., and Friedlaender, G.A.: Clinical biomechanics of the cervical spine, 75-WA/B10-7, New York, 1975, American Society of Mechanical Engineers.

33. Perry, J., and Nickel, V.L.: Total cervical spine fusion for neck paralysis, J. Bone Joint Surg. **41A:**37, 1957.

34. Posner, I., White, A.A., Edwards, W.T., and Hayes, W.C.: A biomechanical analysis of clinical stability of the lumbar and lumbo-sacral spine. Spine. (In press.)

35. Riggins, R.S., and Kraus, J.F.: The risk of neurological damage with fractures of the vertebrae, J. Trauma **17:**126, 1977.

36. Rissanen, P.M.: The surgical anatomy and pathology of the supraspinous and interspinous ligaments of the lumbar spine with special reference to ligament ruptures, Acta Orthop. Scand. Suppl. 46:1, 1960.

37. Roberts, J.B., and Curtiss, P.H.: Stability of the thoracic and lumbar spine in traumatic paraplegia following fracture or fracture-dislocation, J. Bone Joint Surg. **52A:**1115, 1970.

38. Solonen, K.A.: The sacro-iliac joint in the light of anatomical roentgenologic and clinical studies, Acta Orthop. Scand. Suppl. 26:1, 1957.

39. Spence, K.F., Decker, S., and Sell, K.W.: Bursting atlantal fracture associated with rupture of the transverse ligament, J. Bone Joint Surg. **52A:**543, 1970.

40. Steinger, J.K.: Fracture-dislocation of the thoracolumbar spine with special reference to reduction by open and closed operations, J. Bone Joint Surg. **29:**107, 1947.

41. Taylor, A.R.: The mechanism of injury to the spinal cord in the neck without damage to the vertebral column, J. Bone Joint Surg. **33B:**543, 1951.

42. Walheim, G.G., and Olerud, S.: Chronic pelvic instability: new diagnostic techniques, Transactions of the 25th meeting of the Orthopaedic Research Society, **4:**248, 1979.

43. Webb, J.K., Broughton, R.B.K., McSweeny, T., and Park, W.M.: Hidden flexion injury of the cervical spine, J. Bone Joint Surg. **58B:**322, 1976.

44. Weisel, H.: The movement of the sacro-iliac joint, Acta Anat. **23:**80, 1955.

45. Wiesel, S.W., and Rothman, R.H.: Occipitoatlantal hypermobility, Spine **4:**187, 1979.

46. White, A.A., Johnson, R.M., Panjabi, M.M., and Southwick, W.O.: Biomechanics of the axially loaded cervical spine: development of a safe clinical test for ruptured cervical ligaments, J. Bone Joint Surg. **57A:**582, 1975.

47. White, A.A., and Panjabi, M.M.: Clinical biomechanics of the spine, Philadelphia, 1978, J.B. Lippincott.

48. White, A.A., Panjabi, M.M., Hausfeld, J., and Southwick, W.D.: Clinical instability in the thoracic and thoracolumbar spine: review of past and current concepts. Presented at the American Orthopaedic Association meeting, Boca Raton, Florida, 1977.

Index

A

Abduction brace of Roberts for Legg-Calvé-Perthes disease, 75, 76
Abductors, absent or nonfunctioning, causing dislocation of surface replacement of hip, 449, 450
Acetabular component, containment of, to prevent loosening of surface replacement of hip, 452
Acromial osteophytes, 253
Activity
  forces across knee during, 302
  and patellar pain, 347
Adhesions
  intra-articular, soft-tissue release for, 332-333
  knee-joint, arthroscopic resection for, 393-394
Adjustable connecting rod, 113
Age of patient and knee arthroplasty, 314
Alignment in total knee replacement, 398
Allografts
  bone and cartilage, preserved, potential disadvantages of, 34-37
  processing, 52
Ambulation-limiting contractures in Duchenne muscular dystrophy, 19
American Association of Tissue Banks, 37, 45
Anametric Total Knee unit, 299
Anatomy
  of elbow, 185, 188
  of femur, 162
  of humerus, 224
  of long head of biceps, 250
  of pelvis, 165-166
  regional, and external fixation, 120-122
  surgical, and soft-tissue coverage, 144
  of upper extremity, 169-170
Anconeus muscle, 186
Anesthesia
  for knee arthroscopy, 367
  in multiply injured patient, 105-106
  for surgical treatment of muscular dystrophy, 21-22
Angulation deformities of tibia, 88-89
Ankle, stiffness of, prevention of, 158
Anterior compartment syndrome from external fixation of tibia, 157
Anterior and lateral musculotendinous units, transfixion of, from external fixation of tibia, 158
Anterior tibial artery, injury to, from external fixation of tibia, 157-158
Anteroposterior instability
  of elbow, 193
  in recurrent elbow dislocations, chronic, 197-198
Anteversion of femoral neck, excessive, causing loosening of surface replacement of hip, 452-453

Antibiotics
  and allografts, 52
  in bone cement, 407-408
Antigenicity of preserved bone and cartilage allografts, 35-36
Artery(ies)
  injuries to, from external fixation,179
  tibial, anterior, injury to, from external fixation of tibia, 157-158
Arthritic deformity, severe, reconstruction of, 286-297
Arthritic knee
  difficult
    reconstruction of, 277-300
    treatment of, with Variable Axis prosthesis, 286
  nonoperative management of, 277
  treatment of, 284-297
Arthrodesis
  for arthritic knee, 285
  surgical, for arthritic knee, 281
Arthrography in investigation of patellar pain, 346
Arthroplasty
  knee; see Knee, arthroplasty of
  Spherocentric, for arthritic knee, 281-284
  unicompartmental, for arthritic knee, 278
Arthroscopes
  for knee arthroscopy, 358, 360-361
  operating, 358, 361
Arthroscopy
  for chondral defects, 394-395
  in investigation of patellar pain, 346
  knee; see Knee, arthroscopy of
  for lateral retinacular release, 381-385
  for meniscal surgery, 385-395
  for osteochondritis dissecans, 394-395
  for partial meniscectomy, 385-386
  for patellar compression syndrome, 381
  for patellar shaving, 384-385
  for patellar surgery, 381-385
  for resection
    of knee joint adhesions, 393-394
    of meniscal tears, 386-389
  synovectomy via, 392-393
  for "total meniscectomy," 389, 392
Articulated knee prosthesis for treatment of severe mechanical knee joint disease, 277-284
ASIF "tubular" fixator, 114, 115
  application of, 126-131
  for external fixation of tibia, 160-161
Asymptomatic fractures of wires as complications of surface replacement of hip, 445
Atlanta brace for Legg-Calvé-Perthes disease, 75, 76
Atlantoaxial joint
  spinal instability at, 460

Atlantoaxial joint—cont'd
  subluxations and dislocations at, 460, 461-462
Autogenous cancellous bone graft, supplementary, in treatment of infected nonunions and failed septic joints, 177-178
Autopsy for donor of tissue for transplantation, 52
Avulsion, transverse, of supraspinatus tendon, 267
Avulsion fracture of greater tuberosity, rotator cuff tears after, 249

B

Banking of musculoskeletal tissues, guidelines for, 50-53; *see also* Bone banking
Becker form of childhood dystrophy, 2, 4
Biceps, long head of
  anatomy of, 250
  lesions of
    surgery for, 256-257
    treatment of, 255-256
  ruptures of, 250
Biceps tendon
  dislocations of, 250-251
  pathomechanics of, 255
  subluxation of, 251-252
Biceps tendon transfer, 197
Biceps tenosynovitis, 252-255
Bicipital groove osteophytes, 252-253
Bicompartmental knee replacement, 316
Biologic potential of preserved bone and cartilage allografts, 35
Biopsy
  muscle, in diagnosis of muscular dystrophy, 7-10
  synovial, arthroscopy for, 378
Biotrigonometric analysis and practical applications of osteotomies of tibia in children, 83-99
Blisters from proximal realignment of patella, 350
Blood loss in multiply injured patient, 104
Blount's disease
  Langenskiöld's six stages of, 95
  treatment of, 89, 90
Bone
  Cleaning of, before cementation, 410-411
  denuded, soft-tissue coverage of, 177
  erosive defects of, from contiguous neurogenic tumors in neurofibromatosis in childhood, 61
  minimal, resection of, for reconstruction of severe arthritic deformity or failed implant, 287, 289-292
  preparation of, for revision surgery after total hip replacement, 419
Bone banking, 34-53
  background and current methods of, 34-47
Bone block transfer, coracoid, 197
Bone and cartilage allografts, preserved, potential disadvantages of, 34-37
Bone cement
  antibiotic in, 407-408
  choice of, 407
  cylinders of, 408
  fixation with, surgical technique to achieve, 410-413
  good quality, obtaining, 413
  insertion and pressurization of, 411-413
  mechanical strength of, 407-410
  penetration of, 412
  radiopacifier in, 407-408
  surgical guidelines for, 410
  temperature sensitivity of, 409-410
  thickness of, 409
Bone cyst in neurofibromatosis in childhood, 61, 66

Bone deformity complications after supracondylar humeral fractures in children, 229-230
Bone graft
  cancellous, autogenous, supplementary, in treatment of infection nonunions and failed septic joints, 177-178
  osteoperiosteal, 154, 155
  sources of, 152-153
  types of, 153-154
  vascularized, 153-154
Bone grafting
  general principles and use in open fractures, 152-156
  indications for, 154-156
  serial, in treatment of infected nonunions and failed septic joints, 178
Bone growth, disorders of, in neurofibromatosis of childhood, 59, 60
Bone loss and secondary scarring after reconstruction of severe arthritic deformity or failed implant, 292-296
Bone proliferation, subperiosteal, in neurofibromatosis in childhood, 66-67
Bone and soft-tissue procedure, secondary, performed in frame, 143
Bone stock and knee arthroplasty, 315
Bony bridge resection and osteotomy, 97-98
Bony complications of external skeletal fixation, 179-182
Bony defects
  bone grafting for, 154, 156
  tibial, large, management of, 399, 400
Bowing, congenital, and pseudarthrosis in neurofibromatosis in childhood, 59, 61
  surgery for, 62-64
Brace
  abduction, of Roberts for Legg-Calvé-Perthes disease, 75, 76
  Atlanta, for Legg-Calvé-Perthes disease, 75,76
  knee, for patellar pain, 347
  Toronto, for Legg-Calvé-Perthes disease, 73, 75, 76
Bracing
  lower extremity surgery and, 22-25
  for tibial deformity, 88, 89
Bridging of tibial loss, 156
"Broomstick" osteotomy, 91, 93, 94
Bucket-handle tear of meniscus, arthroscopic excision of, 386-389
Burns with fractures
  external fixation for, 177
  multiply injured patient with, 109
Bursitis as complication of surface replacement of hip, 445

C

Café-au-lait spots in neurofibromatosis in childhood, 55
Cameras, television, use of, in knee arthroscopy, 364, 366
Cancellous bone graft, autogenous, supplementary, in treatment of infected nonunions and failed septic joints, 177-178
Cancellous chips and strips for bone grafts, 153
Capitellum, fractures of, 215
Cardiac involvement in muscular dystrophy, 12
Carrier state in muscular dystrophy, 10-11
Cartilage and bone allografts, preserved, potential disadvantages of, 34-37
Cassebaum approach to elbow, 204, 205
Cast, Petri, for Legg-Calvé-Perthes disease, 73, 74
Cellulitis from external fixation, 181
Cement, bone; *see* Bone cement
Cement technique in total knee replacement, 399
Cementation, cleaning of bone before, 410-411
Cementing techniques in hip replacement, improved, 407-413
Cervical spine, lower, instability of 460, 462-470
Cheilotomy for Legg-Calvé-Perthes disease, 80, 81

Childhood, neurofibromatosis in, 54-70
Childhood dystrophy, Becker form of, 2, 4
Children
 medical epicondyle fractures in, 189-191
 osteotomies of tibia in, biotrigonometric analysis and practical applications of, 83-99
 supracondylar humeral fractures in, anterior displaced, 233
 transverse distal humeral epiphyseal fractures in, 234-235
 transverse fractures of distal humerus in, 224-235
 valgus stress in, 190
Chondral defects, arthroscopy for, 394-395
Chondromalacia patellae
 arthroscopy for, 381-385
 definitions of, 342
 patellar pain syndromes and, 342-355
Chondroplasty for patellar pain, 350-351
Circular compression frame, Kronner, 116
Clean wound, obtaining, 152
Cleaning of bone before cementation, 410-411
Clinical instability of spine, 457-458
Closed fractures, external fixation for, 117
Closing wedge osteotomy, 91, 92, 94, 95
Collateral ligament, medial, strain of, 189
Comminuted fracture of ring of C1, 460
Compartment syndromes from external fixation, 179
Compensatory osteotomy, 84-85
Compression frame, circular, Kronner, 116
Condyles, humeral, fractures of, 214
Congenital bowing and pseudarthrosis in neurofibromatosis in childhood, 59, 61
 surgery for, 62-64
Congenital myopathies, 4-5
Connecting rod, adjustable, 113
Consent for tissue donation, 51
Constrained implants for arthritic knee, 286
Contracture
 ambulation-limiting, in Duchenne muscular dystrophy, 19
 flexion
  soft-tissue release for, 331-332
  total knee replacement for, 325-326
 quadriceps, stiff knee and, soft-tissue release for, 332, 333
Coracoid bone block transfer, 197
Cord damage and lower cervical spine instability, 467
Coronoid, fractures of, 215-216
Cortical defects, full-thickness, bone grafting for, 156
Cortical struts for bone grafts, 153
Corticocancellous strips for bone grafts, 153, 154
"Crab meat" lesions from proximal realignment of patella, 350
Creatinine phosphokinase in diagnosis of muscular dystrophy, 6-7
Crests, iliac, as source of bone grafts, 153
Cross-leg pedicle flaps, 150, 151
Cruciate Condylar knee implant, 310, 311
Cruciate ligaments, role of, in knee implant systems, 310
Cultures of allografts, 52
Cutaneous coverage for infected nonunions and failed septic joints, 178
Cutaneous lesions in neurofibromatosis in childhood, 55
Cylinders, bone cement, 408
Cyst
 bone, in neurofibromatosis in childhood, 61, 66
 invasive, formation of, causing loosening of surface replacement of hip, 453

D

Débridement
 of knee, 313-314, 318
 of patella, 353
 in treatment of infected nonunions and failed septic joints, 176-177

Decubiti, pressure, 14
Deep-freezing of allografts, 45, 52
Delayed union from external fixation, 180
Deltoid, detachment of, 245
Derotation osteotomy, 95
Diaphyseal defects, partial-thickness, bone grafting for, 154
Dietary problems in muscular dystrophy, 13
Direct local flaps for rotator cuff tears, 268
Disease
 Blount's
  Langenskiöld's six stages of, 95
  treatment of, 89, 90
 inadvertent transfer of, by preserved bone and cartilage allografts, 36-37, 40-41
 knee joint, severe mechanical, articulated knee prosthesis for, 277-284
 Landouzy-Déjerine, 2-3
  working classification of, 4
 Legg-Calvé-Perthes, treatment of, 73-82
 of muscle, 1-5; *see also* Muscular dystrophy
 neurologic, as contraindication for knee arthroplasty, 314
 von Recklinghausen's; *see* Neurofibromatosis in childhood
Disease process, basic, and knee arthroplasty, 315
Disk space narrowing and instability of lower cervical spine, 467-468
Dislocations
 at atlantoaxial joint, 460, 461-462
 of biceps tendon, 250-251
 as complication of THARIES surface replacement of hip, 435, 440
 elbow, 194-196
  recurrent, chronic anteroposterior instability in, 197-198
 patellar, after total knee replacement, 337-338
 rotator cuff tear after injury without, 239-242
 of shoulder, anterior
  with fracture of greater tuberosity, rotator cuff tear after, 242-244
  rotator cuff tear after, 242
 of surface replacement of hip, 449-451
Displaced supracondylar fractures, anterior, in children, 233
Distal humerus, transverse fractures of, in children, 224-235
Distal radius, fractures of, external fixation for, 173-174
Distal realignment of patella, 352-353
Distant flaps, 150-151
DMD; *see* Duchenne muscular dystrophy
Dome-shaped osteotomy, 91, 93, 94
Donor of tissues for transplantation, selection of, 37-41, 51-52
Duchenne muscular dystrophy, 1-2; *see also* Muscular dystrophy
 ambulation-limiting contractures in, 19
 carrier state for, 10-11
 equinovarus deformity in, 25-26
 genetics of, 5-6
 muscle weakness in, 18-21
 pathomechanics of, 18-21
 posture in, 20-21
 signs of, 2
 working classification of, 4
Dystrophia myotonica, 3-4
 genetics of, 6
 working classification of, 4
Dystrophy
 childhood, Becker form of, 2, 4
 facioscapulohumeral, 2-3
  genetics of, 6
  working classification of, 4
 limb-girdle, 2
  genetics of, 6
  working classification of, 4
 muscular; *see* Muscular dystrophy

E

Effusions, joint, after knee arthroscopy, 377
Elbow
  anatomy of, 185, 188
  anteroposterior instability of, 193
  dislocations of, 194-196
    recurrent, chronic anteroposterior instability in, 197-198
  external fixation of, 172
  in flexion and extension, 187, 189
  fractures about, 183-235
    in adults, 200-223
  instability of, factors influencing, 185-198
  ligaments of, 186
Elbow stress, valgus, 186, 188-189
Electromyography in diagnosis of muscular dystrophy, 7, 8
Electronic-memory image intensifier for tibial osteotomy, 278
Elephantiasis in neurofibromatosis in children, 55, 56
Endoscope, surgery through; *see* Arthroscopy
Enzymes, serum, in diagnosis of muscular dystrophy, 6-7
Epicondyle, medial, fractures of, in children, 189-191
Epiphyseal fractures, humeral, transverse displaced, in children, 234-235
Epiphyseal plus metaphyseal osteotomy, 94, 95, 96
Epiphysiodesis, 91
Equinocavovarus deformity in Duchenne muscular dystrophy, 25-26
Equinus in muscular dystrophy, 24, 26
Erosive defects of bone from contiguous neurogenic tumors in neurofibromatosis in childhood, 61
Established nonunions, bone grafting for, 154
Excision of bucket-handle tear of meniscus, arthroscopic, 386-389
Exercises and patellar pain, 347
External fixators, 112; *see also* External skeletal fixation
  application of, 125, 143
    operating room setup for, 125
    planning of, 125-126
  ASIF "tubular," 114, 115
  classification of, 114-116
  components of, developed during 1930s, 113
  historical perspectives on, 112-114
  pelvic, 108
  pin
    diagram of, 114
    modular, 114, 116
      application of, 132-139
      diagram of, 115
    simple, 114
      application of, 126-131
      diagram of, 115
  pins for, anchoring, in bone, 122, 123
  ring, 116
  for tibia, application of, 159-161
External skeletal fixation, 112-182
  advantages of, 116
  basic concepts of, 118-124
  clinical considerations in, 119-122
  complications of, 179-182
  of elbow, 172
  forces applying at fracture site in, 124
  of forearm, 172
  of fractures of distal radius, 173-174
  frames for, configuration of, 123-124
  for hand fractures, 175
  historical perspectives on, 112-114
  of humerus, 170-171
  indications for, 116-117
  for infected nonunions and failed septic joints, 177
  in integrated treatment plan, 117-118
  introduction to, 112-118

External skeletal fixation—cont'd
  mechanical considerations in, 122-124
  miscellaneous considerations in, 124
  in open fractures
    of femur, 162-164
    of pelvis, 164-169
    to tibia, 156-161
    of upper extremity, 169-175
  pins for; *see* Pins for external fixation
  for thumb metacarpal defect, 175
Extremities; *see* Lower extremity; Upper extremity
Extremity fractures in multiply injured patients, 108-109

F

Facioscapulohumeral dystrophy, 2-3
  genetics of, 6
  working classification of, 4
Failed implant, reconstruction of, 286-297
Failed septic joints and infected nonunions, treatment of, 176-179
Failure, fixation, and techniques of revision surgery in total hip replacement, 414-421
Fat pad syndrome after knee arthroscopy, 377
Femoral head, vascular compromise to, as complication of surface replacement of hip, 446-447
Femoral insertion technique in total hip replacement, 419-421
Femoral neck
  excessive anteversion of, causing loosening of surface replacement of hip, 452-453
  fracture of, as complication of surface replacement of hip, 447-449
Femoral osteotomy for Legg-Calvé-Perthes disease, 77
Femur
  anatomy of, 162
  open fractures of, external fixation in, 162-164
  supracondylar osteotomy of, 91
Fibrous union, apparent, as complication of surface replacement of hip, 445
Fixation
  intramedullary, for lower extremity fractures, 108-109
  skeletal, external, 112-182; *see also* External skeletal fixation
Fixation failure
  and techniques of revision surgery in total hip replacement, 414-421
  of tibial component of total knee replacement, causes and prevention of, 397-400
Fixator, external; *see* External fixators
Fixator frames
  classification of, 123-124
  for external fixation of tibia, designs for, 159, 161
  maintaining, 140-143
  secondary bone and soft-tissue procedures performed in, 143
Flap(s)
  distant, 150-151
    free, 150, 151
  myocutaneous, for soft-tissue coverage, 143-144
  myoplasty
    gastrocnemius, 145-150
    soleus, 144-146
  neurovascular, osteocutaneous, free, 154
  osteocutaneous, free, 154
  pedicle, cross-leg, 150, 151
  for rotator cuff tears, 268, 269
"Flap" tear of meniscus, arthroscopic removal of, 389, 390
Flexion contracture
  soft-tissue release for, 331-332
  total knee replacement for, 325-326
Flexion instability
  soft-tissue release for, 332

Flexion instability—cont'd
    total knee replacement for, 325-326
Flexor of forearm muscle, tear of, 189
Foot deformity in muscular dystrophy, surgical treatment of, 25-26
Forceps for knee arthroscopy, 362-364
Forces
    at fracture site in external fixation, 124
    across knee during activity, 302
    knee-joint, 302
    muscle, and spinal stability, 458-459
Forearm, external fixation of, 172
Forearm muscle, flexor of, tear of, 189
Foreign bodies in knee, arthroscopy to remove, 380
Fracture
    avulsion, of greater tuberosity, rotator cuff tears after, 249
    with burns
        external fixation for, 117
        in multiply injured patient, 109
    of capitellum, 215
    closed, external fixation for, 117
    comminuted, of ring of C1, 460
    of coronoid, 215-216
    of distal humerus, transverse, in children, 224-235
    of distal radius, external fixation of, 173-174
    about elbow, 183-235
        in adults, 200-223
    external fixation for, 122
    extremity, in multiply injured patients, 108-109
    of femoral neck as complication of surface replacement of hip, 447-449
    fragments of, methods to decrease motion between, 123
    of greater tuberosity, anterior dislocation of shoulder with, rotator cuff tear after, 242-244
    hand, external fixation for, 175
    of humeral condyles, 214
    of humerus in children, supracondylar, 224-233
        anterior displaced, 233
    intercondylar T or Y, 202-213
    Jefferson, 460
    medial epicondyle, in children, 189-191
    Monteggia, in adults, 217
    in multiply injured patient, treatment of, 104
    of olecranon, 218-222
    open; *see* Open fractures
    patellar, after total knee replacement, 338
    in patients with muscular dystrophy, 28-29
    pelvic, in multiply injured patient, 107-108
    pelvic-ring, 165, 168, 169
    radial head, 222-223
    rotator cuff tear after injury without, 239-242
    of spine, in multiply injured patient, 106-107
    supracondylar, 200-202
    transverse, distal humeral epiphyseal, in children, 234-235
    of trochlea, 215
    of wires, asymptomatic, as complication of surface replacement of hip, 445
Fracture site, forces applying at, in external fixation, 124
Frame
    compression, Kronner circular, 116
    for external fixator
        configuration for, 123-124
        of femur, 162-164
    fixator; *see* Fixator frames
    Hoffmann; *see* Hoffmann frame
    pelvic, 114
        design of, 164-165
        erection of, 166, 168
    quadrilateral, 115

Free flaps, distant, 150, 151
Free grafts for rotator cuff tears, 268-269
Free osteocutaneous flaps, 154
Free osteocutaneous neurovascular flaps, 154
Free vascularized bone grafts, 154
Freeze-drying of allografts, 45, 52
FSH; *see* Facioscapulohumeral dystrophy
Full-thickness cortical defects, bone grafting for, 156
Full-thickness metaphyseal defects, bone grafting for, 154, 156
Function, loss of, as criterion for performing knee arthroplasty, 313
Fusion, spinal, for scoliosis, 28

G

Gastrocnemius muscle, surgical anatomy of, 144
Gastrocnemius myoplasty flap, 145-150
Genu varum, treatment of, 89
Geopatellar-Geotibial Retainer prosthesis, 279, 280
Gowers' sign, 3
Grafting, bone; *see* Bone grafting
Grafts
    bone; *see* Bone graft
    free, for rotator cuff tears, 268-269
Gravity stress roentgenogram of medial collateral ligament, 191
Groove, bicipital, osteophytes of, 252-253
Growth, bone, disorders of, in neurofibromatosis of childhood, 59, 60
GUEPAR knee replacement, 303, 304

H

Half pins, 119
Halos for spinal fractures, 106-107
Hand, fractures of, external fixation for, 175
Hand-operated instruments for knee arthroscopy, 362-364
Head
    of biceps; *see* Biceps, long head of
    radial, fractures of, 222-223
Heat necrosis from external fixation, 179-180
Heel cord, percutaneous tenotomy of, 23, 24
Hemarthrosis after knee arthroscopy, 377
Herbert knee, 305
Heterotopic ossification
    as complication of surface replacement of hip, 444-445
    after THARIES replacement of hip, 440-441
Hinge osteotomy, 94
Hinged total knee replacements, 302-305
Hip
    infected pseudarthrosis of, with chronic osteomyelitis, 163
    revision surgery of, and controversies in total replacement, 403-453
    surface replacement of
        complications of, 444-453
        indications for, 405-406
        THARIES approach to, 422-442
Hip implant, components of, insertion of, 413
Hip replacement, total; *see* Total hip replacement
Hoffmann frame, 115
    application of, 132-139
    for external fixation of tibia, 159
    for pelvic fixation, 166, 168
Horizontal cleavage tear of meniscus, arthroscopic resection of, 389, 391
Humeral abduction splint, 271
Humeral condyles, fractures of, 214
Humeral epiphyseal fractures in children, transverse distal, 234-235

Humerus
anatomy of, 224
distal, transverse fractures of, in children, 224-235
external fixation of, 170-171
fractures of, in children, supracondylar, anterior displaced, 233
subluxation of, 261, 262
supracondylar fractures of, in children, 224-233
Hyperthermia, malignant, in muscular dystrophy, 21-22
Hypotrophic nonunion, bone grafting for, 154

I
Iliac crests as source of bone grafts, 153
Image intensifier, electronic-memory, for tibial osteotomy, 278
Immobilization of tibia, other methods of, 161
Impingement causing dislocation of surface replacement arthroplasty of hip, 449-451
Implant system, knee, laboratory evaluation of, 307-310
Implants
constrained, for arthritic knee, 286
failed, reconstruction of, 286-297
hip, components of, insertion of, 413
knee; *see* Knee implants
semiconstrained, for arthritic knee, 285-286
Incisions for knee arthroscopy, number and sites of, 375-376
Infected nonunions and failed septic joints, treatment of, 176-179
Infected pseudarthrosis of hip with chronic osteomyelitis, 163
Infection
as contraindication of knee arthroplasty, 314
after knee arthroscopy, 377
involving pins used for external fixation, 140
pin-tract, from external fixation, 180-182
skeletal, external fixation for, 117
after total knee replacement, 339-340
Injury, external fixation "tailored" to, 120
Instability
anteroposterior, in recurrent elbow dislocations, chronic, 197-198
clinical, of spine, 457-458
of elbow
anteroposterior, 193
factors influencing, 185-198
flexion
soft-tissue release for, 332
total knee replacement for, 325-326
knee, total knee replacement for, 324-326
of lower cervical spine, 460, 462-470
of lumbar spine (L1-L5), 475-479
of lumbosacral spine (L5-S1), 479-481
of sacroiliac joints, 481-481
spinal; *see* Spine, instability of
of thoracic and thoracolumbar spine, 470-475
valgus
acute, 188-189
chronic, in adults, 191-192
Instruments for arthroscopy of knee, 360-366
sterilization of, 367, 368
Intercondylar T or Y fractures, 202-213
closed methods of treatment of, 203-204
operative methods for, 204-213
Intra-articular adhesions, soft-tissue release for, 332-333
Intramedullary fixation for lower extremity fractures, 108-109
Intrathoracic meningocele in neurofibromatosis in childhood, 59
Invasive cyst formation causing loosening of surface replacement of hip, 453

Irrigation, knee joint, to remove loose fragments after arthroscopy, 376-377
Irrigation system for knee arthroscopy, 370, 372

J
Jefferson fracture, 460
Joint
atlantoaxial
spinal instability at, 460
subluxation and dislocation at, 460, 461-462
knee; *see* Knee
occipitoatlantal spinal instability at, 459-460
radiocapitellar, in valgus stress, 192, 193
sacroiliac, instability of, 481-482
septic, failed, and infected nonunion, treatment of, 176-179
stiffness of, from external fixation, 180
subtalar, neurofibromatous mass in, 65
uninvolved in external fixation, care of, 140, 141, 142
universal, 113

K
Knee, 275-400
adhesions of, arthroscopic resection for, 393-394
arthritic; *see* Arthritic knee
arthroplasty of; *see also* Total knee replacement
contraindications to, 314
evaluation of patients for, 313-324
other factors in, 314-315
primary considerations in, 313
arthroscopy of
anesthesia for, 367
instruments for, 360-366
sterilization of, 367, 368
joint irrigation after, to remove loose fragments, 376-377
using leg-holding device, 373
methods of positioning and holding knee during, 367-370
numbers and sites of incisions for, 375-376
operative, 357-395
posterior puncture technique for, 373-375
postoperative care after, 377
postoperative problems and management of, 377-378
preoperative instruction and management of, 366-367
to remove loose bodies, 380
for resection of medial synovial shelf, 378-380
for synovial biopsy, 378
types of lesions treated with, 360
débridement of, 313-314, 318
disease of, mechanical, severe articulated knee prosthesis for, 277-284
effusions of, after arthroscopy, 377
forces across, during activity, 302
foreign bodies in, arthroscopy to remove, 380
Herbert, 305
instability of, total knee replacement for, 324-326
irrigation of, to remove loose fragments after arthroscopy, 376-377
lesions of, treated with arthroscopy, 360
long axis of, rotation about, 302
loose bodies in, arthroscopy to remove, 380
normal, motion of, 301
positioning and holding, during arthroscopy, 367-370
reconstruction of, results of, 297-298
scuffing of, after arthroscopy, 377-378
Spherocentric, 305
stiff, and quadriceps contracture, soft-tissue release for, 332, 333
total arthroplasty of, for arthritis, 278-281
Knee braces for patellar pain, 347

Knee designs, total
  mechanical features of, 302-307
  stability characteristics of, 301-312
Knee implant systems
  laboratory evaluation of, 307-310
  role of cruciate ligament in, 310
Knee implants
  for arthritic knee, 285
  Cruciate Condylar, 310, 311
  loosening of, incidence of, 306
  and soft-tissue stability, 312
  tibial plateau design of, 306
  Total Condylar, 310, 311
Knee prosthesis, articulated, for treatment of severe mechanical knee joint disease, 277-284
Knee replacement
  bicompartmental, 316
  GUEPAR, 303, 304
  total, 301-340; *see also* Total knee replacement
  unicompartmental, 315-316, 318
Knee replacement unit, total, nonconstrained, in reconstruction of difficult arthritic knee, 297-300
Knee-ankle-foot orthosis, plastic, 22
Knee-joint forces, 302
Knives for knee arthroscopy, 364
Kronner circular compression frame, 116
Kyphoscoliosis in neurofibromatosis in childhood, 59

L

Laboratory evaluation of knee implant systems, 307-310
Landouzy-Déjerine disease, 2-3
  working classification of, 4
Langenskiöld's six stages of Blount's disease, 95
Lateral and anterior musculotendinous units, transfixion of, from external fixation of tibia, 158
Lateral release for patellar pain, 348
Lateral retinacular release, arthroscopy for, 381-385
Legg-Calvé-Perthes disease
  surgery for, 77-82
  treatment of, 73-82
Leg-holding device for knee arthroscopy, 368, 370, 371
  technique using, 373
Leg-lengthening apparatus, 113
Lesions
  "crab meat," from proximal realignment of patella, 350
  cutaneous, in neurofibromatosis in childhood, 55
  of long head of biceps, 250-257
    surgery for, 256-257
    treatment of, 255-256
  of musculotendinous cuff of shoulder, 239-257
LGD; *see* Limb-girdle dystrophy
Life expectancy, short, as contraindication for knee arthroplasty, 314
"Ligamentotaxis," external fixation for, 117
Ligaments
  cruciate, role of, in knee implant systems, 310
  of elbow, 186
  medial collateral
    repair and reattachment of, 196, 198
    surgery on, 195, 196, 198
Limb lengthening, external fixation for, 117
Limb-girdle dystrophy, 2
  genetics of, 6
  working classification of, 4
Local complications of external skeletal fixation, 179-182
Long head of biceps; *see* Biceps, long head of
Loose bodies
  in knee, arthroscopy to remove, 380

Loose bodies—cont'd
  in olecranon fossa, 191, 192
Loosening
  as complication of surface replacement of hip, 451-453
  of knee implants, incidence of, 306
  of THARIES surface replacement of hip, 435, 438-440
  of total hip replacement
    diagnosis of, 416
    identification, incidence, and significance of 414-416
Lower cervical spine, instability of, 460, 462-470
Lower extremity
  fractures of, in multiply injured patient, 108-109
  full-thickness cortical defects of, bone grafting for, 156
  surgery and bracing of, 22-25
Lumbar spine L1-L5, instability of, 475-479
Lumbosacral spine (L5-S1), instability of, 479-481

M

Malalignment syndromes and patellar incongruence, surgery for, 347-348
Malignant hyperthermia in muscular dystrophy, 21-22
Malunion and knee arthroplasty, 315
Mayo approach to elbow, 204, 206-207
Mechanical knee joint disease, severe, articulated knee prostheses for, 277-284
Medial collateral ligament
  repair and reattachment of, 196, 198
  strain of, 189
  surgery on, 195, 196, 198
Medial epicondyle fractures in children, 189-191
Medial synovial shelf, resection of, arthroscopy for, 378-380
Medical myopathies, 5
Meningocele, intrathoracic, in neurofibromatosis of childhood, 59
Meniscal surgery, arthroscopy for, 385-395
Meniscal tears, classification of, 386
Meniscectomy, arthroscopic
  partial, 385-386
  "total," 389, 392
Meniscus, tears of
  bucket-handle, arthroscopic excision of, 386-389
  horizontal cleavage, arthroscopic resection of, 389, 391
  transverse (radial), arthroscopic resection of, 389, 392
Metabolic myopathies, 5
Metacarpal, thumb, defect of, external fixation for, 175
Metaphyseal defects, bone grafting for, 154, 156
Metaphyseal and epiphyseal osteotomy, 94, 95, 96
Metaphyses as source of bone grafts, 153
Migration, trochanteric, as complication of surface replacement of hip, 445-446
Mobilization of patient after external fixation of pelvis, 168-169
Modular pin fixators, 114, 116
  application of, 132-139
  diagram of, 115
Monteggia fractures in adult, 217
Motion
  in Legg-Calvé-Perthes disease, obtaining, 73-76
  limitation of, after total knee replacement, 338
  of normal knee, 301
Motorized instruments for arthroscopy, 364, 365
Motor-related treatment of muscular dystrophy, 14-29
Multiply injured patient
  anesthesia in, 105-106
  with burns and fractures, 109
  external fixation for, 117
  extremity fractures in, 108-109

Multiply injured patient—cont'd
  management of, 103-109
  nutrition for, 105
  orthopaedic surgical procedures for, timing and staging of,
      104
  pelvic fractures in, 107-108
  spinal fractures in, 106-107
Muscle
  anconeus, 186
  biopsy of, in diagnosis of muscular dystrophy, 7-10
  diseases of, 1-5; *see also* Muscular dystrophy
  exercises for stretching, 16
  forearm, flexor of, tear of, 189
  gastrocnemius, surgical anatomy of, 144
  soleus, surgical anatomy of, 144
Muscle forces and spinal stability, 458-459
Muscle weakness
  in Duchenne muscular dystrophy, 18-21
  progressive, in muscular dystrophy, 14-15, 18-21
Muscular dystrophy
  assessment of, 15
  cardiac involvement in, 12
  carrier state in, 10-11
  common, 1-4
  deformities from, combating, 16-17
  diagnosis of, 1-11
    management, and orthopaedic treatment of, 1-29
  dietary problems in, 13
  Duchenne; *see* Duchenne muscular dystrophy
  electromyography in diagnosis of, 7, 8
  equinus in, 24, 26
  foot deformity in, surgical treatment of, 25-26
  fractures in patients with, 28-29
  general treatment, 11-14
  genetics of, 5-6
  motor-related treatment of, 14-29
  muscle biopsy in diagnosis of, 7-10
  occupational therapy for, 17
  orthopaedic management of, 18-29
  pathomechanics of, 18-21
  physical therapy for, 14-17
  progressive muscular weakness in, 14-15, 18-21
  psychosocial problems in, 13-14
  reproduction and, 14
  respiratory problems with, 12-13
  scoliosis with, surgical treatment of, 27-28
  serum enzymes in diagnosis of, 6-7
  speech problems in, 14
  spinal stabilization in, 28
  surgical treatment of, 21-29
  upper extremities in surgical treatment of, 26-27
  vascular changes in, 14
  wheelchair care of patient with, 17-18
  x-ray features of, 11
Muscular Dystrophy Association, 29
Musculoskeletal tissue
  banking of, guidelines for, 50-53; *see also* Bone banking
  for transplantation, 51-53
Musculotendinous cuff of shoulder, lesions of, 239-257
Musculotendinous units, anterior and lateral, transfixion of,
      from external fixation of tibia, 158
Myocutaneous flaps for soft-tissue coverage, 143-144
Myocutaneous gastrocnemius myoplasty flap, 146-148
Myopathy(ies)
  congenital, 4-5
  medical, 5
  metabolic, 5
  muscle biopsy of, 8

Myoplasty for soft-tissue coverage, 143-144
Myoplasty flap
  gastrocnemius, 145-150
  soleus, 144-146

N

National Conference of Commisioners on Uniform State Laws,
    38
Necrosis
  heat, from external fixation, 179-180
  skin, after total knee replacement, 334-337
Neoplasia in neurofibromatosis in childhood, 67-68
Neoplasms in neurofibromatosis in childhood, 68
Nerve palsy after THARIES surface replacement of hip, 441
Nerve-root damage and instability of lower cervical spine, 467
Neurofibromatosis in childhood, 54-70
  findings in, 55
  genetics of, 54-55
  presenting complaints of, 55
  skeletal manifestations of, 56-68
Neurofibromatous mass in subtalar joint, 65
Neurogenic tumors, contiguous, erosive defects of bone from,
    in neurofibromatosis in childhood, 61
Neurologic disease as contraindication for knee arthroplasty,
    314
Neuropathy, muscle biopsy of, 9, 10
Neurovascular bundle, posterior tibial, injury to, from external
      fixation of tibia, 158
Neurovascular complications of external skeletal fixation, 179
Neurovascular flaps, osteocutaneous, free, 154
Neurovascular "island" flap for rotator cuff tears, 269
Nevus in neurofibromatosis in childhood, 55
Night splints for muscular dystrophy, 16-17
Nodules in neurofibromatosis in childhood, 55
Nonconstrained total knee replacement unit in reconstruction
      of difficult arthritic knee, 297-300
Nonhinged total knee replacements, 305-307
Nonunions
  bone grafting for, 154, 155
  from external fixation, 180
  infected, and failed septic joints, treatment of, 176-179
  trochanteric, as complication of surface replacement of hip,
      445-446
Nutrition for multiply injured patient, 105

O

Occipitoatlantal joint, spinal instability at, 459-460
Occupation of patient and knee arthroplasty, 314-315
Occupational therapy for muscular dystrophy, 17
Olecranon, fractures of, 218-222
Olecranon fossa, loose bodies in, 191, 192
Olecranon process, impingement of, 191
Open fractures
  bone grafting for, 152-156
  external fixation for, 116-117
  of femur, external fixation in, 162-164
  of pelvis, external fixation in, 164-169
  soft-tissue coverage of, 143-152
  of tibia, external fixation for, 156-161
  of upper extremity, external fixation in, 169-175
Opening wedge osteotomy, 91, 92, 93, 94
Operating room personnel during knee arthroscopy, 371-372
Orthopaedic management of muscular dystrophy, 18-29
Orthopaedic surgeon, role of, in trauma team, 103
Orthopaedic surgical procedures for multiply injured patient,
      timing and staging of, 104
Orthopaedics, general, 1-99
Orthosis, knee-ankle-foot, plastic, 22

Ossification, heterotopic
    as complication of surface replacement of hip, 444-445
    after THARIES replacement of hip, 440-441
Osteochondritis dissecans, arthroscopy for, 394-395
Osteocutaneous flaps, free, 154
Osteocutaneous neurovascular flaps, free, 154
Osteomyelitis, chronic, infected pseudarthrosis of hip with,
    163
Osteoperiosteal bone graft, 154, 155
Osteophytes
    acromial, 253
    bicipital groove, 252-253
Osteotomy
    bony bridge resection and, 97-98
    "broomstick," 91, 93, 94
    closing wedge, 91, 92, 94, 95
    compensatory, 84-85
    derotation, 95
    dome-shaped, 91, 93, 94
    epiphyseal and metaphyseal, 94, 95, 96
    gain in length from, 83-84
    hinge, 94
    for Legg-Calvé-Perthes disease
        femoral, 77
        pelvic, 77-78
        Salter, 77-78, 80
        varus, 80
    level of, and amount of restored length, 86
    level to perform, 84-85
    opening wedge, 91, 92, 93, 94
    Roger-Anderson apparatus in, 91, 92
    rotational, 94, 95
    supracondylar, of femur, 91
    supramalleolar, indications for, 91
    tibial
        proximal, for arthritic knee, 277-278, 285
        valgus, 315-316, 317
        varus, 315-316
    of tibias in children, 88-99
        biotrigonometric analysis and practical applications of, 83-
            99
        complications of, 99
        deformity and differential diagnosis in, 88-89
        guidelines for, 94, 99
        indications for, 89-91
        proximal, 91
        techniques for, 91-94, 95-98
    wedge, 85-88
    wedge removed in, determination of, 85-88
Osteotomy site, trochanteric, 424

P

Pain
    as criterion for performing knee arthroplasty, 313
    patellar; *see* Patellar pain
    patellofemoral, diagnosis of, 343-344
Palsy, nerve, after THARIES surface replacement of hip, 441
Partial meniscectomy, arthroscopic, 385-386
Partial-thickness metaphyseal and diaphyseal defects, bone
    grafting for, 154
Patella
    débridement of, 353
    distal realignment of, 352-353
    fracture of, after total knee replacement, 338
    proximal realignment of, 348-350
        results of, 352
    resurfacing of, 353-354
    subluxation or dislocation of, after total knee replacement,
        337-338

Patella pain syndromes and chondromalacia patellae, 342-355
Patellar compression syndrome, arthroscopy for, 381
Patellar incongruence and malalignment syndromes, surgery
    for, 347-348
Patellar pain
    chondroplasty for, 350-351
    investigation of, 343-346
    mechanism of, 346-347
    caused by other syndromes, 353-355
    after total knee replacement, 337-338
    treatment of, 347
        surgical, 347-352
Patellar problems after total knee replacement, 337-338
Patellar shaving, arthroscopy for, 384-385
Patellar surgery, arthroscopy for, 381-385
Patellectomy, 355
Patellofemoral incongruence, 344-346
Patellofemoral pain, diagnosis of, 343-344
Pathologic processes necessitating total knee replacement, 325-
    326
Patient
    mobilization of, after external fixation of pelvis, 168-169
    multiply injured; *see* Multiply injured patient
    selection of, for external skeletal fixation, 119-120
Pedicle advancement for rotator cuff tear, 268, 269
Pedicle flaps, cross-leg, 150, 151
Pelvic external fixator device, 108
Pelvic fractures in multiply injured patient, 107-108
Pelvic frame, 114
    design of, 164-165
    erection of, 166, 168
Pelvic osteotomy for Legg-Calvé-Perthes disease, 77-78
Pelvic-ring fracture, 165, 168, 169
Pelvis
    anatomy of, 165-166
    open fractures of, external fixation in, 164-169
Percutaneous tenotomy of heel cord, 23, 24
Personnel, operating room, during knee arthroscopy, 371-372
Perthes disease; *see* Legg-Calvé-Perthes disease
Petri cast for Legg-Calvé-Perthes disease, 73, 74
Phlebitis after knee arthroscopy, 377
Physical therapy for muscular dystrophy, 14-17
Physiologic effects of trauma, 104-105
Pin fixators
    diagram of, 114
    modular, 114, 116
        application of, 132-139
        diagram of, 115
    simple, 114
        application of, 126-131
        diagram of, 115
Pins
    for external fixation, 119
        anchoring, in bone, 122, 123
        care of, 140, 142
        design and function of, 119
        diameter of, 119
        of femur, 162-163
        of forearm, 172
        of humerus, 170, 171
        infection involving, 140
        of pelvis, 166, 167
        of radius, 173-174
        selection of, 119
        of tibia, 157
            placement of, 159
    half, 119
    placement of, factors affecting, 121-122
    smooth, 119

Pins—cont'd
    threaded, 119
    transfixion, 113, 119
Pin-tract infections for external fixation, 180-182
Pin-tract problems from external fixation, 180
Plastic knee-ankle-foot orthosis, 22
Polymyositis, 5
    muscle biopsy of, 9, 10
Posterior puncture technique for knee arthroscopy, 373-375
Posterior tibial neurovascular bundle, injury to, from external
        fixation of tibia, 158
Posteromedial puncture technique for knee arthroscopy, 373-
        375
Posture in Duchenne muscular dystrophy, 20-21
Preservation of tissues for transplantation, 44-45, 52
Preserved bone and cartilage allografts, potential disadvan-
        tages of, 34-37
Pressure decubiti, 14
Pressurization of bone cement, 411-413
Pressurizer, 412
Probe for knee arthroscopy, 359, 361-362
Pronation with supracondylar humeral fracture in children,
        230-232
Prospective nonunion, bone grafting for, 154, 155
Prostheses
    Geopatellar-Geotibial Retainer, 279, 280
    knee, articulated, for treatment of severe mechanical knee
        joint disease, 277-284
    Spherocentric, 282
    for total knee replacement, design of, 397-398
    Variable Axis, treatment of difficult arthritic knee with, 286,
        290, 291
Protein needs of multiply injured patient, 105
Proximal realignment for patellar pain, 348-350
    results of, 352
Proximal tibial osteotomy, 91
    for arthritic knee, 277-278, 285
Pseudarthrosis
    congenital bowing and, in neurofibromatosis in childhood,
        59, 61
        surgery for, 62-64
    of hip, infected, with chronic osteomyelitis, 163
Psychosocial problems in muscular dystrophy, 13-14
Pulmonary insufficiency from trauma, 104
Pulmonary problems with muscular dystrophy, 12-13
Puncture technique, posterior, for knee arthroscopy, 373-375

Q

Quadriceps contracture, stiff knee and, soft-tissue release for,
        332, 333
Quadriceps reconstruction for patellar pain, 351
Quadrilateral frame, 115
Quality control in banking of musculoskeletal tissues, 51

R

Radial head fractures, 222-223
Radial (transverse) tear of meniscus, arthroscopic resection of,
        389, 392
Radiocapitellar joint in valgus stress, 192, 193
Radiographic analysis of THARIES surface replacement of
        hip, 434
Radiography, stress, in investigation of patellar pain, 346
Radiopacifier in bone cement, 407-408
Radius, distal, fractures of, external fixation of, 173-174
Realignment
    distal, of patella, 352-353
    proximal, for patellar pain, 348-350
        results of, 352

Reconstruction
    of difficult arthritic knee, 277-300
        nonconstrained total knee replacement unit in, 297-300
    knee, results of, 297-298
    quadriceps, for patellar pain, 351
    of severe arthritic deformity or failed implant, 286-297
    soft-tissue, external fixation for, 117
Record keeping
    for banking of musculoskeletal tissues, 51
    in tissue banking, 45, 47, 51
Reduction, loss of, from external fixation, 180
Refracture from external skeletal fixation, 180
Refrigeration of allografts, 45, 52
Release
    lateral, for patellar pain, 348
    retinacular, lateral, arthroscopy for, 381-385
    soft-tissue; *see* Soft-tissue release
Replacement
    of hip
        surface; *see* Surface replacement of hip
        total; *see* Total hip replacement
    knee; *see* Knee replacement; Total knee replacement
Reproduction and muscular dystrophy, 14
Resection
    bony bridge, and osteotomy, 97-98
    of "flap" tears of meniscus, arthroscopic, 389, 390
    of horizontal cleavage tears of meniscus, arthroscopic, 389,
        391
    of knee joint adhesions, arthroscopy for, 393-394
    of medial synovial shelf, arthroscopy for, 378-380
    of minimal bone for reconstruction of severe arthritic defor-
        mity or failed implant, 287, 289-292
    of transverse (radial) tear of meniscus, arthroscopic, 389,
        392
Respiratory problems with muscular dystrophy, 12-13
Retinacular release, lateral, arthroscopy for, 381-385
Revision surgery
    hip, 403-453
    techniques of, fixation failure and, in total hip replacement,
        414-421
    after total hip replacement
        bone preparation and implantation for, 419
        general preparations for, 416-419
Ring fixators, 116
Rod, connecting, adjustable, 113
Roentgen features of muscular dystrophy, 11
Roentgenograms in investigation of patellar pain, 344-346
Roentgenographic measurement of translation by lower cervi-
        cal spine, 465-466
Roger-Anderson apparatus in osteotomies, 91, 92
Rotation about long axis of knee, 302
Rotational osteotomy, 94, 95
Rotational tests of knee implant systems, 307, 308
Rotator cuff, tears of, 239-249, 258-272
    acute, 264
    after anterior dislocation
        with fracture of greater tuberosity, 242-244
        of shoulder, 242
    found at autopsy, 265
    after avulsion fracture of greater tuberosity, 249
    chronic, 265
        with or without history of injury, 244-249
    diagnosis of, 259-264
    after injury without fracture or dislocation, 239-242
    physiology of, 259
    postoperative management of, 272
    spontaneous recovery from, 264
    surgery for, 265-270
    surgical alternatives for mobilizing and repairing, 268

Rotator cuff, tears of—cont'd
  testing for weakness with, 259-260
  variations in pathologic lesions from, 258
Ruptures of long head of biceps, 250

S

Sacroiliac joints, instability of, 481-482
Salter osteotomy for Legg-Calvé-Perthes disease, 77, 78
Scapula, stabilization of, in patients with muscular dystrophy, 26-27
Scarring, secondary, bone loss and, after reconstruction of severe arthritic deformity or failed implant, 292-296
Scintimetry in investigation of patellar pain, 346
Sclerosis of greater humeral tuberosity, 260, 261
Scoliosis
  with muscular dystrophy, surgical treatment of, 27-28
  in neurofibromatosis in childhood, 56-59
Scuffing of knee joint after arthroscopy, 377-378
Secondary bone and soft-tissue procedures performed in frame, 143
Semiconstrained implants for arthritic knee, 285-286
Sepsis
  in multiply injured patient, 105
  after THARIES surface replacement of hip, 440
Septic joints, failed, and infected nonunion, treatment of, 176-179
Serial bone grafting in treatment of infected nonunions and failed septic joints, 178
Serum enzymes in diagnosis of muscular dystrophy, 6-7
Shaving, patellar, arthroscopy for, 384-385
Shear tests of knee implant systems, 307, 309, 310
Shoulder, 237-272
  anterior dislocation of
    with fracture of greater tuberosity, rotator cuff tear after, 242-244
    rotator cuff tear after, 242
  musculotendinous cuff of, lesions of, 239-257
Simple pin fixator, 114
  application of, 126-131
  diagram of, 115
Sinus tract formation after total knee replacement, 337
Skeletal fixation, external, 112-182; *see also* External skeletal fixation
Skeletal infections, external fixation for, 117
Skeletal manifestations of neurofibromatosis in childhood, 56-68
Skin, necrosis of, after total knee replacement, 334-337
Skull traction for spinal fractures, 106-107
Sling, Snyder, for Legg-Calvé-Perthes disease, 73, 74
Smooth pins, 119
Snyder sling for Legg-Calvé-Perthes disease, 73, 74
Soft tissue
  care of, after external fixation, 140, 141
  problems with, after total knee replacement, 334-337
Soft-tissue and bone procedures, secondary, performed in frame, 143
Soft-tissue coverage
  of denuded bone, 177
  for infected nonunions and failed septic joints, 178
  for open fractures, 143-152
  surgical anatomy and, 144
  surgical techniques for, 144-151
Soft-tissue reconstruction, external fixation for, 117
Soft-tissue release
  for arthritic knee, 280
  for flexion contracture, 331-332
  for reconstruction of severe arthritic deformity or failed implant, 286-287, 288

Soft-tissue release—cont'd
  total knee replacement, 326-333
    for varus deformity, 327-331
Soft-tissue stability, knee implant and, 312
Soleus muscle, surgical anatomy of, 144
Soleus myoplasty flap, 144-146
Speech problems in muscular dystrophy, 14
Spherocentric arthroplasty for arthritic knee, 281-284
Spherocentric knee, 305
Spherocentric prosthesis, 282
Spinal deformities in neurofibromatosis in childhood, 56-59
Spinal fusion for scoliosis, 28
Spine, 455-482
  cervical, lower, instability of, 460, 462-470
  clinical instability of, 457-458
  fractures of, in multiply injured patient, 106-107
  instability of
    at atlantoaxial joint, 460
    at occipitoatlantal joint, 459-460
    radiologic interpretation of, 458
  lumbar (L1-L5), instability of, 475-479
  lumbosacral (L5-S1), instability of, 479-481
  stability of
    evaluation and treatment of, 457-482
    muscle forces and, 458-459
  stabilization of, in muscular dystrophy, 28
  thoracic and thoracolumbar, instability of, 470-475
Splint
  humeral abduction, 271
  night, for muscular dystrophy, 16-17
Spondylolisthesis in neurofibromatosis in childhood, 59
Stability of total knee replacement, 398-399
Stability characteristics of total knee designs, 301-312
Sterilization
  of allografts, 52
  of instruments for knee arthroscopy, 367, 368
Stiff knee and quadriceps contracture, soft-tissue release for, 332, 333
Stiffness
  ankle, prevention of, 158
  joint, from external fixation, 180
Storage of tissues for transplantation, 45, 46, 52
Strain, medial collateral ligament, 189
Stress, valgus
  in children, 190
  elbow, 186, 188-189
  radiocapitellar joint in, 192, 193
Stress radiography in investigation of patellar pain, 346
Stress test
  gravity, of medial collateral ligament, 191
  valgus, positive, 195
Stretch test for instability of lower cervical spine, 466-467, 468
Subluxation
  at atlantoaxial joint, 460, 461-462
  of biceps tendon, 251-252
  of humerus, 261, 262
  patellar, after total knee replacement, 337-338
Subperiosteal bone proliferation in neurofibromatosis in childhood, 66-67
Subtalar joint, neurofibromatous mass in, 65
Supination with supracondylar humeral fracture in children, 230-232
Supplementary autogenous cancellous bone graft in treatment of infected nonunions and failed septic joints, 177-178
Supracondylar fractures, 200-202
Supracondylar humeral fractures in children, 224-233
  anterior displaced, 233

Supracondylar osteotomy of femur, 91
Supramalleolar osteotomy, indications for, 91
Supraspinatus tendon, transverse avulsion of, 267
Surface replacement of hip
  complications of, 444-453
  indications for, 405-406
  THARIES approach to, 422-442
Surgeon, orthopaedic, role of, in trauma team, 103
Surgical anatomy and soft-tissue coverage, 144
Syndrome
  anterior compartment, from external fixation of tibia, 157
  compartment, from external fixation, 179
  malalignment, and patellar incongruence, surgery for, 347-348
  patellar compression, arthroscopy for, 381
  patellar pain, and chondromalacia patellae, 342-355
Synovectomy, arthroscopy for, 392-393
Synovial biopsy, arthroscopy for, 378
Synovial shelf, medial, resection of, arthroscopy for, 378-380
Systemic complications
  of external skeletal fixation, 179
  of THARIES surface replacement of hip, 435

T

T fractures, intercondylar, 202-213
Tear
  of flexor of forearm muscle, 189
  of meniscus
    bucket-handle, arthroscopic excision of, 386-389
    classification of, 386
    "flap," arthroscopic removal of, 389, 390
    horizontal cleavage, arthroscopic resection of, 389, 391
    transverse (radial), arthroscopic resection of, 389, 392
  of rotator cuff, 239-249, 258-272; *see also* Rotator cuff, tears of
Television, use of, in knee arthroscopy, 364, 366
Temperature sensitivity of bone cement, 409-410
Tendon
  biceps; *see* Biceps tendon
  supraspinatus, transverse avulsion of, 267
Tenosynovitis, biceps, 252-255
Tenotomy, percutaneous, of heel cord, 23, 24
Test
  gravity stress, of medial collateral ligament, 191
  of knee implant systems
    rotational, 307, 308
    shear, 307, 309, 310
  stress, valgus, positive, 195
  stretch, for instability of lower cervical spine, 466-467, 468
THARIES approach to surface replacement of hip, 422-442
THARIES surface replacement of hip
  complications of, 440-441
    requiring surgery, 435, 436-437
  design and development of, 422-423
  indications and contraindications of, 432
  loosening of, 435, 438-440
  operative technique for, 423-432
  radiographic analysis of, 434
  results of, 433-434
  systemic complications of, 435
  working dimensions of, 431
Thoracic spine fractures in multiply injured patient, 107
Thoracolumbar spine, instability of, 470-475
Threaded pins, 119
Thromboembolism after total knee replacement, 338-339
Thumb metacarpal, defect of, external fixation for, 175
Tibia
  angulation deformities of, 88-89

Tibia—cont'd
  deformity of, bracing for, 88, 89
  external fixator for, application of, 159-161
  large bone defect of, management of, 399, 400
  open fractures of, external fixation for, 156-161
  osteotomies of; *see* Osteotomy, tibial; Osteotomy of tibias in children
  valgus deformity of, treatment of, 91
  varus deformity of, treatment of, 90, 91
Tibial artery, anterior, injury to, from external fixation of tibia, 157-158
Tibial component in total knee replacement, fixation failure of, causes and prevention of, 397-400
Tibial defects, bridging of, 156
Tibial neurovascular bundle, posterior, injury to, from external fixation of tibia, 158
Tibial osteotomy
  proximal, for arthritic knee, 277-278, 285
  valgus, 315-316
  varus, 315-316
Tibial plateau design of knee implant, 306
Tibial tubercle elevation for patellar pain, 354-355
Timing in external fixation, 124
Tissue-banking methodology, 37-47
Tissues
  donation of
    consent for, 51
    reconstruction of cadaver after, 38, 39, 52
  musculoskeletal, banking of, guidelines for, 50-53; *see also* Bone banking
  soft, care of, after external fixation, 140, 141
  for transplantation; *see* Transplantation, tissues for
Toronto brace for Legg-Calvé-Perthes disease, 73, 75, 76
Total Condylar knee implant, 310, 311
Total hip replacement
  controversies in, 403-453
  femoral, insertion techniques for, 419-421
  fixation failure and techniques of revision surgery in, 414-421
  loosening of
    diagnosis of, 416
    identification, incidence, and significance of, 414-416
  revision surgery after
    bone preparation and implantation for, 419
    general preparations for, 416-419
Total knee arthroplasty for arthritic knee, 278-281
Total knee designs
  mechanical features of, 302-307
  stability characteristics of, 301-312
Total knee replacement 301-340; *see also* Knee, arthroplasty of
  alignment in, 398
  cement technique for, 399
  complications after, prevention and management of, 334-340
  fixation failure of tibial component after, 397-400
  hinged, 302-305
  infection after, 339-340
  kinematic features of, 301-302
  limitation of motion after, 338
  mechanical environment for, 301-302
  nonhinged, 305-307
  patellar problems after, 337-338
  pathologic processes necessitating, 325-326
  prosthetic design for, 397-398
  soft-tissue problems after, 334-337
  soft-tissue release and, 326-333, 334
  stability in, 398-399
  surgical technique for, 398-399

Total knee replacement—cont'd
  surgical technique for—cont'd
    principles of, 324
  technique of, 324-333
  thromboembolism after, 338-339
  unconstitutional, results of, 298-299
Total knee replacement unit
  diameter of, 299
  nonconstrained, in reconstruction of difficult arthritic knee, 297-300
"Total" meniscectomy, arthroscopic, 389, 392
Tourniquet for knee arthroscopy, 370-371
Traction skull for spinal fractures, 106-107
Transfer
  biceps tendon, 197
  coracoid bone block, 197
Transfixion of anterior and lateral musculotendinous units from fixation of tibia, 158
Transfixion pin, 113, 119
Transplantation
  musculoskeletal tissues for, 51-53
  tissues for
    distribution and use of, 45
    preservation of, 44-45
    procurement of, 41-44
    record keeping on, 45, 47
    selection of donor for, 37-41
    sources of, 39
    storage of, 45, 46
Transverse avulsion of supraspinatus tendon, 267
Transverse distal humeral epiphyseal fractures in children, 234-235
Transverse fractures of distal humerus in children, 224-235
Transverse (radial) tear of meniscus, arthroscopic resection of, 389, 392
Trauma, 101-182
  physiologic effects of, 104-105
Trauma team, orthopaedic surgeon's role in, 103
Trauma victims; *see* Multiply injured patient
Triangulation
  of instruments in knee arthroscopy, 359, 361
  of oval defect for rotator cuff tear, 268, 270
Trochanteric nonunion or migration as complication of surface replacement of hip, 445-446
Trochanteric osteotomy site, 424
Trochanteric rip-off as complication of surface replacement of hip, 445-446
Trochlea, fractures of, 215
Tubercle, tibial, elevation of, for patellar pain, 354-355
Tuberosity, greater; *see* Greater tuberosity
Tubular fixator, ASIF; *see* ASIF "tubular" fixator
Tumors
  neurogenic, contiguous, erosive defects of bone from, in neurofibromatosis in childhood, 61
  transfer of, by tissue transplantation, 36-37, 40

U

Unconstrained total knee replacements, results of, 298-299
Unicompartmental arthroplasty for arthritic knee, 278

Unicompartmental knee replacement, 315-316, 318
Uniform Anatomic Gift Act, 38
Union
  delayed, from external fixation, 180
  fibrous, apparent, as complication of surface replacement of hip, 445
Universal joint, 113
Upper extremity
  anatomy of, 169-170
  fractures of, in multiply injured patient, treatment of, 109
  full-thickness cortical defects of, bone grafting for, 156
  in muscular dystrophy, surgical treatment of, 26-27
  open fractures of, external fixation in, 169-175

V

Valgus deformity
  soft-tissue release for, 329-331
  from supracondylar humeral fractures in children, 230-232
  of tibia, treatment of, 91
Valgus elbow stress, 186, 188-189
Valgus instability
  acute, 188-189
  chronic, in adults, 191-192
Valgus stress
  in children, 190
  radiocapitellar joint in, 192, 193
Valgus stress test, positive, 195
Valgus tibial osteotomy, 315-316, 317
Van Gorder approach to elbow, 204
Variable Axis prosthesis, treatment of difficult arthritic knee with, 286, 290, 291
Varus deformity
  soft-tissue release for, 327-329
  from supracondylar humeral fractures in children, 230-232
  of tibia, 90, 91
Varus osteotomy for Legg-Calvé-Perthes disease, 80
Varus tibial osteotomy, 315-316
Vascular changes in muscular dystrophy, 14
Vascular compromise to femoral head as complication of surface replacement of hip, 446-447
Vascularized bone grafts, 153-154
von Recklinghausen's disease; *see* Neurofibromatosis in childhood

W

Weakness, muscle; *see* Muscle weakness
Wedge removed in osteotomy, determination of, 85-88
Wedge osteotomy, 85-88
Wheelchair care of patient with muscular dystrophy, 17-18
Wires, asymptomatic fractures of, as complications of surface replacement of hip, 445
Wound, clean, obtaining, 152

X

X-ray features of muscular dystrophy, 11

Y

Y fractures, intercondylar, 202-213